Pregnancy and Birth: Challenges and Concerns

Pregnancy and Birth: Challenges and Concerns

Editor: Cora Bailey

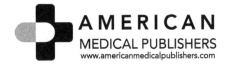

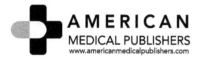

Cataloging-in-Publication Data

Pregnancy and birth : challenges and concerns / edited by Cora Bailey.
   p. cm.
Includes bibliographical references and index.
ISBN 979-8-88740-388-5
1. Pregnancy. 2. Childbirth. 3. Prenatal care. 4. Newborn infants--Care. 5. Labor (Obstetrics).
6. Maternal and infant welfare. I. Bailey, Cora.
RG551 .P74 2023
618.2--dc23

© American Medical Publishers, 2023

American Medical Publishers,
41 Flatbush Avenue,
1st Floor, New York,
NY 11217, USA

ISBN 979-8-88740-388-5 (Hardback)

This book contains information obtained from authentic and highly regarded sources. Copyright for all individual chapters remain with the respective authors as indicated. All chapters are published with permission under the Creative Commons Attribution License or equivalent. A wide variety of references are listed. Permission and sources are indicated; for detailed attributions, please refer to the permissions page and list of contributors. Reasonable efforts have been made to publish reliable data and information, but the authors, editors and publisher cannot assume any responsibility for the validity of all materials or the consequences of their use.

Trademark Notice: Registered trademark of products or corporate names are used only for explanation and identification without intent to infringe.

Contents

Preface VII

Chapter 1 Telomere-Related Disorders in Fetal Membranes Associated with Birth and Adverse Pregnancy Outcomes 1
Jossimara Polettini and Marcia Guimarães da Silva

Chapter 2 The Complement System in the Pathophysiology of Pregnancy and in Systemic Autoimmune Rheumatic Diseases During Pregnancy 10
Cecilia Beatrice Chighizola, Paola Adele Lonati, Laura Trespidi,
Pier Luigi Meroni and Francesco Tedesco

Chapter 3 Occurrence of a RAGE-Mediated Inflammatory Response in Human Fetal Membranes 21
Héléna Choltus, Marilyne Lavergne, Corinne Belville, Denis Gallot,
Régine Minet-Quinard, Julie Durif, Loïc Blanchon and Vincent Sapin

Chapter 4 Dynamic Changes in the Phenotype of Dendritic Cells in the Uterus and Uterine Draining Lymph Nodes After Coitus 33
Ippei Yasuda, Tomoko Shima, Taiki Moriya, Ryoyo Ikebuchi, Yutaka Kusumoto,
Akemi Ushijima, Akitoshi Nakashima, Michio Tomura and Shigeru Saito

Chapter 5 Study of sRAGE, HMGB1, AGE and S100A8/A9 Concentrations in Plasma and in Serum-Extracted Extracellular Vesicles of Pregnant Women with Preterm Premature Rupture of Membranes 45
Damien Bouvier, Yves Giguère, Loïc Blanchon, Emmanuel Bujold, Bruno Pereira,
Nathalie Bernard, Denis Gallot, Vincent Sapin and Jean-Claude Forest

Chapter 6 Fetal Membrane Epigenetics 54
Tamas Zakar and Jonathan W. Paul

Chapter 7 Cortisol Regeneration in the Fetal Membranes, A Coincidental or Requisite Event in Human Parturition? 67
Wang-Sheng Wang, Chun Ming Guo and Kang Sun

Chapter 8 Premature Rupture of Membranes and Severe Weather Systems 77
Mackenzie L. Wheeler and Michelle L. Oyen

Chapter 9 Toxicant Disruption of Immune Defenses: Potential Implications for Fetal Membranes and Pregnancy 82
Sean M. Harris, Erica Boldenow, Steven E. Domino and Rita Loch Caruso

Chapter 10 Innate Immune Mechanisms to Protect Against Infection at the Human Decidual-Placental Interface 92
Regina Hoo, Annettee Nakimuli and Roser Vento-Tormo

Chapter 11 **CD206+ M2-Like Macrophages are Essential for Successful Implantation**...............107
Yosuke Ono, Osamu Yoshino, Takehiro Hiraoka, Erina Sato, Yamato Fukui,
Akemi Ushijima, Allah Nawaz, Yasushi Hirota, Shinichiro Wada, Kazuyuki Tobe,
Akitoshi Nakashima, Yutaka Osuga and Shigeru Saito

Chapter 12 **Progestins Inhibit Interleukin-1β-Induced Matrix Metalloproteinase 1 and Interleukin 8 Expression via the Glucocorticoid Receptor in Primary Human Amnion Mesenchymal Cells**...............117
William Marinello, Liping Feng and Terrence K. Allen

Chapter 13 **The Role(s) of Eicosanoids and Exosomes in Human Parturition**...............129
Eman Mosaad, Hassendrini N. Peiris, Olivia Holland, Isabella Morean Garcia and
Murray D. Mitchell

Chapter 14 **Mechanisms of Key Innate Immune Cells in Early- and Late-Onset Preeclampsia**...............141
Ingrid Aneman, Dillan Pienaar, Sonja Suvakov, Tatjana P. Simic,
Vesna D. Garovic and Lana McClements

Chapter 15 **Proteomic Study of Fetal Membrane: Inflammation-Triggered Proteolysis of Extracellular Matrix May Present a Pathogenic Pathway for Spontaneous Preterm Birth**...............160
Jing Pan, Xiujuan Tian, Honglei Huang and Nanbert Zhong

Chapter 16 **Functional Genomics of Healthy and Pathological Fetal Membranes**...............174
Sarah J. Cunningham, Liping Feng, Terrence K. Allen and Timothy E. Reddy

Chapter 17 **Cholesterol Crystals and NLRP3 Mediated Inflammation in the Uterine Wall Decidua in Normal and Preeclamptic Pregnancies**...............181
Gabriela Brettas Silva, Lobke Marijn Gierman, Johanne Johnsen Rakner,
Guro Sannerud Stødle, Siv Boon Mundal, Astrid Josefin Thaning,
Bjørnar Sporsheim, Mattijs Elschot, Karin Collett, Line Bjørge,
Marie Hjelmseth Aune, Liv Cecilie Vestrheim Thomsen and
Ann-Charlotte Iversen

Chapter 18 **Healing Mechanism of Ruptured Fetal Membrane**...............193
Haruta Mogami and R. Ann Word

Chapter 19 ***In vivo* Assessment of Supra-Cervical Fetal Membrane by MRI 3D CISS**...............198
Wenxu Qi, Peinan Zhao, Wei Wang, Zhexian Sun, Xiao Ma, Hui Wang, Wenjie Wu,
Zichao Wen, Zulfia Kisrieva-Ware, Pamela K. Woodard, Qing Wang,
Robert C. McKinstry and Yong Wang

Chapter 20 **The Role of Danger Associated Molecular Patterns in Human Fetal Membrane Weakening**...............205
Justin G. Padron, Chelsea A. Saito Reis and Claire E. Kendal-Wright

Permissions

List of Contributors

Index

Preface

This book has been an outcome of determined endeavour from a group of educationists in the field. The primary objective was to involve a broad spectrum of professionals from diverse cultural background involved in the field for developing new researches. The book not only targets students but also scholars pursuing higher research for further enhancement of the theoretical and practical applications of the subject.

The term pregnancy refers to the period when one or more fetuses develop inside a woman's womb or uterus. It involves a series of changes that occur in a woman's body as a baby develops within the body. The complete process from conception till birth is completed in about 9 months, which is an average of 266-270 days. The preliminary signs of pregnancy include missed menstrual periods, morning nausea, and feeling of fullness. Enlarged and tender breasts, unusual and persistent fatigue, and frequent urination are some other signs of pregnancy. During the first trimester, all pregnant women experience vomiting and nausea. There are several methods that help in determining pregnancy such as pelvic examination by an obstetrician. The most reliable and affordable method is agglutination test. Prenatal care is important for both mother and fetus. Pregnant women must restrict the consumption of substances like smoking, alcoholic beverages, and non-prescription drugs that harm the fetus. Some of the major challenges that are faced during pregnancy include bladder and bowel changes, hair changes, skin color changes, indigestion, heartburn, leg cramps, etc. This book contains some recent studies on pregnancy and birth. It unravels the recent researches related to the challenges and concerns related to pregnancy and birth. Those in search of information to further their knowledge will be greatly assisted by this book.

It was an honour to edit such a profound book and also a challenging task to compile and examine all the relevant data for accuracy and originality. I wish to acknowledge the efforts of the contributors for submitting such brilliant and diverse chapters in the field and for endlessly working for the completion of the book. Last, but not the least; I thank my family for being a constant source of support in all my research endeavours.

Editor

Telomere-Related Disorders in Fetal Membranes Associated with Birth and Adverse Pregnancy Outcomes

Jossimara Polettini[1]* and Marcia Guimarães da Silva[2]

[1]Universidade Federal da Fronteira Sul (UFFS), Programa de Pós Graduação em Ciências Biomédicas, Faculdade de Medicina, Campus Passo Fundo, Brazil
[2]Universidade Estadual Paulista (UNESP), Faculdade de Medicina, Departamento de Patologia, Botucatu, Brazil

*Correspondence:
Jossimara Polettini
jossimara.polettini@uffs.edu.br

Telomere disorders have been associated with aging-related diseases, including diabetes, vascular, and neurodegenerative diseases. The main consequence of altered telomere is the induction of the state of irreversible cell cycle arrest. Though several mechanisms responsible for the activation of senescence have been identified, it is still unclear how a cell is indeed induced to become irreversibly arrested. Most tissues in the body will experience senescence throughout its lifespan, but intrinsic and extrinsic stressors, such as chemicals, pollution, oxidative stress (OS), and inflammation accelerate the process. Pregnancy is a state of OS, as the higher metabolic demand of the growing fetus results in increased reactive oxygen species production. As a temporary organ in the mother, senescence in fetal membranes and placenta is expected and linked to term parturition (>37 weeks of gestation). However, a persistent, overwhelming, or premature OS affects placental antioxidant capacity, with consequent accumulation of OS causing damage to lipids, proteins, and DNA in the placental tissues. Therefore, senescence and its main inducer, telomere length (TL) reduction, have been associated with pregnancy complications, including stillbirth, preeclampsia, intrauterine growth restriction, and prematurity. Fetal membranes have a notable role in preterm births, which continue to be a major health issue associated with increased risk of neo and perinatal adverse outcomes and/or predisposition to disease in later life; however, the ability to mediate a delay in parturition during such cases is limited, because the pathophysiology of preterm births and physiological mechanisms of term births are not yet fully elucidated. Here, we review the current knowledge regarding the regulation of telomere-related senescence mechanisms in fetal membranes, highlighting the role of inflammation, methylation, and telomerase activity. Moreover, we present the evidences of TL reduction and senescence in gestational tissues by the time of term parturition. In conclusion, we verified that telomere regulation in fetal membranes requires a more complete understanding, in order to support the development of successful effective interventions of the molecular mechanisms that triggers parturition, including telomere signals, which may vary throughout placental tissues.

Keywords: telomere shortening, oxidative stress, parturition, gestation, prematurity, membrane premature rupture

INTRODUCTION

Telomeres are a highly conserved system that plays a central role in maintaining the integrity of the genome and cell. In somatic cells, telomeres reach a critical short length over the lifespan, or under the influence of stressors. Therefore, telomere length (TL) is an important feature of cell aging or senescence, which suggests the idea of a "biological clock," or a marker of cell replication (Hayflick, 1965; Blackburn, 2001).

In pregnancy, senescence has been related to term delivery mechanisms (Menon et al., 2014a; Behnia et al., 2015; Gomez-Lopez et al., 2017). The concept of placental cell aging in term delivery was first proposed in the 1970s; however, only lately has a relatively large number of studies examined the relationship between cell senescence and the consequent morphological changes in pregnancy. Placenta and fetal membranes constitute temporary tissues in the maternal body, and therefore, are "aged" and ready to be eliminated by the time of the term neonate is born. Thus, cellular senescence may be related to gestational complications if the process is activated prematurely (Behnia et al., 2015; Menon, 2016; Cox and Redman, 2017; Arias-Sosa, 2018). One of the main characteristics of senescent cells is the production of inflammatory cytokines, which indicates a possible role of cellular senescence as an effector pathway that converges to trigger parturition. Intrinsic and extrinsic stressors that induce variation in prenatal exposures and maternal states and conditions, such as cigarette smoking, air pollution, diabetes, obesity, oxidative stress, and inflammation are associated with cellular aging, evidenced by the shortening of telomeres in fetal cells (Whiteman et al., 2017). Thus, characteristics of maternal health status and behaviors during pregnancy may influence the individual's susceptibility or propensity to disease in later life. However, few studies have shown a direct correlation between telomere dysfunction specifically in fetal membranes and fetal or developmental programming.

Thus, we begin this review with a brief overview of telomere structure and functions, followed by a description of telomere-related senescence mechanisms and the role of telomere dynamics in pregnancy. We then proceed to discuss the findings regarding fetal membranes telomere-senescence-mediated parturition and adverse gestational outcomes. We conclude by summarizing current knowledge blanks and future research directions.

TELOMERES: STRUCTURE AND FUNCTIONS

Telomeres are nucleoprotein structures at the end of chromosomes that play a vital role in maintaining genomic stability and protecting the chromosomes against fusion and degradation (Blackburn, 1991; Blackburn et al., 2015). In humans, telomeres consist of 2–20 kb of non-coding double-stranded DNA formed by a conserved hexameric (TTAGGG) tandem repeat DNA sequence and a 3' overhang of the G-rich strand, which folds back into the double-stranded DNA, forming a structure known as the t-loop, important for protecting the genome from nucleolytic degradation, unnecessary recombination, repair, and interchromosomal fusion (Lu et al., 2013; Blackburn et al., 2015). Besides having a unique DNA sequence, the protection of chromosomes depends on the association and interaction of human telomeres with the shelterin complex, which contains six specific proteins (TRF1, TRF2, POT1, TIN2, TPP1, and RAP1). This network provides a compact chromatin structure that limits the accessibility of DNA damage repair (DDR) machinery and decreases its mistaken recognition at the telomere region (Bandaria et al., 2016; Fathi et al., 2019) (**Figure 1A**). Since DNA polymerase is unable to fully replicate the 3' end of the DNA strand, telomeres lose part of its sequence with each cell division and reach a critical short length, which, in turn, leads to cellular senescence (Stewart et al., 2003).

Stem cell compartments and embryonic stem cells present telomerase activity; this is a ribonucleoprotein complex, composed of telomerase reverse transcriptase (TERT) and rRNA telomerase component (TERC) subunits and serves as a template for the addition of telomeric repeats to chromosome ends. However, TERT expression and telomerase activity are often very low or undetectable in somatic cells, which explain, in part, the limited capacity of somatic cells to replicate (Rubtsova et al., 2012). Other pathways, such as the alternative lengthening of telomeres (ALT), have been reported in cancer cells (De Vitis et al., 2018). ALT is still not a well-known process, but it is related to telomeric recombination and may be activated when telomerase is repressed. Nonetheless, cultured cells over passages show limited replication capacity, which has been attributed mainly to the shortening of telomeres (Burton and Krizhanovsky, 2014).

Cell aging is a physiological process, as telomeres undergo steady attrition during the proliferation of normal cells; this can be either beneficial or detrimental to the organism. On one hand, it contributes to tumor suppression, limiting tissue damage, and possibly embryonic development, while on the other, it may be associated with aging-related diseases, impaired tissue regeneration, and cellular dysfunction, as well as pregnancy complications (Howcroft et al., 2013; Burton and Krizhanovsky, 2014; Menon et al., 2016; Arias-Sosa, 2018).

TELOMERE-RELATED SENESCENCE MECHANISMS

Replicative senescence is characterized by cellular proliferative capacity, which depends ultimately on progressive telomere shortening to a critically short length, responsible for the limited number of cell divisions (Bekaert et al., 2005). Therefore, TL is one the main inducers of cell aging or senescence, which suggests the idea of a "biological clock," or "Hayflick limit," first described in human fibroblasts cultured *ex vivo* as a proliferative limitation on cells, despite their viability (Hayflick, 1965; Campisi and D'Adda Di Fagagna, 2007; Xu et al., 2013).

The main telomere-related senescence mechanisms include DNA structure dysfunction and modifications. Chromatin and histones structure dysfunction is a key point associated with telomere shortening, which can be triggered by diverse pathways. First, a decrease in histone levels has been observed

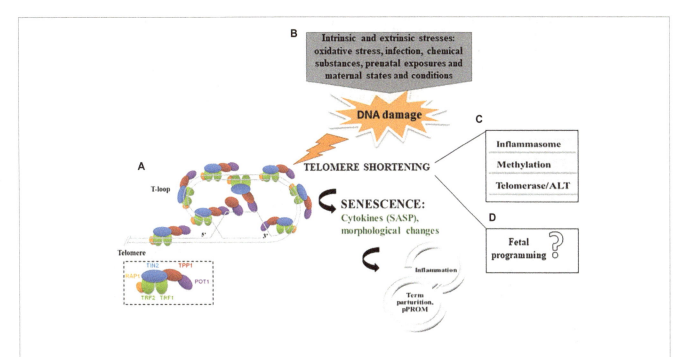

FIGURE 1 | (A) Telomere structure and telomere-binding proteins. The six shelterin proteins are depicted in the small box (Adapted from Lu et al., 2013). (B) Summary of the proposed mechanism for telomere shortening in fetal membranes in parturition. (C) Potential mechanisms of telomere-senescence-mediated parturition and adverse gestational outcomes in fetal membranes. (D) No evidence that telomeres dysfunction in fetal membranes has a direct effect on fetal programing (SASP, senescence-associated secretory phenotypes; ALT, alternative lengthening of telomeres; and pPROM, preterm premature rupture of membranes).

in human senescent fibroblasts compared to levels in younger cells, impairing processes such as replication, transcription, and DNA repair (O'Sullivan et al., 2010; Adams et al., 2013). Moreover, the majority of lysines on histones are physiologically hypoacetylated near telomeres, contributing to the genomic silencing of this region; thus, any histone modifications, such as acetylation, may interfere with the *t*-loop telomere structure. Such modification may also repress hTERT expression in human cells, such that senescence signaling is initiated (Cong and Bacchetti, 2000). Equally, changes in the structural and epigenetic integrity of telomeres throughout population doubling have an impact on core histones and their chaperones, which, in turn, ultimately lead to senescence (O'Sullivan et al., 2010).

Additionally, chromatin structure is also determined by DNA methylation and, although telomere sequence do not contain genes or CpG sequences, the subtelomeres regions (transition regions between the terminal telomeric repeats and the chromosome-specific regions) are notably CpG-rich, therefore, more prone to be physiologically highly methylated (Toubiana and Selig, 2020). Previous studies have shown that aberrant methylation of subtelomeric DNA exists in many diseases, and it has an impact on the TL regulation, as shorter telomeres are significantly associated with decreased methylation levels at most of CpG sites (Buxton et al., 2014; Hu et al., 2019). Changes in the methylation status of different CpG sites are typical in cancer cells (Joyce et al., 2018), but they have also been observed in senescent cells. This has been used by researchers to successfully predict the age of several different tissues and predispositions to aging-related diseases (Bell et al., 2019). This tool using a set of CpG sites is named epigenetic clock, which starts during development when fetal tissues, embryonic, and induced pluripotent stem cells reveal a DNA methylation age (DNAm age) (Horvath, 2013; Bell et al., 2019).

Besides replicative senescence, *stress-induced senescence* demonstrates that the Hayflick limit is no longer a constant but can vary depending on influencers of telomere loss, such as oxidative damage and/or decrease in antioxidative defense. Thus, the mechanisms described above can be influenced by stressors and accelerate the cell aging process. The accumulation of intrinsic and extrinsic stresses is a well-known pathway that triggers telomere dysfunction and impairs telomere end replication (Pickett and Reddel, 2012; Tan and Lan, 2017), mainly through oxidative stress (OS) (von Zglinicki, 2002; Tan and Lan, 2017).

Under conditions of genomic stability, DNA damage activates DDR complex that coordinates repair and cell cycle progression. Since the telomere is a guanine-rich region (triple structure), it is more vulnerable to OS damage compared to the general genome (von Zglinicki et al., 2000; Stewart et al., 2003; Xu et al., 2013); therefore, telomere dysfunction ultimately leads to cell cycle arrest (Rossiello et al., 2014). In mammalian cells, there are two main DDR mechanisms that address double strand breaks (DSBs): homologous recombination (HR) and non-homologous end joining (NHEJ); the latter is related to telomeric DNA. It has been suggested that NHEJ is inhibited by TRF2 shelterin, preventing chromosomal fusions, and, therefore, end-to-end fusion. Conversely, NHEJ is also the main mechanism for DNA ligase N-dependent chromosomal fusions that occur between uncapped telomeres, which suggests a selective regulatory switch, from preventing recombination to promoting it (Evans and Cooke, 2007). OS is known to accelerate telomere attrition *in vitro* and *in vivo*. Pineda-Pampliega et al. (2020) described how oxidative stress shortens telomeres in free-living white stork chicks. According to the authors, the administration of antioxidants had a functional effect on oxidative stress. Furthermore, environmental and behavioral stressors were found to induce OS-induced telomere damage. Exposure to different organic pollutants such as dioxins, furans, and polychlorinated biphenyls (PCBs) through food, water, and air, which occur during the human lifetime, may change TL in peripheral blood leukocytes (Shin et al., 2010; Mitro et al., 2016; Karimi et al., 2020). Serum levels of organochlorine pesticides can be associated with oxidative stress and systemic inflammation that lead to telomere shortening (Karimi et al., 2020). The cellular exposure to non-ortho PCBs and toxic equivalency was associated with increased leukocyte TL in a study population of American adults, contributing population-level findings to the evidence that exposure to environmental contaminants may influence telomere regulation (Mitro et al., 2016). In this same direction, Shin et al. (2010) analyzed the impact of low-dose exposure to persistent pollutants, i.e., lipophilic xenobiotics, on the TL of peripheral blood leukocytes in healthy persons. It was concluded that TL increases with low doses of exposure, suggesting that low doses may act as tumor promoters in carcinogenesis in humans.

Therefore, how does oxidative stress cause telomere shortening? Although there are many suggested pathways for answering this question, the increase of reactive oxygen species and/or decrease in the antioxidant capacity mainly lead to damage in cellular structures, mostly inducing oxidized base in the DNA and consequent DDR defects. Kawanishi and Oikawa (2004) have reported DNA damage caused by the treatment of fibroblast with UVA irradiation, including 8-hydroxy-2'-deoxyguanosine (8-OHdG) formation, specifically at the GGG sequence in the telomere sequence, which was correlated with a decreased in TL. The enzyme responsible for repairing this DNA damage is an 8-oxoG-DNA glycosylase (OGG1), and its action begins by excising the damaged base and subsequent replacement of the modified base (Rosenquist et al., 1997). This local DNA damage can disrupt cell replication; consequently, if the repair mechanism by OGG1 is impaired, a damage to single-stranded DNA strand in the telomere region occurs, which contributes to its shortening. Under the repair failure, mechanisms of DDR by sensor proteins such as the ataxia telangiectasia mutated (ATM) kinase is activated, which regulates the early step(s) of DNA damage signaling, and thereby controls DDR. Persistent DNA damage in response to overwhelming OS causes DNA breaks followed by the phosphorylation of the histone H2AX (γ-H2AX). This *via* induces mechanism of cellular damage involving p53 activation, as well described in cells such as fibroblasts. Alternatively, the route that leads to senescence can be p53-independent, through the activation of mitogen-activated protein kinases (MAPKs) pathway (Iwasa et al., 2003). Salminen et al. (2012) have reported either pathway converges to a downstream activation of NF-κB signaling. In turn, NF-κB system is linked to inflammatory responses in cellular senescence. It is important to note that senescent cells acquire many changes in gene expression, resulting in changes in secreted proteins, such as growth factors, proteases, chemokines, and cytokines, that, together, characterizes the senescence-associated secretory phenotype (SASP; Davalos et al., 2010; Freund et al., 2010; Rodier and Campisi, 2011) (**Figure 2**).

Additionally, a newly discovered telomere-related stressor is sex hormone concentrations, but a direct relation between sex hormones and TL, if any, remains uncertain. Preliminary evidence suggests that sex steroid hormones could be involved in enhancing telomerase activity since serum dihydrotestosterone and estradiol are positively correlated with leukocyte TL independently of age (Yeap et al., 2016, 2020). However, other studies have demonstrated no association of short TL with sex hormones in healthy men and women (Coburn et al., 2018; Gu et al., 2020).

As a result of telomere-related OS disorders, some pathological conditions have been described, including diabetes and vascular disease (Blackburn et al., 2015). Primary cultures of fibroblasts were used to examine the impact of a diabetic environment on telomeres and, under elevated glucose conditions, relative TL loss was observed in this model (Sutanto et al., 2019). On the other hand, type 2 diabetes mellitus patients with non-alcoholic fatty liver disease have a significantly longer leukocyte TL than patients without non-alcoholic fatty liver disease (Zhang et al., 2019). Telomere shortening has been associated with premature vascular aging, which may be involved in lower-extremity amputation in patients with type 1 diabetes at high vascular risk (Sanchez et al., 2020). Of particular interest here, telomere dysfunctions are associated with placental aging in the etiology of parturition and adverse pregnancy outcomes, in which fetal membranes and gestational tissue play a crucial role.

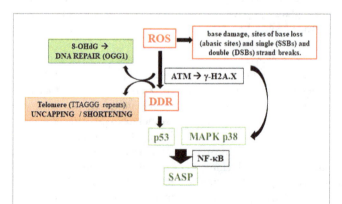

FIGURE 2 | Reactive oxygen species induction of telomere shortening (8-OHdG, 8-hydroxy-2'-deoxyguanosine; OGG1, 8-oxoG-DNA glycosylase; ATM, ataxia telangiectasia mutated kinase; DDR, DNA damage response; MAPK, mitogen-activated protein kinases; and SASP, senescence-associated secretory phenotypes).

FETAL MEMBRANES TELOMERE-SENESCENCE IN PARTURITION AND ADVERSE GESTATIONAL OUTCOMES

In recent years, new evidences have shown that cell senescence is related to term delivery mechanisms (Menon et al., 2014b; Behnia et al., 2015; Gomez-Lopez et al., 2017). The concept of placental cell aging in term delivery was first proposed in the 1970s (Rosso, 1976); however, until recently few studies had reported on cellular senescence related to oxidative stress and its consequent morphological changes (Menon et al., 2012; Polettini et al., 2015b). This process is believed to be physiological since the placenta and fetal membranes constitute temporary tissues in the maternal body, and therefore, would be "aged" and ready to be eliminated after the birth of the neonate (Behnia et al., 2015; Menon, 2016; Cox and Redman, 2017; Arias-Sosa, 2018).

Recent investigations have revealed that term pregnancies are characterized by increased OS that induces DNA damage (Menon, 2016; Cox and Redman, 2017; Arias-Sosa, 2018); therefore, TL is affected. Gestational tissues show evidence of senescence, given that the telomere attrition rate is negatively correlated with gestational age, thus the closer to term, the shorter the telomeres in fetal and placental cells (Gielen et al., 2014; Casavant et al., 2019). Accordingly, recent findings have demonstrated that fetal membranes from term in labor pregnancies had shorter TL than both preterm and term not in labor pregnancies, suggesting the senescence of term placentas along with labor (Menon et al., 2012; Polettini et al., 2015a; Colatto et al., 2020). The same results were observed in fetal membranes and placenta in mouse (Phillippe et al., 2019), providing support for the hypothesis that shorter telomeres at term potentially function as a biologic clock for parturition.

Besides TL analysis, term labor tissues show features and markers of senescence, such as histological enlarged cells and organelles, granulated nuclei, and more intense staining of senescence-associated β-galactosidase (a lysosomal enzyme; Menon et al., 2014a; Behnia et al., 2015) that strengthens the indication of fetal membranes senescence by parturition time. Among the changes in senescent cells, the production of inflammatory mediators is of particular interest (Freund et al., 2010), as they induce parturition. Fetal membranes play a crucial role in this process, as these tissues are in close contact with the amniotic fluid and, consequently, the fetus (Parry and Strauss, 1998). In the third trimester of pregnancy, chorioamniotic cells increase their production of mediators, especially pro-inflammatory cytokines, immunomodulatory cytokines, neutrophil recruitment chemokines, and arachidonic acid metabolites (Kamel, 2010; Hua et al., 2013; Romero et al., 2018). These mediators are essential to stimulate the production of prostaglandins and consequent uterine contractility (Romero et al., 2006).

Therefore, as is well-known, inflammation is a key point in parturition, even in the absence of intrauterine infection, and, in such cases, inflammation may come from the senescence of fetal membranes (Behnia et al., 2016; Martin et al., 2017). Behnia et al. (2015) found higher concentrations of pro-inflammatory SASP markers (granulocyte macrophage colony-stimulating factor and interleukin-6 and -8) in the amniotic fluid of women in labor at term than in women not in labor. Additionally, bioinformatics analysis has shown, under both term and preterm conditions, that maternal exosomes (30–150 nm particles that propagate to distant sites) carry proteins associated with inflammatory and metabolic signaling (Menon et al., 2019). Besides cellular alterations to the pro-inflammatory profile, the inflammasome might be activated during the parturition process by senescent cells with shortened telomeres. Recent findings have revealed telomere dysfunction as a cause of macrophage mitochondrial abnormalities, OS and hyperactivation of the NOD-like receptor family pyrin domain-containing protein 3 (NLRP3) inflammasome (Kang et al., 2018). Likewise, fetal membranes from women who underwent term labor had higher concentrations of NLRP3 (Romero et al., 2018); thus, dysfunctional telomeres might work as a primary factor and cooperate to amplify inflammasome signaling related to parturition signaling. Crosstalk between these pathways may prove to be a key molecular mechanism of immunosenescence that has been reviewed elsewhere (Jose et al., 2017; Ventura et al., 2017) (**Figure 1B**).

In this context, telomere-related cellular aging may be linked to gestational complications if the process is activated prematurely (Biron-Shental et al., 2010; Menon et al., 2012; Smith et al., 2013). Adverse pregnancy outcomes, such as stillbirth, intra uterine growth restriction, and preeclampsia are related to trophoblast dysfunction and attributed to placental villous telomere shortening (Biron-Shental et al., 2014; Ferrari et al., 2016; Paules et al., 2019). As mainly of these adversities are linked to placental dysfunction, the role of senescence in fetal membranes has been poorly investigated in these complications.

One of the firsts reports in fetal membranes demonstrated shorter TL from preterm premature rupture of membranes (pPROM) compared to preterm labor (PTL) with intact membranes pregnancies at the same gestational age, and the first was similar to term (Menon et al., 2012). More recently, structural and histological changes in fetal membranes from women undergoing pPPROM were found to be compatible with senescence, suggesting its role in disrupting membranes remodeling and homeostasis, with overwhelming ROS-associated inflammation (Menon et al., 2014a; Behnia et al., 2015; Menon, 2016; Menon and Richardson, 2017). Mechanistically, telomere shortening in pPROM is likely a result of senescence activators, such as MAPKs, that are increasingly expressed in fetal membranes in pregnant women with pPROM (Lappas et al., 2011). Dutta et al. (2016) have reinforced that prosenescence stress kinase (p38MAPK) activation, OS damage, and signs of senescence are pronounced in fetal membranes from pPROM in comparison with PTL with no rupture of membranes. Accordingly, the induction of OS caused significant protein peroxidation in the amniotic sac in mouse, which was associated with p38MAPK activation and senescence, in addition to increased concentrations of pro-inflammatory cytokines in amniotic fluid (Polettini et al., 2018). Commonly, OS activates a specific p53 transcriptional response in diverse tissues, which regulates the cellular response to DNA damage; however, fetal membranes fail in activating p53 under OS, suggesting a diverse pathway triggering senescence in this tissue (Polettini et al., 2015a) (**Figure 1B**).

Important to note that stressed and injured cells and tissue release stimulatory molecules, such as host-derived damage-associated molecular patterns (DAMPs), that signaling through toll-like receptors (TLRs) and activates cellular response. Therefore, telomere shortening in fetal membranes may also provide additional signs to initiate parturition. In senescent fetal membranes, two DAMPs have been reported, the high mobility group box 1 (HMGB1) and cell-free fetal telomere fragments (Bredeson et al., 2014; Polettini et al., 2015a). Detection of circulating nucleic acids in maternal plasma and serum, such as cell free fetal DNA, has emerged as a predictor marker or monitoring tool for the most common and severe pregnancy complications (Phillippe, 2015). One hypothesis is that DNA telomere fragments from senescent amnion cells are shed into the amniotic fluid, and these fragments can accelerate senescence in healthy gestational tissue, as a fetal signal at term that can cause labor-associated changes (Polettini et al., 2015a). Such observation has been supported by recent *in vitro* experiments, as amniotic cells under OS produce exosomes packed with fetal telomere fragments (Sheller-Miller et al., 2017). The recognition of these molecules was speculating to be through TLR-9 that is known to trigger maternal immune cells activation in response to placenta-derived DNA (Hahn et al., 2014). However, no difference in TLR-9 expression was observed in amnion cells treated with telomere fragments compared to controls (Polettini et al., 2015a). Thus, further experiments are needed to address the specific mechanism by which telomere fragments activate intracellular signaling in fetal and maternal cells.

Regarding methylation, chorionic villi, maternal decidua, fetal membranes, and embryonic tissues have a unique DNAm setting (Robinson and Price, 2015). Particular alterations in DNAm signatures were observed in placentas and fetal membranes with acute chorioamnionitis (Konwar et al., 2018). Moreover, many investigators have described cord blood DNAm related to prematurity and inflammation (Liu et al., 2013; de Goede et al., 2017), but data on telomere-associated methylation are scarce. Wilson et al. (2016) found a correlation between shorter TL and decreased DNAm in genes associated with the telomerase regulation in placentas. The authors have described that almost 20% of the probes within TERT gene showed significant alterations in DNAm associated with TL, but they discuss epigenetic regulation of the TERT is complex, and such changes should be observed throughout the entire TERT gene region in order to elucidate the biological relevance of DNA methylation in this region. In fetal membranes, epigenetic modifications have been described, such as non-coding RNA (lncRNA) that has also been linked to pPROM (Luo et al., 2013). However, as our knowledge, there are yet no studies that have demonstrated telomere-related methylation in fetal membranes and the possible association with parturition and gestational outcomes.

Additionally, low levels of telomerase activity have been associated with TL reduction in the placentas of babies with delayed fetal development in term pregnancies, attributed to accelerated telomere DNA loss and cellular senescence (Davy et al., 2009). Fetal membranes, in particular, maintain characteristics of pluripotent cells; therefore, it would be expected to find telomerase activity in such tissues (Zhou et al., 2013). However, potency, cellular transition capability, and migratory potential are lost in fetal membranes as gestation progresses and/or in response to OS-inducing factors (Richardson and Menon, 2018), and low telomerase activity was detected in fetal membranes regardless term or PTL (Colatto et al., 2020). Accordingly, amniotic fluid derived cells, including amniotic cells, also lack telomerase activity (Chen et al., 2013). Alternatively, ALT can be activated when telomerase is suppressed; however, to date, ALT activity has not been investigated in gestational tissues. ALT regulation is influenced by telomeric repeat-containing RNA (TERRA), a lncRNA, which works as a telomerase-telomere binding inhibitor. In turn, TERRA expression is directly controlled by DNA methylation at the CpG rich gene promoters (Nabetani and Ishikawa, 2011; Coluzzi et al., 2017). In placentas, Novakovic et al. (2016) have demonstrated higher TERRA expression compared to matched somatic cells from cord blood, which was correlated to very low levels of hTERT in first trimester cytotrophoblasts. These data suggest that additional pathways might be involved in TL regulation other than telomerase activity in fetal membranes, but this requires further investigation.

DISCUSSION

A vast literature demonstrates that telomere-dependent replicative senescence in placental and fetal membranes is involved with parturition and gestational adversities. We have summarized that OS, inflammation, methylation, telomerase, and ALT are the main described mechanisms in telomere biology in fetal membranes to date (**Figure 1C**). Diverse DNA methylation are detectable for most cancer-CpG sites beginning 4 years of pre-diagnosis (Joyce et al., 2018); thus, similarly, the understanding of telomere biology, shortening of TL mechanisms, and methylation regulation in fetal membranes might provide early evidences during gestational periods in relation to telomere alterations and the propensity for pregnancy outcomes. Moreover, telomerase and ALT regulation are not fully understood in fetal membranes, which reinforces that further investigation is needed regarding telomere dysfunction in fetal membranes.

The mean TL set during intra uterine development likely has an impact on later extrauterine life, as variation in prenatal exposures and maternal states and conditions may impact fetal developmental trajectories. Subsequently, fetal or developmental programming may influence an individual's susceptibility or propensity for disease in later life (Entringer et al., 2018). A recent systematic review demonstrated that maternal factors such as age, exposure to chemicals (e.g., smoking), and maternal stress during pregnancy and nutritional and sleep disorders are related to the stimulation of telomeres in fetal cells (Whiteman et al., 2017). Also, it has been documented that if TL is reduced in the newborn, the susceptibility to the development of chronic diseases in adulthood is increased (Entringer et al., 2012).

Thus, in terms of fetal programming of the telomere system, the maternal-placental-fetal immune activation, characterized by the increased expression of pro-inflammatory cytokines in response to various adverse conditions during pregnancy, may have the potential to impact fetal TL. Although the maternal and the environmental exposure during the intrauterine period is correlated to the postnatal period, as well as with the outcomes of newborn infants, there is lack of such relation in fetal membranes studies and more studies are required to understand whether telomeres dysfunction in fetal membranes has a direct effect on fetal programing (**Figure 1D**).

Unfortunately, the ability to mediate a delay in parturition during pregnancy complications is limited, and the development of successful effective interventions requires a more complete understanding of the molecular mechanisms that trigger parturition, including telomere signals, which may vary throughout placental tissues.

AUTHOR CONTRIBUTIONS

JP and MGS have equally contributed to this review and approved the submitted version.

REFERENCES

Adams, P. D., Ivanov, A., Pawlikowski, J., Manoharan, I., Tuyn, J. V., Nelson, D. M., et al. (2013). Lysosome-mediated processing of chromatin in senescence. *J. Cell Biol.* 202, 129–143. doi: 10.1083/jcb.201212110

Arias-Sosa, L. A. (2018). Understanding the role of telomere dynamics in normal and dysfunctional human reproduction. *Reprod. Sci.* 26, 6–17. doi: 10.1177/1933719118804409

Bandaria, J. N., Qin, P., Berk, V., Chu, S., and Yildiz, A. (2016). Shelterin protects chromosome ends by compacting telomeric chromatin. *Cell* 164, 735–746. doi: 10.1016/j.cell.2016.01.036

Behnia, F., Sheller, S., and Menon, R. (2016). Mechanistic differences leading to infectious and sterile inflammation. *Am. J. Reprod. Immunol.* 75, 505–518. doi: 10.1111/aji.12496

Behnia, F., Taylor, B. D. B., Woodson, M., Hawkins, H., Kacerovsky, M., Fortunato, S. J. S., et al. (2015). Chorioamniotic membrane senescence: a signal for parturition? *Am. J. Obstet. Gynecol.* 213, 359.e1–359.e16. doi: 10.1016/j.ajog.2015.05.041

Bekaert, S., De Meyer, T., and Van Oostveldt, P. (2005). Telomere attrition as ageing biomarker. *Anticancer Res.* 25, 3011–3021.

Bell, C. G., Lowe, R., Adams, P. D., Baccarelli, A. A., Beck, S., Bell, J. T., et al. (2019). DNA methylation aging clocks: challenges and recommendations. *Genome Biol.* 20:249. doi: 10.1186/s13059-019-1824-y

Biron-Shental, T., Sukenik-Halevy, R., Sharon, Y., and Goldberg-Bittman, L. (2010). Short telomeres may play a role in placental dysfunction in preeclampsia and intrauterine growth restriction. *Am. J. Obstet. Gynecol.* 202, 381.e1–381.e7. doi: 10.1016/j.ajog.2010.01.036

Biron-Shental, T., Sukenik-Halevy, R., Sharon, Y., Laish, I., Fejgin, M. D., and Amiel, A. (2014). Telomere shortening in intra uterine growth restriction placentas. *Early Hum. Dev.* 90, 465–469. doi: 10.1016/j.earlhumdev.2014.06.003

Blackburn, E. H. (1991). Structure and function of telomeres. *Nature* 350, 569–573. doi: 10.1038/350569a0

Blackburn, E. (2001). Switching and signaling at the telomere. *Cell* 106, 661–673. doi: 10.1016/s0092-8674(01)00492-5

Blackburn, E. H., Epel, E. S., and Lin, J. (2015). Human telomere biology: a contributory and interactive factor in aging, disease risks, and protection. *Science* 350, 1193–1198. doi: 10.1126/science.aab3389

Bredeson, S., Papaconstantinou, J., Deford, J. H., Kechichian, T., Syed, T. A., Saade, G. R., et al. (2014). HMGB1 promotes a p38MAPK associated non-infectious inflammatory response pathway in human fetal membranes. *PLoS One* 9:e113799. doi: 10.1371/journal.pone.0113799

Burton, D. G. A., and Krizhanovsky, V. (2014). Physiological and pathological consequences of cellular senescence. *Cell. Mol. Life Sci.* 71, 4373–4386. doi: 10.1007/s00018-014-1691-3

Buxton, J. L., Suderman, M., Pappas, J. J., Borghol, N., McArdle, W., Blakemore, A. I. F., et al. (2014). Human leukocyte telomere length is associated with DNA methylation levels in multiple subtelomeric and imprinted loci. *Sci. Rep.* 4:4954. doi: 10.1038/srep04954

Campisi, J., and D'Adda Di Fagagna, F. (2007). Cellular senescence: when bad things happen to good cells. *Nat. Rev. Mol. Cell Biol.* 8, 729–740. doi: 10.1038/nrm2233

Casavant, S. G., Cong, X., Moore, J., and Starkweather, A. (2019). Associations between preterm infant stress, epigenetic alteration, telomere length and neurodevelopmental outcomes: a systematic review. *Early Hum. Dev.* 131, 63–74. doi: 10.1016/j.earlhumdev.2019.03.003

Chen, Z., Jadhav, A., Wang, F., Perle, M., Basch, R., and Young, B. K. (2013). Senescence and longevity in amniotic fluid derived cells. *Stem Cell Discov.* 3, 47–55. doi: 10.4236/scd.2013.31008

Coburn, S. B., Graubard, B. I., Trabert, B., McGlynn, K. A., and Cook, M. B. (2018). Associations between circulating sex steroid hormones and leukocyte telomere length in men in the National Health and Nutrition Examination Survey. *Andrology* 6, 542–546. doi: 10.1111/andr.12494

Colatto, B. N., Souza, I. F.De, Schinke, L. A. A., Noda-Nicolau, N. M., Silva, M. G., Morceli, G., et al. (2020). Telomere length and telomerase activity in foetal membranes from term and spontaneous preterm births. *Reprod. Sci.* 27, 411–417. doi: 10.1007/s43032-019-00054-z.

Coluzzi, E., Buonsante, R., Leone, S., Asmar, A. J., Miller, K. L., Cimini, D., et al. (2017). Transient ALT activation protects human primary cells from chromosome instability induced by low chronic oxidative stress. *Sci. Rep.* 7:43309. doi: 10.1038/srep43309

Cong, Y. S., and Bacchetti, S. (2000). Histone deacetylation is involved in the transcriptional repression of hTERT in normal human cells. *J. Biol. Chem.* 275, 35665–35668. doi: 10.1074/jbc.C000637200

Cox, L. S., and Redman, C. (2017). The role of cellular senescence in ageing of the placenta. *Placenta* 52, 139–145. doi: 10.1016/j.placenta.2017.01.116

Davalos, A. R., Coppe, J. -P., Campisi, J., and Desprez, P. -Y. (2010). Senescent cells as a source of inflammatory factors for tumor progression. *Cancer Metastasis Rev.* 29, 273–283. doi: 10.1007/s10555-010-9220-9

Davy, P., Nagata, M., Bullard, P., Fogelson, N. S., and Allsopp, R. (2009). Fetal growth restriction is associated with accelerated telomere shortening and increased expression of cell senescence markers in the placenta. *Placenta* 30, 539–542. doi: 10.1016/j.placenta.2009.03.005

de Goede, O. M., Lavoie, P. M., and Robinson, W. P. (2017). Cord blood hematopoietic cells from preterm infants display altered DNA methylation patterns. *Clin. Epigenetics* 9:39. doi: 10.1186/s13148-017-0339-1

De Vitis, M., Berardinelli, F., and Sgura, A. (2018). Telomere length maintenance in cancer: at the crossroad between telomerase and alternative lengthening of telomeres (ALT). *Int. J. Mol. Sci.* 19:606. doi: 10.3390/ijms19020606

Dutta, E. H., Behnia, F., Boldogh, I., Saade, G. R., Menon, R., Taylor, B. D., et al. (2016). Oxidative stress damage-associated molecular signaling pathways differentiate spontaneous preterm birth and preterm premature rupture of the membranes. *Mol. Hum. Reprod.* 22, 143–157. doi: 10.1093/molehr/gav074

Entringer, S., Buss, C., and Wadhwa, P. (2012). Prenatal stress, telomere biology, and fetal programming of health and disease risk. *Sci. Signal.* 5:pt12. doi: 10.1126/scisignal.2003580

Entringer, S., de Punder, K., Buss, C., and Wadhwa, P. D. (2018). The fetal programming of telomere biology hypothesis: an update. *Philos. Trans. R. Soc. B Biol. Sci.* 373:20170151. doi: 10.1098/rstb.2017.0151

Evans, M. D., and Cooke, M. S. (2007). *Oxidative damage to nucleic acids*. 1st Edn. Austin, TX: Landes Bioscience.

Fathi, E., Charoudeh, H. N., Sanaat, Z., and Farahzadi, R. (2019). Telomere shortening as a hallmark of stem cell senescence. *Stem Cell Investig.* 6:7. doi: 10.21037/sci.2019.02.04

Ferrari, F., Facchinetti, F., Saade, G., and Menon, R. (2016). Placental telomere shortening in stillbirth: a sign of premature senescence? *J. Matern. Fetal Med.* 29, 1283–1288. doi: 10.3109/14767058.2015.1046045

Freund, A., Orjalo, A. V., Desprez, P. -Y., and Campisi, J. (2010). Inflammatory networks during cellular senescence: causes and consequences. *Trends Mol. Med.* 16, 238–246. doi: 10.1016/j.molmed.2010.03.003

Gielen, M., Hageman, G., Pachen, D., Derom, C., Vlietinck, R., and Zeegers, M. P. (2014). Placental telomere length decreases with gestational age and is influenced by parity: a study of third trimester live-born twins. *Placenta* 35, 791–796. doi: 10.1016/j.placenta.2014.05.010

Gomez-Lopez, N., Romero, R., Plazyo, O., Schwenkel, G., Garcia-flores, V., Unkel, R., et al. (2017). Preterm labor in the absence of acute histologic chorioamnionitis is characterized by cellular senescence of the chorioamniotic membranes. *Am. J. Obstet. Gynecol.* 217, 592.e1–592.e17. doi: 10.1016/j.ajog.2017.08.008

Gu, D., Li, J., Little, J., Li, H., and Zhang, X. (2020). Associations between serum sex hormone concentrations and telomere length among U.S. adults, 1999-2002. *J. Nutr. Health Aging* 24, 48–54. doi: 10.1007/s12603-019-1291-x

Hahn, S., Giaglis, S., Buser, A., Hoesli, I., Lapaire, O., and Hasler, P. (2014). Cell-free nucleic acids in (maternal) blood: any relevance to (reproductive) immunologists? *J. Reprod. Immunol.* 104-105, 26–31. doi: 10.1016/j.jri.2014.03.007

Hayflick, L. (1965). The limited in vitro lifetime of human diploid cell strains. *Exp. Cell Res.* 37, 614–636. doi: 10.1016/0014-4827(65)90211-9

Horvath, S. (2013). DNA methylation age of human tissues and cell types. *Genome Biol.* 14:R115. doi: 10.1186/gb-2013-14-10-r115

Howcroft, T. K., Campisi, J., Louis, G. B., Smith, M. T., Wise, B., Wyss-Coray, T., et al. (2013). The role of inflammation in age-related disease. *Aging* 5, 84–93. doi: 10.18632/aging.100531

Hu, H., Li, B., and Duan, S. (2019). The alteration of subtelomeric DNA methylation in aging-related diseases. *Front. Genet.* 10:697. doi: 10.3389/fgene.2018.00697

Hua, R., Pease, J. E., Cheng, W., Sooranna, S. R., Viney, J. M., Nelson, S. M., et al. (2013). Human labour is associated with a decline in myometrial chemokine receptor expression: the role of prostaglandins, oxytocin and cytokines. *Am. J. Reprod. Immunol.* 69, 21–32. doi: 10.1111/aji.12025

Iwasa, H., Han, J., and Ishikawa, F. (2003). Mitogen-activated protein kinase p38 defines the common senescence-signalling pathway. *Genes Cells* 8, 131–144. doi: 10.1046/j.1365-2443.2003.00620.x

Jose, S. S., Bendickova, K., Kepak, T., Krenova, Z., and Fric, J. (2017). Chronic inflammation in immune aging: role of pattern recognition receptor crosstalk with the telomere complex? *Front. Immunol.* 8:1078. doi: 10.3389/fimmu.2017.01078

Joyce, B. T., Zheng, Y., Nannini, D., Zhang, Z., Liu, L., Gao, T., et al. (2018). DNA methylation of telomere-related genes and cancer risk. *Cancer Prev. Res.* 11, 511–522. doi: 10.1016/j.physbeh.2017.03.040

Kamel, R. M. (2010). The onset of human parturition. *Arch. Gynecol. Obstet.* 281, 975–982. doi: 10.1007/s00404-010-1365-9

Kang, Y., Zhang, H., Zhao, Y., Wang, Y., Wang, W., He, Y., et al. (2018). Telomere dysfunction disturbs macrophage mitochondrial metabolism and the NLRP3 inflammasome through the PGC-1α/TNFAIP3 axis. *Cell Rep.* 22, 3493–3506. doi: 10.1016/j.celrep.2018.02.071

Karimi, F., Nabizadeh, R., and Yunesian, M. (2020). Association between leukocyte telomere length and serum concentrations of PCBs and organochlorine pesticides. *Arch. Environ. Contam. Toxicol.* 79, 122–130. doi: 10.1007/s00244-020-00732-z

Kawanishi, S., and Oikawa, S. (2004). Mechanism of telomere shortening by oxidative stress. *Ann. N. Y. Acad. Sci.* 1019, 278–284. doi: 10.1196/annals.1297.047

Konwar, C., Price, E. M., Wang, L. Q., Wilson, S. L., Terry, J., and Robinson, W. P. (2018). DNA methylation profiling of acute chorioamnionitis-associated placentas and fetal membranes: insights into epigenetic variation in spontaneous preterm births. *Epigenetics Chromatin* 11:63. doi: 10.1186/s13072-018-0234-9

Lappas, M., Riley, C., Lim, R., Barker, G., Rice, G. E., Menon, R., et al. (2011). MAPK and AP-1 proteins are increased in term pre-labour fetal membranes overlying the cervix: regulation of enzymes involved in the degradation of fetal membranes. *Placenta* 32, 1016–1025. doi: 10.1016/j.placenta.2011.09.011

Liu, Y., Hoyo, C., Murphy, S., Huang, Z., Overcash, F., Thompson, J., et al. (2013). DNA methylation at imprint regulatory regions in preterm birth and infection. *Am. J. Obstet. Gynecol.* 208, 395.e1–395.e7. doi: 10.1016/j.ajog.2013.02.006

Lu, W., Zhang, Y., Liu, D., Songyang, Z., and Wan, M. (2013). Telomeres-structure, function, and regulation. *Exp. Cell Res.* 319, 133–141. doi: 10.1016/j.yexcr.2012.09.005

Luo, X., Shi, Q., Gu, Y., Pan, J., Hua, M., Liu, M., et al. (2013). LncRNA pathway involved in premature preterm rupture of membrane (PPROM): an epigenomic approach to study the pathogenesis of reproductive disorders. *PLoS One* 8:e79897. doi: 10.1371/journal.pone.0079897

Martin, L. F., Moço, N. P., de Lima, M. D., Polettini, J., Miot, H. A., Corrêa, C. R., et al. (2017). Histologic chorioamnionitis does not modulate the oxidative stress and antioxidant status in pregnancies complicated by spontaneous preterm delivery. *BMC Pregnancy Childbirth* 17:376. doi: 10.1186/s12884-017-1549-4

Menon, R. (2016). Human fetal membranes at term: dead tissue or signalers of parturition? *Placenta* 44, 1–5. doi: 10.1016/j.placenta.2016.05.013

Menon, R., Boldogh, I., Hawkins, H. K., Woodson, M., Polettini, J., Syed, T. A., et al. (2014a). Histological evidence of oxidative stress and premature senescence in preterm premature rupture of the human fetal membranes recapitulated in vitro. *Am. J. Pathol.* 184, 1740–1751. doi: 10.1016/j.ajpath.2014.02.011

Menon, R., Bonney, E. A., Condon, J., Mesiano, S., and Taylor, R. N. (2016). Novel concepts on pregnancy clocks and alarms: redundancy and synergy in human parturition. *Hum. Reprod. Update* 22, 535–560. doi: 10.1093/humupd/dmw022

Menon, R., Dixon, C. L., Sheller-Miller, S., Fortunato, S. J., Saade, G. R., Palma, C., et al. (2019). Quantitative proteomics by SWATH-MS of maternal plasma exosomes determine pathways associated with term and preterm birth. *Endocrinology* 160, 639–650. doi: 10.1210/en.2018-00820

Menon, R., Polettini, J., Syed, T. A., Saade, G. R., and Boldogh, I. (2014b). Expression of 8-oxoguanine glycosylase in human fetal membranes. *Am. J. Reprod. Immunol.* 72, 75–84. doi: 10.1111/aji.12220

Menon, R., and Richardson, L. S. (2017). Preterm prelabor rupture of the membranes: a disease of the fetal membranes. *Semin. Perinatol.* 41, 409–419. doi: 10.1053/j.semperi.2017.07.012

Menon, R., Yu, J., Basanta-Henry, P., Brou, L., Berga, S. L., Stephen, J., et al. (2012). Short fetal leukocyte telomere length and preterm prelabor rupture of the membranes. *PLoS One* 7:e31136. doi: 10.1371/journal.pone.0031136

Mitro, S. D., Birnbaum, L. S., Needham, B. L., and Zota, A. R. (2016). Cross-sectional associations between exposure to persistent organic pollutants and leukocyte telomere length among U.S. adults in NHANES, 2001–2002. *Environ. Health Perspect.* 124, 651–658. doi: 10.1289/ehp.1510187

Nabetani, A., and Ishikawa, F. (2011). Alternative lengthening of telomeres pathway: recombination-mediated telomere maintenance mechanism in human cells. *J. Biochem.* 149, 5–14. doi: 10.1093/jb/mvq119

Novakovic, B., Napier, C. E., Vryer, R., Dimitriadis, E., Manuelpillai, U., Sharkey, A., et al. (2016). DNA methylation mediated up-regulation of TERRA non-coding RNA is coincident with elongated telomeres in the human placenta. *Mol. Hum. Reprod.* 22, 791–799. doi: 10.1093/molehr/gaw053

O'Sullivan, R. J., Kubicek, S., Schreiber, S. L., and Karlseder, J. (2010). Reduced histone biosynthesis and chromatin changes arising from a damage signal at telomeres. *Nat. Struct. Mol. Biol.* 17, 1218–1225. doi: 10.1038/nsmb.1897

Parry, S., and Strauss, J. F. (1998). Premature rupture of the fetal membranes. *Mech. Dis.* 338, 663–670.

Paules, C., Dantas, A. P., Miranda, J., Crovetto, F., Eixarch, E., Rodriguez-Sureda, V., et al. (2019). Premature placental aging in term small-for-gestational-age and growth-restricted fetuses. *Ultrasound Obstet. Gynecol.* 53, 615–622. doi: 10.1002/uog.20103

Phillippe, M. (2015). Cell-free fetal DNA, telomeres, and the spontaneous onset of parturition. *Reprod. Sci.* 22, 1186–1201. doi: 10.1177/1933719115592714

Phillippe, M., Sawyer, M. R., and Edelson, P. K. (2019). The telomere gestational clock: increasing short telomeres at term in the mouse. *Am. J. Obstet. Gynecol.* 220, 496.e1–496.e8. doi: 10.1016/j.ajog.2019.01.218

Pickett, H. A., and Reddel, R. R. (2012). The role of telomere trimming in normal telomere length dynamics. *Cell Cycle* 11, 1309–1315. doi: 10.4161/cc.19632

Pineda-Pampliega, J., Herrera-Dueñas, A., Mulder, E., Aguirre, J. I., Höfle, U., and Verhulst, S. (2020). Antioxidant supplementation slows telomere shortening in free-living white stork chicks. *Proc. Biol. Soc.* 287, 20191917. doi: 10.1098/rspb.2019.1917

Polettini, J., Behnia, F., Taylor, B. D., Saade, G. R., Taylor, R. N., and Menon, R. (2015a). Telomere fragment induced amnion cell senescence: a contributor to parturition? *PLoS One* 10:e0137188. doi: 10.1371/journal.pone.0137188

Polettini, J., Dutta, E. H., Behnia, F., Saade, G. R., Torloni, M. R., and Menon, R. (2015b). Aging of intrauterine tissues in spontaneous preterm birth and preterm premature rupture of the membranes: a systematic review of the literature. *Placenta* 36, 969–973. doi: 10.1016/j.placenta.2015.05.003

Polettini, J., Richardson, L. S., and Menon, R. (2018). Oxidative stress induces senescence and sterile inflammation in murine amniotic cavity. *Placenta* 63, 26–31. doi: 10.1016/j.placenta.2018.01.009

Richardson, L., and Menon, R. (2018). Proliferative, migratory, and transition properties reveal metastate of human amnion cells. *Am. J. Pathol.* 188, 2004–2015. doi: 10.1016/j.ajpath.2018.05.019

Robinson, W. P., and Price, E. M. (2015). The human placental methylome. *Cold Spring Harb. Perspect. Med.* 5:a023044. doi: 10.1101/cshperspect.a023044

Rodier, F., and Campisi, J. (2011). Four faces of cellular senescence. *J. Cell Biol.* 192, 547–556. doi: 10.1083/jcb.201009094

Romero, R., Espinoza, J., Kusanovic, J. P., Gotsch, F., Hassan, S., Erez, O., et al. (2006). The preterm parturition syndrome. *BJOG* 113, 17–42. doi: 10.1111/j.1471-0528.2006.01120.x

Romero, R., Xu, Y., Plazyo, O., Chaemsaithong, P., Chaiworapongsa, T., Unkel, R., et al. (2018). A role for the inflammasome in spontaneous labor at term. *Am. J. Reprod. Immunol.* 79:e12440. doi: 10.1111/aji.12440.A

Rosenquist, T. A., Zharkov, D. O., and Grollman, A. P. (1997). Cloning and characterization of a mammalian 8-oxoguanine DNA glycosylase. *Proc. Natl. Acad. Sci. U. S. A.* 94, 7429–7434. doi: 10.1073/pnas.94.14.7429

Rossiello, F., Herbig, U., Longhese, M. P., Fumagalli, M., and d'Adda di Fagagna, F. (2014). Irreparable telomeric DNA damage and persistent DDR signalling as a shared causative mechanism of cellular senescence and ageing. *Curr. Opin. Genet. Dev.* 26, 89–95. doi: 10.1016/j.gde.2014.06.009

Rosso, P. (1976). Placenta as an aging organ. *Curr. Concepts Nutr.* 4, 23–41.

Rubtsova, M. P., Vasilkova, D. P., Malyavko, A. N., Naraikina, Y. V., Zvereva, M. I., and Dontsova, O. A. (2012). Telomere lengthening and other functions of telomerase. *Acta Nat.* 4, 44–61. doi: 10.32607/actanaturae.10630

Salminen, A., Kauppinen, A., and Kaarniranta, K. (2012). Emerging role of NF-κB signaling in the induction of senescence-associated secretory phenotype (SASP). *Cell. Signal.* 24, 835–845. doi: 10.1016/j.cellsig.2011.12.006

Sanchez, M., Hoang, S., Kannengiesser, C., Potier, L., Hadjadj, S., Marre, M., et al. (2020). Leukocyte telomere length, DNA oxidation, and risk of lower-extremity amputation in patients with long-standing type 1 diabetes. *Diabetes Care* 43, 828–834. doi: 10.2337/dc19-0973

Sheller-Miller, S., Urrabaz-Garza, R., Saade, G., and Menon, R. (2017). Damage-associated molecular pattern markers HMGB1 and cell-free fetal telomere fragments in oxidative-stressed amnion epithelial cell-derived exosomes. *J. Reprod. Immunol.* 123, 3–11. doi: 10.1007/s10995-015-1800-4

Shin, J. Y., Choi, Y. Y., Jeon, H. S., Hwang, J. H., Kim, S. A., Kang, J. H., et al. (2010). Low-dose persistent organic pollutants increased telomere length in peripheral leukocytes of healthy Koreans. *Mutagenesis* 25, 511–516. doi: 10.1093/mutage/geq035

Smith, R., Maiti, K., and Aitken, R. J. (2013). Unexplained antepartum stillbirth: a consequence of placental aging? *Placenta* 34, 310–313. doi: 10.1016/j.placenta.2013.01.015

Stewart, S. A., Ben-Porath, I., Carey, V. J., O'Connor, B. F., Hahn, W. C., and Weinberg, R. A. (2003). Erosion of the telomeric single-strand overhang at replicative senescence. *Nat. Genet.* 33, 492–496. doi: 10.1038/ng1127

Sutanto, S. S. I., McLennan, S. V., Keech, A. C., and Twigg, S. M. (2019). Shortening of telomere length by metabolic factors in diabetes: protective effects of fenofibrate. *J. Cell Commun. Signal.* 13, 523–530. doi: 10.1007/s12079-019-00521-x

Tan, R., and Lan, L. (2017). "Induction of site-specific oxidative damage at telomeres by killerred-fused shelretin proteins" in *Telomeres and telomerase: Methods and protocols, methods in molecular biology*. ed. Z. Songyang (Berlin/Heidelberg, Germany: Springer Science+Business Media LLC), 139–146.

Toubiana, S., and Selig, S. (2020). Human subtelomeric DNA methylation: regulation and roles in telomere function. *Curr. Opin. Genet. Dev.* 60, 9–16. doi: 10.1016/j.gde.2020.02.004

Ventura, M. T., Casciaro, M., Gangemi, S., and Buquicchio, R. (2017). Immunosenescence in aging: between immune cells depletion and cytokines up-regulation. *Clin. Mol. Allergy* 15:21. doi: 10.1186/s12948-017-0077-0

von Zglinicki, T. (2002). Oxidative stress shortens telomeres. *Trends Biochem. Sci.* 27, 339–344. doi: 10.1016/S0968-0004(02)02110-2

von Zglinicki, T., Pilger, R., and Sitte, N. (2000). Accumulation of single-strand breaks is the major cause of telomere shortening in human fibroblasts. *Free Radic. Biol. Med.* 28, 64–74. doi: 10.1016/S0891-5849(99)00207-5

Whiteman, V. E., Goswami, A., and Salihu, H. M. (2017). Telomere length and fetal programming: a review of recent scientific advances. *Am. J. Reprod. Immunol.* 77:e12661. doi: 10.1111/aji.12661

Wilson, S. L., Liu, Y., and Robinson, W. P. (2016). Placental telomere length decline with gestational age differs by sex and TERT, DNMT1, and DNMT3A DNA methylation. *Placenta* 48, 26–33. doi: 10.1016/j.placenta.2016.10.001

Xu, Z., Duc, K. D., Holcman, D., and Teixeira, M. T. (2013). The length of the shortest telomere as the major determinant of the onset of replicative senescence. *Genetics* 194, 847–857. doi: 10.1534/genetics.113.152322

Yeap, B. B., Hui, J., Knuiman, M. W., Paul Chubb, S. A., Ho, K. K. Y., Flicker, L., et al. (2020). Associations of plasma IGF1, IGFBP3 and estradiol with leucocyte telomere length, a marker of biological age, in men. *Eur. J. Endocrinol.* 182, 23–33. doi: 10.1530/EJE-19-0638

Yeap, B. B., Knuiman, M. W., Divitini, M. L., Hui, J., Arscott, G. M., Handelsman, D. J., et al. (2016). Epidemiological and mendelian randomization studies of dihydrotestosterone and estradiol and leukocyte telomere length in men. *J. Clin. Endocrinol. Metab.* 101, 1299–1306. doi: 10.1210/jc.2015-4139

Zhang, M., Hu, M. L., Huang, J. J., Xia, S. S., Yang, Y., and Dong, K. (2019). Association of leukocyte telomere length with non-alcoholic fatty liver disease in patients with type 2 diabetes. *Chin. Med. J.* 132, 2927–2933. doi: 10.1097/CM9.0000000000000559

Zhou, K., Koike, C., Yoshida, T., Okabe, M., Fathy, M., Kyo, S., et al. (2013). Establishment and characterization of immortalized human amniotic epithelial cells. *Cell Rep.* 15, 55–67. doi: 10.1089/cell.2012.0021

The Complement System in the Pathophysiology of Pregnancy and in Systemic Autoimmune Rheumatic Diseases During Pregnancy

Cecilia Beatrice Chighizola[1], Paola Adele Lonati[1], Laura Trespidi[2], Pier Luigi Meroni[1] and Francesco Tedesco[1]*

[1] Experimental Laboratory of Immunological and Rheumatologic Researches, Istituto Auxologico Italiano, IRCCS, Milan, Italy,
[2] Department of Obstetrics and Gynaecology, Fondazione Cà Granda, Ospedale Maggiore Policlinico, Milan, Italy

*Correspondence:
Francesco Tedesco
tedesco@units.it

The complement system plays a double role in pregnancy exerting both protective and damaging effects at placental level. Complement activation at fetal-maternal interface participates in protection against infectious agents and helps remove apoptotic and necrotic cells. Locally synthesized C1q contributes to the physiologic vascular remodeling of spiral arteries characterized by loss of smooth muscle cells and transformation into large dilated vessels. Complement activation triggered by the inflammatory process induced by embryo implantation can damage trophoblast and other decidual cells that may lead to pregnancy complications if the cells are not protected by the complement regulators CD55, CD46, and CD59 expressed on cell surface. However, uncontrolled complement activation induces placental alterations resulting in adverse pregnancy outcomes. This may occur in pathological conditions characterized by placental localization of complement fixing antibodies directed against beta2-glycoprotein 1, as in patients with anti-phospholipid syndrome, or circulating immune complexes deposited in placenta, as in patients with systemic lupus erythematosus. In other diseases, such as preeclampsia, the mechanism of complement activation responsible for complement deposits in placenta is unclear. Conflicting results have been reported on the relevance of complement assays as diagnostic and prognostic tools to assess complement involvement in pregnant patients with these disorders.

Keywords: complement, pregnancy, obstetric complications, anti-phospholipid syndrome, systemic lupus erythematosus

INTRODUCTION

Motherhood has become a feasible option in recent years even for women with rheumatic diseases, thanks to the marked improvement in the diagnostic modalities and therapeutic approaches developed in the field of rheumatology. Clinicians devoted to the management of pregnant women with systemic autoimmune rheumatic diseases have accumulated a particular experience in systemic lupus erythematosus (SLE), which disproportionately affects women during childbearing age (1, 2). A unique scenario in the obstetric/rheumatologic field is provided by anti-phospholipid syndrome (APS) that manifests with pregnancy complications and vascular thrombosis. Anti-phospholipid antibodies (aPL) interfere directly with pregnancy progression as documented by the ability of aPL administered to pregnant animals to reproduce the disease, offering an invaluable tool to investigate the pathogenic mechanisms implicated in obstetric complications (3).

Pregnancy has become a relatively frequent condition in SLE and APS women over the last decade and its incidence in patients with these diseases does not appear to be different from that of normal pregnant women. However, despite the progress made in recent years, pregnancies in these conditions are still burdened by a high rate of obstetric complications, mainly in terms of pre-eclampsia, preterm delivery, and intrauterine growth restriction (IUGR) (4) and a tight control is recommended for a positive pregnancy outcome (4, 5). Thus, surrogate biomarkers are highly needed in early gestation to identify women at risk of adverse pregnancy outcome and to monitor progression thanks to serial sampling. Similarly, a better elucidation of the pathogenic steps could lead to the development of more effective targeted therapeutic strategies. In this regard, the complement (C) system has attracted much attention as candidate pathogenic effector of autoimmune and non-autoimmune pregnancy complications and surrogate biomarker to stratify obstetric risk in the general population of pregnant women. Earlier notions on C levels refer to lupus pregnancies, which has become a topic of particular interest following the observation of an association between serum C3 and C4 levels and disease flares in non-gravid patients. *In vivo* APS models have progressively unraveled the importance of C in the pathogenesis of obstetric complications. It is important to emphasize that C is a complex system with a subtle balance between protective and damaging effects. This balance undergoes physiologic modifications during gestation, which may bias the accuracy of results. It is thus timely to review available evidence on the actual and potential relevance of C as pathogenic effector of pregnancy complications and biomarker of obstetric outcome in women with systemic autoimmune rheumatic conditions.

THE COMPLEMENT SYSTEM: A DOUBLE-EDGED SWORD

Complement is a humoral component of the innate immune system that contributes to host defense neutralizing infectious agents, removing immune complexes and clearing apoptotic and necrotic cells. The protective function is accomplished through the action of biologically active products that are released as a result of C activation and exert their effects by enhancing phagocytosis, causing cell cytotoxicity, and promoting inflammation (6). Furthermore, the C system plays an important role in bridging innate and adaptive immunity, as its activation is critical for the development of adaptive immunity (7, 8). C is a versatile system organized to provide protection from a variety of targets using different recognition molecules that sense danger signal coming from foreign agents and altered self and trigger the classical, lectin and alternative activation pathways (9) (**Figure 1**). All pathways converge at the level of C3 and proceed along a common terminal pathway leading to the release of the anaphylotoxins C3a and C5a, cell deposition of C3b and assembly of the terminal C complex. The complex inserts into the cell membrane as membrane attack complex (MAC) forming membrane pores that are responsible for cell lysis. Alternatively, the complex that fails to exert a cytotoxic effect accumulates in blood and extravascular fluids as soluble SC5b-9, which can trigger cytokine synthesis, stimulates inflammation, and induces vascular leakage (10, 11).

Although C is quite selective in focusing the defense activity on dangerous targets recognized by the initiators of the activation pathways, the effector molecules released during the activation process are unable to discriminate between self and non-self and may easily bind to bystander cells. This may happen in physiological conditions, as the C system usually operates at a steady state level of activation, and the split product C3b continuously formed in the circulation and in the extravascular fluid is deposited on the cell surface. As a result, normal cells and tissues are exposed to C attack that may be destructive under conditions of unrestricted C activation. Fortunately, the potential danger that may derive from an undesired C attack is prevented by the protective effect of C regulators and inhibitors present in the fluid phase and widely expressed also on the cell surface (12). These molecules act at various steps of the C sequence and control the function of the system in various ways preventing the assembly of C complexes, favoring their disassembly, and neutralizing the activity of the biologically active products. The membrane–bound regulatory proteins CD46, CD55, and CD59 play a particularly important role in cell protection and may be used by microorganisms and cancer cells to evade C attack. They are often present on the same cells and combine their efforts to control critical steps of C activation at the level of C3 convertases (CD55 and CD46) and MAC assembly (CD59).

The exquisite selectivity of the C system for dangerous targets can be circumvented by C-fixing autoantibodies that react with self-antigens expressed on normal cells and tissues and triggers C activation leading to cell death and tissue damage. However, it is important to emphasize that C activation does not necessarily result in tissue injury, but it may also have beneficial effect contributing for instance to promote angiogenesis and wound healing (13) and also to eliminate inappropriate synaptic connections during development (14).

The role played by the C system in several clinical conditions can now be easily evaluated by functional analysis of the three pathways of C activation and the measurement of activation products recognized by antibodies directed against neoepitopes expressed on cleaved proteins.

THE GROWING IMPORTANCE OF COMPLEMENT IN HEALTHY PREGNANCY

Embryo implantation is a real challenge for the maternal immune system which is confronted with paternal antigens

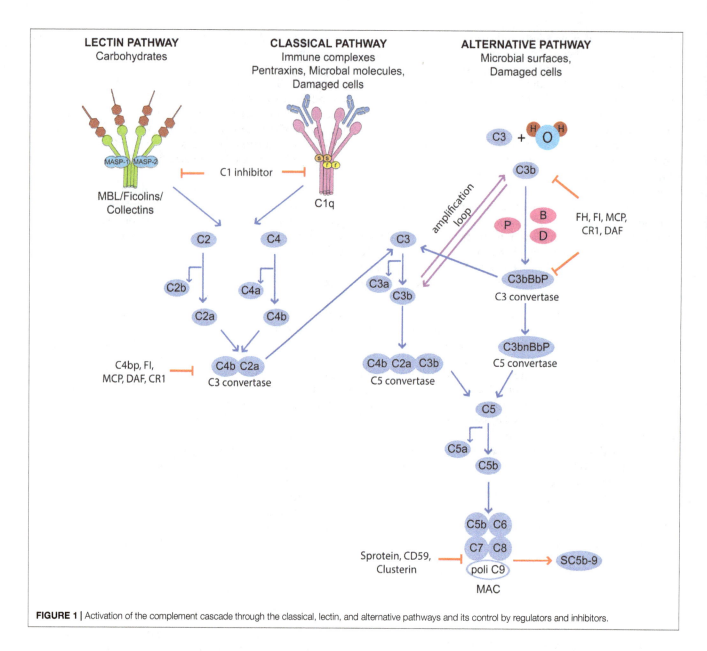

FIGURE 1 | Activation of the complement cascade through the classical, lectin, and alternative pathways and its control by regulators and inhibitors.

expressed on the embryo and the fetus and yet does not mount an immune response leading to its rejection, as it would happen with incompatible organ transplants. Both the trophoblasts that cover the villi bathed into maternal blood and the extravillous trophoblasts invading the maternal decidua represent the main source of these antigens. Villous trophoblasts form a physical double-layer barrier between the fetus and the mother and serve the important function to protect the fetus from maternal immune attack allowing only selective passage of nutrients and defense factors from the mother. Conversely, the extravillous trophoblasts depart from the anchoring villi attached to maternal decidua and contribute to tissue remodeling required for successful implantation. Besides the important role in local defense against infectious agents that may damage the fetus, C has attracted particular attention in recent years for the involvement in the physiologic changes that occur in placenta.

The system is present in the maternal blood that circulates in the intervillous space and may be activated by cell-debris of trophoblasts and possibly immune complexes that have been detected in healthy pregnancy (15). Higher levels of MBL, C4, and C3 and of the activation products C4d, C3a, and SC5b-9 have been reported in pregnant women compared to non-pregnant controls (16), while the circulating levels of C1q do not fluctuate and remain relatively stable throughout normal pregnancy (17, 18). C activation in maternal blood represents a continuous risk for villous trophoblasts and may cause cell damage and impairment of the barrier integrity. This dangerous situation is kept under control by the expression of C regulatory proteins on trophoblast surface including CD55, CD46, and CD59, that act at different steps of the C sequence promoting the decay of the C3 convertases, favoring the inactivation of C3b and C4b and preventing the assembly of C5b-9 (19, 20). C components are also synthesized by different types of cells present in decidua including macrophages, trophoblasts and endothelial cells (21) and form a local system that may operate as a local defense system. Embryo implantation in maternal uterus is associated with an inflammatory-like process induced by proteolytic enzymes that are released by extravillous trophoblast invading the decidua (21). The extensive tissue remodeling caused by trophoblast invasion leads to local recruitment of natural killer cells (NK) and other cells of the innate immune system and activation of the C system, which has limited damaging effect due to the widespread distribution of C regulators. Data collected in recent years have revealed an important role of C1q in the physiological remodeling of decidual spiral artery characterized by partial replacement of endothelial cells by endovascular trophoblasts that migrate upward from the anchoring villi. C1q is synthesized and expressed on the cell surface of both decidual endothelial cells lining the inner side of the spiral arteries and endovascular trophoblasts and serve the important function to establish a molecular bridge between the two cell types (22) (**Figure 2**). The C1q-mediated cellular crosstalk leads to the formation of mosaic vessels with an inner layer formed by the mixture of endothelial cells and trophoblasts. C1q is also synthesized and secreted by the extravillous trophoblasts as soon as they start moving away from the anchoring villi and is required for trophoblast invasion of the decidua (**Figure 2**). By binding to the extracellular matrix, C1q promotes the adhesion and the migration of extravillous trophoblasts that reach the spiral arteries forming cuffs and contribute to the vascular remodeling (23).

COMPLEMENT AND ADVERSE PREGNANCY OUTCOME

Evidence collected over the years has revealed that C plays a dual role during pregnancy. On one hand, the system promotes the physiologic changes at fetal-maternal interface required for a successful pregnancy, and on the other hand it may cause placental damage leading to impairment of the regular progression of gestation. C abnormalities have been reported in several obstetric complications including early pregnancy loss, pre-term birth, and pre-eclampsia. The relevance of C in recurrent miscarriages is supported by data obtained from animal models suggesting a key role for C5a. C activation and interaction of this anaphylatoxin with C5a receptor have been shown to induce the release of soluble vascular endothelial growth factor receptor ultimately resulting in impaired angiogenesis and adverse pregnancy outcomes (24, 25). A role in mediating abortion has also been advocated for anti-C1q antibodies as suggested by the findings that these antibodies administered to pregnant animals induce fetal loss, and that both the prevalence and the titre of anti-C1q antibodies are significantly higher in women with unexplained recurrent pregnancy loss than in healthy parous women (26). Conflicting data have been reported on the circulating levels of C components and C activity in women with early pregnancy loss. While increased levels of C3 and C4 were found in one study and proposed as predictor of fetal loss (27), hypocomplementemia was documented in another study in women with recurrent miscarriages (28). Interestingly, a significant decrease in the placental expression of C regulators

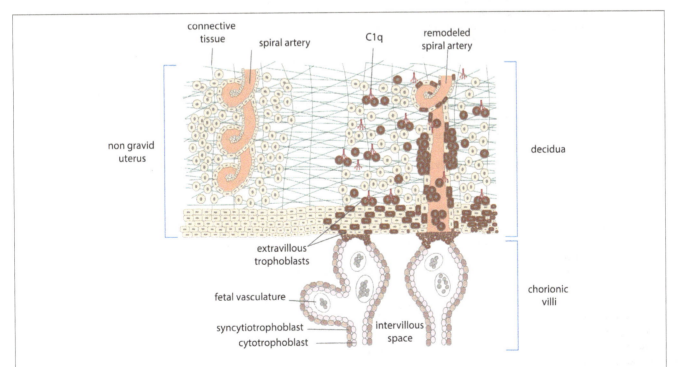

FIGURE 2 | Schematic representation of human placenta showing anchoring villi attached to maternal decidua. Extravillous trophoblasts depart from the villi and invade the decidua surrounding the spiral arteries. Other cells enter the lumen of the arteries as endovasculat trophoblasts and partially replace lining endothelial cells. C1q produced by trophoblasts is used to promote their migration and interaction with endothelial cells.

CD46 and CD55 associated with excessive C activation has been observed after spontaneous abortion, reaffirming the importance of inhibiting C activation to ensure a successful pregnancy (29). Local C activation is supported by the finding of C4d deposits documented by immunohistochemical analysis of the placentae of women with recurrent miscarriages (25). It has been estimated that approximately 20% of otherwise unexplained early pregnancy loss are due to hypocomplementemia (25).

A wealth of data has been collected over several years on the involvement of C in pre-eclampsia, a disorder of pregnancy that affects 3 to 5% of women in the late phase of pregnancy and is characterized by hypertension and proteinuria. Dysregulated angiogenesis is believed to be implicated in the pathogenesis of the disease, as documented by elevated circulating levels of soluble vascular endothelial growth factor receptor 1 (sFlt-1) (30). Animal models have shown that C1q-deficient pregnant mice manifest the key features of human disease such as hypertension, albuminuria, endothelial dysfunction, decreased placental vascular endothelial growth factor, and elevated levels of sFlt-1 providing convincing evidence that C1q protects against pre-eclampsia (31). Consistent with this *in vivo* observation, Agostinis, and colleagues (17) published data indicating that the serum levels of C1q was markedly decreased in both early and late onset forms of pre-eclampsia. Likewise, women with early onset pre-eclampsia are twice as likely to carry deficiency in C4A or C4B suggesting that C4 may also contribute to prevent the onset of pre-eclampsia (32). The reduced concentration of C1q observed in patients with overt pre-eclampsia cannot be used as predictive marker of the disease because the analysis of serum samples collected at an early phase of pregnancy from women who later developed preeclampsia failed to show a decrease in C1q level (17). Mannose binding lectin (MBL) seems to have an opposite effect to that of C1q since the level is elevated in patients with severe pre-eclampsia (33, 34). Furthermore, MBL strongly inhibits the interaction of extravillous trophoblast with C1q and interferes with the process of cell migration (34), suggesting the contribution of MBL to the pathogenesis of the disease.

It has been postulated that C activation following placental ischemia may induce hypertension and impair fetal growth via the endothelin pathway (35). Analysis of C activation products in patients with pre-eclampsia has revealed increased serum levels of C3a, C5a, and SC5b-9 (16, 36, 37) and C activation products have also been detected in the urine of patients with a severe form of the disease as a result of C-mediated renal injury (38). High levels of the activation product of the alternative pathway Bb have been observed in the early phase of pregnancy in women who later developed pre-eclampsia and proposed as an early biomarker of this disease. The finding of high mRNA expression of the membrane C regulators CD55 and CD59 in placenta specimens from pre-eclamptic women has been interpreted as a compensatory attempt to limit local C activation (32). C4d is the C split product most frequently seen in pre-eclamptic placentae, particularly on syncytiotrophoblast, with focal or diffuse staining patterns (39), and the degree of C4d and MAC deposition in the placental tissue is strongly correlated with sFlt1 levels in pre-eclamptic patients (40). Available evidence suggests that activation of the C system is involved in spontaneous preterm birth. Lynch and coworkers (41) measured the circulating levels of Bb, a marker of alternative pathway activation, in pregnant women in the early phase of gestation and found that those with elevated levels were more likely to experience preterm delivery. They propose Bb as a predictor of this adverse pregnancy outcome that develops in late gestation before 34 weeks. An essentially similar conclusion was reached measuring the levels of C3a under the same experimental conditions and again higher levels were associated with preterm birth (42). The increased levels of C5a observed in women with preterm delivery suggest that C5a, by reacting with C5aR, plays a role in the pathogenesis of preterm labor (43).

COMPLEMENT AND OBSTETRIC ANTI-PHOSPHOLIPID SYNDROME

Anti-phospholipid syndrome is an acquired prothrombotic condition characterized by vascular occlusive events occurring in vessels of different size and/or obstetric complications. Adverse pregnancy outcomes include three or more spontaneous abortions before 10 weeks of gestation, one or more unexplained fetal death at or beyond week 10 of gestation, one or more preterm delivery before 34 weeks due to severe pre-eclampsia, HELLP syndrome (hemolytic anemia, elevated liver enzymes, low platelet count) or placental insufficiency. aPL are the serum biomarkers of APS, routinely detected by a functional assay, named lupus anticoagulant (LA), and two solid phase assays identifying IgG and IgM antibodies against cardiolipin (aCL) and beta2-glycoprotein I (anti-β2GPI). β2GPI, the main antigenic target of aPL, is a five domain (D) glycoprotein comprising four C control protein (CCP)-like domains (DI-DIV) and one domain (44) with a large lysine loop which allows β2GPI to interact with anionic phospholipids and other molecules on cell surfaces, coagulation factors, platelets, and complement (45). Antibodies against β2GPI co-localize with their target antigen on trophoblasts and decidual endothelial cells in immunized animals that had received fluorescein-labeled β2GPI (46) and interfere with pregnancy progression by impairing the function of the developing placenta. The antibodies exert their effect on the maternal side, promoting a negative imbalance of angiogenic factors that inhibits endometrial angiogenesis. Furthermore, they act on trophoblasts inducing apoptosis and inhibiting the secretion of β human chorionic gonadotropin and matrix metalloproteinases (MMP) required for invasion of decidua, and in complex with β2GPI activate the classical pathway of the C cascade (47). Several clinical studies have examined the activation of the C system in pregnant patients with APS and its contribution to pregnancy complications. Decreased serum levels of C4 and C3 have been reported in approximately one third of patients with APS (48) and the follow-up of these patients throughout pregnancy revealed that the C4 and C3 levels remained persistently low compared to the values of control pregnant women when normalized for the trimester of gestation (49). As shown in **Table 1**, lower levels of C3 and C4 were found to correlate with adverse obstetric outcomes in some studies (50, 51), but not in others (49, 52). Data obtained from a prospective

TABLE 1 | Studies assessing the correlation of C3 and C4 serum levels with obstetric outcome in pregnant women with anti-phospholipid syndrome.

Author, year	Number of APS patients/ pregnancies	Study design	Timing of C testing	Control group	Main findings
Ruffatti, 2011 (50)	114/114 All PAPS	Retrospective	Baseline and at the end of pregnancies	None	- Hypocomplementemia was associated with adverse pregnancy outcome at univariate analysis.
De Carolis, 2012 (51)	47/47 PAPS/SAPS (No SLE)	Prospective	Within 20 gestational weeks	None	- Hypocomplementemia was associated with fetal loss and preterm delivery at univariate analysis. - Women with hypocomplementemia had lower neonatal birth weight. - Hypocomplementemia was not associated with PE and IUGR at univariate analysis.
Reggia, 2012 (49)	45/57 PAPS	Retrospective	I-II-III trimester	49 women with UCTD/SjS 175 healthy pregnant women	- Hypocomplementemia was not associated with adverse pregnancy outcome in PAPS women. - Women with PAPS had lower C3 and C4 than healthy women, but similar to UCTD and SjS.
Deguchi, 2017 (52)	69/81 PAPS/SAPS (mainly SLE)	Retrospective	NS	None	- Hypocomplementemia was not associated with pregnancy loss, premature delivery and IUGR. - Hypocomplementemia was associated with hypertension at multivariate analysis.

PAPS, primary anti-phospholipid syndrome; SAPS, secondary anti-phospholipid syndrome; C, complement; NS, not specified; SLE, systemic lupus erythematosus; UCTD, undifferentiated connective tissue disease; SjS, Sjögren syndrome; PE, pre-eclampsia; and IUGR, intra-uterine growth restriction.

study of APS pregnant women led De Carolis et al. (51) to suggest that reduced C3 and C4 levels should be regarded as predictors of lower neonatal birth weight and preterm delivery. A multicenter study performed in Japan showed that low levels of C3 and C4 represent a risk factor for hypertensive disorders of pregnancy (52). Evaluation of biologically active circulating products of the C system in APS pregnant patients offers more direct insights on C activation in this clinical condition. Blood samples from 161 aPL positive women including 60 with SLE were analyzed for the presence of Bb and SC5b-9 and increased levels of both activation products were found in all patients with adverse obstetric outcome (53). This finding has been confirmed by a more recent study, reporting higher C5a and C5b-9 levels in APS pregnant patients with pregnancy complications compared to healthy pregnant women (54). More convincing evidence supporting the role of C in inducing aPL-dependent placental damage and pregnancy failure has been obtained from the immunohistochemical analysis of placental tissue for C deposits. The presence of C4d in placentae from APS women has been documented at the fetal-maternal interface, in particular on syncytiotrophoblast basement membrane, and to some extent also on extravillous trophoblasts of the basal plate by three groups (55–57). C4 deposits were found to be associated with intrauterine fetal death (55) and placental abnormalities including decidual vasculopathy, increased syncytial knots, and villous infarcts (57). Two groups have documented deposits of C5b-9 mainly localized on extravillous trophoblasts of placentae from aPL-positive women and observed no difference in the staining intensity between APS and control groups (56, 57). These findings are in contrast with the data obtained by Scambi et al. who reported higher levels of C5b-9 solubilized from APS placentae compared to controls, in particular in APS patients who experienced a pregnancy complication (54). Our group has conducted a prospective study on 13 APS patients with medium to high titers of anti-β2GPI antibodies and positive LA who had pregnancies that resulted in one abortion, four fetal losses, and eight preterm deliveries (58). Histological and immunohistochemical analysis revealed placental abnormalities characterized by decidual vasculopathy and intervillous thrombi and deposition of IgG, IgM, C1q, C4, and C3 suggesting C activation through the classical pathway. Interestingly, C5b-9 was detected in all placentae and was localized on the surface of syncytiotrophoblasts, intervillous fibrin and decidual vessels supporting its contribution to tissue damage. Taken together, these findings suggest that complement activation is involved in placental pathology acting both on villous trophoblast and on endothelial cells of decidual vessels (**Figure 3**). Animal models of APS developed by infusing patient's IgG have provided key information on the role played by the C system in eliciting placental abnormalities and adverse pregnancy outcomes. Mice deficient in C3, C4, C5, and factor B were found to be resistant to aPL-induced fetal loss (59–61) and similar results were obtained using a C3 convertase inhibitor, a C5a receptor antagonist or anti-C5 antibodies (60). C5a has been identified as the main mediator of fetal injury by interacting with C5aR expressed on polymorphonuclear leukocytes and by stimulating the release of tissue factor and tumour necrosis factor (TNF)-α, which in turn promotes inflammation (62, 63). Given the growing evidence implicating C activation as key contributor to the pathogenesis of the clinical manifestations of APS, C inhibitors have been considered good candidates for the therapy of APS. Although the neutralizing anti-C5 antibody eculizumab has been used successfully in treating patients with catastrophic APS and in preventing re-thrombosis in patients undergoing surgical intervention (58, 64), very few information is available on its use in APS pregnant patients except for an anecdotal report of a patient who received eculizumab to prevent severe pregnancy complications (65). A non-C fixing anti-β2GPI monoclonal antibody that was shown to prevent fetal loss in aPL-treated pregnant mice offers an alternative therapeutic approach (66). The advantage of this antibody is to target the β2GPI protein constitutively expressed on villous and extravillous trophoblasts as well as on the endothelium of decidual vessels with relatively high affinity and to compete with antibodies from APS patients.

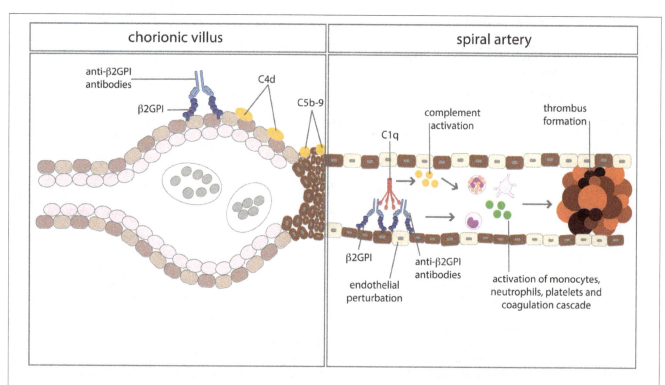

FIGURE 3 | Complement-mediated biological effects at placental level in anti-phospholipid syndrome. Complement activated by antibodies interacting with β2GPI bound to trophoblasts and vascular endothelium of decidual vessels leads to cell damage and promotion of thrombus formation.

COMPLEMENT AND SYSTEMIC LUPUS ERYTHEMATOSUS IN PREGNANCY

Systemic lupus erythematosus is a complex multisystem autoimmune disease with a highly heterogeneous presentation ranging from laboratory abnormalities to multi-organ inflammation and failure and characterized by the production of autoantibodies directed against double stranded DNA and several other autoantigens. The clinical manifestations of SLE are underpinned by several etiopathogenic mechanisms, such as deregulated production of autoantibodies against cellular constituents, abnormal cytokine release, innate, and adaptive immune alterations. Impaired clearance of apoptotic debris is believed to mediate sustained antigen presentation to B cells, ultimately resulting in exaggerated autoantibody production (67). C activated by immune complexes formed in the circulation and at tissue level following interaction of autoantibodies with their target antigen is involved in the pathogenesis of the clinical manifestations of SLE. Some of these autoantibodies are directed against C components, as is the case of anti-C1q antibodies detected in nearly one third of patients with lupus nephritis and thought to have important pathogenic effects in the development of the disease (68). Immune complexes containing anti-C1q antibodies were found to be more potent C activators than classical immune complexes (69). Deposits of C components and C activation products including the terminal complex have been documented in the kidney of SLE patients co-localized with immune complexes suggesting the involvement of C in tissue damage (70). Data accumulated over several years have shown that C plays a paradoxical role in SLE. On the one hand, C activated by immune complexes stimulates inflammation, and causes tissue lesions. The important role played by C is suggested by the beneficial effect of eculizumab in patients with severe lupus nephritis resistant to conventional therapy (71, 72). Further evidence supporting the contribution of C activation to SLE pathogenesis is provided by lupus-prone mouse models, such as NZB/W and MRL/lpr mice, that share with the human disease similar features including autoantibodies production, hypocomplementemia, circulating and glomerular-bound immune complexes, and severe nephritis (73). Treatment of these mice with anti-C5 monoclonal antibodies resulted in improvement of nephritis, reduced proteinuria and prolonged survival (74). On the other hand, C deficiency is now recognized to be a risk factor for SLE development, based on the finding that genetic deficiencies of the early components of the classical pathway from C1q to C4 are associated with the onset of SLE (75). C1q-deficient individuals have the highest susceptibility to SLE due to the role of C1q in the removal of apoptotic cells. The disease occurs in up to 55–75% of individuals with this genetic defect and presents with characteristic clinical features including early age of onset, no gender predilection, low frequency of anti-dsDNA antibodies, prominent photosensitivity, and fewer renal symptoms (76). Given this background, it is not surprising that the C system has attracted particular attention as an important marker of disease activity in SLE patients. It's long been known that C activation in SLE is accompanied by a secondary reduction in circulating C levels and increase in C split products. Importantly, the decrease in C1q, C3, and C4 levels correlates with disease activity and precedes clinically evident flare (77), even though the decrease in C levels are not invariably associated with disease flares (78). Despite the technical and biological limitations, measurements of C3 and C4 have been included not only in the recent classification criteria for SLE, but also in the disease activity indexes such as SLEDAI (79). Recently, C deposition on immune cells was proposed as a more robust method to diagnose and monitor SLE and a panel of parameters including C4d-deposition on B cells and erythrocytes was suggested (80, 81).

Pregnancies in patients with SLE have always been regarded to be at risk, even though the rates of fetal loss and maternal mortality have steadily decreased over the years (82). However, pregnant women with SLE still display an increased hazard of premature delivery and IUGR irrespectively of disease activity, while the odds for pre-eclampsia is elevated in women with active disease only (83). Hypocomplementemia during gestation has been identified as one of the multiple predictors of poor pregnancy outcome in SLE pregnancies including high disease activity in the 6 months before conception, use of anti-hypertensive medications, non-white ethnicity, aPL positivity, and a history of nephritis or active nephritis at conception. Data on C levels in SLE pregnant women vary considerably in different studies, depending on the composition of the study cohort. Thus, hypocomplementemia is prevalent in certain disease manifestations, such as lupus nephritis. C4 level is a more reliable marker of renal involvement in SLE since low C4 at baseline and a history of previous kidney disease have been found to be independently associated with a higher risk of developing active nephritis in pregnancy (84). Pregnant women with lupus nephritis display significantly lower levels of C3 and C4 more often than other SLE subjects (85). Data on the association of C levels with poor pregnancy outcome can be obtained from studies that assess several clinical and laboratory variables of SLE as predictors of adverse obstetric outcomes, but there is no universal agreement on the clinical significance of complement levels as biomarkers in lupus pregnancies. Indeed, few authors deny a predictive role for C3 and C4 whereas in other studies low C3 and/or C4 levels have been associated with adverse pregnancy outcomes such as spontaneous abortion, premature birth and stillbirth (86–88). Unfortunately, a control group of healthy pregnant women was not included in these studies, and the C levels were not normalized for the gestational age, thus limiting the conclusions on the relationship between C3 and C4 levels and pregnancy outcomes. Changes in C levels were evaluated in 386 SLE patients throughout gestation in the PROMISSE study, and a smaller increase in C3 levels in the second and third trimesters was observed in women with adverse obstetric outcome compared to women with uneventful pregnancy, though the difference was not significant (87). Because of the well-known fluctuation of C levels throughout pregnancy, it is not surprising that low C values may not correlate with disease activity in pregnant patients with SLE except when they are lower than those expected in normal pregnant women at the same gestational age (89, 90). The C activation products Ba, Bb and SC5b-9 represent more sensitive indicators of C activation and may be useful to predict and diagnose flares in pregnant SLE patients (89). In the PROMISSE cohort, these markers of C activation (Bb and SC5b-9) were detected in the circulation in early gestation among those SLE/aPL + women who later developed pregnancy complications (53). Analysis of placentae from aPL-negative SLE patients by Matrai and colleagues revealed signs of tissue malperfusion, infarction and intervillous thrombi and increased deposits of C4d and C5b-9 on syncytiotrophoblasts and extravillous trophoblasts compared to controls (56). The extent of C4d deposition was found to be inversely correlated with low placental and birth weight (91).

CONCLUSION

Complement is a versatile system that shows exquisite adaptation to environmental changes and is able to recognize dangerous exogenous and endogenous agents and structures. Besides exerting protective functions, C is now recognized to promote functions unrelated to host defense including tissue repair and remodeling. Data collected in recent years have shown that C plays an important role in the structural organization of placenta at fetal-maternal interface contributing to vascular remodeling of spiral arteries in maternal decidua, a critical process required for the regular progression of pregnancy. However, placenta is not exempt from potential damage that may derive from activation products released as a result of general or local C activation leading to adverse pregnancy outcomes. C exerts a direct damaging effect in clinical situation such as APS as suggested by the failure of antibodies to induce fetal loss in C-deficient animals or treated with neutralizing antibodies to C components. The finding of C components at placental level both in APS patients and in animal models further supports the involvement of C in the onset of placental alterations and has both diagnostic and therapeutic implications. Measurement of C levels is routinely performed in many obstetrics/rheumatology joint clinics to monitor APS pregnancies, but hypocomplementemia does not seem to be a reliable marker to predict pregnancy loss in these patients. More sophisticated and sensitive methods have been proposed to monitor C activation, as is the case of cell-bound C split products. The recent report of a higher percentage of C4-positive B lymphocytes, erythrocytes, and platelets in patients with obstetric and thrombotic manifestations compared to controls (92) suggests that this assay may be an interesting tool to explore C activation in pregnant women with APS or SLE. Preventive treatment with neutralizing antibodies or other reagents aimed at controlling C activation is a promising therapeutic approach in APS. Indeed, heparin currently used as treatment of choice for pregnant APS women together with low dose aspirin was shown to inhibit C activation and to prevent cell binding of β2GPI as a result of interaction with the heparin-binding site located on DV (93). C is most likely involved in the adverse pregnancy outcome observed in patients with SLE, a prototypical C-mediated disease. Currently, measurement of C levels is requested by the obstetricians to differentiate between nephritis and pre-eclampsia in SLE patient with proteinuria. C3 and C4 levels normally rise in patients with pre-eclampsia, while drops in C3 and C4 levels, coupled with a rising anti-dsDNA titre, are more likely associated with disease flares (94). However, despite many studies conducted to identify predictors of adverse outcome in lupus pregnancies, there are no clear data supporting the association between fluctuation of C levels and disease flare during gestation. Conclusive data on C-mediated tissue damage associated with adverse pregnancy outcomes can be provided by the histological analysis of placenta samples from patients. To be informative, the results should be compared with those of healthy controls of the same gestational age as the phenotype changes with the progression of gestation. To date, C4d has emerged as the most interesting biomarker of C activation in placenta specimens. This is not surprising since C4d, like C3d, binds covalently to the target cell surface and, being highly stable, acts as a fingerprint of C-mediated activation leading to tissue injury. In conclusion, there are indications to suggest that C is involved in complicated pregnancies, although the precise mechanism by which C is activated is not always clear and remains to be determined.

AUTHOR CONTRIBUTIONS

PM and FT designed the study. CC, PL, and LT retrieved the relevant literature. CC and FT drafted the manuscript. PL prepared the figures. PM, LT, and FT revised the literature critically for important intellectual content. All authors approved the final version of the article.

REFERENCES

Andreoli L, Fredi M, Nalli C, Reggia R, Lojacono A, Motta M, et al. Pregnancy implications for systemic lupus erythematosus and the antiphospholipid syndrome. *J Autoimmun.* (2012) 38:J197–208. doi: 10.1016/j.jaut.2011.11.010

Ostensen M, Andreoli L, Brucato A, Cetin I, Chambers C, Clowse ME, et al. State of the art: reproduction and pregnancy in rheumatic diseases. *Autoimmun Rev.* (2015) 14:376–86. doi: 10.1016/j.autrev.2014.12.011

Meroni PL, Borghi MO, Raschi E, Tedesco F. Pathogenesis of antiphospholipid syndrome: understanding the antibodies. *Nat Rev Rheumatol.* (2011) 7:330–9. doi: 10.1038/nrrheum.2011.52

Jain V, Gordon C. Managing pregnancy in inflammatory rheumatological diseases. *Arthritis Res Ther.* (2011) 13:206. doi: 10.1186/ar3227

Andreoli L, Bertsias GK, Agmon-Levin N, Brown S, Cervera R, Costedoat-Chalumeau N, et al. EULAR recommendations for women's health and the management of family planning, assisted reproduction, pregnancy and menopause in patients with systemic lupus erythematosus and/or antiphospholipid syndrome. *Ann Rheum Dis.* (2017) 76:476–85. doi: 10.1136/annrheumdis-2016-209770

Merle NS, Noe R, Halbwachs-Mecarelli L, Fremeaux-Bacchi V, Roumenina LT. Complement system part II: role in immunity. *Front Immunol.* (2015) 6:257. doi: 10.3389/fimmu.2015.00257

Dunkelberger JR, Song WC. Complement and its role in innate and adaptive immune responses. *Cell Res.* (2010) 20:34–50. doi: 10.1038/cr.2009.139

Freeley S, Kemper C, Le Friec G. The "ins and outs" of complement-driven immune responses. *Immunol Rev.* (2016) 274:16–32. doi: 10.1111/imr.12472

Reis ES, Mastellos DC, Hajishengallis G, Lambris JD. New insights into the immune functions of complement. *Nat Rev Immunol.* (2019) 19:503–16. doi: 10.1038/s41577-019-0168-x

Bossi F, Fischetti F, Pellis V, Bulla R, Ferrero E, Mollnes TE, et al. Platelet-activating factor and kinin-dependent vascular leakage as a novel functional activity of the soluble terminal complement complex. *J Immunol.* (2004) 173:6921–7. doi: 10.4049/jimmunol.173.11.6921

Dobrina A, Pausa M, Fischetti F, Bulla R, Vecile E, Ferrero E, et al. Cytolytically inactive terminal complement complex causes transendothelial migration of polymorphonuclear leukocytes in vitro and in vivo. *Blood.* (2002) 99:185–92. doi: 10.1182/blood.v99.1.185

Zipfel PF, Skerka C. Complement regulators and inhibitory proteins. *Nat Rev Immunol.* (2009) 9:729–40. doi: 10.1038/nri2620

Bossi F, Tripodo C, Rizzi L, Bulla R, Agostinis C, Guarnotta C, et al. C1q as a unique player in angiogenesis with therapeutic implication in wound healing. *Proc Natl Acad Sci USA.* (2014) 111:4209–14. doi: 10.1073/pnas.1311968111

Stevens B, Allen NJ, Vazquez LE, Howell GR, Christopherson KS, Nouri N, et al. The classical complement cascade mediates CNS synapse elimination. *Cell.* (2007) 131:1164–78. doi: 10.1016/j.cell.2007.10.036

Girardi G, Prohaszka Z, Bulla R, Tedesco F, Scherjon S. Complement activation in animal and human pregnancies as a model for immunological recognition. *Mol Immunol.* (2011) 48:1621–30. doi: 10.1016/j.molimm.2011.04.011

Derzsy Z, Prohaszka Z, Rigo J Jr., Fust G, Molvarec A. Activation of the complement system in normal pregnancy and preeclampsia. *Mol Immunol.* (2010) 47:1500–6. doi: 10.1016/j.molimm.2010.01.021

Agostinis C, Stampalija T, Tannetta D, Loganes C, Vecchi Brumatti L, De Seta F, et al. Complement component C1q as potential diagnostic but not predictive marker of preeclampsia. *Am J Reprod Immunol.* (2016) 76:475–81. doi: 10.1111/aji.12586

Jia K, Ma L, Wu S, Yang W. Serum levels of complement factors C1q, Bb, and H in normal pregnancy and severe Pre-Eclampsia. *Med Sci Monit.* (2019) 25:7087–93. doi: 10.12659/MSM.915777

Holmes CH, Simpson KL, Okada H, Okada N, Wainwright SD, Purcell DF, et al. Complement regulatory proteins at the feto-maternal interface during human placental development: distribution of CD59 by comparison with membrane cofactor protein (CD46) and decay accelerating factor (CD55). *Eur J Immunol.* (1992) 22:1579–85. doi: 10.1002/eji.1830220635

Tedesco F, Narchi G, Radillo O, Meri S, Ferrone S, Betterle C. Susceptibility of human trophoblast to killing by human complement and the role of the complement regulatory proteins. *J Immunol.* (1993) 151:1562–70.

Bulla R, Bossi F, Tedesco F. The complement system at the embryo implantation site: friend or foe? *Front Immunol.* (2012) 3:55. doi: 10.3389/fimmu.2012.00055

Bulla R, Agostinis C, Bossi F, Rizzi L, Debeus A, Tripodo C, et al. Decidual endothelial cells express surface-bound C1q as a molecular bridge between endovascular trophoblast and decidual endothelium. *Mol Immunol.* (2008) 45:2629–40. doi: 10.1016/j.molimm.2007.12.025

Agostinis C, Bulla R, Tripodo C, Gismondi A, Stabile H, Bossi F, et al. An alternative role of C1q in cell migration and tissue remodeling: contribution to trophoblast invasion and placental development. *J Immunol.* (2010) 185:4420– 9. doi: 10.4049/jimmunol.0903215

Girardi G, Yarilin D, Thurman JM, Holers VM, Salmon JE. Complement activation induces dysregulation of angiogenic factors and causes fetal rejection and growth restriction. *J Exp Med.* (2006) 203:2165–75. doi: 10.1084/jem.20061022

Girardi G. Complement activation, a threat to pregnancy. *Semin Immunopathol.* (2018) 40:103–11. doi: 10.1007/s00281-017-0645-x

Ohmura K, Oku K, Kitaori T, Amengual O, Hisada R, Kanda M, et al. Pathogenic roles of anti-C1q antibodies in recurrent pregnancy loss. *Clin Immunol.* (2019) 203:37–44. doi: 10.1016/j.clim.2019.04.005

Sugiura-Ogasawara M, Nozawa K, Nakanishi T, Hattori Y, Ozaki Y. Complement as a predictor of further miscarriage in couples with recurrent miscarriages. *Hum Reprod.* (2006) 21:2711–4. doi: 10.1093/humrep/del229

Micheloud D, Sarmiento E, Teijeiro R, Jensen J, Rodriguez Molina JJ, Fernandez-Cruz E, et al. Hypocomplementemia in the absence of autoantibodies in women with recurrent pregnancy loss. *Allergol Immunopathol.* (2007) 35:90–4. doi: 10.1157/13106775

Banadakoppa M, Chauhan MS, Havemann D, Balakrishnan M, Dominic JS, Yallampalli C. Spontaneous abortion is associated with elevated systemic C5a and reduced mRNA of complement inhibitory proteins in placenta. *Clin Exp Immunol.* (2014) 177:743–9. doi: 10.1111/cei.12371

Wikstrom AK, Larsson A, Eriksson UJ, Nash P, Norden-Lindeberg S, Olovsson M. Placental growth factor and soluble FMS-like tyrosine kinase-1 in early-onset and late-onset preeclampsia. *Obstet Gynecol.* (2007) 109:1368–74. doi: 10.1097/01.AOG.0000264552.85436.a1

Singh J, Ahmed A, Girardi G. Role of complement component C1q in the onset of preeclampsia in mice. *Hypertension*. (2011) 58:716–24. doi: 10.1161/HYPERTENSIONAHA.111.175919

Lokki AI, Heikkinen-Eloranta J, Jarva H, Saisto T, Lokki ML, Laivuori H, et al. Complement activation and regulation in preeclamptic placenta. *Front Immunol*. (2014) 5:312. doi: 10.3389/fimmu.2014.00312

Than NG, Romero R, Erez O, Kusanovic JP, Tarca AL, Edwin SS, et al. A role for mannose-binding lectin, a component of the innate immune system in pre- eclampsia. *Am J Reprod Immunol*. (2008) 60:333–45. doi: 10.1111/j.1600-0897.2008.00631.x

Agostinis C, Bossi F, Masat E, Radillo O, Tonon M, De Seta F, et al. MBL interferes with endovascular trophoblast invasion in pre- eclampsia. *Clin Dev Immunol*. (2012) 2012:484321. doi: 10.1155/2012/484321

Regal JF, Lund JM, Wing CR, Root KM, McCutcheon L, Bemis LT, et al. Interactions between the complement and endothelin systems in normal pregnancy and following placental ischemia. *Mol Immunol*. (2019) 114:10–8. doi: 10.1016/j.molimm.2019.06.015

Haeger M, Bengtson A, Karlsson K, Heideman M. Complement activation and anaphylatoxin (C3a and C5a) formation in preeclampsia and by amniotic fluid. *Obstet Gynecol*. (1989) 73:551–6.

Denny KJ, Coulthard LG, Finnell RH, Callaway LK, Taylor SM, Woodruff TM. Elevated complement factor C5a in maternal and umbilical cord plasma in preeclampsia. *J Reprod Immunol*. (2013) 97:211–6. doi: 10.1016/j.jri.2012.11.006

Burwick RM, Fichorova RN, Dawood HY, Yamamoto HS, Feinberg BB. Urinary excretion of C5b-9 in severe preeclampsia: tipping the balance of complement activation in pregnancy. *Hypertension*. (2013) 62:1040–5. doi: 10.1161/HYPERTENSIONAHA.113.01420

Buurma A, Cohen D, Veraar K, Schonkeren D, Claas FH, Bruijn JA, et al. Preeclampsia is characterized by placental complement dysregulation. *Hypertension*. (2012) 60:1332–7. doi: 10.1161/HYPERTENSIONAHA.112.194324

Yonekura Collier AR, Zsengeller Z, Pernicone E, Salahuddin S, Khankin EV, Karumanchi SA. Placental sFLT1 is associated with complement activation and syncytiotrophoblast damage in preeclampsia. *Hypertens Pregnancy*. (2019) 38:193–9. doi: 10.1080/10641955.2019.1640725

Lynch AM, Gibbs RS, Murphy JR, Byers T, Neville MC, Giclas PC, et al. Complement activation fragment Bb in early pregnancy and spontaneous preterm birth. *Am J Obstet Gynecol*. (2008) 199:354.e1–8. doi: 10.1016/j.ajog.2008.07.044

Lynch AM, Gibbs RS, Murphy JR, Giclas PC, Salmon JE, Holers VM. Early elevations of the complement activation fragment C3a and adverse pregnancy outcomes. *Obstet Gynecol*. (2011) 117:75–83. doi: 10.1097/AOG.0b013e3181fc3afa

Lappas M, Woodruff TM, Taylor SM, Permezel M. Complement C5A regulates prolabor mediators in human placenta. *Biol Reprod*. (2012) 86:190. doi: 10.1095/biolreprod.111.098475

de Groot PG, Meijers JC. beta(2)-Glycoprotein I: evolution, structure and function. *J Thromb Haemost*. (2011) 9:1275–84. doi: 10.1111/j.1538-7836.2011.04327.x

McDonnell T, Wincup C, Buchholz I, Pericleous C, Giles I, Ripoll V, et al. The role of beta-2-glycoprotein I in health and disease associating structure with function: more than just APS. *Blood Rev*. (2020) 39:100610. doi: 10.1016/j.blre.2019.100610

Agostinis C, Biffi S, Garrovo C, Durigutto P, Lorenzon A, Bek A, et al. In vivo distribution of beta2 glycoprotein I under various pathophysiologic conditions. *Blood*. (2011) 118:4231–8. doi: 10.1182/blood-2011-01-333617

Chighizola CB, Andreoli L, Gerosa M, Tincani A, Ruffatti A, Meroni PL. The treatment of anti-phospholipid syndrome: A comprehensive clinical approach. *J Autoimmun*. (2018) 90:1–27. doi: 10.1016/j.jaut.2018.02.003

Tabacco S, Giannini A, Garufi C, Botta A, Salvi S, Del Sordo G, et al. Complementemia in pregnancies with antiphospholipid syndrome. *Lupus*. (2019) 28:1503–9. doi: 10.1177/0961203319882507

Reggia R, Ziglioli T, Andreoli L, Bellisai F, Iuliano A, Gerosa M, et al. Primary anti- phospholipid syndrome: any role for serum complement levels in predicting pregnancy complications? *Rheumatology*. (2012) 51:2186–90. doi: 10.1093/rheumatology/kes225

Ruffatti A, Tonello M, Visentin MS, Bontadi A, Hoxha A, De Carolis S, et al. Risk factors for pregnancy failure in patients with anti-phospholipid syndrome treated with conventional therapies: a multicentre, case-control study. *Rheumatology*. (2011) 50:1684–9. doi: 10.1093/rheumatology/ker139

De Carolis S, Botta A, Santucci S, Salvi S, Moresi S, Di Pasquo E, et al. Complementemia and obstetric outcome in pregnancy with antiphospholipid syndrome. *Lupus*. (2012) 21:776–8. doi: 10.1177/09612033 12444172

Deguchi M, Yamada H, Sugiura-Ogasawara M, Morikawa M, Fujita D, Miki A, et al. Factors associated with adverse pregnancy outcomes in women with antiphospholipid syndrome: a multicenter study. *J Reprod Immunol*. (2017) 122:21–7. doi: 10.1016/j.jri.2017.08.001

Kim MY, Guerra MM, Kaplowitz E, Laskin CA, Petri M, Branch DW, et al. Complement activation predicts adverse pregnancy outcome in patients with systemic lupus erythematosus and/or antiphospholipid antibodies. *Ann Rheum Dis*. (2018) 77:549–55. doi: 10.1136/annrheumdis-2017- 212224

Scambi C, Ugolini S, Tonello M, Bortolami O, De Franceschi L, Castagna A, et al. Complement activation in the plasma and placentas of women with different subsets of antiphospholipid syndrome. *Am J Reprod Immunol*. (2019) 82:e13185. doi: 10.1111/aji.13185

Cohen D, Buurma A, Goemaere NN, Girardi G, le Cessie S, Scherjon S, et al. Classical complement activation as a footprint for murine and human antiphospholipid antibody-induced fetal loss. *J Pathol*. (2011) 225:502–11. doi: 10.1002/path.2893

Matrai CE, Rand JH, Baergen RN. Absence of distinct immunohistochemical distribution of annexin A5, C3b, C4d, and C5b-9 in placentas from patients with antiphospholipid antibodies, preeclampsia, and systemic lupus erythematosus. *Pediatr Dev Pathol*. (2019) 22:431–9. doi: 10.1177/1093526619836025

Shamonki JM, Salmon JE, Hyjek E, Baergen RN. Excessive complement activation is associated with placental injury in patients with antiphospholipid antibodies. *Am J Obstet Gynecol*. (2007) 196:167.e1–167.e5. doi: 10.1016/j.ajog.2006.10.879

Tedesco F, Borghi MO, Gerosa M, Chighizola CB, Macor P, Lonati PA, et al. Pathogenic role of complement in antiphospholipid syndrome and therapeutic implications. *Front Immunol*. (2018) 9:1388. doi: 10.3389/fimmu.2018.01388

Holers VM, Girardi G, Mo L, Guthridge JM, Molina H, Pierangeli SS, et al. Complement C3 activation is required for antiphospholipid antibody-induced fetal loss. *J Exp Med*. (2002) 195:211–20. doi: 10.1084/jem.200116116

Girardi G, Berman J, Redecha P, Spruce L, Thurman JM, Kraus D, et al. Complement C5a receptors and neutrophils mediate fetal injury in the antiphospholipid syndrome. *J Clin Invest*. (2003) 112:1644–54. doi: 10.1172/JCI18817

Thurman JM, Kraus DM, Girardi G, Hourcade D, Kang HJ, Royer PA, et al. A novel inhibitor of the alternative complement pathway prevents antiphospholipid antibody-induced pregnancy loss in mice. *Mol Immunol*. (2005) 42:87–97. doi: 10.1016/j.molimm.2004.07.043

Berman J, Girardi G, Salmon JE. TNF-alpha is a critical effector and a target for therapy in antiphospholipid antibody-induced pregnancy loss. *J Immunol*. (2005) 174:485–90. doi: 10.4049/jimmunol.174.1.485

Salmon JE, Girardi G. Antiphospholipid antibodies and pregnancy loss: a disorder of inflammation. *J Reprod Immunol*. (2008) 77:51–6. doi: 10.1016/j.jri.2007.02.007

Meroni PL, Macor P, Durigutto P, De Maso L, Gerosa M, Ferraresso M, et al. Complement activation in antiphospholipid syndrome and its inhibition to prevent rethrombosis after arterial surgery. *Blood*. (2016) 127:365–7. doi: 10.1182/blood-2015-09-672139

Gustavsen A, Skattum L, Bergseth G, Lorentzen B, Floisand Y, Bosnes V, et al. Effect on mother and child of eculizumab given before caesarean section in a patient with severe antiphospholipid syndrome: a case report. *Medicine*. (2017) 96:e6338. doi: 10.1097/MD.0000000000 006338

Agostinis C, Durigutto P, Sblattero D, Borghi MO, Grossi C, Guida F, et al. A non-complement-fixing antibody to beta2 glycoprotein I as a novel therapy for antiphospholipid syndrome. *Blood*. (2014) 123:3478–87. doi: 10.1182/blood-2013-11-537704

Tsokos GC, Lo MS, Costa Reis P, Sullivan KE. New insights into the immunopathogenesis of systemic lupus erythematosus. *Nat Rev Rheumatol*. (2016) 12:716–30. doi: 10.1038/nrrheum.2016.186

Siegert C, Daha M, Westedt ML, van der Voort E, Breedveld F. IgG autoantibodies against C1q are correlated with nephritis, hypocomplementemia, and dsDNA antibodies in systemic lupus erythematosus. *J Rheumatol*. (1991) 18:230–4.

Orbai AM, Truedsson L, Sturfelt G, Nived O, Fang H, Alarcon GS, et al. Anti- C1q antibodies in systemic lupus erythematosus. *Lupus*. (2015) 24:42–9. doi: 10.1177/0961203314547791

Biesecker G, Katz S, Koffler D. Renal localization of the membrane attack complex in systemic lupus erythematosus nephritis. *J Exp Med*. (1981) 154:1779–94. doi: 10.1084/jem.154.6.1779

Pickering MC, Ismajli M, Condon MB, McKenna N, Hall AE, Lightstone L, et al. Eculizumab as rescue therapy in severe resistant lupus nephritis. *Rheumatology*. (2015) 54:2286–8. doi: 10.1093/rheumatology/kev307

Coppo R, Peruzzi L, Amore A, Martino S, Vergano L, Lastauka I, et al. Dramatic effects of eculizumab in a child with diffuse proliferative lupus nephritis resistant to conventional therapy. *Pediatr Nephrol.* (2015) 30:167–72. doi: 10.1007/s00467-014-2944-y

Bao L, Cunningham PN, Quigg RJ. Complement in lupus nephritis: new perspectives. *Kidney Dis.* (2015) 1:91–9. doi: 10.1159/000431278

Wang Y, Hu Q, Madri JA, Rollins SA, Chodera A, Matis LA. Amelioration of lupus-like autoimmune disease in NZB/WF1 mice after treatment with a blocking monoclonal antibody specific for complement component C5. *Proc Natl Acad Sci USA.* (1996) 93:8563–8. doi: 10.1073/pnas.93.16.8563

Trouw LA, Pickering MC, Blom AM. The complement system as a potential therapeutic target in rheumatic disease. *Nat Rev Rheumatol.* (2017) 13:538–47. doi: 10.1038/nrrheum.2017.125

Macedo AC, Isaac L. Systemic lupus erythematosus and deficiencies of early components of the complement classical pathway. *Front Immunol.* (2016) 7:55. doi: 10.3389/fimmu.2016.00055

Swaak AJ, Groenwold J, Bronsveld W. Predictive value of complement profiles and anti-dsDNA in systemic lupus erythematosus. *Ann Rheum Dis.* (1986) 45:359–66. doi: 10.1136/ard.45.5.359

Sandhu V, Quan M. SLE and serum complement: causative, concomitant or coincidental? *Open Rheumatol J.* (2017) 11:113–22. doi: 10.2174/1874312901711010113

Aringer M, Costenbader K, Daikh D, Brinks R, Mosca M, Ramsey-Goldman R, et al. 2019 European league against rheumatism/american college of rheumatology classification criteria for systemic lupus erythematosus. *Ann Rheum Dis.* (2019) 78:1151–9. doi: 10.1136/annrheumdis-2018-214819

Batal I, Liang K, Bastacky S, Kiss LP, McHale T, Wilson NL, et al. Prospective assessment of C4d deposits on circulating cells and renal tissues in lupus nephritis: a pilot study. *Lupus.* (2012) 21:13–26. doi: 10.1177/0961203311422093

Putterman C, Furie R, Ramsey-Goldman R, Askanase A, Buyon J, Kalunian K, et al. Cell-bound complement activation products in systemic lupus erythematosus: comparison with anti-double-stranded DNA and standard complement measurements. *Lupus Sci Med.* (2014) 1:e000056. doi: 10.1136/lupus-2014-000056

Mehta B, Luo Y, Xu J, Sammaritano L, Salmon J, Lockshin M, et al. Trends in maternal and fetal outcomes among pregnant women with systemic lupus erythematosus in the United States: a cross-sectional analysis. *Ann Intern Med.* (2019) 171:164–71. doi: 10.7326/M19-0120

Skorpen CG, Lydersen S, Gilboe IM, Skomsvoll JF, Salvesen KA, Palm O, et al. Influence of disease activity and medications on offspring birth weight, preeclampsia and preterm birth in systemic lupus erythematosus: a population-based study. *Ann Rheum Dis.* (2018) 77:264–9. doi: 10.1136/annrheumdis-2017-211641

Buyon JP, Kim MY, Guerra MM, Lu S, Reeves E, Petri M, et al. Kidney outcomes and risk factors for nephritis (Flare/De Novo) in a multiethnic cohort of pregnant patients with lupus. *Clin J Am Soc Nephrol.* (2017) 12:940–6. doi: 10.2215/CJN.11431116

Mok CC. Epidemiology and survival of systemic lupus erythematosus in Hong Kong Chinese. *Lupus.* (2011) 20:767–71. doi: 10.1177/0961203310388447

Al Arfaj AS, Khalil N. Pregnancy outcome in 396 pregnancies in patients with SLE in Saudi Arabia. *Lupus.* (2010) 19:1665–73. doi: 10.1177/0961203310378669

Buyon JP, Kim MY, Guerra MM, Laskin CA, Petri M, Lockshin MD, et al. Predictors of pregnancy outcomes in patients with lupus: a cohort study. *Ann Intern Med.* (2015) 163:153–63. doi: 10.7326/M14-2235

Clowse ME, Wallace DJ, Weisman M, James A, Criscione-Schreiber LG, Pisetsky DS. Predictors of preterm birth in patients with mild systemic lupus erythematosus. *Ann Rheum Dis.* (2013) 72:1536–9. doi: 10.1136/annrheumdis-2012-202449

Abramson SB, Buyon JP. Activation of the complement pathway: comparison of normal pregnancy, preeclampsia, and systemic lupus erythematosus during pregnancy. *Am J Reprod Immunol.* (1992) 28:183–7. doi: 10.1111/j.1600-0897.1992.tb00787.x

Buyon JP, Tamerius J, Ordorica S, Young B, Abramson SB. Activation of the alternative complement pathway accompanies disease flares in systemic lupus erythematosus during pregnancy. *Arthritis Rheum.* (1992) 35:55–61. doi: 10.1002/art.1780350109

Minamiguchi S, Mikami Y, Nakajima N, Salah A, Kondoh E, Tatsumi K, et al. Complement split product C4d deposition in placenta in systemic lupus erythematosus and pregnancy-induced hypertension. *Pathol Int.* (2013) 63:150–7. doi: 10.1111/pin.12041

Lonati PA, Scavone M, Gerosa M, Borghi MO, Pregnolato F, Curreli D, et al. Blood cell-bound C4d as a marker of complement activation in patients with the antiphospholipid syndrome. *Front Immunol.* (2019) 10:773. doi: 10.3389/fimmu.2019.00773

Girardi G, Redecha P, Salmon JE. Heparin prevents antiphospholipid antibody-induced fetal loss by inhibiting complement activation. *Nat Med.* (2004) 10:1222–6. doi: 10.1038/nm1121

Mok CC, Wong RW. Pregnancy in systemic lupus erythematosus. *Postgrad Med J.* (2001) 77:157–65. doi: 10.1136/pmj.77.905.157

Occurrence of a RAGE-Mediated Inflammatory Response in Human Fetal Membranes

Héléna Choltus[1†], Marilyne Lavergne[1], Corinne Belville[1], Denis Gallot[1,2], Régine Minet-Quinard[1,3], Julie Durif[3], Loïc Blanchon[1] and Vincent Sapin[1,3]*

[1] CNRS, INSERM, GReD, Université Clermont Auvergne, Clermont-Ferrand, France, [2] CHU de Clermont-Ferrand, Obstetrics and Gynecology Department, Clermont-Ferrand, France, [3] CHU de Clermont-Ferrand, Biochemistry and Molecular Genetic Department, Clermont-Ferrand, France

*Correspondence:
Vincent Sapin
vincent.sapin@uca.fr

†ORCID:
Héléna Choltus
orcid.org/0000-0002-7557-7029

Context: Sterile inflammation has been shown to play a key role in the rupture of the fetal membranes (FMs). Moreover, an early and exacerbated runaway inflammation can evolve into a preterm premature rupture of membranes and lead to potential preterm birth. In this context, we investigated the receptor for advanced glycation end products (RAGE), an axis implied in physiological sterile inflammation, in conjunction with two major ligands: AGEs and High-Mobility Group Box 1 (HMGB1). Our first objective was to determine the spatiotemporal expression profiles of the different actors of the RAGE-signaling axis in human FMs, including its intracellular adaptors Diaphanous-1 and Myd88. Our second goal was to evaluate the functionality of RAGE signaling in terms of FMs inflammation.

Methods: The presence of the actors (RAGE, HMGB1, Myd88, and Diaphanous-1) at the mRNA level was investigated by reverse transcription quantitative polymerase chain reaction (RT-qPCR) in the human amnion and choriodecidua at the three trimesters and at term. Measurements were conducted at two distinct zones: the zone of intact morphology (ZIM) and the zone of altered morphology (ZAM). Then, proteins were quantified using Western blot analysis, and their localization was evaluated by immunofluorescence in term tissues. In addition, pro-inflammatory cytokine secretion was quantified using a Multiplex assay after the treatment of amnion and choriodecidua explants with two RAGE ligands (AGEs and HMGB1) in the absence or presence of a RAGE inhibitor (SAGEs).

Results: The FMs expressed the RAGE-signaling actors throughout pregnancy. At term, RNA and protein overexpression of the RAGE, HMGB1, and Diaphanous-1 were found in the amnion when compared to the choriodecidua, and the RAGE was overexpressed in the ZAM when compared to the ZIM. The two RAGE ligands (AGEs and HMGB1) induced differential cytokine production (IL1β and TNFα) in the amnion and choriodecidua.

Conclusion: Considered together, these results indicate that RAGE signaling is present and functional in human FMs. Our work opens the way to a better understanding of FMs weakening dependent on a RAGE-based sterile inflammation.

Keywords: fetal membranes, RAGE, alarmins, sterile inflammation, rupture of fetal membranes

INTRODUCTION

Fetal membranes are an essential actor in human parturition; if they do not achieve their missions, the childbirth can be impacted (Naeye and Peters, 1980; Romero et al., 2006; Menon, 2016; Menon and Richardson, 2017). These fetal tissues consist of two layers: the amnion, which is the innermost layer directly in contact with the amniotic fluid (AF), and the chorion, which adheres to the maternal decidua. This 9-month organ participates in the correct development of the fetus by providing AF homeostasis as well as physical and microbial barriers during pregnancy; however, they also play a role in parturition by their programmed rupture at term (after 37 weeks gestation) (Buhimschi et al., 2004; Moore et al., 2006; King et al., 2007; Prat et al., 2012). In this way, FMs undergo progressive weakening leading to this physiologic rupture of membranes (ROM) thanks to several mechanisms, such as apoptosis, senescence, or inflammation (Parry and Strauss, 1998; Menon et al., 2019).

Recently, an increasing number of studies have shown the implication of one key phenomenon in the FMs weakening: sterile inflammation (Girard et al., 2014; Romero et al., 2014, 2015). This concept is dependent on specific molecules called alarmins or "damage-associated molecular patterns" (DAMPs), which are released and recognized by pattern recognition receptors (PRRs) leading to a microbial-free inflammatory response or a "sterile" inflammation. Examples of DAMPs include high-mobility group box 1 (HMGB1) protein, the S100 protein family, uric acid, cell-free DNA, and advanced glycation end-products (AGEs), and examples of PRRs include toll-like receptors, scavenger receptors, NOD-like receptors, and the receptor for AGEs (Taglauer et al., 2014; Nadeau-Vallée et al., 2016; Brien et al., 2019). It has been determined that AF contains many of these alarmins, which induce pro-inflammatory cytokine release by activating various cellular pathways (Holmlund et al., 2007; Jakobsen et al., 2012; Bredeson et al., 2014; Menon and Moore, 2020). Lappas and colleagues demonstrated an induction of cytokine release (IL1β, IL6, IL8, TNFα) by FMs in response to AGEs (Lappas et al., 2007).

However, it still remains unclear how this phenomenon works exactly or which receptor translates this inflammatory signaling to the FMs to prepare for a successful ROM that does not occur before 37 weeks. In the case of early activation, preterm prelabor rupture of the membranes (pPROM) can occur. pPROM affects 3–4% of all pregnancies and leads to 30–40% of all preterm births. Yearly, there are about 15 million cases of preterm birth worldwide. It is important to note that this problem is associated with the rise of perinatal mortality, morbidity, and developmental troubles (Schreiber and Benedetti, 1980; Silverman and Wojtowycz, 1998; Fujimoto et al., 2002; England et al., 2013; Lorthe, 2018; Bouvier et al., 2019; Shiqiao et al., 2019). Thus, it is essential to better understand the ROM to improve pPROM diagnostics and clinical care.

In this study, we decided to investigate the implication of one actor: RAGE (Neeper et al., 1992; Brett et al., 1993). Originally discovered in 1992 as a new member of the immunoglobulin superfamily of receptors, the RAGE is a 55 kDa cell surface receptor that interacts with several ligands (including AGEs and HMGB1) implicated in the pathogenesis of many inflammatory diseases (Kierdorf and Fritz, 2013; Ray et al., 2016; Hudson and Lippman, 2018). Indeed, the RAGE is known to activate pro-inflammatory pathways and the release of cytokines and has been described as participating in the weakening of FMs (Rzepka et al., 2015). Plus, lower concentrations of a soluble RAGE, a competitive RAGE isoform lacking the intracellular domain, has been discovered in the maternal serum of patients suffering from pPROM (Hájek et al., 2008). Furthermore, even if the expression of the RAGE has been outlined in the placental sphere, little is known about the RAGE in FMs and even less on the action and physiopathology of the RAGE in terms of the ROM (Yan et al., 2018). Plus, it is well known that RAGE signaling activity relies on its interaction with intracellular adaptors proteins such as Diaphanous-1, Myd88, and TIR adaptor protein (TIRAP) (Hudson et al., 2008; Sakaguchi et al., 2011). Thus, this study intends to provide more information about the RAGE axis actors in the FMs and determine if a RAGE-dependent inflammatory response can specifically occur in the amnion or choriodecidua when exposed to alarmins such as HMGB1 and AGEs.

MATERIALS AND METHODS

Chemicals

HMGB1 (SRP6265, 10 µg/mL in phosphate-buffered saline 1X) was purchased from Sigma-Aldrich (Saint-Quentin-Fallavier, France) and AGE-bovine serum albumin (10 mg/mL, ab51995) from Abcam (Paris, France). Semi-synthetic glycosaminoglycan ethers (SAGEs) (GM-1111, 10 mg/mL in water), used for the RAGE inhibition, were kindly gifted by GlycoMira Therapeutics (Salt Lake City, UT, United States) (Zhang et al., 2011). Cell culture medium and antibiotics (streptomycin, penicillin, amphotericin B) were obtained from Fisher Scientific (Illkirch-Graffenstaden, France). Fetal bovine serum (FBS) was purchased from Eurobio Scientific (Les Ulis, France). Collagen I was obtained from Stemcell Technologies (Grenoble, France). Superscript IV first-strand-synthesis system, Taq DNA polymerase recombinant (10342020), and Pierce BCA protein assay kit (23225) were obtained from Fisher Scientific.

Tissue Collection

Full-term FMs were collected from non-smoking women with healthy pregnancies from vaginal or scheduled cesarean deliveries (breech presentation, scarred wombs) (Centre Hospitalier Universitaire Estaing, Clermont-Ferrand, France) after obtaining informed consent. Gestational ages were 39.08 ± 0.11 weeks, mean maternal ages were 35.30 ± 0.94 years, and maternal body mass index (BMI) was 26.64 ± 6.65. The selected FMs were collected from singleton pregnant women who had no underlying diseases and no gestational diabetes or clinical chorioamnionitis (defined by maternal fever, uterine tenderness, and/or purulent amniotic fluid). The research protocol was approved by the institutional regional ethics committee (DC-2008-558). The amnion was dissociated from the choriodecidua. The zone of altered morphology (ZAM, with the thread) and the zone of intact morphology (ZIM, away from the thread) were also distinguished. Indeed a suture sewn placed onto the FMs (from cesarean deliveries) in front of the cervix by the midwife allowed us to identify ZAM; then, a 4-cm-diameter circle was cut and considered as ZAM, and explants localized places away from circle boundary were considered as ZIM.

Concerning samples used for RAGE axis actor exploration throughout the pregnancy, first-trimester membranes ($N = 3$) were obtained following aspiration after voluntary termination of pregnancy. Second-trimester membranes were harvested after medical termination of pregnancy ($N = 3$). Eligible cases corresponded to lethal fetal anomalies that had no impact on the FMs (e.g., severe cardiac anomalies or brain damage). Then, preterm third-trimester membranes ($N = 3$) were collected from pregnancies after cesarean births. The amnion was dissociated from the choriodecidua except for trimester 1 samples.

Tissue Culture

Explants (dissociated) of the amnion and choriodecidua were cultivated (5% CO_2, 95% humidified air, 37°C) in Dulbecco's modified eagle medium/nutrient mixture F-12 (DMEM-F12- GlutaMAX) supplemented with 10% FBS, 100 μg/ml of streptomycin, 100 U/ml of ampicillin, and 25 μg/ml amphotericin B. Explants were 2 cm^2 in size, obtained 2 cm away from the pre-placental edge and prepared by dissection. Tissue fragments were transferred (in duplicate) to 24-well culture plates and incubated in cell media at 37°C for 1 h before treatment.

Tissue Explant Treatment

Explants were treated with AGEs (150, 250, and 500 μg/ml) or HMGB1 (100, 200, and 300 ng/ml) in the absence or presence of SAGEs (500 μg/ml) for 18 h (cell medium collection for cytokine release assay). In addition, an internal control was performed by treating explants with a combination of lipopolysaccharide (LPS) (10 μg/ml) and TNFα (100 ng/ml) to validate inflammatory reactivity of FMs samples used. FMs were validated when there was a release response of at least one cytokine.

RT-PCR and Quantitative RT-PCR

After the disruption step with Precellys homogenizer (Bertin Technologies, Montigny-le-Bretonneux, France) using ceramic beads (KT03961, Ozyme, Saint-Cyr-l'École, France), total RNAs were extracted from human amnion or choriodecidua using RNAzol® RT (RN190, Molecular Research Center, Cincinnati, OH, United States). The reverse transcription was made from 1 μg of RNA using a Superscript IV first-strand-synthesis system for reverse transcription polymerase chain reaction (RT-PCR). PCR experiments were performed using specific oligonucleotides (**Table 1**). Results were analyzed on a 2% agarose gel and verified by DNA sequencing. RAGE, HMGB1, Myd88, and Diaphanous-1 expression was assessed by quantitative RT-PCR (RT-qPCR) performed using LightCycler® 480 SYBR Green I Master (Roche, Meylan, France). Transcript quantification was performed twice on at least four independent experiments. Results were normalized to the geometric mean of the human housekeeping genes RPL0 (36b4) and RPS17 (acidic ribosomal phosphoprotein P0 and ribosomal protein S17, respectively) as recommended by the MIQE guidelines (Bustin et al., 2009).

Western Blot Analysis

After the preliminary tissue homogenization previously described, total proteins were extracted from human amnion and choriodecidua (total, ZIM, or ZAM) with a plasma membrane protein extraction kit (BioVision, Lyon, France), and protein sample concentrations were measured using a Pierce BCA protein assay kit. For Western blot analysis, proteins were resolved on a 4–15% Mini-PROTEAN® TGX Stain-Free™ Precast Gel (Bio-Rad, Marnes-la-Coquette, France) to perform total protein normalization (Gilda and Gomes, 2013). Before transfer, stain-free imaging was completed. This technology utilizes a proprietary trihalo compound to enhance natural protein fluorescence by covalently binding to tryptophan residues with a brief UV activation (Bio-Rad). Then, the transfer was performed on nitrocellulose membrane (Bio-Rad) and saturated over 1 h 30 min with 5% skimmed milk in tris-buffered saline (TBS) 1X. Antibody against the RAGE (1/1000, AF1179, R&D Systems, Noyal-Châtillon-sur-Seiche, France), HMGB1 (1/10000, ab79823, Abcam), Myd88 (1/1000, ab133739, Abcam), and Diaphanous-1 (1/5000, ab1173, Abcam) were diluted in 5% skimmed milk-TBS 1X-TWEEN® 20 0.1% and incubated overnight at 4°C. The next day, the membrane was washed three times with TBS 1X/TWEEN® 20 0.1% and incubated at room temperature with a horseradish peroxidase coupled secondary antibody anti-goat or anti-rabbit (1/5000 or 1/10,000, respectively, BI 2403 or BI 2407, Abliance, Compiègne, France) for 1 h 30 min. The revelation was completed using an ECL clarity kit for Western blot on the ChemiDoc™ imaging system (Bio-Rad). Image Lab Software (Bio-Rad) was used for quantification. Results are expressed as a mean of at least three independent experiments.

Supernatant Protein Concentration

Before the Multiplex assays were completed, the supernatants of the treated explants were concentrated into 2 kDa centrifugal filter units (Vivacon® 500, Sartorius, Aubagne, France) for protein concentration and purification, following the manufacturer's instructions.

Cytokine Multiplex Assay

The release of TNFα, IL1β, IL6, and IL8 in the culture media was tested using a MILLIPLEX MAP Human Cytokine/Chemokine Magnetic Bead Panel Milliplex® MAP Kit (Merck Millipore, Molsheim, France) based on the Luminex® xMAP® technology, according to the manufacturer's instructions (Biosource International). Finally, cytokine concentrations were normalized to total protein concentration, and the ratio "treated/untreated" was reported.

Cellular Distress Determination

For the evaluation of the treatment impact on cell suffering, the release of the intracellular enzyme lactate dehydrogenase

TABLE 1 | Forward and reverse primer sequences used for RT-PCR and RT-qPCR amplification of human genes.

Gene	Sequence 5'-3' (F: forward, R: reverse)	Product size (bp)	Hybridation temperature (°C)
hsRAGE	F: TGTGCTGATCCTCCCTGAGA R: CGAGGAGGGGCCAACTGCA	139	61
hsRPL0/36B4	F: AGGCTTTAGGTATCACCACT R: GCAGAGTTTCCTCTGTGATA	219	61
hsRSP17	F: TGCGAGGAGATCGCCATTATC R: AAGGCTGAGACCTCAGGAAC	169	61
hsMyd88	F: GCAGGAGGAGGCTGAGAAGC R: CGGATCATCTCCTGCACAAACT	167	63
hsDia-1	F: AGAGCCACACTTCCTTTCCATC R: TCAATCTCAATCTGGAGGTGCC	167	61
hsHMGBI	F: ACCTATATCCCTCCCAAAGGG R: TTTTTGGGCGATACTCAGAGCA	109	61

(LDH) into the cell media was quantified on a machine automate (Siemens Vista, Paris, France) using an enzymatic assay, following the manufacturer's recommendations.

Immunofluorescence

After permeabilization in PBS 1X/FBS 10%/Triton 0.1% over 1 h 30 min, the primary antibody against the RAGE (1/100, ab37647, Abcam) was applied on the FM sections overnight at 4°C. After three washes in permeabilization buffer, secondary antibody anti-rabbit Alexa Fluor 488 (1/1000, A21206, Life Technologies) was incubated for 2 h at room temperature. Slides were washed three times in TWEEN® PBS 1X and incubated with Hoechst (15 min, dilution in PBS 1X 1/10,000; bisBenzimide H, 33258, Sigma-Aldrich). Finally, slides were mounted with CitiFluor™ Tris-MWL 4–88 (Electron Microscopy Science) and examined under an Apotome Zeiss Imager microscope (magnification ×200). For negative controls, incubation without the primary antibody was performed.

Statistical Analysis

The data expressed as mean ± standard error of the mean (SEM) are an average of duplicates or triplicates of at least three independent experiments. The comparison of means was performed by non-parametric test (Kruskal–Wallis one-way ANOVA test followed by a Dunn's post-test for comparison of more than two conditions), or a Wilcoxon signed-rank test (comparing a fold change to one) using PRISM software 5.02 (GraphPad Software Inc.). For all studies, values were considered significantly different at $p < 0.05(*)$, $p < 0.01(**)$, and $p < 0.001(***)$.

RESULTS

Are RAGE Axis Actors Expressed in Fetal Membranes During Pregnancy?

We investigated the mRNA expression profile of the RAGE, its adaptors and one ligand (HMGB1) in FMs on amnion and choriodecidua samples throughout pregnancy (first trimester: 1 to 13 weeks of gestation (WG); second trimester: 14–26 WG; third trimester: 27–37 WG; at term: 38–40 WG, by cesarean or vaginal delivery). RT-PCR experiments revealed that FMs expressed the RAGE, HMGB1, Myd88, and Diaphanous-1 in both layers, the amnion and choriodecidua in each of the stages considered (Figure 1A). No significant difference in RAGE expression was revealed by RT-qPCR between trimesters (data not shown). Plus, RAGE protein expression was also demonstrated in both layers obtained after vaginal delivery or caesarean section with the separate consideration of the ZIM and ZAM (Figure 1B).

Is the RAGE Axis Actor Expression Layer- or Zone-Dependent at Term?

Based on RT-qPCR analysis at term, we revealed an overexpression of RAGE (Figure 2A, left panel) and HMGB1 (Figure 2A, right panel) in the amnion compared to the choriodecidua in consideration of the ZAM. Moreover, RAGE expression was also area-dependent: it was found to be significantly more expressed in the rupture zone (ZAM) than in the ZIM. These results were confirmed at the protein level for both using western blot analysis (Figure 2B, upper panel for representative experiment and Figure 2B, lower panel for quantification).

Furthermore, considering that the RAGE requires intracellular adaptor binding to induce a cellular response, we also investigated the expression of Diaphanous-1, Myd88, and TIR adaptor protein (TIRAP). First, TIRAP was found at very low levels for mRNA and not detected by immunoblot in both layers (data not shown). Furthermore, we revealed that Diaphanous-1 is overexpressed in the amnion for mRNA (only in ZAM) and protein level in both zones (Figures 3A,B, left panels). Plus, we found a Myd88 protein overexpression in the choriodecidua in comparison to the amnion in the ZAM (Figures 3A,B, right panels).

Are the Amnion or Choriodecidua Able to Trigger an Inflammatory Response to Alarmins?

Before further investigation, cell toxicity that may have been caused by the induction of AGEs and HMGB1 treatments in the amnion and choriodecidua explants was checked. This was done using LDH release measurements in the culture media after 18 h of alarmin treatment and revealed no cell toxicity for each condition (three concentrations tested for each one; Figure 4). Then, we performed a dose response effect of AGEs and HMGB1 on cytokine release after 18 h

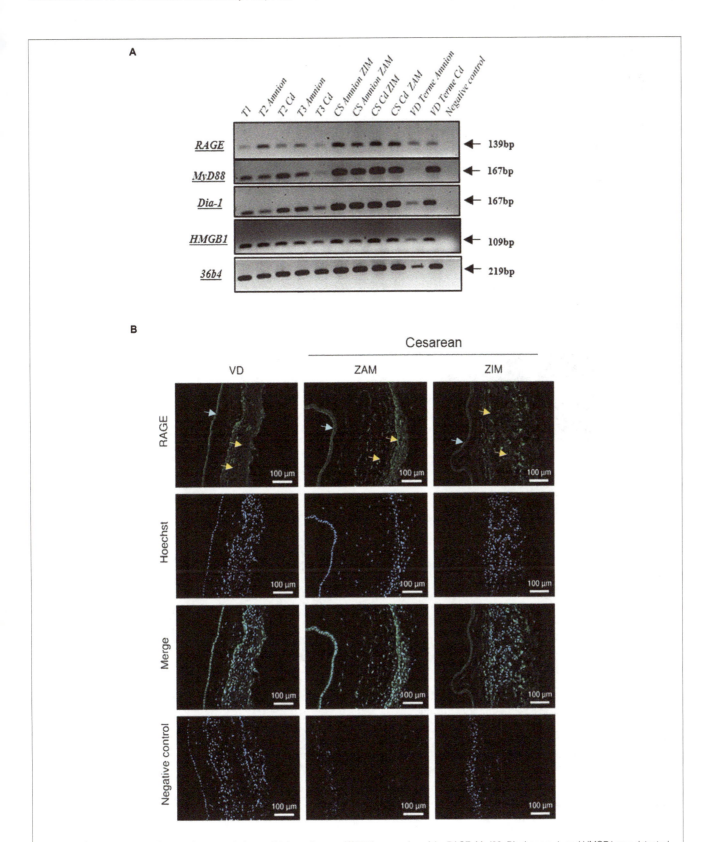

FIGURE 1 | Expression of RAGE-signaling actors in human fetal membranes. **(A)** RNA expression of the RAGE, Myd88, Diaphanous-1, and HMGB1 was detected by RT-PCR on the amnion and choriodecidua (Cd) samples from the different trimesters (T1, T2, and T3), caesarean (CS), or vaginal (VD) delivery at term. Negative controls were performed in the absence of cDNA. **(B)** RAGE protein localization in human fetal membranes at term was investigated by immunofluorescence (green staining, Alexa488) on sections from vaginal delivery (VD) or caesarean (ZIM and ZAM) at magnification ×200. Cyan arrows indicate amniotic epithelium and yellow designate choriodecidua. Nuclei were counterstained with Hoechst (blue). Negative controls consisted of primary antibody-free incubation.

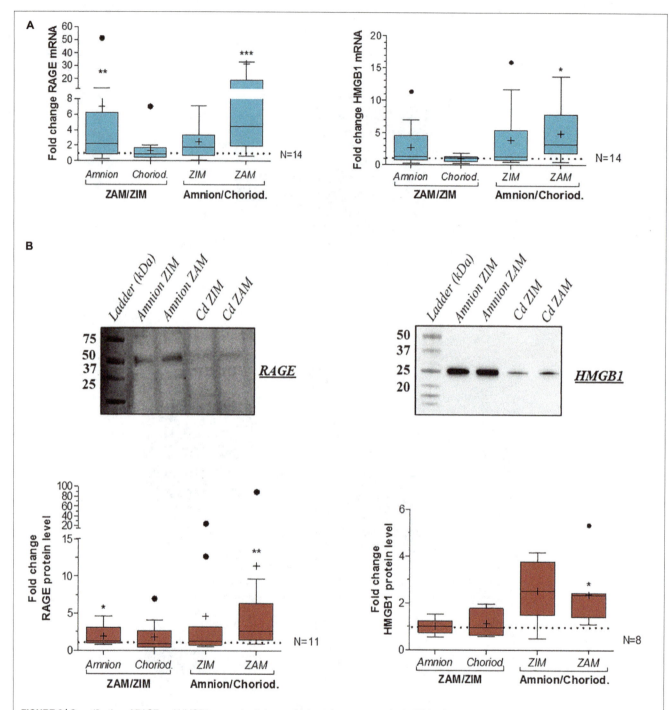

FIGURE 2 | Quantification of RAGE and HMGB1 expression in human fetal membranes at term in the ZIM and ZAM. RAGE and HMGB1 expression were quantified by RT-qPCR ($N = 14$) (A) and Western blot (respectively, $N = 11$ and $N = 8$) (B) on the amnion and choriodecidua (Cd) at term in the ZIM and ZAM. To highlight an area (ZAM vs. ZIM) or tissue (Amnion vs. Choriodecidua) effect, ZAM is reported on ZIM (ZAM/ZIM in left panel) in both amnion and choriodecidua, and amnion is reported on choriodecidua (amnion/choriodecidua in right panel) in both ZIM and ZAM. Statistical fold change analysis was performed by a Wilcoxon signed-rank test comparing to one. * means $p < 0.05$, ** means $p < 0.01$, *** means $p < 0.001$. Results are presented in Tukey boxes, and means are indicated by "+." Representative Western blot membranes indicate the band that was quantified proteins (RAGE: 50 kDa and HMGB1 at 25 kDa).

of treatment on both the amnion and choriodecidua. First, in the amnion (**Figure 5**, upper left panel), we observed that AGEs did not stimulate IL8 release, but increased TNFα in the same way for all concentrations (150, 250, and 500 μg/ml) and IL1β (more at 150 than 500 μg/ml). Finally, we found that AGEs also induced IL6 release at 150 μg/ml. For the choriodecidua (**Figure 5**, upper right panel), the same responses as the amnion were found for IL8 and TNFα, and IL1β was

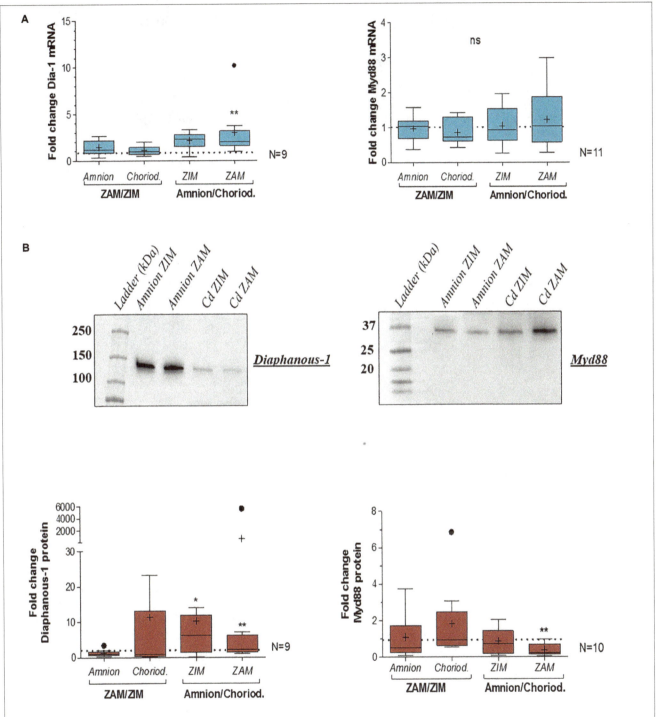

FIGURE 3 | Quantification of RAGE-signaling adaptors in human fetal membranes at term in the ZIM and ZAM. Myd88 and Diaphanous-1 expressions were quantified by RT-qPCR (respectively, $N = 11$ and $N = 9$) (A) and Western blot ($N = 9$ and $N = 10$) (B) on the amnion and choriodecidua (Cd) at term in the ZIM and ZAM. To highlight an area (ZAM vs. ZIM) or tissue (amnion vs. choriodecidua) effect, ZAM is reported on ZIM (ZAM/ZIM in left panel) in both amnion and choriodecidua, and amnion is reported on choriodecidua (amnion/choriodecidua in right panel) in both ZIM and ZAM. Statistical fold change analysis was performed by a Wilcoxon signed-rank test comparing to one. * means $p < 0.05$, ** means $p < 0.01$. Results are presented in Tukey boxes, and means are indicated by "+." Representative Western blot membranes indicate the band that was quantified (Diaphanous-1 was detected around 150 kDa and Myd88 at 37 kDa).

increased regardless of the dose (more with 500 µg/ml). By contrast, induction was not relevant for IL6 at any concentration. A second time, we demonstrated that HMGB1 (**Figure 5**, lower panel) stimulated TNFα release in both tissues (at 200 and 300 ng/ml) and IL1β at the same doses but only in the amnion. Any significant induction could be reported by

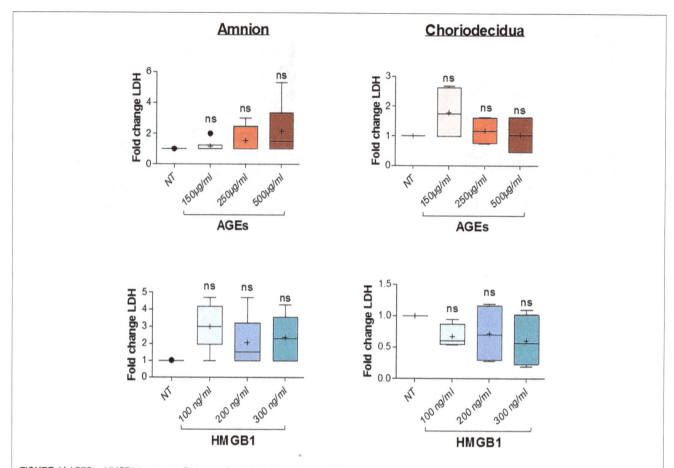

FIGURE 4 | AGES or HMGB1 treatment effects on cell toxicity in the amnion and choriodecidua explants. Toxicity was evaluated by LDH release measurement in culture supernatants after 18 h of treatment with a dose effect of AGEs (150, 250, and 500 μg/ml) or HMGB1 (100, 200, and 300 ng/ml; N = 3 in duplicate). Statistical analysis was performed using a Kruskal–Wallis one-way ANOVA test followed by a Dunn's post-test and showed no significant difference. Results are presented in Tukey boxes, and means are indicated by "+."

HMGB1 treatment for IL8 and IL6. Regarding our results, and in accordance with those already described in previous articles (Lappas et al., 2007; Plazyo et al., 2016), 500 μg/ml of AGEs and 200 ng/ml of HMGB1 were kept for the following SAGEs blocking experiments.

Does Blocking the RAGE Modulate the Inflammatory Response Induced by Alarmins in Fetal Membranes?

Finally, to investigate whether AGEs and HMGB1 alarmins induce a RAGE-dependent inflammatory response, we measured pro-inflammatory cytokine release in the amnion and choriodecidua co-treated with or without SAGEs (a RAGE inhibitor) for 18 h. Results demonstrated a significant lower TNFα release induction by AGEs (**Figure 6**, upper panel) and HMGB1 (**Figure 6**, lower panel) when the RAGE was inhibited by SAGEs in the amnion and choriodecidua. Plus, we noticed that AGEs and HMGB1 stimulated IL1β secretion in both layers, but in the presence of SAGEs, this induction was not any more significant for HMGB1. Finally, we found no impact on either IL8 or IL6.

DISCUSSION

Since these last years, more and more studies have underlined the importance of sterile inflammation in the weakening of FMs as a key event of the ROM (hopefully after 37 weeks of gestation). It is now considered that AF is a source of specific molecules called alarmins (or DAMPs), which are endogenously expressed and produced when cells are suffering. For example, HMGB1 is normally a nuclear protein implicated in DNA reparation, but when cells are in danger, HMGB1 is released and becomes an alarmin, triggering an inflammatory cascade. As another kind of DAMPs, AGEs are formed by the non-enzymatic Maillard reaction, between sugars and proteins, lipids, or nucleic acids (John and Lamb, 1993), and many inflammatory diseases are linked to an accumulation of these AGEs in tissues (Kang et al., 2012; Guedes-Martins et al., 2013; Wautier et al., 2014). Above all, both AGEs and HMGB1 have been described as activating inflammatory response in gestational tissues (placenta, FMs, umbilical cord) and were found to be increased in cases of pPROM. Indeed, HMGB1 has been found to be more elevated in the AF due to a release caused by damaged FMs occurring during intra-amniotic inflammation found during preterm birth

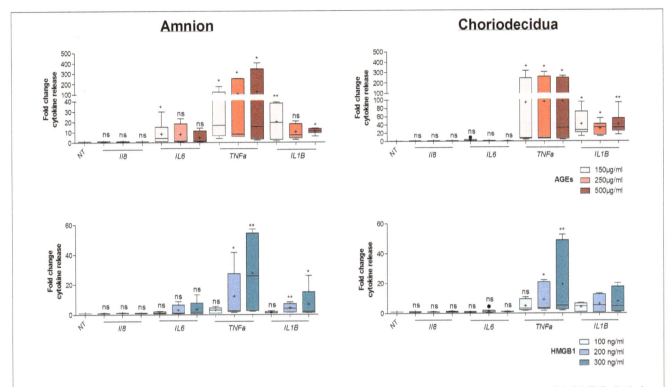

FIGURE 5 | Dose response effect on cytokine release by AGEs and HMGB1 into fetal membrane explants. Evaluation of cytokine release (IL8, IL6, TNFα, IL1β) after 18 h of dose effect treatment of AGEs (150, 250, and 500 μg/ml) and HMGB1 (100, 200, and 300 ng/ml) on the amnion or choriodecidua explants was evaluated by Multiplex assay (N = 3 in duplicate). Statistical analysis was performed using a Kruskal–Wallis one-way ANOVA test followed by a Dunn's post-test. * means $p < 0.05$, ** means $p < 0.01$. Results are presented in Tukey boxes, and means are indicated by "+."

(Bredeson et al., 2014; Baumbusch et al., 2016). This could be an exacerbation of inflammatory processes mediated by HMGB1, a major player in labor events (Stephen et al., 2015). In addition, AGEs levels in maternal plasma were described as more important during the first trimester for pregnancies with preterm labor or pPROM (Kansu-Celik et al., 2019). However, there is still a lack of knowledge about which receptor recognizes these alarmins and causes inflammation in the FMs. Some studies have described an overexpression of the RAGE in the placenta and maternal serum in cases of pPROM and also a progressive increase of the soluble isoform of RAGE (sRAGE), acting as a decoy, during pregnancy and then finally decreasing at term (Romero et al., 2008; Yan et al., 2018). Moreover, plasmatic sRAGE levels were found to be lower in patients with pPROM, suggesting an over-activation of the RAGE pathway (Hájek et al., 2008). In this way, our work aimed to enlighten the implication of the RAGE in sterile inflammation in FMs.

The expression of the RAGE in FMs has already been described at term but had not been described during the different trimesters of pregnancy. Presently, we conducted a global exploration of the RAGE axis in both FMs layers (amnion and choriodecidua). First, we proved that FMs not only expressed the RAGE and HMGB1 during all three trimesters of pregnancy, but it also expressed Diaphanous-1 and Myd88, two intracellular adaptors required for inflammatory activity of the RAGE. After that, we observed the presence of the RAGE protein in the amniotic epithelium, the layer directly exposed to AF alarmins and also in all choriodecidua. Thus, we found a differential RNA and protein expression between not only the amnion and choriodecidua and also between the ZAM and the rest of the FMs, the ZIM. Indeed, we showed the overexpression of the RAGE in the amnion compared to the choriodecidua and, above all, in the ZAM compared to the ZIM. These findings strengthen the idea of RAGE participation and importance in the ROM process as previously suggested (Rzepka et al., 2015). Plus, we demonstrated HMGB1 levels to be more important in the amnion. This was not very surprising; indeed, literature already described an increase in sterile inflammation linked with HMGB1 on the fetal side of the FMs, more precisely, in the amnion epithelial cells (Romero et al., 2011). But our work brings the first data on RAGE adaptors in fetal membranes and this is not negligible. In fact, it is currently well known that the RAGE is deficient in intrinsic tyrosine kinase activity and requires intracellular adaptors to induce cell signaling cascades. In this way, a yeast-two-hybrid experiment was achieved and identified a binding partner of RAGE cytosolic domain, the protein Diaphanous-1. Meanwhile, there is no proof that Diaphanous-1 is required for all RAGE induced-transduction cascades; however, some studies reported its implication in protein/signal pathway stimulation triggered by RAGE ligands (Xu et al., 2010; Touré et al., 2012). Hudson et al. (2008) also demonstrated that downregulation of Diaphanous-1 expression by RNA interference inhibited RAGE-mediated activation of Rac-1 and Cdc42 and, in parallel, RAGE ligand-stimulated inflammatory, vascular, and cell migration

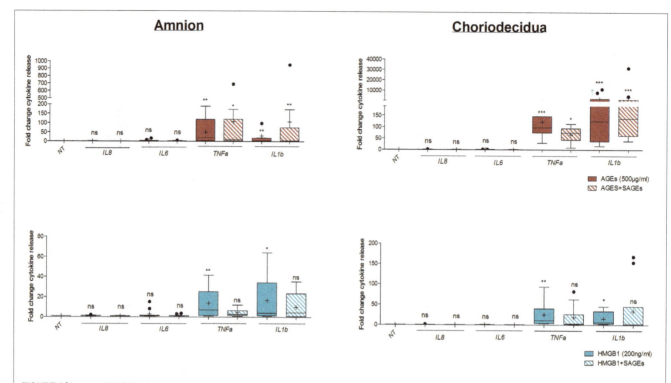

FIGURE 6 | Impact of RAGE inhibition on the induction of inflammatory response by AGEs and HMGB1 alarmins in the amnion and choriodecidua. Pro-inflammatory cytokine (IL8, IL6, TNFα, IL1β) secretion was quantified by Multiplex assay after 18 h of treatment with AGEs (500 μg/ml) or HMGB1 (200 ng/ml) in the presence or absence of RAGE inhibitor, SAGEs (500 μg/ml) (N = 5 in duplicate). Each treated condition was reported to corresponding not treated (NT) either without SAGEs or with SAGEs, which were both fixed to one. Statistical analysis was performed using a Kruskal–Wallis one-way ANOVA test followed by a Dunn's post-test. * means $p < 0.05$, ** means $p < 0.01$, *** means $p < 0.001$. Results are presented in Tukey boxes, and means are indicated by "+."

responses. Diaphanous-1 aside, the RAGE owns other adaptor proteins, such as TIRAP or MyD88, shared with the toll-like receptors TLR2 and TLR4. The Sakaguchi group revealed that ligand binding leads to phosphorylation of the RAGE cytoplasmic domain by protein kinase Cζ (pSer391), promoting TIRAP and MyD88 interaction. Furthermore, blocking TIRAP and MyD88 considerably abolished ligand-activated RAGE inflammatory signaling (Akt, p38 MAP kinase, NFκB) (Sakaguchi et al., 2011). In our study, we demonstrated an overexpression of Diaphanous-1 in the amnion, unlike Myd88, which was found to be expressed more in the choriodecidua. These data may suggest a layer-specific signaling couple, RAGE/Diaphanous-1 in the amnion and RAGE/Myd88 in the choriodecidua. Additionally, considering that RAGE and TLR2/4 partly share an intracellular signaling pathway, including MyD88 binding, we could suppose cooperation between RAGE and TLRs in immune response in choriodecidua, explaining why MyD88 was overexpressed in this layer, closer to the genito-urinary microbiota. Indeed, fetal membranes are already known to respond to different types of bacteria by modifications of TLR expression patterns (Abrahams et al., 2013).

As previously stated, AGEs or HMGB1 have been described as inducing cytokine release (IL6, IL8, TNFα, IL1β) in the FMs but without making a distinction between both layers. To investigate a possible differential response to ligands between the amnion and choriodecidua, we decided to perform our treatments with a dissociation of these two sheets using either AGEs or HMGB1. First, we confirmed results from previous studies with TNFα and IL1β release in response to AGEs and HMGB1 in both the amnion and choriodecidua (Lappas et al., 2007; Bredeson et al., 2014; Plazyo et al., 2016). In addition to such results, we did not find the same results for IL8 and IL6 with their release not being stimulated by any dose except for IL6 in the amnion by AGEs at 150 μg/ml. This contrast with previous results can be explained by the use of different concentrations of alarmins. For example, the Lappas group used concentrations of 1 mg/ml of AGEs, and those used for HMGB1 were between 10 ng and 50 μg/ml for Plazyo and colleagues and 1 and 50 ng/ml by the Bredeson team. Then, in our study, for IL6 release, we dissociated layers and could, therefore, hypothesize that only the amnion produces such interleukin in response to AGEs or to HMGB1.

Finally, the major finding of this study was that RAGE inhibition by SAGEs decreased or aborted the TNFα release for both alarmins, indicating that RAGE is required for FMs to initiate this cytokine production. However, contrary to choriodecidua, in amnion, it seems RAGE is not the only actor needed in TNFα release induction because the induction was diminished and not aborted. Globally, this result is of primary importance, as TNFα could activate NFκB complex and the production of the granulocyte macrophage colony-stimulating factor (GM-CSF), which is described to be the critical intermediate for FMs weakening by the intervention of specific proteases (Kumar et al., 2014). The release of IL1β was only inhibited by SAGEs when tissues were treated by HMGB1 and not by AGEs. Considered together, the results obtained in our work proved for the first time that the RAGE is directly implied in the inflammatory response in human FMs in a ligand and layer-dependent manner.

Our study constitutes the direct evidence of RAGE action in FMs weakening, which is an essential process for the ROM, adding a feature of the pathophysiological partition of the RAGE in the story of childbirth. Further studies are required to elucidate which intracellular pathway, among NFκB and MAPK kinases, for example, leads to this RAGE-dependent cytokine release in FMs, but also which cellular type inside the amnion or choriodecidua has the ability to react to the presence of alarmins.

ETHICS STATEMENT

The Institutional Local Ethics Committee, structure of the University Hospital of Clermont-Ferrand (specialized for Human clinical questions) approved this study and the research protocol. Healthy fetal membranes were collected after receiving oral informed consent (according to the French law named "Huriet-n°88–1138" which considers placenta and fetal membranes as chirurgical wastes) from the patients in the "Centre Hospitalier Universitaire Estaing" (Clermont-Ferrand, France).

AUTHOR CONTRIBUTIONS

HC designed and performed the experiments, and wrote the manuscript. ML and CB helped HC to carry out some experiments. JD helped with Multiplex assays. RM-Q performed lactate dehydrogenase assays. DG allowed HC to obtain human fetal membranes from patients in the Centre Hospitalier Universitaire Estaing (Clermont-Ferrand, France). VS and LB supervised the project.

REFERENCES

Abrahams, V. M., Potter, J. A., Bhat, G., Peltier, M. R., Saade, G., and Menon, R. (2013). Bacterial modulation of human fetal membrane toll-like receptor expression. *Am. J. Reprod. Immunol.* 69, 33–40. doi: 10.1111/aji.12016

Baumbusch, M. A., Buhimschi, C. S., Oliver, E. A., Zhao, G., Thung, S., Rood, K., et al. (2016). High Mobility Group-Box 1 (HMGB1) levels are increased in amniotic fluid of women with intra-amniotic inflammation-determined preterm birth, and the source may be the damaged fetal membranes. *Cytokine* 81, 82–87. doi: 10.1016/j.cyto.2016.02.013

Bouvier, D., Forest, J.-C., Blanchon, L., Bujold, E., Pereira, B., Bernard, N., et al. (2019). Risk factors and outcomes of preterm premature rupture of membranes in a cohort of 6968 pregnant women prospectively recruited. *J. Clin. Med.* 8:1987. doi: 10.3390/jcm8111987

Bredeson, S., Papaconstantinou, J., Deford, J. H., Kechichian, T., Syed, T. A., Saade, G. R., et al. (2014). HMGB1 promotes a p38MAPK associated non-infectious inflammatory response pathway in human fetal membranes. *PLoS One* 9:e113799. doi: 10.1371/journal.pone.0113799

Brett, J., Schmidt, A. M., Yan, S. D., Zou, Y. S., Weidman, E., Pinsky, D., et al. (1993). Survey of the distribution of a newly characterized receptor for advanced glycation end products in tissues. *Am. J. Pathol.* 143, 1699–1712.

Brien, M.-E., Baker, B., Duval, C., Gaudreault, V., Jones, R. L., and Girard, S. (2019). Alarmins at the maternal-fetal interface: involvement of inflammation in placental dysfunction and pregnancy complications 1. *Can. J. Physiol. Pharmacol.* 97, 206–212. doi: 10.1139/cjpp-2018-0363

Buhimschi, I. A., Jabr, M., Buhimschi, C. S., Petkova, A. P., Weiner, C. P., and Saed, G. M. (2004). The novel antimicrobial peptide β3-defensin is produced by the amnion: a possible role of the fetal membranes in innate immunity of the amniotic cavity. *Am. J. Obstet. Gynecol.* 191, 1678–1687. doi: 10.1016/j.ajog.2004.03.081

Bustin, S. A., Benes, V., Garson, J. A., Hellemans, J., Huggett, J., Kubista, M., et al. (2009). The MIQE guidelines: minimum information for publication of quantitative real-time PCR experiments. *Clin. Chem.* 55, 611–622. doi: 10.1373/clinchem.2008.112797

England, M., Benjamin, A., and Abenhaim, H. (2013). Increased risk of preterm premature rupture of membranes at early gestational ages among maternal cigarette smokers. *Am. J. Perinatol.* 30, 821–826. doi: 10.1055/s-0032-1333408

Fujimoto, T., Parry, S., Urbanek, M., Sammel, M., Macones, G., Kuivaniemi, H., et al. (2002). A single nucleotide polymorphism in the matrix metalloproteinase-1 (MMP-1) promoter influences amnion cell MMP-1 expression and risk for preterm premature rupture of the fetal membranes. *J. Biol. Chem.* 277, 6296–6302. doi: 10.1074/jbc.M107865200

Gilda, J. E., and Gomes, A. V. (2013). Stain-Free total protein staining is a superior loading control to β-actin for Western blots. *Anal. Biochem.* 440, 186–188. doi: 10.1016/j.ab.2013.05.027

Girard, S., Heazell, A. E. P., Derricott, H., Allan, S. M., Sibley, C. P., Abrahams, V. M., et al. (2014). Circulating cytokines and alarmins associated with placental inflammation in high-risk pregnancies. *Am. J. Reprod. Immunol.* 72, 422–434. doi: 10.1111/aji.12274

Guedes-Martins, L., Matos, L., Soares, A., Silva, E., and Almeida, H. (2013). AGEs, contributors to placental bed vascular changes leading to preeclampsia. *Free Radic. Res.* 47, 70–80. doi: 10.3109/10715762.2013.815347

Hájek, Z., Germanová, A., Koucký, M., Zima, T., Kopecký, P., Vítková, M., et al. (2008). Detection of feto-maternal infection/inflammation by the soluble receptor for advanced glycation end products (sRAGE): results of a pilot study. *J. Perinat. Med.* 36, 399–404. doi: 10.1515/JPM.2008.080

Holmlund, U., Wähämaa, H., Bachmayer, N., Bremme, K., Sverremark-Ekström, E., and Palmblad, K. (2007). The novel inflammatory cytokine high mobility group box protein 1 (HMGB1) is expressed by human term placenta. *Immunology* 122, 430–437. doi: 10.1111/j.1365-2567.2007.02662.x

Hudson, B. I., Kalea, A. Z., Del Mar Arriero, M., Harja, E., Boulanger, E., D'Agati, V., et al. (2008). Interaction of the RAGE cytoplasmic domain with diaphanous-1 is required for ligand-stimulated cellular migration through activation of Rac1 and Cdc42. *J. Biol. Chem.* 283, 34457–34468. doi: 10.1074/jbc.M801465200

Hudson, B. I., and Lippman, M. E. (2018). Targeting RAGE signaling in inflammatory disease. *Annu. Rev. Med.* 69, 349–364. doi: 10.1146/annurev-med-041316-085215

Jakobsen, T. R., Clausen, F. B., Rode, L., Dziegiel, M. H., and Tabor, A. (2012). High levels of fetal DNA are associated with increased risk of spontaneous preterm delivery. *Prenat. Diagn.* 32, 840–845. doi: 10.1002/pd.3917

John, W. G., and Lamb, E. J. (1993). The Maillard or browning reaction in diabetes. *Eye* 7(Pt 2), 230–237. doi: 10.1038/eye.1993.55

Kang, R., Tang, D., Lotze, M. T., and Zeh, H. J. III (2012). AGER/RAGE-mediated autophagy promotes pancreatic tumorigenesis and bioenergetics through the IL6-pSTAT3 pathway. *Autophagy* 8, 989–991. doi: 10.4161/auto.20258

Kansu-Celik, H., Tasci, Y., Karakaya, B. K., Cinar, M., Candar, T., and Caglar, G. S. (2019). Maternal serum advanced glycation end products level as an early marker for predicting preterm labor/PPROM: a prospective preliminary study. *J. Matern. Fetal. Neonatal. Med.* 32, 2758–2762. doi: 10.1080/14767058.2018.1449202

Kierdorf, K., and Fritz, G. (2013). RAGE regulation and signaling in inflammation and beyond. *J. Leukocyte Biol.* 94, 55–68. doi: 10.1189/jlb.1012519

King, A. E., Paltoo, A., Kelly, R. W., Sallenave, J.-M., Bocking, A. D., and Challis, J. R. G. (2007). Expression of natural antimicrobials by human placenta and fetal membranes. *Placenta* 28, 161–169. doi: 10.1016/j.placenta.2006.01.006

Kumar, D., Moore, R. M., Nash, A., Springel, E., Mercer, B. M., Philipson, E., et al. (2014). Decidual GM-CSF is a critical common intermediate necessary for thrombin and TNF induced in-vitro fetal membrane weakening. *Placenta* 35, 1049–1056. doi: 10.1016/j.placenta.2014.10.001

Lappas, M., Permezel, M., and Rice, G. E. (2007). Advanced glycation endproducts mediate pro-inflammatory actions in human gestational tissues via nuclear factor- B and extracellular signal-regulated kinase 1/2. *J. Endocrinol.* 193, 269–277. doi: 10.1677/JOE-06-0081

Lorthe, E. (2018). Épidémiologie, facteurs de risque et pronostic de l'enfant. RPC: rupture prématurée des membranes avant terme CNGOF. *Gynécol. Obstét. Fertil. Sénol.* 46, 1004–1021. doi: 10.1016/j.gofs.2018.10.019

Menon, R. (2016). Human fetal membranes at term: dead tissue or signalers of parturition? *Placenta* 44, 1–5. doi: 10.1016/j.placenta.2016.05.013

Menon, R., and Moore, J. J. (2020). Fetal membranes, not a mere appendage of the placenta, but a critical part of the fetal-maternal interface controlling parturition. *Obstet. Gynecol. Clin. North Am.* 47, 147–162. doi: 10.1016/j.ogc.2019.10.004

Menon, R., and Richardson, L. S. (2017). Preterm prelabor rupture of the membranes: a disease of the fetal membranes. *Semin. Perinatol.* 41, 409–419. doi: 10.1053/j.semperi.2017.07.012

Menon, R., Richardson, L. S., and Lappas, M. (2019). Fetal membrane architecture, aging and inflammation in pregnancy and parturition. *Placenta* 79, 40–45. doi: 10.1016/j.placenta.2018.11.003

Moore, R. M., Mansour, J. M., Redline, R. W., Mercer, B. M., and Moore, J. J. (2006). The physiology of fetal membrane rupture: insight gained from the determination of physical properties. *Placenta* 27, 1037–1051. doi: 10.1016/j.placenta.2006.01.002

Nadeau-Vallée, M., Obari, D., Palacios, J., Brien, M. -È, Duval, C., Chemtob, S., et al. (2016). Sterile inflammation and pregnancy complications: a review. *Reproduction* 152, R277–R292. doi: 10.1530/REP-16-0453

Naeye, R. L., and Peters, E. C. (1980). Causes and consequences of premature rupture of fetal membranes. *Lancet* 1, 192–194. doi: 10.1016/s0140-6736(80)90674-1

Neeper, M., Schmidt, A. M., Brett, J., Yan, S. D., Wang, F., Pan, Y. C., et al. (1992). Cloning and expression of a cell surface receptor for advanced glycosylation end products of proteins. *J. Biol. Chem.* 267, 14998–15004.

Parry, S., and Strauss, J. F. (1998). Premature rupture of the fetal membranes. *New Engl. J. Med.* 338, 663–670. doi: 10.1056/NEJM199803053381006

Plazyo, O., Romero, R., Unkel, R., Balancio, A., Mial, T. N., Xu, Y., et al. (2016). HMGB1 induces an inflammatory response in the chorioamniotic membranes that is partially mediated by the inflammasome. *Biol. Reprod.* 95, 130–130. doi: 10.1095/biolreprod.116.144139

Prat, C., Blanchon, L., Borel, V., Gallot, D., Herbet, A., Bouvier, D., et al. (2012). Ontogeny of aquaporins in human fetal membranes1. *Biol. Reprod.* 86:48. doi: 10.1095/biolreprod.111.095448

Ray, R., Juranek, J. K., and Rai, V. (2016). RAGE axis in neuroinflammation, neurodegeneration and its emerging role in the pathogenesis of amyotrophic lateral sclerosis. *Neurosci. Biobehav. Rev.* 62, 48–55. doi: 10.1016/j.neubiorev.2015.12.006

Romero, R., Chaiworapongsa, T., Savasan, Z. A., Xu, Y., Hussein, Y., Dong, Z., et al. (2011). Damage-associated molecular patterns (DAMPs) in preterm labor with intact membranes and preterm PROM: a study of the alarmin HMGB1. *J. Matern. Fetal Neonatal Med.* 24, 1444–1455. doi: 10.3109/14767058.2011.591460

Romero, R., Espinoza, J., Hassan, S., Gotsch, F., Kusanovic, J. P., Avila, C., et al. (2008). Soluble receptor for advanced glycation end products (sRAGE) and endogenous secretory RAGE (esRAGE) in amniotic fluid: modulation by infection and inflammation. *J. Perinat. Med.* 36, 388–398. doi: 10.1515/JPM.2008.076

Romero, R., Espinoza, J., Kusanovic, J. P., Gotsch, F., Hassan, S., Erez, O., et al. (2006). The preterm parturition syndrome. *BJOG* 113(Suppl. 3), 17–42. doi: 10.1111/j.1471-0528.2006.01120.x

Romero, R., Miranda, J., Chaemsaithong, P., Chaiworapongsa, T., Kusanovic, J. P., Dong, Z., et al. (2015). Sterile and microbial-associated intra-amniotic inflammation in preterm prelabor rupture of membranes. *J. Matern. Fetal Neonatal Med.* 28, 1394–1409. doi: 10.3109/14767058.2014.958463

Romero, R., Miranda, J., Chaiworapongsa, T., Korzeniewski, S. J., Chaemsaithong, P., Gotsch, F., et al. (2014). Prevalence and clinical significance of sterile intra-amniotic inflammation in patients with preterm labor and intact membranes. *Am. J. Reprod. Immunol.* 72, 458–474. doi: 10.1111/aji.12296

Rzepka, R., Dołęgowska, B., Rajewska, A., Kwiatkowski, S., Sałata, D., Budkowska, M., et al. (2015). Soluble and endogenous secretory receptors for advanced glycation end products in threatened preterm labor and preterm premature rupture of fetal membranes. *Biomed. Res. Int.* 2015, 1–10. doi: 10.1155/2015/568042

Sakaguchi, M., Murata, H., Yamamoto, K., Ono, T., Sakaguchi, Y., Motoyama, A., et al. (2011). TIRAP, an adaptor protein for TLR2/4, transduces a signal from RAGE phosphorylated upon ligand binding. *PLoS One* 6:e23132. doi: 10.1371/journal.pone.0023132

Schreiber, J., and Benedetti, T. (1980). Conservative management of preterm premature rupture of the fetal membranes in a low socioeconomic population. *Am. J. Obstet. Gynecol.* 136, 92–96. doi: 10.1016/0002-9378(80)90572-4

Shiqiao, H., Bei, X., Yudi, G., and Lei, J. (2019). Assisted reproductive technology is associated with premature rupture of membranes. *J. Matern. Fetal Neonatal Med.* doi: 10.1080/14767058.2019.1610738 [Epub ahead of print].

Silverman, R. K., and Wojtowycz, M. (1998). Risk factors in premature rupture of membranes. *Prim. Care Update OB GYNS* 5:181. doi: 10.1016/s1068-607x(98)00092-4

Stephen, G. L., Lui, S., Hamilton, S. A., Tower, C. L., Harris, L. K., Stevens, A., et al. (2015). Transcriptomic profiling of human choriodecidua during term labor: inflammation as a key driver of labor. *Am. J. Reprod. Immunol.* 73, 36–55. doi: 10.1111/aji.12328

Taglauer, E. S., Wilkins-Haug, L., and Bianchi, D. W. (2014). Review: cell-free fetal DNA in the maternal circulation as an indication of placental health and disease. *Placenta* 35(Suppl.), S64–S68. doi: 10.1016/j.placenta.2013.11.014

Touré, F., Fritz, G., Li, Q., Rai, V., Daffu, G., Zou, Y. S., et al. (2012). The formin mDia1 mediates vascular remodeling via integration of oxidative & signal transduction pathways. *Circ. Res.* 110, 1279–1293. doi: 10.1161/CIRCRESAHA.111.262519

Wautier, M.-P., Tessier, F. J., and Wautier, J.-L. (2014). [Advanced glycation end products: a risk factor for human health]. *Ann. Pharm. Fr.* 72, 400–408. doi: 10.1016/j.pharma.2014.05.002

Xu, Y., Toure, F., Qu, W., Lin, L., Song, F., Shen, X., et al. (2010). Advanced glycation end product (AGE)-receptor for AGE (RAGE) signaling and up-regulation of Egr-1 in hypoxic macrophages. *J. Biol. Chem.* 285, 23233–23240. doi: 10.1074/jbc.M110.117457

Yan, H., Zhu, L., Zhang, Z., Li, H., Li, P., Wang, Y., et al. (2018). HMGB1-RAGE signaling pathway in pPROM. *Taiwanese J. Obstet. Gynecol.* 57, 211–216. doi: 10.1016/j.tjog.2018.02.008

Zhang, J., Xu, X., Rao, N. V., Argyle, B., McCoard, L., Rusho, W. J., et al. (2011). Novel sulfated polysaccharides disrupt cathelicidins, inhibit RAGE and reduce cutaneous inflammation in a mouse model of rosacea. *PLoS One* 6:e16658. doi: 10.1371/journal.pone.0016658

Dynamic Changes in the Phenotype of Dendritic Cells in the Uterus and Uterine Draining Lymph Nodes After Coitus

Ippei Yasuda[1,2], Tomoko Shima[1], Taiki Moriya[2], Ryoyo Ikebuchi[2,3], Yutaka Kusumoto[2], Akemi Ushijima[1], Akitoshi Nakashima[1], Michio Tomura[2]* and Shigeru Saito[1]*

[1] Department of Obstetrics and Gynecology, University of Toyama, Toyama, Japan, [2] Laboratory of Immunology, Faculty of Pharmacy, Osaka Ohtani University, Osaka, Japan, [3] Research Fellow of Japan Society for the Promotion of Science, Tokyo, Japan

*Correspondence:
Michio Tomura
michio.tomura@gmail.com
Shigeru Saito
s30saito@med.u-toyama.ac.jp

Dendritic cells (DCs) are essential for successful embryo implantation. However, the properties of uterine DCs (uDCs) during the implantation period are not well characterized. In this study, we investigated the dynamic changes in the uDC phenotypes during the period between coitus and implantation. In virgin mice, we evaluated the expressions of CD103 and XCR1, this is the first report to demonstrate uDCs expressing CD103 in XCR1$^+$cDC1s and XCR1$^+$cDC2s. On day 0.5 post coitus (pc), the number of uterine CD11c$^+$CD103$^-$MHC classII^{high}CD86^{high}–mature DCs rapidly increased and then decreased to non-pregnancy levels on days 1.5 and 2.5 pc. On day 3.5 pc just before implantation, the number of CD11c$^+$CD103$^+$MHC class II^{dim}CD86^{dim}–immature DCs increased in the uterus. The increase in mature uDCs on day 1.5 pc was observed in both allogeneic- and syngeneic mating, suggesting that sexual intercourse, or semen, play a role in this process. Meanwhile, the increase in immature uDCs on day 3.5 pc was only observed in allogeneic mating, suggesting that allo-antigens in the semen contribute to this process. Next, to understand the turnover and migration of uDCs, we monitored DC movement in the uterus and uterine draining lymph nodes (dLNs) using photoconvertible protein Kikume Green Red (KikGR) mice. On day 0.5 pc, uDCs were composed of equal numbers of remaining DCs and migratory DCs. However, on day 3.5 pc, uDCs were primarily composed of migratory DCs, suggesting that most of the uDCs migrate from the periphery just before implantation. Finally, we studied the expression of PD-L2—which induces immunoregulation—on DCs. On day 3.5 pc, PD-L2 was expressed on CD103$^+$-mature and CD103$^-$-mature DCs in the uterus. However, PD-L2 expression on CD103$^-$-immature DCs and CD103$^+$-immature DCs was very low. Furthermore, both remaining and migratory DCs in the uterus and uterus-derived-DCs in the dLNs on day 3.5 pc highly expressed PD-L2 on their surface. Therefore, our study findings provide a better understanding of the dynamic changes occurring in uterine DCs and dLNs in preparation for implantation following allogeneic- and syngeneic mating.

Keywords: feto-maternal tolerance, Kikume Green Red (KikGR), PD-L2, photoconvertible protein, tolerogenic dendritic cells, uterus

INTRODUCTION

Dendritic cells (DCs) play an essential role in successful implantation and placentation in allogeneic- and syngeneic pregnancy (1–4). Moreover, uterus-resident DCs have been proposed to contribute to feto-maternal tolerance by regulating T cell activation (1, 5–8). Uterine DCs (uDCs) take up paternal antigens and present them to T cells in the draining lymph node (dLN), thereby inducing the regulatory T cells (Tregs) at the feto-maternal interface (5, 7, 9–13). The essential role of uDCs in the maintenance of feto-maternal tolerance during pregnancy has been examined. For instance, IDO-expressing DCs and plasmacytoid DCs (pDCs) act as tolerogenic DCs (tDCs) (4). These tDCs have been shown to possess the capability of immunoregulation by inducing Tregs, as well as T cell, anergy and deletion (6, 14, 15). However, few reports have examined the characteristics of uDC subsets in murine pregnancy (2, 4, 16–22).

Based on their morphological features and functions, DCs can be classified into conventional DCs (cDCs) and pDCs (4, 23–26). While each DC subset can present antigens to $CD4^+$ T cells, $CD103^+$ DCs can also present antigens to $CD8^+$ T cells (23). Each DC subset is reported as tDC in food tolerance and tumor immunity (4, 15, 16, 27–31), however, little is known on the type of DC phenotype that increases in the uterus before implantation.

Transient inflammation in the uterine cervix and endometrium is observed after coitus-induced dynamic changes in immune cells (32–34). After insemination, neutrophils migrate rapidly into the uterus and are immediately decreased to non-pregnant levels by day 1.5 post coitus (pc) (35). Subsequently, DCs and macrophages migrate into the uterine endometrium to clear semen debris and make the uterus sterile (33). However, little is known about the phenotype, subsets, and spatiotemporal features of uDCs, as well as the migration of DCs between the uterus and the draining para-aortic lymph nodes. Hence, in the current study we aimed to investigate the dynamic changes in uDCs during allogenic- and syngeneic mating, from coitus to before implantation. To this end, we examined the surface markers of uDCs via flow cytometry, and migration of DCs using mouse line expressing photoconvertible fluorescent protein Kikume Green Red (KikGR) (36–38). We found that approximately 75% of uDCs were transformed to migratory DCs from day 2.5 to 3.5 pc. These migratory DCs may, therefore, play important roles in successful implantation.

RESULTS

Uterine DCs Are Increased Following Coitus and Just Before Implantation

To clarify the dynamic changes in uDC phenotype from coitus to implantation, we analyzed the time course for the classification of uDC subsets in allogeneic pregnancy (**Figure 1A**). Uterine DCs were identified as propidium iodide (PI)$^-$ $CD45^+$ Gr-1$^-$ F4/80$^-$ $CD11c^+$ MHC class II$^{low-high}$ B220$^-$ cells ($CD11c^+$ DCs) (**Figure 1B** and **Supplementary Figure 1A**). We then subdivided them into $CD103^-$ $CD11b^{-/+}$ ($CD103^-$ DCs) and $CD103^+$ $CD11b^{-/+}$ ($CD103^+$ DCs) cells (**Figure 1B** and **Supplementary Figure 1B**). Moreover, uterine pDCs were identified as PI$^-$ $CD45^+$ Gr-1$^-$ F4/80$^-$ $CD11c^+$ PDCA-1$^+$ $CD11b^-$ $Ly6C^+$ $B220^+$ cells.

Compared to the non-mated control virgin mice, the total number of uDCs were increased on days 0.5 and 1.5 pc (9.7 and 4.9-folds, respectively), and returned to the non-pregnancy level on day 2.5 pc (1.7-fold), followed by an additional increase on day 3.5 pc (6.6-fold) (**Figure 1C**). The proportion of each DC subset in virgin mice showed that the majority of uDCs were $CD103^-$ DCs (79.0%), followed by $CD103^+$ DCs (17.8%), while pDCs (3.3%) were in minority (**Supplementary Figure 1C**). Hence the number of $CD103^-$ DCs was similar to that of $CD11c^+$ DCs (**Figure 1C**). Meanwhile, although the proportion of $CD103^+$ DCs was smaller than $CD103^-$ DCs, similar changes were observed in the time course (**Figure 1C**). Additionally, pDCs increased in number beginning on day 1.5 pc, however, continued to only represent a minor population (**Figure 1C**).

Presence of CD103-Expressing uDCs in XCR1$^+$-cDC1s and XCR1$^-$-cDC2s

Recently, the characteristics of different DC subsets have been classified (26, 39). Therefore, here we sought to examine the expression of CD64, CD26, XCR1, and SIRPα to compare the presence of different DC subsets. First, we confirmed the exclusion of macrophages by staining for F4/80 and CD64 expression (**Supplementary Figure 2A**). From the total F4/80$^+$ cell population, F4/80$^+$ CD64$^+$ cells accounted for 68%, while F4/80$^+$ CD64$^+$ cells accounted for 12.5% of the total CD64$^+$ cell population, indicating that F4/80$^+$ gating effectively excluded most of the macrophages (**Supplementary Figure 2B**). Next, we confirmed the proportion of DCs by examining CD26 expression (**Supplementary Figures 2C,D**). The expression of CD26 in $CD11c^+$ DCs, $CD103^-$ DCs, and $CD103^+$ DCs was 69, 54.5, and 95.3%, respectively (**Supplementary Figure 2D**). These results indicate that PI$^-$ $CD45^+$ Gr-1$^-$ F4/80$^-$ $CD11c^+$ MHC class II$^+$ B220$^-$ cells may be considered as DCs in the uterus. Moreover, although both CD103 and XCR1 have commonly served as markers of cDC1s, CD103 expression was also recently detected in cDC2s (26). Therefore, we further confirmed the DC subset be detecting XCR1 and SIRPα expression (**Supplementary Figure 2E**). In the $CD11c^+$ DC population, the proportion of XCR1$^+$ DCs and $CD103^+$ DCs was 13.5 and 43%, respectively (**Supplementary Figures 2E,F**). Conversely, CD103 expression was detected in 13.1% of $CD103^+$ XCR1$^+$ DCs, and in 34.7% of $CD103^+$ XCR1$^-$ DCs (**Supplementary Figures 2E,G**), indicating the presence of CD103 in both cDC1s and cDC2s in the uterus.

Mature DCs Increase After Coitus and Decrease to Non-pregnancy Levels Just Before Implantation

We then subdivided each DC subset into $CD86^{low}$ MHC class II^{low}-immature DCs and $CD86^{high}$ MHC class II^{high}-mature DCs

---

Abbreviations: cDCs, conventional DCs; DCs, dendritic cells; dLN, draining lymph node; KikGR, Kikume Green Red; LNDCs, lymph node DCs; MPA, medroxyprogesterone; pc, post coitus; pDCs, plasmacytoid DCs; PI, propidium iodide; tDCs, tolerogenic DCs; Tregs, regulatory T cells; tSNE, t-distributed stochastic neighbor embedding; uDCs, uterine dendritic cells.

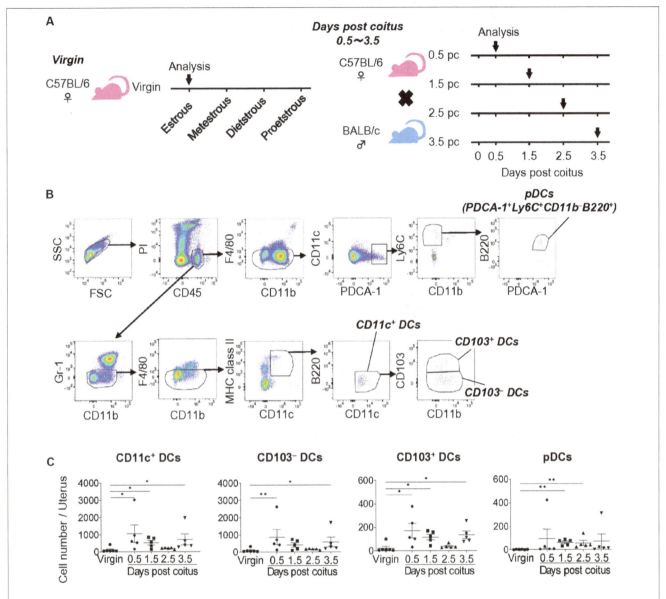

FIGURE 1 | Cell numbers of uDCs after coitus in allogeneic mating. **(A)** Experimental time course. The DCs in the uterus in non-mated control virgin mice and mice on days 0.5, 1.5, 2.5, and 3.5 pc were analyzed by flow cytometry. **(B)** Gating strategy was used to identify CD103$^-$ DCs, CD103$^+$ DCs, and pDCs in the uterus. **(C)** Graphs show number of CD11c$^+$ DCs and each DC subset in the uterus at each time point. A minimum of five samples from each time point were analyzed. Data represent mean ± SEM and are representative of three independent experiments. Statistical comparisons were performed using Kruskal-Wallis test with Dunn's multiple comparisons test (**$P < 0.01$, *$P < 0.05$).

(**Figure 2A**) (15). The frequency of mature DCs among CD11c$^+$-total DCs increased at days 0.5 and 1.5 pc compared to that in virgin mice, and then returned to the level observed in virgin mice on days 2.5 and 3.5 pc (**Figures 2B,D,E**). Meanwhile, the frequency of CD11c$^+$-immature DCs increased on day 3.5 pc compared to that in virgin mice (**Figures 2B,C,E**). CD103$^-$-mature DCs also increased at days 0.5 and 1.5 pc, however, the frequency of CD103$^+$-mature DCs and pDCs did not change on days 0.5 and 1.5 pc. Hence, the increased number of mature uDCs on days 0.5 and 1.5 pc was likely due to increased CD103$^-$ DCs. Moreover, the frequency of CD103$^+$-immature uDCs on day 3.5 pc was significantly elevated compared to that in virgin mice,

suggesting that an increase in immature uDCs on day 3.5 was due to increased CD103$^+$ DCs.

Characterization of uDCs Using t-Distributed Stochastic Neighbor Embedding (tSNE)

To define the specific DC subset present during the implantation period, we next analyzed the time course of uDC subsets via dimensionality reduction analysis, using tSNE. The pooled data for individual CD11c$^+$ DCs and pDCs within the uterus across each time point ($n = 26$) was concatenated and

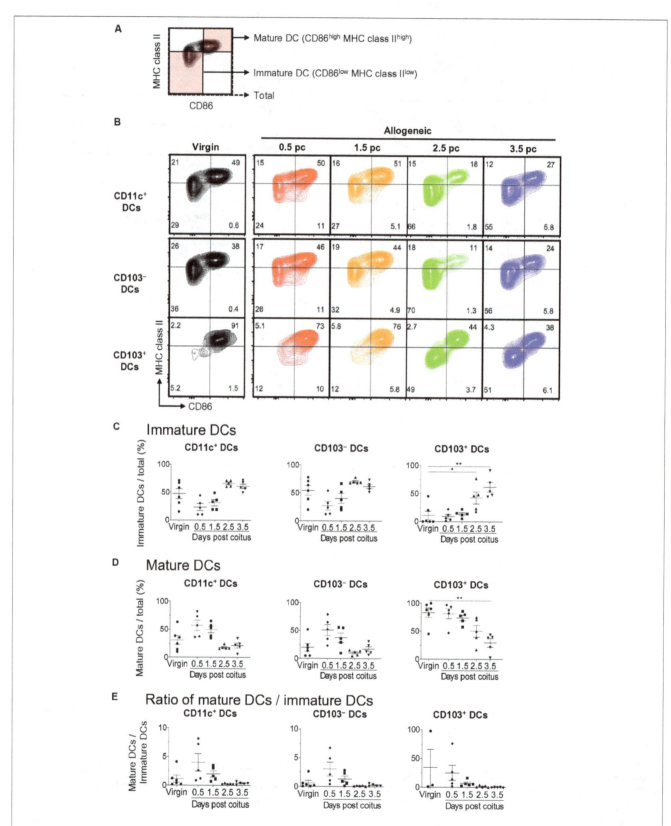

FIGURE 2 | Time course for uterine immature and mature DCs after coitus in allogeneic mating. **(A,B)** Flow cytometry contour plots show immature DCs and mature DCs based on the expression of CD86 and MHC class II **(A)**, and representative plots in proportion to those within each DC subset at each time point **(B)**. **(C–E)** Graphs show the proportion of immature DCs **(C)** and mature DCs **(D)** out of the total DCs, and ratio of mature DCs/immature DCs **(E)** in each DC subset at each time point. A minimum of five samples from each time point were analyzed. Data represent mean ± SEM **(C–E)** and are representative of three independent experiments. Statistical comparisons were performed using the Kruskal-Wallis test with Dunn's multiple comparisons test (**$P < 0.01$, *$P < 0.05$).

visualized as a two-dimensional map by tSNE (**Supplementary Figure 3**). Results show that the clusters of each DC subset—particularly those of CD103$^+$ DCs—were clearly divided into two clusters, MHC class II^{high} CD86^{high} and MHC class II^{dim} CD86^{dim} (**Supplementary Figure 3A**). The changes in distribution demonstrate (**Supplementary Figures 3B,D,E**) that the primary clusters in virgin mice consisted of cluster 6 made up of CD103$^+$ mature DCs (**Supplementary Figures 3A,C**), clusters 8, 9, and 10 comprised of DCs without any specific surface markers, and cluster 12 made up of CD11b$^+$ DCs. After coitus, the increased clusters on days 0.5 and 1.5 pc appeared as cluster 11 (**Supplementary Figures 3D-F**), which contained CD11c$^+$ CD86^{high} MHC class II^{high} Ly6C$^-$ PDCA-1^{dim} CD11b$^+$ CD103$^-$-mature DCs (**Supplementary Figures 3A,C**). Interestingly, new clusters on days 2.5 and 3.5 pc appeared as cluster 7 (**Supplementary Figures 3D-F**), containing CD11c$^+$ CD86^{dim} MHC class II^{dim} Ly6C$^-$ PDCA-1^{dim} CD11b$^-$ CD103$^+$-immature DCs (**Supplementary Figures 3A,C**). These results indicate that these newly appearing DCs before implantation are primarily CD103$^+$ immature DCs.

Differences in uDC Populations Between Allogeneic- and Syngeneic Mating

To examine the differences in the uDC populations in response to paternal antigens, we analyzed the characteristics of uDCs between virgin, allogeneic-, and syngeneic mating on days 1.5 and 3.5 pc (**Figure 3A**). The increase in uDCs on day 1.5 pc was observed in both allogeneic- and syngeneic mating (**Figure 3B**). There were no significant changes in the number or frequencies of uDCs between allogeneic- and syngeneic mating on day 1.5 pc (**Figures 3B-E**). However, an increase in CD103$^-$- and CD103$^+$-immature uDCs was observed in allogeneic mating, but not in syngeneic mating on day 3.5 pc (**Figures 3C-E**). These results suggest that the induction of immature DCs in the uterus before implantation is dependent on paternal antigens.

Immature uDCs Are Increased Among the Infiltrating and Pre-existing DCs Just Before Implantation

Although the migration and pre-existence of uDCs using CFSE labeling in non-pregnant mice has been reported, little is known regarding how resident and migratory uDCs contribute to successful implantation (1). Thus, we elucidated the turnover of uDCs in KikGR mice (**Figure 4A** left). All DCs in the uterus were converted to KikGR-red immediately after photoconversion (**Supplementary Figures 4A-D**). Consequently, under such photoconversion conditions, we analyzed the KikGR-red remaining DCs and non-photoconverted KikGR-green migratory DCs at 24 h after photoconversion of the uterus with KikGR mice from day 0.5 to 1.5 pc, from 1.5 to 2.5 pc, and from 2.5 to 3.5 pc (**Figure 4A** right). This protocol allowed us to monitor the uDC turnover for 24 h on each gestational day. Results show that migratory DCs consisted of equal numbers of immature and mature DCs, with no change the proportion of immature/mature DCs in the migratory DCs over time (**Supplementary Figures 5B, 6A,B** and **Figure 4B**). In general, infiltrating DCs—which are of the immature phenotype—migrate to peripheral organs and are subsequently matured. Thus, equal proportions of mature and immature phenotypes in infiltrating DCs at 24 h from coitus to before implantation implies that the maturation rate of infiltrating DCs is not altered drastically. Alternatively, the remaining DCs were predominantly of the mature phenotype throughout the period after coitus, and just before implantation, with the proportion of mature DCs in the remaining DCs observed to gradually decrease (**Supplementary Figures 5B, 6C** and **Figure 4C**). During the analysis of changes due to cell turnover, the time course study revealed that the proportion of remaining DCs in the uterus gradually decreased by day 3.5 pc (**Figure 4D**). These results indicate that increased immature uDCs before implantation primarily make up the infiltrating DCs.

DC Subsets of Uterine dLNs After Coitus to Just Before Implantation

It has been reported that paternal antigen-specific Tregs increase in the dLNs before implantation (13, 40). Uterus-derived DCs would then stimulate the paternal antigen-specific Tregs by presenting paternal antigens. Thus, it is important to understand dynamic changes in the migratory patterns of uDCs to dLN from coitus to before implantation. To this end, we analyzed the time course of MHC class II^{high} DCs in dLNs (**Supplementary Figure 7A**). Compared with virgin mice, the total number of migratory DCs in dLNs from day 0.5, 1.5, 2.5, and 3.5 pc were increased by 2.5, 14.4, 8.3, and 18.6-fold, respectively (**Supplementary Figure 7B**). In the changes of each DC subset, CD103$^-$ DCs, CD103$^+$ DCs, and pDCs levels were significantly increased on day 3.5 pc compared to those in virgin mice (**Supplementary Figure 7B**). Meanwhile, CD103$^+$ DCs accounted for a minor population in dLNs throughout this period. To clarify the dynamic changes of migratory uDCs in the dLNs, we next analyzed the migration of uDCs using KikGR mice (**Figure 4A**). No KikGR-red DCs were detected in the dLNs immediately after photoconversion, indicating that photoconversion was restricted to the uterus (**Supplementary Figures 4C,D**). However, 24 h after photoconversion, we detected KikGR-red DCs in migratory DCs (CD11c$^+$ MHC class II^{high}) (**Figure 4E**), but not in lymph node DCs (LNDCs) (CD11c$^+$ MHC class II^{int}) (**Supplementary Figure 7C**), suggesting that uterine migratory DCs were exclusively CD11c$^+$ MHC class II^{high}. Furthermore, the time course study revealed that the migration of KikGR-red uterus-derived total DCs, CD103$^-$ DCs, and CD103$^+$ DCs in the dLNs showed an increasing trend by day 3.5 pc (**Figure 4E**).

PD-L2$^+$ Expression on DCs

PD-L2 has been implicated to play a critical role in immune tolerance by negatively regulating the T cell immune response (27, 41). To clarify its contribution to tolerogenic conditioning, we analyzed PD-L2 expression on DCs (**Figure 5A**) and found that it was not expressed on mature and immature uDCs in virgin mice (**Figures 5B,C**). However, more than 30% of CD103$^+$- and CD103$^-$-mature DCs, but not immature DCs,

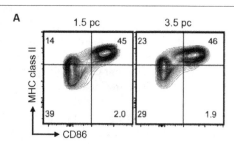
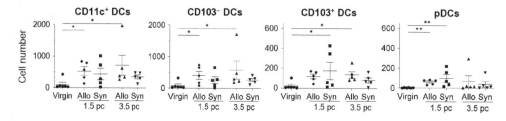
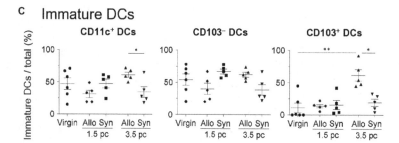
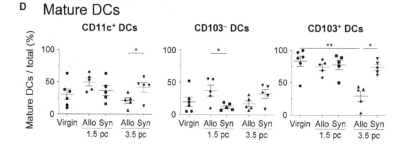
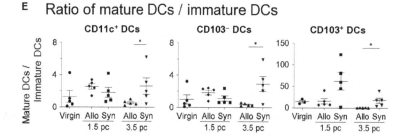

FIGURE 3 | Comparison of uDC phenotype between allogeneic- and syngeneic mating. **(A)** Flow cytometry contour plots show immature DCs and mature DCs in syngeneic mating on days 1.5 and 3.5 pc. **(B,C)** Graphs show total DC number **(B)**, proportion of immature DCs **(C)** and mature DCs **(D)** out of the total DCs, and the ratio of mature DCs/immature DCs within each DC subset **(E)** in virgin, allogeneic-, and syngeneic mating mice at each time point. A minimum of five samples from each time point were analyzed. Data represent mean ± SEM **(B,C)** and are representative of three independent experiments. Statistical comparisons were performed using Mann-Whitney U-test (**$P < 0.01$, *$P < 0.05$).

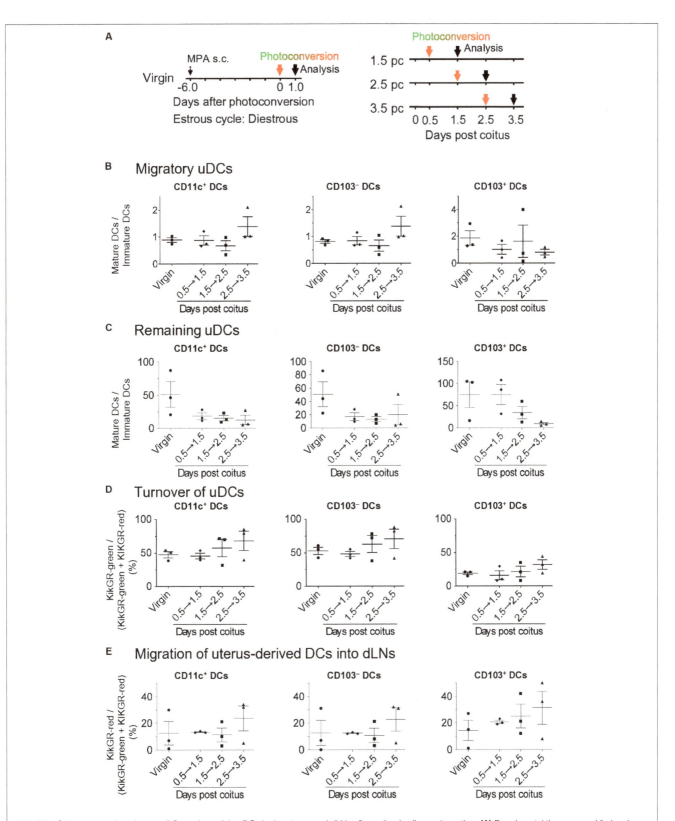

FIGURE 4 | Time course for migratory DCs and remaining DCs in the uterus and dLNs after coitus in allogeneic mating. (A) Experimental time course. Virgin mice were synchronized at the diestrous stage, and the uteri of mice after coitus in allogeneic mating were photoconverted on days 0.5, 1.5, and 2.5 pc. The DCs in the uteri and dLNs were analyzed 24 h after photoconversion. (B–E) Graphs show the ratio of mature DCs/immature DCs (B,C) in each DC subset labeled with KikGR-green (B) and KikGR-red (C), and proportion of each DC subset labeled with KikGR-green in the uterus, (D) and KikGR-red within MHC class II high DC subset in the dLNs (E) out of the total DCs 24 h after photoconversion. Three samples from each time point were analyzed. Data represent mean ± SEM (B–E) and are representative of three independent experiments. Statistical comparisons were performed using the Kruskal-Wallis test with Dunn's multiple comparisons test.

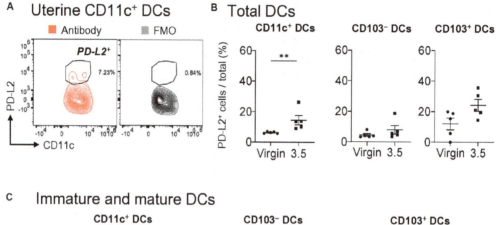
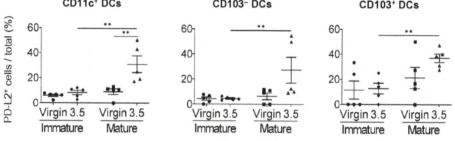
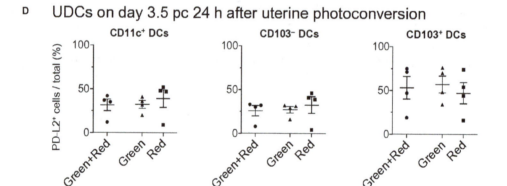
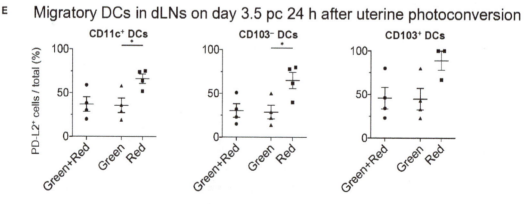

FIGURE 5 | Expression of PD-L2 in uDCs increased immediately before implantation. **(A)** Flow cytometry contour plots show expressions of PD-L2 in uterine $CD11c^+$ DCs with fluorescence minus one (FMO). **(B,C)** Proportion of $PD-L2^+$ DCs of total DCs **(B)**, immature DCs, and mature DCs **(C)** in allogeneic mating at each time point. **(D,E)** Proportion of $PD-L2^+$ DCs within the uterus **(D)** and dLNs **(E)** in allogeneic mating 24 h after uterine photoconversion on day 3.5 pc. A minimum of five **(B,C)** and four **(D,E)** samples from each time point were analyzed. Data represent mean ± SEM **(B,C)** and are representative of three independent experiments. Statistical comparisons were performed using Mann-Whitney U-test **(B,C)** and Kruskal-Wallis test with Dunn's multiple comparisons test **(D,E)** (**$P < 0.01$, *$P < 0.05$).

expressed PD-L2 on day 3.5 pc in allogeneic mating (**Figure 5C**). Moreover, we examined results for day 3.5 pc—24 h after uterine photoconversion—to clarify the type of DCs expressing PD-L2. However, no clear differences were observed in PD-L2 expression between the migratory DCs and remaining DCs in the uterus on day 3.5 pc (**Figure 5D**). Meanwhile, a significant increase was observed in the expression of PD-L2 on uterus-derived $CD11c^+$ DCs and $CD103^-$ DCs in the uterine dLNs (**Figure 5E**), suggesting that the DCs expressing PD-L2 in uterine dLNs were actually migratory DCs from the uterus.

DISCUSSION

In this study, we showed that there is a transient increase in $CD11c^+$ $CD86^{high}$ MHC class II^{high} $Ly6C^-$ $PDCA-1^{dim}$ $CD11b^+$ $CD103^-$-mature uDCs on day 0.5 pc, and $CD11c^+$ $CD86^{dim}$ MHC class II^{dim} $Ly6C^-$ $PDCA-1^{dim}$ $CD11b^-$ $CD103^+$-immature uDCs on day 3.5 pc. The mature DCs were observed following allogeneic- and syngeneic mating on day 1.5 pc, suggesting that sexual intercourse itself, or semen, induced accumulation of mature DCs in the uterus after coitus. After seminal priming, semen stimulates uterine inflammation through the γδ T cells/IL-17A axis (35). Moderate inflammation is proposed to play an important role in successful implantation (32). Additionally, even mechanical injury of the endometrium can contribute to the receptivity of uterus for implantation with the accumulation of DCs (42, 43). It is proposed that moderate inflammation also contributes to the infiltration of DCs to the uterus, which induces feto-maternal tolerance by recognition of paternal antigens (32, 33, 44). Our study showed that paternal antigens did not affect the increase in uDCs on day 0.5 pc as the increased uDCs on day 1.5 pc were observed in both allogeneic- and syngeneic mating. Hence, the increase in mature uDCs might play a role in successful implantation and decidualization in allogeneic- and syngeneic mating. However, the role of inflammation in successful implantation remains unknown. Moreover, further investigations are required to confirm the role of uDCs on day 1.5 pc in the process of implantation.

The migration and pre-existence of uDCs using CFSE labeling in non-pregnant mice has been reported, however, little is known about the process by which resident and migratory uDCs contribute to successful implantation (1). Our study was the first to show turnover in the uterus and migration of uDCs to the dLNs using KikGR mice. We found that half of uDCs interchanged from day 0.5 to 1.5 pc. Interestingly, uterine remaining DCs were almost mature DCs, and an equal number of immature and mature made up the migratory DC population on day 1.5 pc. In general, infiltrating DCs—which are immature phenotype—migrate to peripheral organs and are subsequently matured. After coitus uDCs are almost matured for 24 h. Importantly, we revealed that uDCs before implantation consist of two types, namely immature DCs and $CD103^-$- and $CD103^+$-mature DCs expressing PD-L2. Immature DCs, which have been previously reported (1, 45), have low antigen presenting capacity. These immature uDCs regulate maternal T cell-activation against fetal antigens and induce paternal antigen-specific Tregs in vitro via seminal plasma (13). Our data showed that the frequency of immature uDCs was significantly higher in allogeneic mating as compared to that in syngeneic mating on day 3.5 pc, suggesting that immature uDCs may prevent rejection of the semi-allogenetic fetus by regulating the maternal immune system. Interestingly, our data showed that approximately 68% of uDCs were transformed to migratory DCs from day 2.5 to 3.5 pc. These migratory DCs may play important roles in successful implantation by regulating decidualization and angiogenesis, as these DCs regulate the activation of T cells (1, 2, 5–8). Additionally, we observed the presence of immature uDCs immediately before implantation originating from migratory DCs, however, it was unclear the origins of these immature DCs, which must be investigated in future. Similarly, the mechanism by which DCs migrate from the periphery to the uterus should also be characterized.

Immature DCs are typically reported to be tDCs (1, 45), however, another type of uDCs found on day 3.5 pc were the $CD103^-$- and $CD103^+$-mature DCs expressing PD-L2 (**Figures 5B,C**). We showed that a large proportion of the uterus-remaining mature DCs express PD-L2 immediately before implantation. These PD-L2-expressing cells may stimulate effector T cells with an inhibitory signal via the PD-L2/PD1 pathway, thereby inhibiting their effector T cell functions allowing for successful implantation during allogeneic pregnancy. However, it has been reported that the number of paternal antigen-specific Tregs increase in the dLNs before implantation during allogeneic, but not syngeneic mating (13, 40). The DCs in the dLNs that migrated from the uterus were of the $CD103^-$- and $CD103^+$-mature phenotype, suggesting that they could take up the paternal allo-antigen from the semen and migrate to the dLNs, wherein they could effectively stimulate both the paternal allo-antigen-specific-$CD4^+$, and -$CD8^+$ effector T cells, as well as the Tregs in dLNs before implantation (23).

Although few reports have detailed DC subtypes in the uterus, we evaluated not only $CD103^-$ DCs, $CD103^+$ DCs, and pDCs in allogeneic- and syngeneic pregnancy, but also $XCR1^+$ DCs and $XCR1^-$ DCs in virgin mice. To our knowledge, this is the first study reporting CD103-expressing uDCs in cDC2s. Thus far, many reports on cDCs have shown cDC1s and cDC2s as $CD103^+$ DCs and $CD11b^+$ DCs, respectively (46–50) and, like the DC classification of intestines (26, 39, 51), it would be necessary to investigate the expressions of XCR1 and SIRPα before detecting the expression of CD103, although, the distribution of cDC1s and cDC2s in the uterus was not determined in our present study. Additionally, as a limitation of this study, the functional analysis of migratory DCs was not examined, thus, further examination will be required to determine the relative abundance of proliferation, activation markers, and functional analysis of the uterine cDC1s and cDC2s. During DC turnover analysis we did not examine uterine photoconversion from day 0 to 1.0 pc, as there was a limitation of natural sexual intercourse after photoconversion. In addition, as a topic for further study, we plan to examine the role of sperm and seminal plasma in the induction of DC differentiation. Further research is also required to investigate the induction of Tregs and anti-inflammatory cytokines, or tolerogenic functions of each DC subset, as well as the properties of human uDC subsets associated with implantation failure.

In conclusion, we comprehensively demonstrated the coitus-induced uDC dynamics associated with preparing tolerogenic conditions in the uterus and dLNs at the time of implantation. Importantly, we revealed that uDCs before implantation consist of two types of DCs: the immature DCs, as it has been previously proposed, as well as the $CD103^-$- and $CD103^+$-mature DCs expressing PD-L2, which may present paternal allo-antigens to $CD4^+$ and $CD8^+$ T cells with an inhibitory signal, thereby inhibiting their effector T cell functions. Our findings deepen the current understanding regarding the reproductive immune response before implantation, and may serve to provide new targets for the prevention of implantation failure.

MATERIALS AND METHODS

Mice

C57BL/6 and BALB/c mice were purchased from CLEA Japan. Knock-in mice carrying KikGR cDNA under the CAG promoter (KikGR mice) were generated as previously described (36, 37). Mice were bred and maintained in a specific pathogen-free facility at Osaka Ohtani University. All animal procedures were performed in accordance with the institutional guidelines of the Animal Research Committee of Osaka Ohtani University. C57BL/6 female mice aged 8–10 weeks were mated with BALB/c or C57BL/6 male mice. KikGR knock-in C57BL/6 female mice aged 8–10 weeks were mated with BALB/c male mice. The presence of vaginal plugs was determined the next morning and females were then separated from the males. The presence of vaginal plugs marked day 0.5 of pregnancy. Pregnant mice were euthanized on days 0.5, 1.5, 2.5, and 3.5 pc. Six days before photoconversion, non-pregnant virgin mice were synchronized in the diestrous stage via subcutaneous injection with 2 mg medroxyprogesterone (MPA) (Tokyo Chemical Industry, Osaka, Japan).

Photoconversion

During photoconversion of the uterus, non-photoconverted regions were protected from light using aluminum foil, while the region of the uterus targeted for photoconversion was exposed to violet light (405 nm, 100 mW/cm^2) for 2 min from the front and behind following laparotomy. Following photoconversion, the abdominal wall was closed. To keep the exposed tissues moist during exposure to light, warmed PBS was applied to the region of photoconversion. To prevent hypothermia, mice were warmed with a heater during the perioperative stages.

Reagents, Antibodies, and Flow Cytometric Analysis

Mononuclear cells were isolated from dLNs and the uterus on days 0.5, 1.5, 2.5, and 3.5 pc. Resected uteri were minced with scissors, and the tissues were then passed through a 100-μm cell strainer. The antibodies used were as follows: purchased from BD, eBioScience, or BioLegend: FITC-conjugated anti-I-A/I-E (clone M5/114.15.2), plycoerythrin (PE)-conjugated anti-CD103 (clone 2E7), PE-Dazzle594-conjugated anti-CD11c (clone N418), PE-cyanine5-conjugated anti-CD45R/B220 and streptavidin (clone RA3-6B2), PE-cyanine7-conjugated anti-Gr-1 and I-A/I-E (clone RB-6-8C5, and M5/114.15.2, respectively), allophycocyanin (APC)-conjugated anti-PDCA-1, CD26,and SIRPα (clone 927, H194-112, and P84, respectively), Alexa Flour 700-conjugated anti-CD45 (clone 30-F11), APC-cyanine7-conjugated anti-F4/80 and CD45 (clone BM8 and 30-F11, respectively), APC-R700-conjugated anti-CD103 (clone M290), Brilliant Violet (BV) 421-conjugated anti-CD86, CD64, and XCR1 (clone GL-1, X54-5/7.1, and ZET, respectively), Pacific blue-conjugated anti-CD11b (clone M1/70), BV510-conjugated anti-Ly6C, CD45, and CD11c (clone HK1.4, 30-F11, and N418, respectively), and biotin-conjugated anti-CD273 (clone TY25). For flow cytometric analysis, cells were washed with Dulbecco's PBS supplemented with 2% fetal calf serum (FCS), and 0.02% sodium azide. Next, cells were incubated with 2.4G2 hybridoma culture supernatant to block Fc binding. Dead cells were labeled with PI. Stained samples were acquired using SP6800 (SONY, Tokyo, Japan). KikGR-green and red signals were detected using 530/60 and 595/50 bandpass filters, respectively. Flow cytometry data were analyzed using the FlowJo software (Tree Star, Ashland, OR, United States).

Data Analysis

Dimensionality reduction was performed using tSNE analysis, followed by FlowJo. First, we exported PI^- $CD45^+$ $Gr-1^-$ $F4/80^-$ $CD11c^+$ MHC class II^+ $B220^-$ ($CD11c^+$ DCs) and PI^- $CD45^+$ $Gr-1^-$ $F4/80^-$ $CD11c^+$ $PDCA-1^+$ $CD11b^-$ $Ly6C^+$ $B220^+$ (pDCs) compartments from each dataset, and the cell numbers were adjusted to be the same as those in the minimal sample for each gestational age, including a minimum of five uterine samples. Next, the data was concatenated and visualized as a two-dimensional map by tSNE.

Mann-Whitney U-test and Kruskal-Wallis test with Dunn's multiple comparisons test were performed using GraphPad Prism version 8.4.3 (GraphPad Software, San Diego, CA, United States). Data in bar graphs represent mean ± standard error of mean (SEM). P-values <0.05 were considered to be statistically significant.

ETHICS STATEMENT

The animal study was reviewed and approved by Osaka Ohtani University.

AUTHOR CONTRIBUTIONS

IY designed the study, performed the experiments, analyzed the data, and wrote the manuscript. TM, RI, YK, AU, TS, and AN performed the experiments and analyzed the data. MT, TS, AN, and SS designed the study and wrote the manuscript. All authors read and approved the final version of the manuscript.

ACKNOWLEDGMENTS

We thank Shinji Imai for performing a portion of the flow cytometric analysis, and Editage (www.editage.com) for English language editing.

REFERENCES

Collins MK, Tay CS, Erlebacher A. Dendritic cell entrapment within the pregnant uterus inhibits immune surveillance of the maternal/fetal interface in mice. *J Clin Invest.* (2009) 119:2062–73. doi: 10.1172/JCI38714

Plaks V, Birnberg T, Berkutzki T, Sela S, BenYashar A, Kalchenko V, et al. Uterine DCs are crucial for decidua formation during embryo implantation in mice. *J Clin Invest.* (2008) 118:3954–65. doi: 10.1172/JCI36682

Krey G, Frank P, Shaikly V, Barrientos G, Cordo-Russo R, Ringel F, et al. In vivo dendritic cell depletion reduces breeding efficiency, affecting implantation and early placental development in mice. *J Mol Med.* (2008) 86:999–1011. doi: 10.1007/s00109-008-0379-2

Fang WN, Shi M, Meng CY, Li DD, Peng JP. The balance between conventional DCs and plasmacytoid DCs is pivotal for immunological tolerance during pregnancy in the mouse. *Sci Rep.* (2016) 6:26984. doi: 10.1038/srep26984

Blois SM, Kammerer U, Alba Soto C, Tometten MC, Shaikly V, Barrientos G, et al. Dendritic cells: key to fetal tolerance? *Biol Reprod.* (2007) 77:590–8. doi: 10.1095/biolreprod.107.060632

Steinman RM, Hawiger D, Nussenzweig MC. Tolerogenic dendritic cells. *Annu Rev Immunol.* (2003) 21:685–711. doi: 10.1146/annurev.immunol.21.120601.141040

Tagliani E, Erlebacher A. Dendritic cell function at the maternal-fetal interface. *Expert Rev Clin Immunol.* (2011) 7:593–602. doi: 10.1586/eci.11.52

Oderup C, Cederbom L, Makowska A, Cilio CM, Ivars F. Cytotoxic T lymphocyte antigen-4-dependent down-modulation of costimulatory molecules on dendritic cells in CD4+ CD25+ regulatory T-cell-mediated suppression. *Immunology.* (2006) 118:240–9. doi: 10.1111/j.1365-2567.2006.02362.x

Tsuda S, Nakashima A, Shima T, Saito S. New paradigm in the role of regulatory T cells during pregnancy. *Front Immunol.* (2019) 10:573. doi: 10.3389/fimmu.2019.00573

Remes Lenicov F, Rodriguez Rodrigues C, Sabatte J, Cabrini M, Jancic C, Ostrowski M, et al. Semen promotes the differentiation of tolerogenic dendritic cells. *J Immunol.* (2012) 189:4777–86. doi: 10.4049/jimmunol.1202089

Rieger L, Honig A, Sutterlin M, Kapp M, Dietl J, Ruck P, et al. Antigen-presenting cells in human endometrium during the menstrual cycle compared to early pregnancy. *J Soc Gynecol Investig.* (2004) 11:488–93. doi: 10.1016/j.jsgi.2004.05.007

Hsu P, Santner-Nanan B, Dahlstrom JE, Fadia M, Chandra A, Peek M, et al. Altered decidual DC-SIGN+ antigen-presenting cells and impaired regulatory T-cell induction in preeclampsia. *Am J Pathol.* (2012) 181:2149–60. doi: 10.1016/j.ajpath.2012.08.032

Shima T, Nakashima A, Yasuda I, Ushijima A, Inada K, Tsuda S, et al. Uterine CD11c+ cells induce the development of paternal antigen-specific Tregs via seminal plasma priming. *J Reprod Immunol.* (2020) 141:103165. doi: 10.1016/j.jri.2020.103165

Ghaebi M, Nouri M, Ghasemzadeh A, Farzadi L, Jadidi-Niaragh F, Ahmadi M, et al. Immune regulatory network in successful pregnancy and reproductive failures. *Biomed Pharmacother.* (2017) 88:61–73. doi: 10.1016/j.biopha.2017.01.016

Vendelova E, Ashour D, Blank P, Erhard F, Saliba AE, Kalinke U, et al. Tolerogenic transcriptional signatures of steady-state and pathogen-induced dendritic cells. *Front Immunol.* (2018) 9:333. doi: 10.3389/fimmu.2018.00333

Blois SM, Alba Soto CD, Tometten M, Klapp BF, Margni RA, Arck PC. Lineage, maturity, and phenotype of uterine murine dendritic cells throughout gestation indicate a protective role in maintaining pregnancy. *Biol Reprod.* (2004) 70:1018–23. doi: 10.1095/biolreprod.103.022640

Li Y, Lopez GE, Vazquez J, Sun Y, Chavarria M, Lindner PN, et al. Decidual-placental immune landscape during syngeneic murine pregnancy. *Front Immunol.* (2018) 9:2087. doi: 10.3389/fimmu.2018.02087

Keenihan SN, Robertson SA. Diversity in phenotype and steroid hormone dependence in dendritic cells and macrophages in the mouse uterus. *Biol Reprod.* (2004) 70:1562–72. doi: 10.1095/biolreprod.103.024794

Habbeddine M, Verbeke P, Karaz S, Bobe P, Kanellopoulos-Langevin C. Leukocyte population dynamics and detection of IL-9 as a major cytokine at the mouse fetal-maternal interface. *PLoS One.* (2014) 9:e107267. doi: 10.1371/journal.pone.0107267

Zhao H, Kalish F, Schulz S, Yang Y, Wong RJ, Stevenson DK. Unique roles of infiltrating myeloid cells in the murine uterus during early to midpregnancy. *J Immunol.* (2015) 194:3713–22. doi: 10.4049/jimmunol.1401930

Blois SM, Freitag N, Tirado-Gonzalez I, Cheng SB, Heimesaat MM, Bereswill S, et al. NK cell-derived IL-10 is critical for DC-NK cell dialogue at the maternal-fetal interface. *Sci Rep.* (2017) 7:2189. doi: 10.1038/s41598-017-02333-8

Negishi Y, Ichikawa T, Takeshita T, Takahashi H. Miscarriage induced by adoptive transfer of dendritic cells and invariant natural killer T cells into mice. *Eur J Immunol.* (2018) 48:937–49. doi: 10.1002/eji.201747162

Takenaka MC, Quintana FJ. Tolerogenic dendritic cells. *Semin Immunopathol.* (2017) 39:113–20. doi: 10.1007/s00281-016-0587-8

Durai V, Murphy KM. Functions of murine dendritic cells. *Immunity.* (2016) 45:719–36. doi: 10.1016/j.immuni.2016.10.010

Ban YL, Kong BH, Qu X, Yang QF, Ma YY. BDCA-1+, BDCA-2+ and BDCA-3+ dendritic cells in early human pregnancy decidua. *Clin Exp Immunol.* (2008) 151:399–406. doi: 10.1111/j.1365-2249.2007.03576.x

Guilliams M, Dutertre CA, Scott CL, McGovern N, Sichien D, Chakarov S, et al. Unsupervised high-dimensional analysis aligns dendritic cells across tissues and species. *Immunity.* (2016) 45:669–84. doi: 10.1016/j.immuni.2016.08.015

Marinelarena A, Bhattacharya P, Kumar P, Maker AV, Prabhakar BS. Identification of a novel OX40L(+) dendritic cell subset that selectively expands regulatory T cells. *Sci Rep.* (2018) 8:14940. doi: 10.1038/s41598-018-33307-z

Sun CM, Hall JA, Blank RB, Bouladoux N, Oukka M, Mora JR, et al. Small intestine lamina propria dendritic cells promote de novo generation of Foxp3 T reg cells via retinoic acid. *J Exp Med.* (2007) 204:1775–85. doi: 10.1084/jem.20070602

Scott CL, Aumeunier AM, Mowat AM. Intestinal CD103+ dendritic cells: master regulators of tolerance? *Trends Immunol.* (2011) 32:412–9. doi: 10.1016/j.it.2011.06.003

Ahmadabad HN, Salehnia M, Saito S, Moazzeni SM. Decidual soluble factors, through modulation of dendritic cells functions, determine the immune response patterns at the feto-maternal interface. *J Reprod Immunol.* (2016) 114:10–7. doi: 10.1016/j.jri.2016.01.001

Svajger U, Rozman P. Induction of tolerogenic dendritic cells by endogenous biomolecules: an update. *Front Immunol.* (2018) 9:2482. doi: 10.3389/fimmu.2018.02482

Dekel N, Gnainsky Y, Granot I, Mor G. Inflammation and implantation. *Am J Reprod Immunol.* (2010) 63:17–21. doi: 10.1111/j.1600-0897.2009.00792.x

Robertson SA, Sharkey DJ. Seminal fluid and fertility in women. *Fertil Steril.* (2016) 106:511–9. doi: 10.1016/j.fertnstert.2016.07.1101

Kammerer U, Eggert AO, Kapp M, McLellan AD, Geijtenbeek TB, Dietl J, et al. Unique appearance of proliferating antigen-presenting cells expressing DC-SIGN (CD209) in the decidua of early human pregnancy. *Am J Pathol.* (2003) 162:887–96. doi: 10.1016/S0002-9440(10)63884-9

Song ZH, Li ZY, Li DD, Fang WN, Liu HY, Yang DD, et al. Seminal plasma induces inflammation in the uterus through the gammadelta T/IL-17 pathway. *Sci Rep.* (2016) 6:25118. doi: 10.1038/srep25118

Tomura M, Hata A, Matsuoka S, Shand FH, Nakanishi Y, Ikebuchi R, et al. Tracking and quantification of dendritic cell migration and antigen trafficking between the skin and lymph nodes. *Sci Rep.* (2014) 4:6030. doi: 10.1038/srep06030

Nakanishi Y, Ikebuchi R, Chtanova T, Kusumoto Y, Okuyama H, Moriya T, et al. Regulatory T cells with superior immunosuppressive capacity emigrate from the inflamed colon to draining lymph nodes. *Mucosal Immunol.* (2018) 11:437–48. doi: 10.1038/mi.2017.64

Futamura K, Sekino M, Hata A, Ikebuchi R, Nakanishi Y, Egawa G, et al. Novel full-spectral flow cytometry with multiple spectrally-adjacent fluorescent proteins and fluorochromes and visualization of in vivo cellular movement. *Cytometry A.* (2015) 87:830–42. doi: 10.1002/cyto.a.22725

Bosteels C, Neyt K, Vanheerswynghels M, van Helden MJ, Sichien D, Debeuf N, et al. Inflammatory type 2 cDCs acquire features of cDC1s and macrophages to orchestrate immunity to respiratory virus infection. *Immunity.* (2020) 52:1039-56.e9. doi: 10.1016/j.immuni.2020.04.005

Shima T, Inada K, Nakashima A, Ushijima A, Ito M, Yoshino O, et al. Paternal antigen-specific proliferating regulatory T cells are increased in uterine-draining lymph nodes just before implantation and in pregnant uterus just after implantation by seminal plasma-priming in allogeneic mouse pregnancy. *J Reprod Immunol.* (2015) 108:72-82. doi: 10.1016/j.jri.2015. 02.005

Chen C, Qu QX, Huang JA, Zhu YB, Ge Y, Wang Q, et al. Expression of programmed-death receptor ligands 1 and 2 may contribute to the poor stimulatory potential of murine immature dendritic cells. *Immunobiology.* (2007) 212:159-65. doi: 10.1016/j.imbio.2007.01.004

Barash A, Dekel N, Fieldust S, Segal I, Schechtman E, Granot I. Local injury to the endometrium doubles the incidence of successful pregnancies in patients undergoing in vitro fertilization. *Fertil Steril.* (2003) 79:1317-22. doi: 10.1016/s0015-0282(03)00345-5

Raziel A, Schachter M, Strassburger D, Bern O, Ron-El R, Friedler S. Favorable influence of local injury to the endometrium in intracytoplasmic sperm injection patients with high-order implantation failure. *Fertil Steril.* (2007) 87:198-201. doi: 10.1016/j.fertnstert.2006.05.062

Saito S, Shima T, Nakashima A, Inada K, Yoshino O. Role of paternal antigen-specific Treg cells in successful implantation. *Am J Reprod Immunol.* (2016) 75:310-6. doi: 10.1111/aji.12469

Kim BJ, Choi YM, Rah SY, Park DR, Park SA, Chung YJ, et al. Seminal CD38 is a pivotal regulator for fetomaternal tolerance. *Proc Natl Acad Sci USA.* (2015) 112:1559-64. doi: 10.1073/pnas.1413493112

Flores-Langarica A, Cook C, Muller Luda K, Persson EK, Marshall JL, Beristain-Covarrubias N, et al. Intestinal CD103(+)CD11b(+) cDC2 conventional dendritic cells are required for primary CD4(+) T and B cell responses to soluble flagellin. *Front Immunol.* (2018) 9:2409. doi: 10.3389/fimmu.2018.02409

Ohta T, Sugiyama M, Hemmi H, Yamazaki C, Okura S, Sasaki I, et al. Crucial roles of XCR1-expressing dendritic cells and the XCR1-XCL1 chemokine axis in intestinal immune homeostasis. *Sci Rep.* (2016) 6:23505. doi: 10.1038/srep23505

Zeng R, Bscheider M, Lahl K, Lee M, Butcher EC. Generation and transcriptional programming of intestinal dendritic cells: essential role of retinoic acid. *Mucosal Immunol.* (2016) 9:183-93. doi: 10.1038/mi.2015.50

Scott CL, Tfp ZM, Beckham KS, Douce G, Mowat AM. Signal regulatory protein alpha (SIRPalpha) regulates the homeostasis of CD103(+) CD11b(+) DCs in the intestinal lamina propria. *Eur J Immunol.* (2014) 44:3658-68. doi: 10.1002/eji.201444859

Stary G, Olive A, Radovic-Moreno AF, Gondek D, Alvarez D, Basto PA, et al. VACCINES. A mucosal vaccine against *Chlamydia trachomatis* generates two waves of protective memory T cells. *Science.* (2015) 348:aaa8205. doi: 10.1126/science.aaa8205

Becker M, Guttler S, Bachem A, Hartung E, Mora A, Jakel A, et al. Ontogenic, phenotypic, and functional characterization of XCR1(+) dendritic cells leads to a consistent classification of intestinal dendritic cells based on the expression of XCR1 and SIRPalpha. *Front Immunol.* (2014) 5:326. doi: 10.3389/fimmu.2014.00326

Study of sRAGE, HMGB1, AGE and S100A8/A9 Concentrations in Plasma and in Serum-Extracted Extracellular Vesicles of Pregnant Women with Preterm Premature Rupture of Membranes

Damien Bouvier[1,2]*, Yves Giguère[3,4], Loïc Blanchon[2], Emmanuel Bujold[3,5], Bruno Pereira[6], Nathalie Bernard[3], Denis Gallot[2,7], Vincent Sapin[1,2] and Jean-Claude Forest[3,4]

[1] Biochemistry and Molecular Genetic Department, Centre Hospitalier Universitaire (CHU) Clermont-Ferrand, Clermont-Ferrand, France, [2] Faculty of Medicine, CNRS 6293, INSERM 1103, GReD, Université Clermont Auvergne, Clermont-Ferrand, France, [3] Centre de Recherche du Centre Hospitalier Universitaire (CHU) de Québec-Université Laval, Québec City, QC, Canada, [4] Department of Molecular Biology, Medical Biochemistry and Pathology, Faculty of Medicine, Université Laval, Québec City, QC, Canada, [5] Department of Obstetrics and Gynecology, Faculty of Medicine, Université Laval, Québec City, QC, Canada, [6] Biostatistics Unit Direction de la Recherche Clinique et des Innovations (DRCI), Centre Hospitalier Universitaire (CHU) Clermont-Ferrand, Clermont-Ferrand, France, [7] Department of Obstetrics and Gynecology, Centre Hospitalier Universitaire (CHU) Clermont-Ferrand, Clermont-Ferrand, France

*Correspondence:
Damien Bouvier
dbouvier@chu-clermontferrand.fr

Preterm premature rupture of membranes (PPROM), defined as rupture of fetal membranes prior to 37 weeks of gestation, complicates approximately 2–4% of pregnancies and is responsible for 40% of all spontaneous preterm births. PPROM arises from complex pathophysiological pathways with a key actor: inflammation. Sterile inflammation is a feature of senescence-associated fetal membrane maturity. During specific steps of sterile inflammation, cells also release highly inflammatory damage-associated molecular pattern markers (DAMPs), such as high-mobility group box 1 (HMGB1) or S100A8/A9, known to link and activate the receptor for advanced glycation end products (RAGE). The objective of this study was to measure longitudinally during pregnancy concentrations of the soluble form of RAGE (sRAGE) and its main ligands (AGE, HMGB1, S100A8/A9) in blood specimens. We studied 246 pregnant women (82 with PPROM and 164 matched control pregnant women without complications) from a cohort of 7,866 pregnant women recruited in the first trimester and followed during pregnancy until delivery. sRAGE, AGE, HMGB1, and S100A8/A9 concentrations were measured in plasma and in serum-extracted extracellular vesicles from first trimester (T1), second trimester (T2), and delivery (D). In plasma, we observed, in both PPROM and control groups, (i) a significant increase of HMGB1 concentrations between T1 vs. T2, T1 vs. D, but not between T2 vs. D; (ii) a significant decrease of sRAGE concentrations between T1 and T2 and a significant increase between T2 and D; (iii) a significant decrease of AGE from T1 to D; (iv) no significant variation of S100A8/A9 between trimesters. In intergroup comparisons (PPROM vs. control group), there were no significant differences in time variation taking into account the matching effects.

There was a correlation between plasma and serum-extracted extracellular vesicle concentrations of sRAGE, AGE, HMGB1, and S100A8/A9. Our results suggest that the rupture of fetal membranes (physiological or premature) is accompanied by a variation in plasma concentrations of sRAGE, HMGB1, and AGE. The study of RAGE and its main ligands in extracellular vesicles did not give additional insight into the pathophysiological process conducting to PPROM.

Keywords: preterm premature rupture of membranes, extracellular vesicles, soluble receptor for advanced glycation end products, advanced glycation end products, high-mobility group box 1, S100A8/A9

INTRODUCTION

Preterm premature rupture of membranes (PPROM), defined as rupture of fetal membranes prior to 37 weeks of gestation, complicates approximately 2–4% of all pregnancies and is responsible for 40–50% of all preterm births (Naeye and Peters, 1980; Mercer et al., 2000). PPROM arises from complex, multifaceted pathophysiological pathways where the inflammation axis plays a major role (Menon and Richardson, 2017). Indeed, recent reports indicated that PPROM may be associated with sterile inflammation in the fetal membranes (Romero et al., 2015). In support of this hypothesis, it has been shown that histological chorioamnionitis in the presence of a negative amniotic fluid culture increases the risk of preterm birth (Park et al., 2017). Sterile inflammation is a feature of senescence-associated fetal membranes maturity and is characterized mostly by the presence of inflammatory biomarkers, growth factors, and matrix degrading enzymes (Coppe et al., 2008). During the specific steps of sterile inflammation, senescent, stressed, or necrotic cells release highly inflammatory damage-associated molecular pattern markers (DAMPs) (Menon and Richardson, 2017). High-mobility group box 1 (HMGB1) is one of the DAMPs that have been linked to parturition (Sheller-Miller et al., 2017; D'Angelo et al., 2018). In a mouse model, intra-amniotic administration of HMGB1 induces spontaneous preterm labor and birth (Gomez-Lopez et al., 2016). Moreover, it was observed that HMGB1 induces an inflammatory response, partially mediated by the inflammasome, in the fetal membranes (Plazyo et al., 2016). This intra-amniotic inflammasome activation was highlighted *in vivo* in human (Gomez-Lopez et al., 2019). HMGB1 is a known ligand of receptor for advanced glycation end products (RAGE), and the RAGE system is associated with pregnancy complications as preeclampsia or PPROM (Naruse et al., 2012; Rzepka et al., 2015). Moreover, AGEs could be implicated in PPROM with blood levels significantly higher in pregnant women complicated with PPROM (Kansu-Celik et al., 2019). Calprotectin (or S100A8/A9) is also a known ligand of RAGE (Pruenster et al., 2016) implicated in some pregnancy pathologies as preeclampsia (Pergialiotis et al., 2016).

Extracellular vesicles are a heterogeneous group of cell-derived membranous structures comprising exosomes (50–150 nm) and microvesicles (50–500 nm up to 1 μm), which originate from the endosomal system or which are shed from the plasma membrane, respectively (van Niel et al., 2018). The study of maternal plasma exosomes determines pathways associated with PPROM including non-specific inflammation or oxidative stress (Menon et al., 2019). The RAGE system (receptor and ligands) has not been specifically studied in maternal blood exosomes. However, some DAMPs, such as HMGB1 have been identified as present in oxidative-stressed amnion epithelial cell-derived exosomes (Sheller-Miller et al., 2017). Furthermore, *in vitro*, amnion epithelial cell exosomes lead to an increased inflammatory response in maternal uterine cells, suggesting that fetal cell exosomes may act as a signal to parturition in choriodecidua and migrate into the maternal circulation (Hadley et al., 2018). Combining maternal characteristics and environmental and clinical known risk factors (Bouvier et al., 2019) to candidate biomarkers may in the future result in proposing a clinically predictive model identifying asymptomatic women at higher risk of PPROM.

In this context, taking advantage of a large cohort of pregnant women recruited prospectively at the beginning of pregnancy, we investigated the changes in the concentrations of the soluble form of RAGE (sRAGE) and its main ligands (AGE, HMGB1, S100A8/A9) in plasma and in the serum-extracted extracellular vesicles from first trimester to delivery to better understand the potential role of the RAGE system in PPROM.

MATERIALS AND METHODS

Study Design and Participants

This is a case/control study of sRAGE, HMGB1, AGE, and S100A8/A9 concentrations in plasma samples and serum-extracted exosomes of pregnant women with PPROM from an already constituted prospective biobank for which blood samples were collected [research program funded by the CIHR Institute of Human Development, Child and Youth Health Initiative (Grant Number: NRFHPG-)]. The biobank includes samples from 7,866 pregnant women recruited at the CHU de Québec-Université Laval between April 2005 and March 2010 and followed during pregnancy until delivery (Forest et al., 2014). Participants gave their informed written consent, and the study was approved by the Ethics Committee of the CHU de Québec [initial approval date: November 9, 2004, project 5-04-10-01 [95.05.17], SC12-01-159]. Cases were selected from all pregnant women with PPROM for whom three successive blood samples were collected and then frozen: one during the first trimester (T1), one during the second trimester (T2), and one at delivery (D). In the control group, we selected pregnant women (two control for one case) with delivery at term (after 37 weeks of gestation) and for whom three plasma and serum samples were collected and then frozen (T1, T2, and D). Women in the control group were matched with those in the case group on the following criteria: maternal age (±5 years), gestational age at T1 sample (±1 week), gestational age at T2 sample (±3 weeks), storage time at -80°C (±6 months). A total of 246 pregnant women (82 with PPROM and 164 matched control pregnant women) were selected.

Serum Extracellular Vesicle Extraction

For total extracellular vesicles from 30 to 120 nm isolation from 738 serum samples (three samples T1, T2, and D for 246 women), we used a kit (ref 4478360) from Invitrogen™ (Carlsbad, California, United States) using 450 μl of serum and following the manufacturer's instructions. Then, for extraction of total proteins from extracellular vesicles, we used Invitrogen™ kit (ref 4478545) following the manufacturer's instructions. The assay of total proteins in the extracellular vesicle extracts was carried out using a Vista® analyzer (Siemens, Munich, Germany). The assay of apolipoprotein B (Apo B) in 16 extracellular vesicle extracts (eight from the control group and eight from the PPROM group) was carried out using a Vista® analyzer (Siemens, Munich, Germany).

ELISA of Soluble Receptor for Advanced Glycation End Products, High-Mobility Group Box 1, Advanced Glycation End Products, and S100A8/A9

The concentrations of sRAGE, HMGB1, AGE, and S100A8/A9 in 738 plasma samples (three samples T1, T2, and D for 246 women) and in 738 serum-extracted extracellular vesicle samples (three samples T1, T2, and D for 246 women) was measured by the ELISA method using MyBioSource® kits (San Diego, California, United States) following the manufacturer's instructions (ref MBS2515963, MBS024146, MBS2000151, and MBS7606803, respectively). The concentrations of sRAGE, HMGB1, AGE, and S100A8/A9 of each serum extracellular vesicle sample were normalized against total protein concentrations.

Statistics

Statistical analyses were performed using Stata software, Version 13 (StataCorp, College Station, Texas, United States). All tests were two-sided, with a Type I error set at 0.05. Continuous data were expressed as mean and standard deviation (SD) or median and interquartile range (IQR) according to statistical distribution. The assumption of normality was assessed by using the Shapiro–Wilk test. The comparisons between the PPROM and control groups, for non-repeated data, were performed using Student t-test or Mann–Whitney test when the assumptions of t-test were not met for continuous parameters. Chi-square test or, if applicable, Fisher's exact test were applied for categorical variables. The relation between continuous variables (AGEs, sRAGE, HMGB1, S100A8/A9 concentrations) in serum-extracted extracellular vesicles and in plasma was analyzed estimating correlation coefficients, Pearson or Spearman according to the statistical distribution and applying a Sidak's type I error correction to take into account multiple comparisons. These correlations' results were illustrated with a color-coded heat map.

Random-effects models for repeated data were performed to compare the evolution of AGEs, sRAGE, HMGB1, and S100A8/A9 plasma concentrations and serum-extracted extracellular vesicle concentrations between groups (PPROM and controls). The following fixed effects were measured: time (T1, T2, D), group and $time \times group$ interaction, taking into account between- and within-participant variability (subject as random-effect). The normality of residuals from these models was studied using the Shapiro–Wilk test. When appropriate, a logarithmic transformation was proposed to achieve the normality of dependent outcome. A Sidak's type I error correction was applied to perform multiple comparisons.

RESULTS

Description of the Cohort

Of the 7,866 pregnant women recruited for the biobank, 189 women presented a PPROM (2.4%). Of these, 82 fulfilled the criteria of disposing of three blood samples. Therefore, a total of 246 pregnant women (82 with PPROM and 164 matched control pregnant women, 1:2 ratio) were selected. No significant differences ($p = 0.7$) were observed between the mean age of mothers in the control group (29.5 years, SD: 4.1) and the PPROM group (29.3 years, SD: 4.2) (**Table 1**). Some risk factors of PPROM were found significantly higher in the PPROM group as nulliparity, past history of PPROM, gestational diabetes mellitus, smoking during pregnancy (**Table 1**). A significant difference ($p < 0.001$) for the gestational age at delivery was expectedly observed between the PPROM group [36 weeks, interquartile range (IQR): 35.1–36.4] and the control group (38.7 weeks, IQR: 38.1–39.3) (**Table 1**).

Assays in Plasma

A significant decrease of median concentrations of AGEs in both PPROM and control groups was observed between T1 and T2, T2 and D, and T1 and D (see p^1 and p^2 in **Table 2** for the PPROM and control group, respectively; **Figure 1A**). These variations in

TABLE 1 | Characteristics of the case (PPROM) and control groups.

		PPROM group	Control group	p
n		82	164	/
Mean age of mothers (SD) in years		29.3 (4.2)	29.5 (4.1)	0.7
Nulliparity in%		58.5	43.3	0.02
Past history of PPROM in%		15.6	0	<0.001
Gestational diabetes mellitus in%		14.6	6.7	0.04
Smokers during pregnancy in%		21.3	11.7	0.04
Median gestational age (IQR) in weeks	First trimester	15.1 (14–16.6)	15 (14–15.6)	0.37
	Second trimester	27.9 (26.1–28.5)	27.9 (26.2–28.4)	0.97
	Delivery	36 (35.1–36.4)	38.7 (38.1–39.3)	<0.001

IQR, interquartile range; PPROM, preterm premature rupture of membranes; SD, standard deviation.

TABLE 2 | Median AGEs, sRAGE, HMGB1, and S100A8/A9 plasma concentrations from 82 women in the PPROM group and 164 women in the control group at three points: first trimester (T1), second trimester (T2), and delivery (D).

	PPROM group (n = 82)		Control group (n = 164)		p³	p⁴
	Median (IQR)	p¹ T1 vs. T2 T2 vs. D D vs. T1	Median (IQR)	p² T1 vs. T2 T2 vs. D D vs. T1		
AGEs (ng/ml)						
First trimester	3,569 (2,665–4,532)	0.04	3,651 (2,951–4,345)	<0.001	0.16	0.41
Second trimester	3,313 (2,676–4,232)	<0.001	3,353 (2,692–4,125)	<0.001	0.17	0.76
Delivery	2,885 (2,284–3,818)	<0.001	2,993 (2,439–3,694)	<0.001	0.97	0.43
sRAGE (pg/ml)						
First trimester	1,819 (915–3,234)	0.001	1,873 (1,170–3,402)	<0.001	0.33	0.55
Second trimester	1,556 (808–2,625)	<0.001	1,719 (971–2,670)	<0.001	0.65	0.30
Delivery	2,178 (1,092–3,721)	0.06	2,418 (1,432–3,665)	<0.001	0.15	0.21
HMGB1 (ng/ml)						
First trimester	22.3 (14.1–33.9)	<0.001	19.1 (13–31.3)	<0.001	0.65	0.32
Second trimester	30.4 (22.6–44.3)	0.24	30.4 (21.5–40.7)	0.09	0.86	0.29
Delivery	27.8 (20.5–37.7)	<0.001	27.7 (19–38.9)	<0.001	0.78	0.26
S100A8/A9 (ng/ml)						
First trimester	332 (157–865)	0.77	344 (168–692)	0.61	0.98	0.68
Second trimester	344 (216–644)	0.14	325 (204–678)	0.55	0.33	0.64
Delivery	297 (163–568)	0.24	316 (157–673)	0.93	0.31	0.23

p^1 and p^2: intragroup comparison between T1, T2, and D in the PPROM group (p^1) and in the control group (p^2) (random-effects models for repeated measures). p^3: intergroup comparison: interaction time × group, taking into account the matching effect (random-effects models for repeated measures). p^4: comparison (of medians) between the PPROM group and the control group, taking into account the matching effect. AGEs, advanced glycation end products; HMGB1, high-mobility group box 1; IQR, interquartile range; PPROM, preterm premature rupture of membranes; sRAGE, soluble receptor of advanced glycation end products.

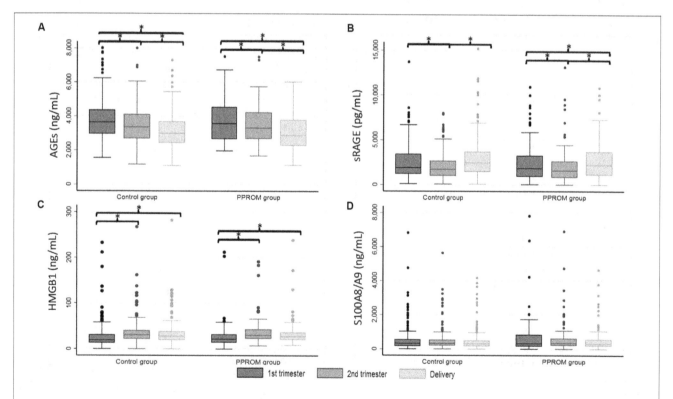

FIGURE 1 | Box plot of AGEs **(A)**, sRAGE **(B)**, HMGB1 **(C)**, and S100A8/A9 **(D)** plasma median concentrations from 82 women in the PPROM group and 164 women in the control group at three points: first trimester, second trimester, and delivery. *$p < 0.05$ (random-effects for repeated measures). AGEs, advanced glycation end products; HMGB1, high-mobility group box 1; PPROM, preterm premature rupture of membranes; sRAGE, soluble receptor of advanced glycation end products.

concentrations observed during pregnancy were not significantly different between the PPROM and control groups (see p^3 in **Table 2**). Similarly, for each sampling time (T1, T2, D), the medians of plasma concentrations are not significantly different between the PPROM and control groups (see p^4 in **Table 2**).

For sRAGE in both PPROM and control groups, a significant decrease of median concentration between T1 and T2 and then a significant increase between T2 and D were observed (see p^1 and p^2 in **Table 2** for the PPROM and control group, respectively; **Figure 1B**). At delivery, the sRAGE concentration was significantly higher than at T1 in the control group ($p < 0.001$) but not in PPROM ($p = 0.06$). These variations in concentrations observed during pregnancy were not significantly different between the PPROM and control groups (see p^3 in **Table 2**). Similarly, for each sampling time (T1, T2, D), the medians of plasma concentrations were not significantly different between the PPROM and control groups (see p^4 in **Table 2**).

For HMGB1 in both PPROM and control groups, a significant increase of median concentration was observed between T1 and T2 (and also T1 and D) followed by a stagnation between T2 and D (see p^1 and p^2 in **Table 2** for the PPROM and control groups, respectively; **Figure 1C**). These variations in concentrations observed during pregnancy were not significantly different between the PPROM and control groups (see p^3 in **Table 2**). Similarly, for each sampling time (T1, T2, D), the medians of plasma concentrations were not significantly different between the PPROM and control groups (see p^4 in **Table 2**).

For S100A8/A9, in both PPROM and control groups, no significant variations of median concentrations were observed between T1, T2, and D (see p^1 and p^2 in **Table 2** for the PPROM and control groups, respectively, see p^3 in **Table 2** and **Figure 1D**). Similarly, for each sampling time (T1, T2, D), the medians of plasma concentrations were not significantly different between the PPROM and control groups (see p^4 in **Table 2**).

Assays in Serum-Extracted Extracellular Vesicles

Similar results as those obtained in plasma are presented in **Table 3** were observed. The variations of concentration during pregnancy were similar as in plasma (see p^1 and p^2 in **Table 3** for the PPROM and control groups, respectively; **Figure 2**). For all four markers (AGEs, sRAGE, HMGB1, and S100A8/A9) measured in serum-extracted extracellular vesicles, the variations in concentration observed during pregnancy were not significantly different between the PPROM group and the control group (see p^3 in **Table 3**). Similarly, for each sampling time (T1, T2, D), the medians of serum-extracted extracellular vesicles concentrations were not significantly different between the two groups (see p^4 in **Table 3**). Moreover, AGEs, sRAGE, HMGB1, and S100A8/A9 concentrations were significantly correlated between the plasma and the serum-extracted extracellular vesicles for both the PPROM group (expect for AGEs at delivery) and the control group (**Figure 3**).

The assay of Apo B in 16 extracellular vesicles extracts (eight from the control group and eight from the PPROM group) was carried out. The results were found to be below or at the lower limit of linearity (<0.26 g/L).

TABLE 3 | Median AGEs, sRAGE, HMGB1, and S100A8/A9 serum-extracted extracellular vesicle concentrations from 82 women in the PPROM group and 164 women in the control group at three points: first trimester (T1), second trimester (T2), and delivery (D).

	PPROM group (n = 82)		Control group (n = 164)		p^3	p^4
	Median (IQR)	p^1 T1 vs. T2 T2 vs. D D vs. T1	Median (IQR)	p^2 T1 vs. T2 T2 vs. D D vs. T1		
AGEs (μ g/g of protein)						
First trimester	97.4 (64.7–117.5)	0.01	90 (66.3–115.1)	0.20	0.53	0.40
Second trimester	83.3 (61.2–107)	0.77	86.3 (63–110.3)	0.97	0.85	0.89
Delivery	81.4 (59.4–105.2)	0.01	81.6 (60.1–101.6)	0.22	0.41	0.91
sRAGE (ng/g of protein)						
First trimester	43.3 (30.6–57.3)	0.004	40.6 (30.3–57.6)	< 0.001	0.42	0.92
Second trimester	36.7 (29.6–48.8)	0.07	34.7 (27.9–48.4)	0.06	0.73	0.43
Delivery	40.1 (32.3–54.2)	0.29	37.9 (27.4–51.7)	0.001	0.25	0.27
HMGB1 (μ g/g of protein)						
First trimester	3.4 (1.8–4.7)	< 0.001	2.8 (1.8–4.6)	0.001	0.23	0.59
Second trimester	4.1 (2.4–6.2)	< 0.001	3.5 (2.1–5.2)	< 0.001	0.21	0.11
Delivery	3.2 (1.8–4.4)	0.63	2.9 (1.7–4.7)	0.64	0.95	0.66
S100A8/A9 (μ g/g of protein)						
First trimester	125 (93–174)	0.008	123 (86–186)	0.84	0.11	0.80
Second trimester	143 (107–226)	0.001	140 (95–205)	0.25	0.11	0.16
Delivery	127 (91–183)	0.39	119 (85–191)	0.34	0.99	0.89

p^1 and p^2: intragroup comparison between T1, T2, and D in the PPROM group (p^1) and in the control group (p^2). p^3: intergroup comparison: interaction time × group, taking into account the matching effect (random-effects models for repeated measures). p^4: comparison (of medians) between the PPROM group and the control group, taking into account the matching effect (random-effects models for repeated measures). AGEs, advanced glycation end products; HMGB1, high-mobility group box 1; IQR, interquartile range; PPROM, preterm premature rupture of membranes; sRAGE, soluble receptor of advanced glycation end products.

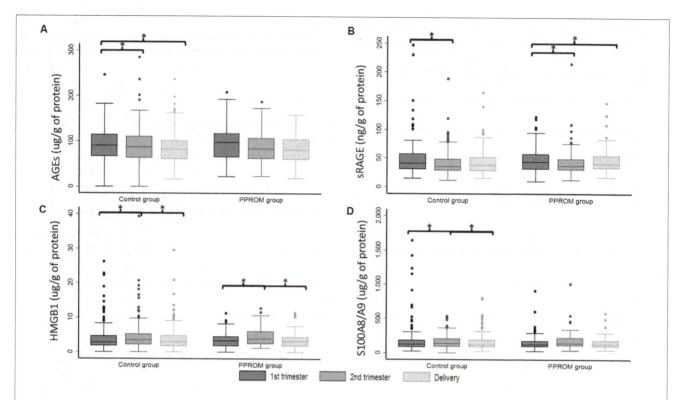

FIGURE 2 | Box plot of AGEs **(A)**, sRAGE **(B)**, HMGB1 **(C)**, and S100A8/A9 **(D)** serum-extracted extracellular vesicle median concentrations from 82 women in the PPROM group and 164 women in the control group at three points: first trimester, second trimester, and delivery. $*p < 0.05$ (random-effects for repeated measures). AGEs, advanced glycation end products; HMGB1, high-mobility group box 1; PPROM, preterm premature rupture of membranes; sRAGE, soluble receptor of advanced glycation end products.

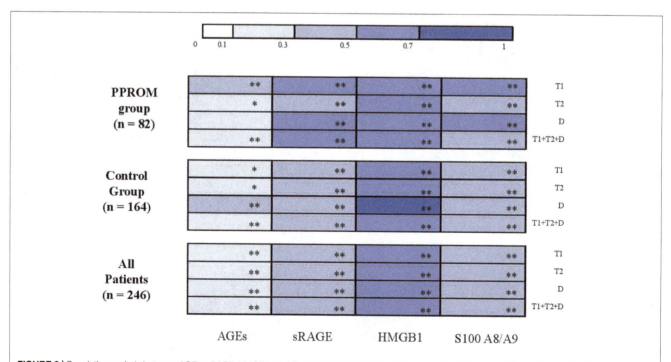

FIGURE 3 | Correlation analysis between AGEs, sRAGE, HMGB1, and S100A8/A9 concentrations in serum-extracted extracellular vesicles and in plasma (color-coded heat map plot). AGEs, advanced glycation end products; D, delivery; HMGB1, high-mobility group box 1; PPROM, preterm premature rupture of membranes; sRAGE, soluble receptor of advanced glycation end products; T1, first trimester; T2, second trimester. $*p < 0.05$; $**p < 0.001$.

DISCUSSION

We studied for the first time, on a large number of pregnant women (with and without PPROM), the kinetics from the first trimester to delivery of the plasma concentrations (and serum-extracted exosomes) of four major actors of the RAGE system: sRAGE and three of its ligands, HMGB1, AGEs, and S100A8/9. Among the 189 women with PPROM (2.4% of the cohort), 82 had three blood samples during their pregnancies and were matched to normal controls in a ratio of 1–2. Despite the potential bias linked to the matching criteria, we identified the clinical known risk factors for PPROM as described in a previous study (Bouvier et al., 2019).

There were no significant differences in the serum concentration of total circulating extracellular vesicles between pregnant women with and without PPROM. However, it was proposed that the study of maternal plasma-extracted exosomes could determine pathways associated with PPROM including non-specific inflammation or oxidative stress (Menon et al., 2019). The specific study of biomarkers of the RAGE system in serum-extracted extracellular vesicles of pregnant women was relevant to identify an earlier signal of suffering from the fetal membranes. In this study, we observed that this is not the case and that the concentrations are strongly correlated to those of "total serum," for the studied actors of RAGE signaling, in contrast to the cellular networks in the work of Menon's team. Flow cytometry could have been used to determine whether RAGE or studied DAMPs are present on the surface of or inside the extracellular vesicles, but this was not available in our current setting. Another limitation of the study is the absence of characterization of the extracellular vesicles extracted from the serum (van Niel et al., 2018) and of the study of the cellular or tissue origin of these vesicles. Measurement of Apo B below or at the lower limit of linearity (<0.26 g/L) confirmed the absence of contamination of the preparations of extracellular vesicles.

So far, studies on blood levels of sRAGE as PPROM or prematurity risk factor show discordant results (Hajek et al., 2008; Germanova et al., 2010; Bastek et al., 2012; Rzepka et al., 2016). In our study, no differences in plasma sRAGE concentrations were observed between the control and PPROM groups, as already described (Hajek et al., 2008; Rzepka et al., 2016). Indeed, Rzepka et al. (2016) found the same results and found the endogenous secretory RAGE (esRAGE) more interesting as a potential biomarker of PPROM. Bastek et al. (2012) found lower serum concentrations of sRAGE in women who gave birth prematurely including spontaneous premature labor with intact membranes and thus confirmed results of a smaller study (Germanova et al., 2010). Conversely, Hajek et al. (2008) found, in a pilot study, higher values of serum concentrations of sRAGE in women who gave birth prematurely. In our study, an interesting kinetics is observed with a decrease of sRAGE plasma concentration between T1 and T2, and then an increase between T2 and D. Germanova et al. (2010) described exactly the opposite but on a smaller cohort of 79 women with only 25 measurements per trimester. These different conclusions could be due to the presence of different size of cohorts, type of circulating RAGE, and various assays used to measure sRAGE.

Concerning the RAGE ligands in plasma, we observed no differences in S100A8/19 concentrations between the PPROM group and the control group and no variations during pregnancy. Also, we found no differences in plasma AGE concentrations between the PPROM and control groups. These results are in contradiction with those of a recent study on a small cohort of 46 pregnant women (nine with PPROM and 37 without PPROM) where the blood concentration of AGEs at T1 was higher in women with PPROM (Kansu-Celik et al., 2019). Noteworthy, a decrease in the serum concentration of AGEs during pregnancy was also observed in a previous study where the kinetics were studied between the second trimester and delivery (Quintanilla-Garcia et al., 2018). In our study, no differences in plasma HMGB1 concentrations were observed between the PPROM and control groups. However, variations in plasma HMGB1 concentrations during pregnancy were observed with a significant increase between T1 and T2 and then stagnation between T2 and D in both PPROM and control groups. It was previously observed that senescent fetal membranes contribute to sterile inflammation by generation of DAMPs, like HMGB1 (Menon et al., 2016). Also, an increase in the expression of HMGB1, with activation of the RAGE pathway, in the placenta of women with PPROM has been demonstrated (Yan et al., 2018). Our results show the same kinetics in women with PPROM and in control women. HMGB1 has a physiological implication and can be at the "frontiers in physiology." Based on our blood results, the mechanistic link between the increases in plasma concentrations of HMGB1 and sRAGE and the decrease in the plasma concentration of AGEs should be further investigated. It has been reported that the sRAGE-AGE complex becomes degraded in the spleen or liver (Ramasamy et al., 2008).

CONCLUSION

In conclusion, our results suggest that the rupture of fetal membranes (physiological or premature) may be related to RAGE activation possibly by the ligand HMGB1. If a more important production of HMGB1 occurring during pregnancy with PPROM could not be detected directly by a higher concentration of HGMB1 in PPROM vs. control group, an indirect proof by the different kinetics of sRAGE between first trimester and delivery could be proposed.

ETHICS STATEMENT

The studies involving human participants were reviewed and approved by the Ethics Committee of the CHU de Québec. The patients/participants provided their written informed consent to participate in this study.

AUTHOR CONTRIBUTIONS

DB analyzed and interpreted the data and wrote the initial version of the manuscript. J-CF and YG were in charge of the research program on pregnancy complications, designed the study, and assisted with the interpretation of the data and writing of the manuscript. NB and EB supervised the trial and data collection. DB and NB carried out serum exosome extractions and all assays. BP provided statistical advice for the study design and analyzed the data. VS, LB, and DG experts in PPROM, reviewed the manuscript, assisted with the interpretation of the data. All authors substantially contributed to its revision.

ACKNOWLEDGMENTS

The authors thank the research nurses for the recruitment of participants and retrieval of data from the medical records. The authors also thank all study participants.

REFERENCES

Bastek, J. A., Brown, A. G., Foreman, M. N., McShea, M. A., Anglim, L. M., Adamczak, J. E., et al. (2012). The soluble receptor for advanced glycation end products can prospectively identify patients at greatest risk for preterm birth. *J. Maern. Fetal Neonatal. Med.* 25, 1762–1768. doi: 10.3109/14767058.2012.663825

Bouvier, D., Forest, J. C., Blanchon, L., Bujold, E., Pereira, B., Bernard, N., et al. (2019). Risk factors and outcomes of preterm premature rupture of membranes in a cohort of 6968 pregnant women prospectively recruited. *J. Clin. Med.* 8:E1987. doi: 10.3390/jcm8111987

Coppe, J. P., Patil, C. K., Rodier, F., Sun, Y., Munoz, D. P., Goldstein, J., et al. (2008). Senescence-associated secretory phenotypes reveal cell-nonautonomous functions of oncogenic RAS and the P53 tumor suppressor. *PLoS Biol.* 6:2853–2868. doi: 10.1371/journal.pbio.0060301

D'Angelo, G., Marseglia, L., Granese, R., Di Benedetto, A., Giacobbe, P., Impellizzeri, A., et al. (2018). Different concentration of human cord blood HMGB1 according to delivery and labour: a pilot study. *Cytokine* 108, 53–56. doi: 10.1016/j.cyto.2018.03.019

Forest, J. C., Theriault, S., Masse, J., Bujold, E., and Giguere, Y. (2014). Soluble fms-like tyrosine kinase-1 to placental growth factor ratio in mid-pregnancy as a predictor of preterm preeclampsia in asymptomatic pregnant women. *Clin. Chem. Lab. Med.* 52, 1169–1178. doi: 10.1515/cclm-2013-0955

Germanova, A., Koucky, M., Hajek, Z., Parizek, A., Zima, T., and Kalousova, M. (2010). Soluble receptor for advanced glycation end products in physiological and pathological pregnancy. *Clin. Biochem.* 43, 442–446. doi: 10.1016/j.clinbiochem.2009.11.002

Gomez-Lopez, N., Romero, R., Maymon, E., Kusanovic, J. P., Panaitescu, B., Miller, D., et al. (2019). Clinical chorioamnionitis at term IX: in vivo evidence of intra-amniotic inflammasome activation. *J. Perinat. Med.* 47, 276–287. doi: 10.1515/jpm-2018-0271

Gomez-Lopez, N., Romero, R., Plazyo, O., Panaitescu, B., Furcron, A. E., Miller, D., et al. (2016). Intra-amniotic administration of hmgb1 induces spontaneous preterm labor and birth. *Am. J. Reprod. Immunol.* 75, 3–7. doi: 10.1111/aji.12443

Hadley, E. E., Sheller-Miller, S., Saade, G., Salomon, C., Mesiano, S., Taylor, R. N., et al. (2018). Amnion epithelial cell-derived exosomes induce inflammatory changes in uterine cells. *Am. J. Obstet. Gynecol.* 219, 478.e1–478.e21. doi: 10.1016/j.ajog.2018.08.021

Hajek, Z., Germanova, A., Koucky, M., Zima, T., Kopecky, P., Vitkova, M., et al. (2008). Detection of feto-maternal infection/inflammation by the soluble receptor for advanced glycation end products (SRAGE): results of a pilot study. *J. Perinat. Med.* 36, 399–404. doi: 10.1515/JPM.2008.080

Kansu-Celik, H., Tasci, Y., Karakaya, B. K., Cinar, M., Candar, T., and Caglar, G. S. (2019). Maternal serum advanced glycation end products level as an early marker for predicting preterm labor/PPROM: a prospective preliminary study. *J. Matern. Fetal Neonatal. Med.?* 32, 2758–2762. doi: 10.1080/14767058.2018.1449202

Menon, R., Behnia, F., Polettini, J., Saade, G. R., Campisi, J., and Velarde, M. (2016). Placental membrane aging and HMGB1 signaling associated with human parturition. *Aging* 8, 216–230. doi: 10.18632/aging.100891

Menon, R., Dixon, C. L., Sheller-Miller, S., Fortunato, S. J., Saade, G. R., Palma, C., et al. (2019). Quantitative proteomics by SWATH-MS of maternal plasma exosomes determine pathways associated with term and preterm birth. *Endocrinology* 160, 639–650. doi: 10.1210/en.2018-00820

Menon, R., and Richardson, L. S. (2017). Preterm prelabor rupture of the membranes: a disease of the fetal membranes. *Semin. Perinatol.* 41, 409–419. doi: 10.1053/j.semperi.2017.07.012

Mercer, B. M., Goldenberg, R. L., Meis, P. J., Moawad, A. H., Shellhaas, C., Das, A., et al. (2000). The preterm prediction study: prediction of preterm premature rupture of membranes through clinical findings and ancillary testing. The National Institute of Child Health and Human Development Maternal-Fetal Medicine Units Network. *Am. J. Obstet. Gynecol.* 183, 738–745. doi: 10.1067/mob.2000.106766

Naeye, R. L., and Peters, E. C. (1980). Causes and consequences of premature rupture of fetal membranes. *Lancet* 1, 192–194. doi: 10.1016/s0140-6736(80)90674-1

Naruse, K., Sado, T., Noguchi, T., Tsunemi, T., Yoshida, S., Akasaka, J., et al. (2012). Peripheral RAGE (Receptor for Advanced Glycation Endproducts)-ligands in normal pregnancy and preeclampsia: novel markers of inflammatory response. *J. Reprod. Immunol.* 93, 69–74. doi: 10.1016/j.jri.2011.12.003

Park, J. W., Park, K. H., and Jung, E. Y. (2017). Clinical significance of histologic chorioamnionitis with a negative amniotic fluid culture in patients with preterm labor and premature membrane rupture. *PLoS One* 12:e0173312. doi: 10.1371/journal.pone.0173312

Pergialiotis, V., Prodromidou, A., Pappa, E., Vlachos, G. D., Perrea, D. N., and Papantoniou, N. (2016). An Evaluation of calprotectin as serum marker of preeclampsia: a systematic review of observational studies. *Inflamm. Res.* 65, 95–102. doi: 10.1007/s00011-015-0903-0

Plazyo, O., Romero, R., Unkel, R., Balancio, A., Mial, T. N., Xu, Y., et al. (2016). HMGB1 induces an inflammatory response in the chorioamniotic membranes that is partially mediated by the inflammasome. *Biol. Reprod.* 95:130. doi: 10.1095/biolreprod.116.144139

Pruenster, M., Vogl, T., Roth, J., and Sperandio, M. (2016). S100A8/A9: from basic science to clinical application. *Pharmacol. Ther.* 167, 120–131. doi: 10.1016/j.pharmthera.2016.07.015

Quintanilla-Garcia, C. V., Uribarri, J., Fajardo-Araujo, M. E., Barrientos-Romero, J. J., Romero-Gutierrez, G., Reynaga-Ornelas, M. G., et al. (2018). Changes in circulating levels of carboxymethyllysine, Soluble receptor for advanced glycation end products (sRAGE), and inflammation markers in women during normal pregnancy. *J. Matern. Fetal Neonatal. Med.* 25, 1–6. doi: 10.1080/14767058.2018.1481948

Ramasamy, R., Yan, S. F., Herold, K., Clynes, R., and Schmidt, A. M. (2008). Receptor for advanced glycation end products: fundamental roles in the inflammatory response: winding the way to the pathogenesis of endothelial dysfunction and atherosclerosis. *Ann. N. Y. Acad. Sci.* 1126, 7–13. doi: 10.1196/annals.1433.056

Romero, R., Miranda, J., Chaemsaithong, P., Chaiworapongsa, T., Kusanovic, J. P., Dong, Z., et al. (2015). Sterile and microbial-associated intra-amniotic inflammation in preterm prelabor rupture of membranes. *J. Matern. Fetal Neonatal. Med.* 28, 1394–1409. doi: 10.3109/14767058.2014.958463

Rzepka, R., Dolegowska, B., Rajewska, A., Kwiatkowski, S., Salata, D., Budkowska, M., et al. (2015). Soluble and endogenous secretory receptors for advanced glycation end products in threatened preterm labor and preterm premature rupture of fetal membranes. *BioMed Res. Int.* 2015:568042. doi: 10.1155/2015/568042

Rzepka, R., Dolegowska, B., Rajewska, A., Salata, D., Budkowska, M., Kwiatkowski, S., et al. (2016). Diagnostic potential of evaluation of SDF-1alpha and SRAGE levels in threatened premature labor. *Biomed. Res. Int.* 2016:2719460. doi: 10.1155/2016/2719460

Sheller-Miller, S., Urrabaz-Garza, R., Saade, G., and Menon, R. (2017). Damage-associated molecular pattern markers HMGB1 and cell-free fetal telomere fragments in oxidative-stressed amnion epithelial cell-derived exosomes. *J. Reprod. Immunol.* 123, 3–11. doi: 10.1016/j.jri.2017.08.003

van Niel, G., D'Angelo, G., and Raposo, G. (2018). Shedding light on the cell biology of extracellular vesicles. *Nat. Rev. Mol. Cell Biol.* 19, 213–228. doi: 10.1038/nrm.2017.125

Yan, H., Zhu, L., Zhang, Z., Li, H., Li, P., Wang, Y., et al. (2018). HMGB1-RAGE Signaling Pathway in PPROM. *Taiwan J. Obstet. Gynecol.* 57, 211–216. doi: 10.1016/j.tjog.2018.02.008

Fetal Membrane Epigenetics

Tamas Zakar[1,2,3,4*] *and Jonathan W. Paul*[2,3,4]

[1] Department of Maternity & Gynaecology, John Hunter Hospital, New Lambton Heights, NSW, Australia, [2] School of Medicine and Public Health, Faculty of Health and Medicine, The University of Newcastle, Callaghan, NSW, Australia, [3] Priority Research Centre for Reproductive Science, The University of Newcastle, Callaghan, NSW, Australia, [4] Hunter Medical Research Institute, New Lambton Heights, NSW, Australia

*Correspondence:
Tamas Zakar
Tamas.Zakar@newcastle.edu.au

The characteristics of fetal membrane cells and their phenotypic adaptations to support pregnancy or promote parturition are defined by global patterns of gene expression controlled by chromatin structure. Heritable epigenetic chromatin modifications that include DNA methylation and covalent histone modifications establish chromatin regions permissive or exclusive of regulatory interactions defining the cell-specific scope and potential of gene activity. Non-coding RNAs acting at the transcriptional and post-transcriptional levels complement the system by robustly stabilizing gene expression patterns and contributing to ordered phenotype transitions. Here we review currently available information about epigenetic gene regulation in the amnion and the chorion laeve. In addition, we provide an overview of epigenetic phenomena in the decidua, which is the maternal tissue fused to the chorion membrane forming the anatomical and functional unit called choriodecidua. The relationship of gene expression with DNA (CpG) methylation, histone acetylation and methylation, micro RNAs, long non-coding RNAs and chromatin accessibility is discussed in the context of normal pregnancy, parturition and pregnancy complications. Data generated using clinical samples and cell culture models strongly suggests that epigenetic events are associated with the phenotypic transitions of fetal membrane cells during the establishment, maintenance and termination of pregnancy potentially driving and consolidating the changes as pregnancy progresses. Disease conditions and environmental factors may produce epigenetic footprints that indicate exposures and mediate adverse pregnancy outcomes. Although knowledge is expanding rapidly, fetal membrane epigenetics is still in an early stage of development necessitating further research to realize its remarkable basic and translational potential.

Keywords: amnion, chorion, decidua, chromatin modifications, non-coding RNAs, human pregnancy, parturition

INTRODUCTION

Current consensus defines an epigenetic trait as "a stably heritable phenotype resulting from changes in a chromosome without alterations in the DNA sequence." (Berger et al., 2009) The fetal membranes and the adjacent decidua adopt a phenotype in early gestation that supports pregnancy by preserving the integrity of the gestational sac, reducing myometrial contractility and controlling maternal innate and adaptive immunity to tolerate the semi-allogenic fetus. These protective characteristics are maintained stably throughout pregnancy despite the massive growth of the gestational sac. At term, a phenotype transition occurs that promotes membrane rupture, myometrial contractions, inflammation and lowered immune tolerance (Menon et al., 2016, 2019). The changes trigger birth. Similar changes can be elicited by pathological conditions, such as genital tract infection, pre-eclampsia and uterine overdistension, often inducing birth before term (Romero et al., 2014).

Epigenetic events establish, sustain and adjust chromatin structure in a cell-specific fashion through DNA methylation, post-translational histone modifications and regulatory non-coding RNAs. The resulting chromatin landscapes determine cell-specific gene expression patterns, which determine tissue phenotypes (Roadmap Epigenomics Consortium et al., 2015). Evidence is accumulating that characteristic chromatin modification patterns and non-coding RNA transcriptomes occur in the fetal membrane and decidua cells and change dynamically during normal and pathological pregnancies. This suggests that the mechanisms driving the phenotype transformations during gestation and at birth are, at least partially, epigenetic. This article summarizes information about epigenetic processes and associated phenotype changes in the amnion, chorion laeve and the decidua and consider their significance in normal pregnancies, during labor and in pregnancy disorders.

AMNION

In primates, amnion epithelial cells differentiate from epiblasts at about Day 8 of pregnancy, which is prior to gastrulation (Enders et al., 1986; Sasaki et al., 2016). The pluripotent epiblast phenotype is preserved throughout pregnancy to a substantial degree, as evidenced by the ability of amnion cells to differentiate to cells of all three germ layers *in vitro* under appropriate conditions (Easley et al., 2012). During the most of the gestation, the amnion exhibits characteristics that are anti-inflammatory and smooth muscle relaxant in agreement with a role in protecting the pregnancy (Carvajal et al., 2006; Silini et al., 2013). Furthermore, the mechanical strength of the gestational sac is provided by the strong collagenous ("compact") layer of the amnion membrane, which is maintained by the fibroblastic (mesenchymal) cells of the connective tissue underlying the epithelial layer. There is now evidence that the mesenchymal cells may be derived from the epithelial cells that undergo reversible epithelial-to-mesenchymal cell transformation (EMT) allowed by their phenotypic plasticity. There is also evidence that EMT in the amnion occurs increasingly with advancing gestation and in response to the proinflammatory cytokine, TNFα, or oxidative stress, which intensifies remodeling and results in the mechanical weakening of the membrane (Janzen et al., 2017; Richardson et al., 2020). Moreover, amnion mesenchymal cells respond strongly to proinflammatory stimuli, further promoting membrane rupture and the production of uterotonic factors including prostaglandins (Whittle et al., 2000; Sato et al., 2016). Thus, controlled and properly timed phenotype transitions of the amnion cells are critical for both maintaining pregnancy and triggering birth. Epigenetic events impacting on gene expression patterns are believed to contribute to the gestational transformations of amnion cells, which is stimulating interest in the topic.

DNA Methylation

Methylation of cytosines at the 5th position in the CpG motifs of DNA (5meCpG) is the most thoroughly studied epigenetic chromatin modification. CpG methylation is traditionally considered to silence genes by promoting closed chromatin structure or recruitment of repressor complexes to gene regulatory regions (Jones, 2012). There are about 28 million CpG sites in the human genome and more than 80% of these are methylated (Breiling and Lyko, 2015; Lövkvist et al., 2016). The density of DNA methylation in particular chromatin regions depends on the frequency of CpG dinucleotides, which varies substantially in the genome. Recent global analyses of CpG methylation levels have indicated, however, that the relationship of DNA methylation to gene activity depends on the genomic context. For example, higher CpG frequency regions, called CpG islands (Gardiner-Garden and Frommer, 1987), are generally unmethylated in promoters, and CpG sites are highly methylated in the transcribed regions of active genes. Low CpG density promoters and regulatory regions may exhibit variable methylation associated with variable gene activity, which is often tissue-specific and change with cellular differentiation (Jones, 2012).

Although DNA CpG methylation is considered a stable and mitotically heritable epigenetic modification, it undergoes turnover catalyzed by DNA methylating and demethylating enzyme systems (Schubeler, 2015; Kim and Costello, 2017). DNA methylation in human cells is performed by a family of DNA methyl transferases (DNMTs), which includes DNMT1, DNMT3A, -3B, and DNMT3L. DNMT1 is generally responsible for "maintenance" methylation during the S- (DNA-replicating) phase of the cell cycle because of its selectivity toward hemi-methylated CpG motifs in the nascent double-stranded DNA. DNMT3A and -3B perform "*de novo*" methylation at unmethylated CpG sites. DNMT3L is a catalytically inactive essential cofactor of DNMT3A and -3B. The characteristics of DNA methyltransferases have been extensively studied and reviewed in the literature (Tajima et al., 2016; Gowher and Jeltsch, 2018). DNMTs (except for DNMT3L) are expressed in the amnion and the decidua (Grimaldi et al., 2012; Mitchell et al., 2013) and are discussed in later sections. A group of 5meCpG-binding proteins (MBDs) recognize and functionally interpret DNA methylation patterns as signals for gene repression in most genomic contexts (Du et al., 2015). The mechanisms include heterochromatin formation, establishment of repressive histone modifications, nucleosome remodeling and extension of methylated DNA regions. Of the 11 MBD proteins identified so far (Du et al., 2015) one, MBD5, has been reported in decidualizing endometrial cells (Grimaldi et al., 2012). MBD proteins and their roles as methylated DNA readers is a major unexplored area of fetal membrane epigenetics.

The elucidation of the biochemical mechanisms that erase the 5meCpG modification was challenging because of the large energy barrier obstructing the direct enzymatic removal of the

5-methyl group. The best characterized removal pathway is initiated by the oxidative modification of the 5-methyl group producing 5-hydroxymethyl cytosine (5-hmC). The reaction is catalyzed by the Ten-Eleven Translocation group of dioxygenases (TET-1, -2, and -3), which use molecular oxygen and 2-oxoglutarate as co-substrates. TETs can oxidize 5-hmC further to 5-formyl and 5-carboxyl cytosine, which are detected by the base excision DNA repair (BER) system eventually replacing 5meC with unmodified cytosine in the CpG motifs (Kohli and Zhang, 2013; Bochtler et al., 2017). The central role of 5-hmC in DNA demethylation is reinforced by the inefficiency of DNMT1 to recognize 5-hmCpG for maintenance methylation, which results in the "passive" loss of methylation of the affected 5meCpGs during replication (Hashimoto et al., 2012; Kohli and Zhang, 2013). Thus, 5-hmC is generated from 5meC and as a consequence its incidence is lower than that of 5meC in somatic cells (Globisch et al., 2010). Its presence, however, indicates sites of dynamic DNA methylation in the genome such as poised enhancers, low- and intermediate CpG density promoters and bivalent promoters that are subject to developmental regulation (Yu et al., 2012; Gao and Das, 2014). Finally, proteins that bind 5-hmCpGs with high affinity and may function as epigenetic readers of 5-hmCpG and its oxidized derivatives have been discovered (Spruijt et al., 2013) suggesting that these modified bases may carry epigenetic information in addition to their role in 5meCpG turnover.

DNA methylation in the fetal membranes has been studied so far using traditional techniques that do not discriminate between 5meC and 5-hmC such as bisulfite conversion (Huang et al., 2010) or have no verified selectivity between the two modified bases (e.g., enzyme-based assays). These studies are mostly descriptive, and the results are reported in terms of CpG methylation. The main findings are summarized and discussed in the following sections.

Genome-Wide Profiling

CpG methylation has been profiled genome-wide in the amnion using the Illumina Infinium HumanMethylation27k BeadChip (HM27k) array (Eckmann-Scholz et al., 2012). The array features probes targeting over 25,000 CpG sites preferentially in promoter CpG islands with approximately 2–3 sites per gene. The probed CpGs showed bimodal distribution with either high or low levels of methylation in cells isolated from mid-trimester amniocentesis samples and expanded in culture. Such distribution is expected in somatic cells (Pidsley et al., 2016). Methylation patterns distinguished amnion-derived cells and villous chorion samples at similar gestational age as determined by principal component analysis (PCA) and hierarchical clustering (Eckmann-Scholz et al., 2012). However, amniotic fluid may contain cells from fetal skin, airways and intestine, potentially confounding the characterization of cells originating from amnion tissue. In another study (Kim et al., 2013), amnion tissue samples from women after term and preterm labor and term not in labor were processed for methylation analysis with the HM27k array. PCA analysis robustly separated the amnion samples according to the presence or absence of labor, but not according to gestational age. Nevertheless, more than 60 genes were found to be differentially methylated at term labor versus preterm labor and term not in labor versus term labor ($p < 0.0001$), with no overlap among the top 15 differentially methylated genes in the two comparisons. Yoo et al. (2018) used the more advanced HM450 BeadChip (HM450k) containing over 485,000 probes offering a much wider genomic coverage that includes CpG islands, shores and shelves, gene bodies, untranslated regions and enhancers (Pidsley et al., 2016). Amnion tissues after term and preterm delivery were compared and methylation differences were matched to differential gene expression determined by whole transcriptome sequencing. Nearly 36,000 differentially methylated CpG sites and over 1,000 differentially expressed genes were found, of which, 71 genes exhibited reciprocal changes of expression and CpG methylation in either direction. Two genes related to cell adhesion, integrin subunit alpha 11 (*ITGA11*) and trombospondin-2 (*THBS2*), were selected for verification using bisulfite pyrosequencing and real-time RT-PCR with independently collected samples. Both genes showed lower methylation and higher expression preterm than at term. Although this study used genome-wide discovery approaches to find previously discovered and expected relationships between gene methylation and expression, it has confirmed that CpG methylation in the amnion is dynamic and related to transcriptional activity at a subset of genes linked to tissue function.

Pre-eclampsia is a severe pregnancy complication characterized by hypertension, proteinuria and maternal inflammatory reactions. Its pathogenesis is unclear but abnormal placentation, angiogenic imbalance and endothelial dysfunction are well-documented attributes of the condition. DNA methylation has been studied in the early onset form (<34 weeks of gestation) of the disease using formaldehyde-fixed, paraffin-embedded full thickness fetal membrane samples that included amnion, chorion and attached decidua (Ching et al., 2014). CpG methylation profiling with the HM450k system showed nearly 10,000 differentially methylated CpG sites with mostly increased methylation in pre-eclampsia. Differentially methylated CpGs in gene-annotated genomic regions revealed decreased methylation in promoters and increased methylation within gene bodies, consistent with widespread transcriptional activation. A number of these genes and associated pathways have been found previously to be activated in pre-eclamptic placentae. Promoter hypomethylation has also been found in several pri-microRNA (pri-miRNA) genes, indicating the epigenetic regulation of miRNA expression. Thorough bioinformatic analysis has established the fetal membranes/decidua as epigenetic responders to the pre-eclamptic condition, but tissue-specific responses remained uncharacterized because of the use of unseparated full thickness membrane samples. Suzuki et al. (2016) addressed cellular heterogeneity in the amnion by performing whole genome bisulfite sequencing with separated amnion epithelial and mesenchymal cells. They found cell-specific methylation patterns and identified one CpG site (in an intron of the *SIPA1L1* gene) with a robust cell type-specific methylation difference, which could be used as a marker to correct for the variable cell type composition in amnion tissue samples. Genome wide methylation analysis was conducted with an assay called HELP-tagging, which utilized the methylation sensitive restriction enzyme, *Hpa*II. With this assay the authors surveyed the methylation state of over 545,000 CpG sites in normal versus pre-eclamptic amnion samples (62, overall) and found 4,058 differentially methylated sites in 3,035 genes. Methylation of 123, 85, and 99 sites were influenced by systolic blood pressure, proteinuria grade and the combination of the two, respectively, in regression models. RNAseq with a subset of samples revealed that 41 genes were differentially expressed in pre-eclampsia; however, none of the differentially methylated sites were in the vicinity of the differentially expressed genes, indicating the complexity of 5meCpG-mediated gene regulation. Overall, the presence of pre-eclampsia-associated epigenetic "signatures" in the amnion is remarkable, because this tissue is not a prime player in the disease. It appears, however, that epigenetic plasticity makes the amnion a useful surrogate to report the effects of adverse intrauterine conditions on fetal tissues in general, which may impact on disease susceptibility later in life.

Candidate Genes

Methylation analysis of candidate genes having well-established functions is a straightforward approach to explore the role of DNA methylation in gene regulation with physiological relevance. Wang et al. (2008) examined the methylation of the *MMP1* gene promoter in the amnion in normal pregnancies and in cases of preterm pre-labor rupture of the membranes (pPROM). Matrix metalloproteases (MMPs), such as MMP1, have a key role in breaking down the collagen matrix of the amnion contributing to membrane rupture at term and preterm birth. The *MMP1* proximal promoter contains no CpG island, only 14 sporadic CpG sites, which are fairly highly methylated ($\approx$50%) in amnion samples, as determined by clonal bisulfite sequencing. Treatment of primary cultures of amnion mesenchymal cells with the DNA-demethylating agent, 5-aza-3′-deoxycytidine (5-AZA), increased *MMP1* expression and decreased the methylation of one CpG motif at 1,538 bases upstream of the transcription initiation site. Interestingly, the methylation level of this site was significantly lower in amnion samples from deliveries complicated by pPROM compared to normal term controls. This group also described a previously undetected polymorphism in the *MMP1* promoter that generated a new CpG site as a minor allele. The presence of this CpG reduced *MMP1* promoter activity in amnion mesenchymal cells and even more so when it was methylated. *In vivo*, this site was always methylated and, remarkably, was significantly protective of pPROM in an African American population. This study illustrates that epigenetic and genetic differences may combine forming complex patterns of regulation that can be understood by analyses involving both levels. In the case of *MMP1*, the effect of DNA methylation on gene activity interacted with the polymorphism of the promoter shaping the impact on fetal membrane integrity and the risk of pPROM.

TIMP1 is a protease inhibitor protein that interacts with MMPs to control extracellular matrix remodeling. The *TIMP1* proximal promoter contains no CpG island and the 25 CpG sites around the transcriptional start site (−275)–(+279) are highly methylated in the amnion of female fetuses compared to males, as shown by Vincent et al. (2015), using the Sequenom Epityper technology. This is not surprising, since the gene is located in the X chromosome and one copy is in the hypermethylated homologous X chromosome in females. Notably, however, *TIMP1* mRNA abundance was higher in female than in male amnions and mRNA expression did not change with spontaneous labor despite a significant decrease of promoter methylation. Lipopolysaccharide (LPS) treatment of amnion explants increased methylation without effect on expression. Pre-treatment with the DNA demethylating agent, 5-AZA (5 uM, 48 h), did not affect *TIMP1* mRNA, or *TIMP1* promoter methylation levels in male or female amnions but sensitized the tissues to respond to LPS with increased *TIMP1* expression. These data suggest that *TIMP1* promoter methylation is dynamic but not linked to the level of gene activity in the amnion. Responsiveness to LPS might be influenced by methylation possibly at remote sites *in trans*.

Methylation of candidate genes in the amnion has been assessed in two further studies using the Methyl-Profiler PCR system (Mitchell et al., 2013; Sykes et al., 2015). The Methyl-Profiler (or MethylScreen) technology employs methylation-dependent and methylation sensitive restriction enzymes to probe the methylation density of pre-selected DNA sequences (Holemon et al., 2007). Labor-associated inflammatory genes (*PTGS2*, *BMP2*, *NAMPT/PBEF*, *CXCL2*), steroid receptor genes (*ESR1*, *PGR*, *NR3C1/GR*) and renin-angiotensin system components (*ACE*, *ATP6AP2/PRR*, *AGTR1*, *CTSD*, *KLK1*) were examined with the technique for promoter methylation density in amnion samples from early gestation (11–17 weeks) and after term delivery with or without labor. With the exception of *KLK1* (kallikrein 1), the proximal promoters of these genes have relatively high CpG density overlapping with CpG islands. Methylation densities of these promoters showed bimodal distribution with either highly methylated or sparsely methylated copies. The distributions did not change with gestational age or with labor but varied between genes and among individuals. Furthermore, the distribution of highly versus sparsely methylated promoter copies did not correlate with expression levels but correlated significantly between individuals. This suggests that the methylation of these promoters was established in early pregnancy (before 11–17 weeks) in a gene-specific fashion under the influence of individual conditions and was maintained until after delivery. In agreement with this, the expression of the DNMTs, DNMT1 and -3a, were highest in early pregnancy and decreased by term. Interestingly, the low CpG *KLK1* promoter exhibited intermediate methylation density in some of the samples and a loss of methylation at term, indicating dynamic methylation without a significant influence on expression level.

Histone Modifications

Covalent post-translational modifications of histones, which include acetylation, methylation, phosphorylation, ubiquitination, and sumoylation, are pervasive throughout the chromatin and are organized in patterns characteristic of genomic features, such as promoters, enhancers, transcribed sequences and heterochromatin regions (Roadmap Epigenomics Consortium et al., 2015). They contribute to functional states such as open or closed chromatin, active or repressed genes, poised or operative enhancers. Recent evidence also indicates that modified histones are involved in directing DNA methyltransferases to chromatin regions where DNA methylation occurs during replication and cell differentiation (Fu et al., 2020). For example, DNMT3A and -3B contain PWWP domains that bind trimethylated lysine-36 in histone 3 (H3K36me3) (Rona et al., 2016), potentially directing these enzymes to exonic sequences of transcribed genes that are highly methylated and rich in H3K36me3. In addition, targeting of DNA methylation to heterochromatic regions through interactions between DNMT3A/B and methylated H3K9, or the lysine methyltransferase establishing this gene silencing modification (G9a), or chromodomain (methyl-lysine binding) proteins associating with methylated H3K9, has been reported but the molecular mechanisms are still unclear (Rose and Klose, 2014). Moreover, DNMT3 proteins contain ADD domains, which specifically recognize unmethylated H3K4 (H3K4me0), potentially explaining the antagonism between DNA methylation and H3K4 methylation genome wide (Fu et al., 2020). Even maintenance methylation by DNMT1 has been shown to depend on histone modifications such as H3K9 methylation and H3K27 ubiquitination [reviewed by Rose and Klose (2014)].

Despite their significance in epigenetic regulation, histone modifications are still scantly characterized in the fetal membranes. For example, genome-wide screens performed routinely using chromatin immunoprecipitation with antibodies selective for modified histones (ChIP-seq) have not been published with amnion or chorion to inform about gestational changes or pathological alterations. Studies employing ChIP combined with PCR, however, have demonstrated the presence of histone modifications in the promoter regions of a few labor-associated genes in the amnion. Gene activating histone-3 and -4 acetylation (H3ac, H4ac) and histone-3, lysine-4 demethylation (H3K4me2) have been reported at the promoter of the *PTGS2* gene, which encodes a key enzyme of prostaglandin biosynthesis (Mitchell et al., 2008, 2011). Further, H4ac levels were significantly elevated at term labor when *PTGS2* expression increased (Mitchell et al., 2008). Histone-3, lysine-4 trimethylation (H3K4me3) and histone-3, lysine-27 trimethylation (H3K27me3), which are activating and repressive chromatin marks, respectively, were assessed at the promoters of *PTGS2* and two other inflammatory genes, *NAMPT/PBEF*/visfatin and *BMP2*, in amnion tissues collected in early pregnancy (10–18 weeks) and at term (Mitchell et al., 2019). The expression of these genes increased robustly at the end of gestation. Both histone modifications were present at the promoters, and sequential double ChIP showed that the same promoter copies were marked by H3K4me3 as well as H3K27me3, indicating epigenetic "bivalence." Remarkably, bivalence was significantly reduced at term by the loss of the repressive H3K27me3 mark, indicating a shift toward a state poised for expression. H3K4 methyl transferases and H3K27me3 demethylases were expressed increasingly in the tissues with advancing pregnancy, potentially mediating the changes in histone methylation. This study suggests that an epigenetic process activating bivalently marked genes participates in the mechanism stimulating labor at term. The concept, however, has to be corroborated by the genome-wide profiling of H3K4me3 and H3K27me3 levels at gene regulatory regions in fetal membrane cells collected at different times during gestation.

Histone deacetylases are a diverse group of chromatin-modifying enzymes comprising 18 members classified into four groups (Seto and Yoshida, 2014). They are excellent drug targets, and histone deacetylase inhibitors and activators of varying isoform selectivity can be used as tools to explore the involvement of histone acetylation in gene expression control. Using this approach, Poljak et al. (2014) determined that Class II histone deacetylases may participate in the up-regulation of matrix metalloprotease-9 (MMP9) expression by ILβ in cultured amnion cells, while Class III histone deacetylases inhibit it. Similarly, the histone deacetylase inhibitor, TSA (Trichostatin A), reduced ILβ-stimulated PTGS2 expression in amnion explants supporting a role of histone acetylation in the action of the cytokine (Mitchell, 2006). The involvement of histone acetylation in these activities still needs to be confirmed by demonstrating cognate operational changes in acetyl histone levels at the gene regulatory regions since many non-histone proteins are also acetylated and are substrates for histone deacetylases (Seto and Yoshida, 2014). Therefore, drugs interfering with protein acetylation may cause global changes in the acetyl-proteome of the cells with functional consequences not necessarily mediated by histone acetylation-dependent epigenetic events (Norris et al., 2009; Orren and Machwe, 2019). An example for this has been found in the pregnant human myometrium, where TSA treatment *ex vivo* preserves progesterone receptor expression in its non-laboring state (Ilicic et al., 2017) potentially by epigenetic mechanisms (Ke et al., 2016; Ilicic et al., 2019) and reduces contractility by an extranuclear action that increases heat shock protein 20 acetylation promoting actin depolymerization and relaxation (Karolczak-Bayatti et al., 2011).

Non-coding RNAs

Transcription is not restricted to chromatin regions encoding protein-coding genes, but it is widespread throughout the genome. The resulting non-coding RNAs vary in size and function (Kung et al., 2013). The long non-coding RNA class, called lncRNAs, are over 200 bases long and have been implicated in epigenetic regulation by recruiting chromatin modifying protein complexes to the DNA regions to which they are tethered by complementary sequences. A well-characterized example is Xist RNA, which directs polycomb-regulatory complex-2 (PRC2) (catalyzing H3K27me3-dependent repression) to the X chromosome during X chromosome inactivation [reviewed by Kung et al. (2013)]. Long ncRNAs have been implicated in a range of reproductive disorders via epigenetic mechanisms (Shen and Zhong, 2015). Profiling of lncRNAs in (villous) placenta using a dedicated microarray covering over 33,000 (curated) lncRNAs (Arraystar Human LncRNA Array v2.0) revealed numerous differentially expressed lncRNAs in association with term and preterm birth and pPROM in two studies (Luo et al., 2013, 2015).

Ten differentially expressed natural antisense lncRNAs have been paired with differential mRNA expression from the same loci arguing for functional relationships (Luo et al., 2015). It will be important to extend these studies to the fetal membranes since integrated lncRNA, chromatin modification and gene expression profiling could reveal lncRNA-mediated epigenetic events involved in normal birth, pPROM and immune regulation in tissues covering most of the maternal-fetal interface.

A distinct group of lncRNAs, called pri-miRNAs, is processed into small, 22 nucleotides long RNA fragments, called micro-RNAs (miRNAs). Micro-RNAs act as guides to direct protein complexes to mRNAs or non-coding RNAs by sequence recognition (Hammond, 2015). Depending on the degree of complementarity, this results in (m)RNA degradation and/or the inhibition of mRNA translation to proteins. By conservative estimate, there are 2,300 human miRNAs validated to date (Alles et al., 2019). Because of the tolerant complementarity, a particular miRNA may be predicted to target numerous, possibly hundreds, of mRNA species or non-coding RNAs and a particular RNA species can concurrently interact with several miRNAs. Micro-RNAs, therefore, are proposed to have homeostatic roles providing robustness to cell phenotypes by dampening the effects of stochastic fluctuations of transcription (O'brien et al., 2018). Remarkably, the miR-200 family and the ZEB transcription factors were proposed to participate in a bi-stable double negative feedback loop that controls epithelial-mesenchymal transition in epithelial cell lines. The phenotype switch may be triggered by TGFβ and is reinforced by DNA methylation at the miR-200c~141 promoters (Gregory et al., 2011). This interaction is just one example of the crosstalk between the micro-RNA and chromatin modification aspects of epigenetic regulation. Genes encoding micro-RNAs both at intergenic and intronic locations are subject to regulation by DNA methylation and histone modifications. The control is reciprocal, since DNMTs, TATs and histone modifying enzymes are targeted by micro-RNAs in normal and diseased (e.g., cancerous) cells (Chhabra, 2015; Yao et al., 2019). In the amnion, TGFβ-driven epithelial-mesenchymal transition occurs reversibly during gestation and apparently irreversibly at labor leading to membrane rupture (Janzen et al., 2017). Many molecular details of this process have been determined recently (Richardson et al., 2020); however, the contribution of epigenetic mechanisms, including miRNAs, is still unknown despite numerous possibilities identified in cancer cells undergoing analogous changes of phenotype (Serrano-Gomez et al., 2016). Epigenetic regulation underpinning the epithelial-mesenchymal transition of amnion cells is a promising new frontier of fetal membrane research.

Micro-RNAs in the Fetal Membranes

Montenegro et al. (2007) have profiled miRNAs in chorioamnionic membrane samples (with attached decidua) using the TaqMan MicroRNA qRT-PCR Assays Human Panel (Applied Biosystems–Early Access kit), which assays 157 miRNAs. Most (>150) of the tested miRNAs were detected, of which 13 had decreased levels with advancing pregnancy in women after preterm birth without histological chorioamnionitis. No differences were detected with term labor. In a subsequent study by the same group (Montenegro et al., 2009), 455 miRNAs were tested using the miRCURY LNA (Exiqon) microarray (v.8.1). Here, 39 differentially expressed miRNAs were found and most (79.5%) showed lower expression at term labor compared to preterm labor. One of them, miR-338, was verified experimentally in decidual cells to target *PLA2G4B* mRNA, which encodes a phospholipase involved in prostaglandin biosynthesis. They have also demonstrated a marked down-regulation of *Dicer*, a key enzyme of miRNA biogenesis, with advancing pregnancy in agreement with a widespread reduction of miRNA levels. This finding suggests that the homeostatic role of miRNAs, which is to stabilize a transcriptome that maintains the pregnancy-supporting phenotype of the membranes, is weakened at term, thus facilitating the transition to a labor-promoting state. An even higher number of miRNAs (875 miRNAs included in the miRCURY Array v.11 from Exiqon) have been tested in isolated amnion tissues at term and after preterm labor (Kim et al., 2011). This analysis found 32 differentially expressed miRNAs between the placental and extra-placental (reflected) regions of the amnion with 31 exhibiting lower levels in the reflected part. Moreover, down-regulation of the miR-143/miR-145 cluster has been verified by qRT-PCR in the reflected amnion at term labor and miR-143 has been shown to target *PTGS2* mRNA in a transfection assay with amnion mesenchymal cells. Collectively, the above series of studies suggests that a widespread decrease in miRNA expression plays a role in the labor-promoting proinflammatory switch in the fetal membranes at term. Post-transcriptional de-repression of genes of the prostaglandin biosynthetic pathway has been identified by targeted experiments as part of this process.

The miRNA profile of term amnion has been examined in obese women (with pre-pregnancy body-mas index >30) by Nardelli et al. (2014) using the TaqMan human MicroRNA Panel v.1.0, which contains 365 miRNAs. Seventy one percent of the tested miRNAs were detected in the amnions, of which 7 miRNAs were found only in obese women. The study also found 25 miRNAs that were differentially expressed in obese versus non-obese mothers. Further, Enquobahrie et al. (2015) explored the association of 8 preselected miRNAs with preterm birth of various clinical presentations (spontaneous, pPROM, pre-eclampsia) in the amnion and the chorion leave, based on the involvement of these miRNAs in placental pathologies (Enquobahrie et al., 2015). The two fetal membrane tissues expressed these miRNAs differentially, and miR-210 and miR-233 levels in the amnion, but not in the chorion leave, were inversely associated with preterm birth risk. These pioneering studies indicate that unfavorable conditions affect miRNA expression in the amnion, which may contribute to adverse pregnancy outcomes.

DECIDUA

The decidua is the endometrium of pregnancy and, being a maternal tissue, is not part of the *fetal* membranes by strict definition. It forms the maternal side of the maternal-fetal contact zone, however, and is fused with the chorion leave so intimately that it is practically impossible to separate them completely, even with sharp dissection (Mitchell and Powell, 1984). The close contact predicts functional interactions, which warrants including an overview of the epigenetics of the human decidua in this chapter to provide context for the anatomical unit often referred to as the "choriodecidua." We focus on decidual stromal cells acknowledging that the decidua in pregnancy contains a complex and dynamic array of leukocytes (Gomez-Lopez et al., 2010), which are also subject to epigenetic regulation (Kim et al., 2012; Walsh et al., 2017). Comprehensive reviews, including the epigenetic aspects of decidual differentiation, have been published (Guo, 2012; Gao and Das, 2014; Liu et al., 2019).

DNA Methylation

Differentiation of the endometrium to decidua involves the transformation of endometrial stromal cells to decidual cells (Zhu et al., 2014), which has similarities to mesenchymal-to-epithelial phenotype transition (Zhang et al., 2013). It occurs in the non-pregnant uterus during the progesterone-dominated secretory phase of the menstrual cycle and its proper execution is essential for successful pregnancy. The role of DNA methylation in the process was explored initially by determining the expression of DNMTs in the endometrium during the menstrual cycle and in *in vitro* models, where decidual differentiation was induced by combined progestogen (progesterone, P4 or medroxyprogesterone acetate, MPA) and estradiol (E2) or cAMP treatments of cultured endometrial stromal cells (Yamagata et al., 2009; Vincent et al., 2011; Grimaldi et al., 2012; Logan et al., 2013). These studies showed down-regulation of DNA methyl transferase expression during decidualization. Likewise, 5-AZA (a DNA methyl transferase inhibitor) treatment fostered a phenotype in the endometrial culture system reminiscent of the decidual state (Logan et al., 2010). In spite of these observations, no change in the global level of DNA methylation has been detected (Grimaldi et al., 2012), suggesting that DNA methylation changes during decidual transformation may involve alterations of methylation pattern rather than changing the overall methylation degree. CpG site-specific methylation during decidualization *in vivo* has been investigated using the Illumina HM27k array (Houshdaran et al., 2014). The top 10% of probes reporting variable CpG methylation (2,578 probes) effectively separated samples from the proliferative and secretory phases of the cycle by unsupervised cluster analysis. Differential methylation analysis, however, identified just 66 CpGs with altered methylation, with several of them associated with genes important in endometrial biology. The follow-up study using primary endometrial fibroblasts decidualized *in vitro* by P4 and E2 indicated methylation changes at several CpGs and associated genes detected *in vivo* (Houshdaran et al., 2014). In a similar study, Maekawa et al. (2019) used the more comprehensive HM450k array and found only 23 differentially methylated CpGs after MPA + E2 treatment without change in the expression of the associated genes. Moreover, the DNA methylation status of the decidual marker genes *PRL* and *IGFBP1* showed no change after differentiation induced by MPA + E2, as determined by bisulfite (clonal) sequencing. Collectively, these data suggest that DNA methylation dynamics is slight in the decidua and the involvement of CpG methylation in the decidualization process is subtle. Other epigenetic processes, such as histone modifications, may play a more predominant role.

Histone Modifications

Decidual transformation of endometrial stromal cells *in vivo* and *in vitro* is associated with the decreasing expression of EZH2, which is the catalytic component of the histone methyltransferase complex, PRC2 (Grimaldi et al., 2011). PRC2 methylates the lysine-27 residue of histone-3, establishing the repressive H3K27me3 modification. Reduced EZH2 activity was accompanied by lowered H3K27me3 levels at the *PRL* and *IGFBP1* genes and the increased expression of the gene products, prolactin and insulin-like growth factor-binding protein 1, which are the best characterized markers of decidualization. However, the global H3K27me3 level remained unaltered after EZH2 down-regulation, indicating the locus selectivity of the histone modification changes (Grimaldi et al., 2011). Genome-wide survey of H3K27me3-marked sites by chromatin immunoprecipitation coupled to microarray promoter analysis (ChIP-chip technology, using the NimbleGen Human ChIP-chip 3 × 720 K RefSeq promoter array) confirmed the global rearrangement of the H3K27me3 pattern. Upon decidual transformation, H3K27-acetylation, which is the alternative modification of the H3K27 sites marking active gene promoters and enhancers, exhibited a marked global increase, including the *PRL* and *IGFBP1* genes, indicating widespread gene activation (Grimaldi et al., 2011). Subsequent studies in essence confirmed these findings by both genome-wide and candidate gene approaches (Tamura et al., 2014, 2018; Katoh et al., 2018) and implicated another gene-activating histone modification, H3K4me3, in the transformation process. Further, insulin signaling was one of the major pathways associated with genes up-regulated by the two activating histone modifications (Tamura et al., 2014). Following up on this line of investigations, Jozaki et al. (2019) determined that decidualization was dependent on the availability of glucose for the endometrial cells. In low glucose medium acetylation of the *FOXO1* promoter regions and expression of *PRL* and *IGFBP1* were suppressed. FOXO1 is a transcription factor with pivotal involvement in decidualization (Grinius et al., 2006; Park et al., 2016). Remarkably, glucose up-regulated *FOXO1* expression and promoter H3K27 acetylation in the decidualizing endometrial stromal cells, which in turn induced *PRL* and *IGFBP1* expression associated with promoter H3K27 acetylation (Jozaki et al., 2019). Although the histone acetyl transferase(s) that function in the glucose sensing mechanism were not identified, the results further support the fundamental role of epigenetic histone modifications in decidual transformation.

At term, the decidua acquires a pro-inflammatory phenotype (Norwitz et al., 2015) that involves the emergence of myofibroblast cells (Nancy et al., 2018). Nuclear accumulation of the H3K27me3 demethylase, lysine demethylase 6A (KDM6A), has been detected concomitantly with this process, which suggests that epigenetic mechanisms, including the removal of the suppressive H3K27me3 mark, take part in the transition

(Nancy et al., 2018). Very recently, a comprehensive analysis of chromatin landscape changes has been reported in endometrial fibroblasts decidualized *in vitro* (Sakabe et al., 2020). Chromatin accessibility using the ATAC-seq technique, ChIP-seq with H3K4me1, H3K27ac, and H3K4me3 antibodies, and promoter capture Hy-C to detect distant regulatory elements, were integrated and matched with RNA-seq data in this large-scale genome-wide study. In general agreement with previous findings, the results showed extensive changes during decidual transformation, particularly at enhancer sites marked with H3K4me1 and H3K27ac. Importantly, these chromatin data were also integrated with a genome-wide association study (GWAS) dataset that involved 43,568 women and explored genetic associations with gestational duration and preterm birth (Zhang et al., 2017). The computational integration of the GWAS with the functionally annotated chromatin regions in decidualized cells increased the heritability estimates of gestational duration and resulted in the discovery of additional non-coding chromatin loci and associated genes, such as the gene encoding the transcription factor, Heart And Neural Crest Derivatives Expressed 2 (HAND2), potentially linked to gestational length (Marinić et al., 2020). From the epigenetic perspective, these studies have revealed that epigenetically controlled genomic loci involved in decidual transformation are critical for determining gestational length in women.

Non-coding RNAs

Information about miRNAs controlling endometrial receptivity and decidualization has been reviewed previously, highlighting the Let-7, miR-200, miR-181, miR-542, and miR-30 family and miR-17-92 cluster members in these events (Liu et al., 2016, 2019). Steady expression of Let-7 miRNA isoforms has also been reported in late gestation fetal membranes/decidua (Chan et al., 2013). In decidualization models of human endometrial stromal cells *in vitro*, two microarray analyses tested 435 (Qian et al., 2009) and 1,205 (Tochigi et al., 2017) human miRNAs for differential expression. In the former study, 16 and 33 miRNAs were found to be up- and down-regulated, respectively, while in the latter study, 1 was shown up-regulated and 5 down-regulated under similar threshold criteria. There was no overlap between the two differential expression datasets. Likewise, miR-181a up-regulation was found critical for decidual transformation in one study (Zhang et al., 2015), while miR-181, -183, and -200 family members were found down-regulated in decidualized cells other investigations (Qian et al., 2009; Estella et al., 2012) reporting that reduced hsa-miR-222 expression was particularly crucial (Qian et al., 2009). Jimenez et al. (2016) described the participation of up-regulated miR-200 in decidualization *in vitro*, and potentially *in vivo*, as part of the miR-200/ZEB regulatory network (Gregory et al., 2011), which confirms that endometrial stromal cells undergo mesenchymal-to-epithelial transition during decidual transformation (Zhang et al., 2013). Furthermore, *in vitro* decidualization also appear to involve the induction of the long intergenic non-coding RNA, LINC00473 (Liang et al., 2016). Further work shall reconcile the incongruous data from different laboratories and reveal a consistent picture about the participation of particular RNA species in decidual cell differentiation and function. The importance of short and long non-coding RNAs in these processes, however, is beyond doubt.

At term labor, down-regulation of microRNAs targeting inflammatory genes has been detected in (unseparated) choriodecidua samples leaving the contribution of the maternal (decidua) and the fetal (chorion laeve) components to be determined (Montenegro et al., 2009; Stephen et al., 2015).

Finally, there is considerable interest in defining the role of decidual non-coding-RNAs in the pathogenesis of early pregnancy loss (Dong et al., 2014; Wang et al., 2015; Hong et al., 2018; Zhao et al., 2018), pre-eclampsia (Zhao et al., 2014; Lv et al., 2018; Tong et al., 2018; Moradi et al., 2019) and in the establishment of the persistent decidual phenotype after implantation (Lv et al., 2016; Wang et al., 2016). Alterations of miRNA profiles have been demonstrated under these conditions, but the detailed discussion of these aspects of miRNA involvement are beyond the scope of this review.

DISCUSSION

The information currently available about epigenetic events in the fetal membranes and the decidua establishes structural changes of the chromatin as an important contributor to gene regulation in these tissues throughout pregnancy and in labor. The major types of chromatin modifications, such as DNA (CpG) methylation and histone modifications, have been found and many of them located in genome-wide and candidate gene-focused studies. Alterations in modification levels and patterns have been detected in association with gestational age, labor status and pathological conditions. Long and short non-coding RNAs (miRNAs), which represent a separate, but connected, branch of epigenetic regulation, have also been described and studied in detail. **Figure 1** illustrates the overall gestational dynamics of DNA methylation, histone modifications and microRNA expression in the amnion and the decidua as deduced from the currently available data. The periods around implantation, early pregnancy and preparation for birth are the most active for epigenetic events to occur. Environmental and disease-associated inputs can impinge upon the fetal membranes throughout pregnancy, but epigenetic mechanisms are most likely to be influenced at these dynamic periods. Acknowledging all the advances and the increasing pace of new discoveries it remains clear that fetal membrane epigenetics is still in an early stage of development. Some critical gaps of knowledge and foreseeable future directions are indicated in the preceding sections and several more are outlined below.

- Most data about epigenetic events in the fetal membranes describe associations between chromatin modifications, non-coding RNAs and outcomes related to various physiological or pathological states of pregnancy. Associations do not prove causation; therefore, inferences about epigenetic involvement remain tentative. Evidence supporting functional roles can be generated by interventional studies that target components of the epigenetic machinery using inhibitors of chromatin

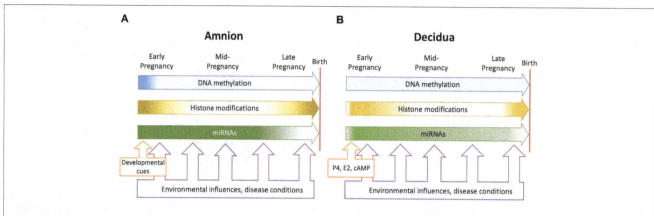

FIGURE 1 | Overall dynamics of epigenetic events in the amnion **(A)** and the decidua **(B)** during pregnancy. The blue, orange, and green block arrows indicate DNA methylation, histone modifications and miRNAs, respectively. Shading denotes changing levels and shifting genome-wide distributions. In the amnion, DNA methylation and histone modification patterns are established in early gestation to support pregnancy. Histone modification patterns change at term when labor-associated inflammatory genes are activated, and tissue remodeling occurs. Micro-RNAs stabilize the protective transcriptome until term, when levels decline concomitantly with inflammatory gene activation. In the decidua, hormonal influences (progesterone, estrogens, and cAMP signaling) trigger differentiation to the pregnancy-protective phenotype. The process involves major changes in histone modifications and miRNA expression but relatively modest alterations in DNA methylation. At term, histone modifications change, and key miRNAs decline to foster a proinflammatory and labor-promoting phenotype. Environmental adversities and disease conditions may be present throughout pregnancy but most likely impact on epigenetic events during periods of dynamic change. The resulting epigenetic "footprints" may influence gene expression patterns contributing to fetal membrane disfunction and may signify fetal exposure to unfavorable intrauterine conditions.

modifying enzymes and specially designed epigenetic chemical probes (Wu et al., 2019). A few of these studies have been published with fetal membrane cells or tissues so far (Mitchell, 2006; Logan et al., 2010; Poljak et al., 2014) and the results highlight the need for careful consideration of off-target effects and toxicity. Other options including the genetic manipulation of chromatin modifying enzyme and/or epigenetic reader levels and activity still need to be exploited in fetal membrane research. Correlations with polymorphisms of epigenetic effector genes may provide corroborating, but still associative, evidence for epigenetic involvement in fetal membrane regulation. Polymorphisms of the DNMT3B and DNMT3L genes were found to associate with familial preterm birth and birth weight, respectively, but fetal membrane involvement (e.g., associations with pPROM) was not reported (Haggarty et al., 2013; Barisic et al., 2020).

- Fetal membrane tissues *in vivo* are subject to environmental exposures and lifestyle conditions such as smoking, diet, toxic substances and effects of social stress. Epigenetic mechanisms mediate the long term (even transgenerational) effects of these exposures and conditions as determined in animal models (Suter and Aagaard-Tillery, 2009). Furthermore, a subset of the epigenetic changes have been proposed to be of adaptive nature predicting future environmental challenges (Duncan et al., 2014). "Metastable epialleles," which are genomic loci that function as epigenetic sensors of the environment, are critical in the process. Metastable epigenetic loci have been found in animals (Rakyan et al., 2002), for example, the *agouti* locus in mice (Dolinoy et al., 2007) and were tentatively identified in humans (Waterland et al., 2010; Dominguez-Salas et al., 2014). Smoking, nutrition and vitamin C intake significantly alter the incidence of pPROM indicating their impacts on fetal membrane function (Siega-Riz et al., 2003; Kyrklund-Blomberg et al., 2005; Nabet et al., 2007; Myhre et al., 2013), but the epigenetic aspects of these effects remain to be explored.
- Epigenetic events in the chorion leave are much less studied than in the amnion and the decidua. The chorion leave constitutes the fetal side of the maternal-fetal contact zone and a role in establishing and maintaining the maternal tolerance of the fetus is implied by its location (Kim et al., 2015). Chorion leave trophoblasts have a phenotype distinct from villous trophoblasts (e.g., chorion leave trophoblasts do not form syncytia) and possess a unique DNA methylation pattern (Eckmann-Scholz et al., 2012; Robinson and Price, 2015). Understanding the epigenetic aspects of fetal membrane function will require the characterization of chorion leave cell chromatin structure on a level with the other fetal membrane components.
- The amnion, chorion and decidua contain several types of cells, and experimental results with tissue samples represent a sum generated by heterogeneous cell mixtures that often vary in proportions. Chromatin modification patterns are cell specific, and epigenetic differences predominant in a particular cell type may be masked by the average. Analysis of isolated individual cell types or correction for cellular heterogeneity using cell-specific markers are approaches that can alleviate the problem of variable cell composition and increase the robustness of results. Importantly, the expanding suite of single cell epigenomic techniques (Clark et al., 2016) offers exciting new possibilities to analyze the composition and phenotype dynamics of fetal membrane cell populations and will very likely become a major research direction in the future.

- To identify chromatin loci where epigenetic alterations occur during pregnancy, labor and pathological conditions will require the generation and bioinformatic integration of genome-wide DNA methylation and histone modification datasets, as these modifications buttress the chromatin together and function in a combined fashion (Roadmap Epigenomics Consortium et al., 2015). Inclusion of transcriptomic, chromatin accessibility (Buenrostro et al., 2015) and chromatin conformation capture (Kempfer and Pombo, 2020) data in the integrative analyses are expected to inform about the functional impact of chromatin modification changes. These approaches are technically complex and computationally demanding, but also extremely informative, as has been demonstrated recently with decidual cells (Sakabe et al., 2020).
- Lastly, it is important to emphasize that advanced, genome-wide approaches and the more traditional analysis of individual candidate genes supplement each other and pursuing them in combination can result in optimal outcomes. Validation of key findings in genome-wide screens, and mechanistic studies in culture systems in general benefit from focusing on genes and regulatory regions pinpointed by genomic scale analyses. Emerging unexplored epigenetic mechanisms like non-cytosine DNA methylation (Ji et al., 2018) and protein mediated inheritance (Harvey et al., 2018) are exciting future directions in fetal membrane research.

AUTHOR CONTRIBUTIONS

TZ conceptualized the work and drafted the manuscript. JP provided intellectual input, edited the manuscript drafts, and finalized the figure designs. Both authors contributed to the article and approved the submitted version.

REFERENCES

Alles, J., Fehlmann, T., Fischer, U., Backes, C., Galata, V., Minet, M., et al. (2019). An estimate of the total number of true human miRNAs. *Nucleic Acids Res.* 47, 3353–3364. doi: 10.1093/nar/gkz097

Barisic, A., Kolak, M., Peterlin, A., Tul, N., Gasparovic Krpina, M., Ostojic, S., et al. (2020). DNMT3B rs1569686 and rs2424913 gene polymorphisms are associated with positive family history of preterm birth and smoking status. *Croat. Med. J.* 61, 8–17. doi: 10.3325/cmj.2020.61.8

Berger, S. L., Kouzarides, T., Shiekhattar, R., and Shilatifard, A. (2009). An operational definition of epigenetics. *Genes Dev.* 23, 781–783. doi: 10.1101/gad.1787609

Bochtler, M., Kolano, A., and Xu, G. L. (2017). DNA demethylation pathways: additional players and regulators. *Bioessays* 39, 1–13.

Breiling, A., and Lyko, F. (2015). Epigenetic regulatory functions of DNA modifications: 5-methylcytosine and beyond. *Epigenetics Chromatin* 8:24.

Buenrostro, J. D., Wu, B., Chang, H. Y., and Greenleaf, W. J. (2015). ATAC-seq: a method for assaying chromatin accessibility genome-wide. *Curr. Protoc. Mol. Biol.* 109, 21.29.1–21.29.9.

Carvajal, J. A., Vidal, R. J., Cuello, M. A., Poblete, J. A., and Weiner, C. P. (2006). Mechanisms of paracrine regulation by fetal membranes of human uterine quiescence. *J. Soc. Gynecol. Investig.* 13, 343–349. doi: 10.1016/j.jsgi.2006.04.005

Chan, H. W., Lappas, M., Yee, S. W., Vaswani, K., Mitchell, M. D., and Rice, G. E. (2013). The expression of the let-7 miRNAs and Lin28 signalling pathway in human term gestational tissues. *Placenta* 34, 443–448. doi: 10.1016/j.placenta.2013.02.008

Chhabra, R. (2015). miRNA and methylation: a multifaceted liaison. *Chembiochem* 16, 195–203. doi: 10.1002/cbic.201402449

Ching, T., Song, M. A., Tiirikainen, M., Molnar, J., Berry, M., Towner, D., et al. (2014). Genome-wide hypermethylation coupled with promoter hypomethylation in the chorioamniotic membranes of early onset pre-eclampsia. *Mol. Hum. Reprod.* 20, 885–904. doi: 10.1093/molehr/gau046

Clark, S. J., Lee, H. J., Smallwood, S. A., Kelsey, G., and Reik, W. (2016). Single-cell epigenomics: powerful new methods for understanding gene regulation and cell identity. *Genome Biol.* 17:72.

Dolinoy, D. C., Das, R., Weidman, J. R., and Jirtle, R. L. (2007). Metastable epialleles, imprinting, and the fetal origins of adult diseases. *Pediatr. Res.* 61, 30R–37R.

Dominguez-Salas, P., Moore, S. E., Baker, M. S., Bergen, A. W., Cox, S. E., Dyer, R. A., et al. (2014). Maternal nutrition at conception modulates DNA methylation of human metastable epialleles. *Nat. Commun.* 5:3746.

Dong, F., Zhang, Y., Xia, F., Yang, Y., Xiong, S., Jin, L., et al. (2014). Genome-wide miRNA profiling of villus and decidua of recurrent spontaneous abortion patients. *Reproduction* 148, 33–41. doi: 10.1530/rep-14-0095

Du, Q., Luu, P. L., Stirzaker, C., and Clark, S. J. (2015). Methyl-CpG-binding domain proteins: readers of the epigenome. *Epigenomics* 7, 1051–1073. doi: 10.2217/epi.15.39

Duncan, E. J., Gluckman, P. D., and Dearden, P. K. (2014). Epigenetics, plasticity, and evolution: how do we link epigenetic change to phenotype? *J. Exp. Zool. B Mol. Dev. Evol.* 322, 208–220. doi: 10.1002/jez.b.22571

Easley, C. A. T., Miki, T., Castro, C. A., Ozolek, J. A., Minervini, C. F., Ben-Yehudah, A., et al. (2012). Human amniotic epithelial cells are reprogrammed more efficiently by induced pluripotency than adult fibroblasts. *Cell. Reprogram.* 14, 193–203. doi: 10.1089/cell.2011.0106

Eckmann-Scholz, C., Bens, S., Kolarova, J., Schneppenheim, S., Caliebe, A., Heidemann, S., et al. (2012). DNA-methylation profiling of fetal tissues reveals marked epigenetic differences between chorionic and amniotic samples. *PLoS One* 7:e39014. doi: 10.1371/journal.pone.0039014

Enders, A. C., Schlafke, S., and Hendrickx, A. G. (1986). Differentiation of the embryonic disc, amnion, and yolk sac in the rhesus monkey. *Am. J. Anat.* 177, 161–185. doi: 10.1002/aja.1001770205

Enquobahrie, D. A., Hensley, M., Qiu, C., Abetew, D. F., Hevner, K., Tadesse, M. G., et al. (2015). Candidate gene and microRNA expression in fetal membranes and preterm delivery risk. *Reprod. Sci.* 23, 731–737. doi: 10.1177/1933719115612925

Estella, C., Herrer, I., Moreno-Moya, J. M., Quinonero, A., Martinez, S., Pellicer, A., et al. (2012). miRNA signature and Dicer requirement during human endometrial stromal decidualization in vitro. *PLoS One* 7:e41080. doi: 10.1371/journal.pone.0041080

Fu, K., Bonora, G., and Pellegrini, M. (2020). Interactions between core histone marks and DNA methyltransferases predict DNA methylation patterns observed in human cells and tissues. *Epigenetics* 15, 272–282. doi: 10.1080/15592294.2019.1666649

Gao, F., and Das, S. K. (2014). Epigenetic regulations through DNA methylation and hydroxymethylation: clues for early pregnancy in decidualization. *Biomol. Concepts* 5, 95–107. doi: 10.1515/bmc-2013-0036

Gardiner-Garden, M., and Frommer, M. (1987). CpG islands in vertebrate genomes. *J. Mol. Biol.* 196, 261–282. doi: 10.1016/0022-2836(87)90689-9

Globisch, D., Munzel, M., Muller, M., Michalakis, S., Wagner, M., Koch, S., et al. (2010). Tissue distribution of 5-hydroxymethylcytosine and search for active demethylation intermediates. *PLoS One* 5:e15367. doi: 10.1371/journal.pone.0015367

Gomez-Lopez, N., Guilbert, L. J., and Olson, D. M. (2010). Invasion of the leukocytes into the fetal-maternal interface during pregnancy. *J. Leukoc. Biol.* 88, 625–633. doi: 10.1189/jlb.1209796

Gowher, H., and Jeltsch, A. (2018). Mammalian DNA methyltransferases: new discoveries and open questions. *Biochem. Soc. Trans.* 46, 1191–1202. doi: 10.1042/bst20170574

Gregory, P. A., Bracken, C. P., Smith, E., Bert, A. G., Wright, J. A., Roslan, S., et al. (2011). An autocrine TGF-beta/ZEB/miR-200 signaling network regulates establishment and maintenance of epithelial-mesenchymal transition. *Mol. Biol. Cell* 22, 1686–1698. doi: 10.1091/mbc.e11-02-0103

Grimaldi, G., Christian, M., Quenby, S., and Brosens, J. J. (2012). Expression of epigenetic effectors in decidualizing human endometrial stromal cells. *Mol. Hum. Reprod.* 18, 451–458. doi: 10.1093/molehr/gas020

Grimaldi, G., Christian, M., Steel, J. H., Henriet, P., Poutanen, M., and Brosens, J. J. (2011). Down-regulation of the histone methyltransferase EZH2 contributes to the epigenetic programming of decidualizing human endometrial stromal cells. *Mol. Endocrinol.* 25, 1892–1903. doi: 10.1210/me.2011-1139

Grinius, L., Kessler, C., Schroeder, J., and Handwerger, S. (2006). Forkhead transcription factor FOXO1A is critical for induction of human decidualization. *J. Endocrinol.* 189, 179–187. doi: 10.1677/joe.1.06451

Guo, S. W. (2012). The endometrial epigenome and its response to steroid hormones. *Mol. Cell. Endocrinol.* 358, 185–196. doi: 10.1016/j.mce.2011.10.025

Haggarty, P., Hoad, G., Horgan, G. W., and Campbell, D. M. (2013). DNA methyltransferase candidate polymorphisms, imprinting methylation, and birth outcome. *PLoS One* 8:e68896. doi: 10.1371/journal.pone.0068896

Hammond, S. M. (2015). An overview of microRNAs. *Adv. Drug Deliv. Rev.* 87, 3–14. doi: 10.1007/978-3-319-03725-7_1

Harvey, Z. H., Chen, Y., and Jarosz, D. F. (2018). Protein-based inheritance: epigenetics beyond the chromosome. *Mol. Cell* 69, 195–202. doi: 10.1016/j.molcel.2017.10.030

Hashimoto, H., Liu, Y., Upadhyay, A. K., Chang, Y., Howerton, S. B., Vertino, P. M., et al. (2012). Recognition and potential mechanisms for replication and erasure of cytosine hydroxymethylation. *Nucleic Acids Res.* 40, 4841–4849. doi: 10.1093/nar/gks155

Holemon, H., Korshunova, Y., Ordway, J. M., Bedell, J. A., Citek, R. W., Lakey, N., et al. (2007). MethylScreen: DNA methylation density monitoring using quantitative PCR. *Biotechniques* 43, 683–693. doi: 10.2144/000112597

Hong, L., Yu, T., Xu, H., Hou, N., Cheng, Q., Lai, L., et al. (2018). Down-regulation of miR-378a-3p induces decidual cell apoptosis: a possible mechanism for early pregnancy loss. *Hum. Reprod.* 33, 11–22. doi: 10.1093/humrep/dex347

Houshdaran, S., Zelenko, Z., Irwin, J. C., and Giudice, L. C. (2014). Human endometrial DNA methylome is cycle-dependent and is associated with gene expression regulation. *Mol. Endocrinol.* 28, 1118–1135. doi: 10.1210/me.2013-1340

Huang, Y., Pastor, W. A., Shen, Y., Tahiliani, M., Liu, D. R., and Rao, A. (2010). The behaviour of 5-hydroxymethylcytosine in bisulfite sequencing. *PLoS One* 5:e8888. doi: 10.1371/journal.pone.0008888

Ilicic, M., Zakar, T., and Paul, J. W. (2017). Modulation of progesterone receptor isoform expression in pregnant human myometrium. *Biomed Res. Int.* 2017:4589214.

Ilicic, M., Zakar, T., and Paul, J. W. (2019). Epigenetic regulation of progesterone receptors and the onset of labour. *Reprod. Fertil. Dev.* 31, 1035–1038. doi: 10.1071/rd18392

Janzen, C., Sen, S., Lei, M. Y., Gagliardi De Assumpcao, M., Challis, J., and Chaudhuri, G. (2017). The role of epithelial to mesenchymal transition in human amniotic membrane rupture. *J. Clin. Endocrinol. Metab.* 102, 1261–1269.

Ji, P., Wang, X., Xie, N., and Li, Y. (2018). N6-Methyladenosine in RNA and DNA: an epitranscriptomic and epigenetic player implicated in determination of stem cell fate. *Stem Cells Int.* 2018:3256524.

Jimenez, P. T., Mainigi, M. A., Word, R. A., Kraus, W. L., and Mendelson, C. R. (2016). miR-200 regulates endometrial development during early pregnancy. *Mol. Endocrinol.* 30, 977–987. doi: 10.1210/me.2016-1050

Jones, P. A. (2012). Functions of DNA methylation: islands, start sites, gene bodies and beyond. *Nat. Rev. Genet.* 13, 484–492. doi: 10.1038/nrg3230

Jozaki, K., Tamura, I., Takagi, H., Shirafuta, Y., Mihara, Y., Shinagawa, M., et al. (2019). Glucose regulates the histone acetylation of gene promoters in decidualizing stromal cells. *Reproduction* 157, 457–464. doi: 10.1530/rep-18-0393

Karolczak-Bayatti, M., Sweeney, M., Cheng, J., Edey, L., Robson, S. C., Ulrich, S. M., et al. (2011). Acetylation of heat shock protein 20 (Hsp20) regulates human myometrial activity. *J. Biol. Chem.* 286, 34346–34355. doi: 10.1074/jbc.m111.278549

Katoh, N., Kuroda, K., Tomikawa, J., Ogata-Kawata, H., Ozaki, R., Ochiai, A., et al. (2018). Reciprocal changes of H3K27ac and H3K27me3 at the promoter regions of the critical genes for endometrial decidualization. *Epigenomics* 10, 1243–1257. doi: 10.2217/epi-2018-0006

Ke, W., Chen, C., Luo, H., Tang, J., Zhang, Y., Gao, W., et al. (2016). Histone deacetylase 1 regulates the expression of progesterone receptor a during human parturition by occupying the progesterone receptor a promoter. *Reprod. Sci.* 23, 955–964. doi: 10.1177/1933719115625848

Kempfer, R., and Pombo, A. (2020). Methods for mapping 3D chromosome architecture. *Nat. Rev. Genet.* 21, 207–226. doi: 10.1038/s41576-019-0195-2

Kim, C. J., Romero, R., Chaemsaithong, P., and Kim, J. S. (2015). Chronic inflammation of the placenta: definition, classification, pathogenesis, and clinical significance. *Am. J. Obstet. Gynecol.* 213(4 Suppl.), S53–S69.

Kim, J., Pitlick, M. M., Christine, P. J., Schaefer, A. R., Saleme, C., Comas, B., et al. (2013). Genome-wide analysis of DNA methylation in human amnion. *ScientificWorldJournal* 2013:678156.

Kim, M., and Costello, J. (2017). DNA methylation: an epigenetic mark of cellular memory. *Exp. Mol. Med.* 49:e322. doi: 10.1038/emm.2017.10

Kim, S. Y., Romero, R., Tarca, A. L., Bhatti, G., Kim, C. J., Lee, J., et al. (2012). Methylome of fetal and maternal monocytes and macrophages at the feto-maternal interface. *Am. J. Reprod. Immunol.* 68, 8–27. doi: 10.1111/j.1600-0897.2012.01108.x

Kim, S. Y., Romero, R., Tarca, A. L., Bhatti, G., Lee, J., Chaiworapongsa, T., et al. (2011). miR-143 regulation of prostaglandin-endoperoxidase synthase 2 in the amnion: implications for human parturition at term. *PLoS One* 6:e24131. doi: 10.1371/journal.pone.0024131

Kohli, R. M., and Zhang, Y. (2013). TET enzymes, TDG and the dynamics of DNA demethylation. *Nature* 502, 472–479. doi: 10.1038/nature12750

Kung, J. T., Colognori, D., and Lee, J. T. (2013). Long noncoding RNAs: past, present, and future. *Genetics* 193, 651–669. doi: 10.1534/genetics.112.146704

Kyrklund-Blomberg, N. B., Granath, F., and Cnattingius, S. (2005). Maternal smoking and causes of very preterm birth. *Acta Obstet. Gynecol. Scand.* 84, 572–577. doi: 10.1111/j.0001-6349.2005.00848.x

Liang, X. H., Deng, W. B., Liu, Y. F., Liang, Y. X., Fan, Z. M., Gu, X. W., et al. (2016). Non-coding RNA LINC00473 mediates decidualization of human endometrial stromal cells in response to cAMP signaling. *Sci. Rep.* 6:22744.

Liu, H., Huang, X., Mor, G., and Liao, A. (2019). Epigenetic modifications working in the decidualization and endometrial receptivity. *Cell. Mol. Life Sci.* 77, 2091–2101. doi: 10.1007/s00018-019-03395-9

Liu, W., Niu, Z., Li, Q., Pang, R. T., Chiu, P. C., and Yeung, W. S. (2016). MicroRNA and embryo implantation. *Am. J. Reprod. Immunol.* 75, 263–271.

Logan, P. C., Ponnampalam, A. P., Rahnama, F., Lobie, P. E., and Mitchell, M. D. (2010). The effect of DNA methylation inhibitor 5-Aza-2'-deoxycytidine on human endometrial stromal cells. *Hum. Reprod.* 25, 2859–2869. doi: 10.1093/humrep/deq238

Logan, P. C., Ponnampalam, A. P., Steiner, M., and Mitchell, M. D. (2013). Effect of cyclic AMP and estrogen/progesterone on the transcription of DNA methyltransferases during the decidualization of human endometrial stromal cells. *Mol. Hum. Reprod.* 19, 302–312. doi: 10.1093/molehr/gas062

Lövkvist, C., Dodd, I. B., Sneppen, K., and Haerter, J. O. (2016). DNA methylation in human epigenomes depends on local topology of CpG sites. *Nucleic Acids Res.* 44, 5123–5132. doi: 10.1093/nar/gkw124

Luo, X., Pan, J., Wang, L., Wang, P., Zhang, M., Liu, M., et al. (2015). Epigenetic regulation of lncRNA connects ubiquitin-proteasome system with infection-inflammation in preterm births and preterm premature rupture of membranes. *BMC Pregnancy Childbirth* 15:35. doi: 10.1186/s12884-015-0460-0

Luo, X., Shi, Q., Gu, Y., Pan, J., Hua, M., Liu, M., et al. (2013). LncRNA pathway involved in premature preterm rupture of membrane (PPROM): an epigenomic approach to study the pathogenesis of reproductive disorders. *PLoS One* 8:e79897. doi: 10.1371/journal.pone.0079897

Lv, H., Tong, J., Yang, J., Lv, S., Li, W. P., Zhang, C., et al. (2018). Dysregulated pseudogene HK2P1 may contribute to preeclampsia as a competing endogenous RNA for hexokinase 2 by impairing decidualization. *Hypertension* 71, 648–658. doi: 10.1161/hypertensionaha.117.10084

Lv, Y., Gao, S., Zhang, Y., Wang, L., Chen, X., and Wang, Y. (2016). miRNA and target gene expression in menstrual endometria and early pregnancy decidua. *Eur. J. Obstet. Gynecol. Reprod. Biol.* 197, 27–30. doi: 10.1016/j.ejogrb.2015.11.003

Maekawa, R., Tamura, I., Shinagawa, M., Mihara, Y., Sato, S., Okada, M., et al. (2019). Genome-wide DNA methylation analysis revealed stable DNA methylation status during decidualization in human endometrial stromal cells. *BMC Genomics* 20:324. doi: 10.1186/s12864-019-5695-0

Marinić, M., Mika, K., Chigurupati, S., and Lynch, V. J. (2020). Evolutionary transcriptomics implicates HAND2 in the origins of implantation and regulation of gestation length. *bioRxiv* [Preprint]. doi: 10.1101/2020.06.15.152868 bioRxiv: 2020.2006.2015.152868,

Menon, R., Bonney, E. A., Condon, J., Mesiano, S., and Taylor, R. N. (2016). Novel concepts on pregnancy clocks and alarms: redundancy and synergy in human parturition. *Hum. Reprod. Update* 22, 535–560. doi: 10.1093/humupd/dmw022

Menon, R., Richardson, L. S., and Lappas, M. (2019). Fetal membrane architecture, aging and inflammation in pregnancy and parturition. *Placenta* 79, 40–45. doi: 10.1016/j.placenta.2018.11.003

Mitchell, B. F., and Powell, W. A. (1984). Progesterone production by human fetal membranes: an in vitro incubation system for studying hormone production and metabolism. *Am. J. Obstet. Gynecol.* 148, 303–309. doi: 10.1016/s0002-9378(84)80073-3

Mitchell, C., Johnson, R., Bisits, A., Hirst, J., and Zakar, T. (2011). PTGS2 (prostaglandin endoperoxide synthase-2) expression in term human amnion in vivo involves rapid mRNA turnover, polymerase-II 5′-pausing, and glucocorticoid transrepression. *Endocrinology* 152, 2113–2122. doi: 10.1210/en.2010-1327

Mitchell, C. M., Hirst, J. J., Mitchell, M. D., Murray, H. G., and Zakar, T. (2019). Genes upregulated in the amnion at labour are bivalently marked by activating and repressive histone modifications. *Mol. Hum. Reprod.* 25, 228–240. doi: 10.1093/molehr/gaz007

Mitchell, C. M., Johnson, R. F., Giles, W. B., and Zakar, T. (2008). Prostaglandin H synthase-2 gene regulation in the amnion at labour: histone acetylation and nuclear factor kappa B binding to the promoter in vivo. *Mol. Hum. Reprod.* 14, 53–59. doi: 10.1093/molehr/gam086

Mitchell, C. M., Sykes, S. D., Pan, X., Pringle, K. G., Lumbers, E. R., Hirst, J. J., et al. (2013). Inflammatory and steroid receptor gene methylation in the human amnion and decidua. *J. Mol. Endocrinol.* 50, 267–277. doi: 10.1530/jme-12-0211

Mitchell, M. D. (2006). Unique suppression of prostaglandin h synthase-2 expression by inhibition of histone deacetylation, specifically in human amnion but not adjacent choriodecidua. *Mol. Biol. Cell* 17, 549–553. doi: 10.1091/mbc.e05-08-0818

Montenegro, D., Romero, R., Kim, S. S., Tarca, A. L., Draghici, S., Kusanovic, J. P., et al. (2009). Expression patterns of microRNAs in the chorioamniotic membranes: a role for microRNAs in human pregnancy and parturition. *J. Pathol.* 217, 113–121. doi: 10.1002/path.2463

Montenegro, D., Romero, R., Pineles, B. L., Tarca, A. L., Kim, Y. M., Draghici, S., et al. (2007). Differential expression of microRNAs with progression of gestation and inflammation in the human chorioamniotic membranes. *Am. J. Obstet. Gynecol.* 197, 289.e1–289.e6.

Moradi, M. T., Rahimi, Z., and Vaisi-Raygani, A. (2019). New insight into the role of long non-coding RNAs in the pathogenesis of preeclampsia. *Hypertens. Pregnancy* 38, 41–51. doi: 10.1080/10641955.2019.1573252

Myhre, R., Brantsaeter, A. L., Myking, S., Eggesbo, M., Meltzer, H. M., Haugen, M., et al. (2013). Intakes of garlic and dried fruits are associated with lower risk of spontaneous preterm delivery. *J. Nutr.* 143, 1100–1108. doi: 10.3945/jn.112.173229

Nabet, C., Lelong, N., Ancel, P. Y., Saurel-Cubizolles, M. J., and Kaminski, M. (2007). Smoking during pregnancy according to obstetric complications and parity: results of the EUROPOP study. *Eur. J. Epidemiol.* 22, 715–721. doi: 10.1007/s10654-007-9172-8

Nancy, P., Siewiera, J., Rizzuto, G., Tagliani, E., Osokine, I., Manandhar, P., et al. (2018). H3K27me3 dynamics dictate evolving uterine states in pregnancy and parturition. *J. Clin. Invest.* 128, 233–247. doi: 10.1172/jci95937

Nardelli, C., Iaffaldano, L., Ferrigno, M., Labruna, G., Maruotti, G. M., Quaglia, F., et al. (2014). Characterization and predicted role of the microRNA expression profile in amnion from obese pregnant women. *Int. J. Obes.* 38, 466–469. doi: 10.1038/ijo.2013.121

Norris, K. L., Lee, J. Y., and Yao, T. P. (2009). Acetylation goes global: the emergence of acetylation biology. *Sci. Signal.* 2:pe76. doi: 10.1126/scisignal.297pe76

Norwitz, E. R., Bonney, E. A., Snegovskikh, V. V., Williams, M. A., Phillippe, M., Park, J. S., et al. (2015). Molecular regulation of parturition: the role of the decidual clock. *Cold Spring Harb. Perspect. Med.* 5:a023143. doi: 10.1101/cshperspect.a023143

O'brien, J., Hayder, H., Zayed, Y., and Peng, C. (2018). Overview of microRNA biogenesis, mechanisms of actions, and circulation. *Front. Endocrinol.* 9:402. doi: 10.3389/fendo.2018.00402

Orren, D. K., and Machwe, A. (2019). Lysine acetylation of proteins and its characterization in human systems. *Methods Mol. Biol.* 1983, 107–130. doi: 10.1007/978-1-4939-9434-2_7

Park, Y., Nnamani, M. C., Maziarz, J., and Wagner, G. P. (2016). Cis-regulatory evolution of forkhead box O1 (FOXO1), a terminal selector gene for decidual stromal cell identity. *Mol. Biol. Evol.* 33, 3161–3169. doi: 10.1093/molbev/msw193

Pidsley, R., Zotenko, E., Peters, T. J., Lawrence, M. G., Risbridger, G. P., Molloy, P., et al. (2016). Critical evaluation of the Illumina methylationEPIC beadchip microarray for whole-genome DNA methylation profiling. *Genome Biol.* 17:208.

Poljak, M., Lim, R., Barker, G., and Lappas, M. (2014). Class I to III histone deacetylases differentially regulate inflammation-induced matrix metalloproteinase 9 expression in primary amnion cells. *Reprod. Sci.* 21, 804–813. doi: 10.1177/1933719113518990

Qian, K., Hu, L., Chen, H., Li, H., Liu, N., Li, Y., et al. (2009). Hsa-miR-222 is involved in differentiation of endometrial stromal cells in vitro. *Endocrinology* 150, 4734–4743. doi: 10.1210/en.2008-1629

Rakyan, V. K., Blewitt, M. E., Druker, R., Preis, J. I., and Whitelaw, E. (2002). Metastable epialleles in mammals. *Trends Genet.* 18, 348–351. doi: 10.1016/s0168-9525(02)02709-9

Richardson, L. S., Taylor, R. N., and Menon, R. (2020). Reversible EMT and MET mediate amnion remodeling during pregnancy and labor. *Sci. Signal.* 13:eaay1486. doi: 10.1126/scisignal.aay1486

Roadmap Epigenomics Consortium, Kundaje, A., Meuleman, W., Ernst, J., Bilenky, M., Yen, A., et al. (2015). Integrative analysis of 111 reference human epigenomes. *Nature* 518, 317–330.

Robinson, W. P., and Price, E. M. (2015). The human placental methylome. *Cold Spring Harb. Perspect. Med.* 5:a023044. doi: 10.1101/cshperspect.a023044

Romero, R., Dey, S. K., and Fisher, S. J. (2014). Preterm labor: one syndrome, many causes. *Science* 345, 760–765. doi: 10.1126/science.1251816

Rona, G. B., Eleutherio, E. C. A., and Pinheiro, A. S. (2016). PWWP domains and their modes of sensing DNA and histone methylated lysines. *Biophys. Rev.* 8, 63–74. doi: 10.1007/s12551-015-0190-6

Rose, N. R., and Klose, R. J. (2014). Understanding the relationship between DNA methylation and histone lysine methylation. *Biochim. Biophys. Acta* 1839, 1362–1372. doi: 10.1016/j.bbagrm.2014.02.007

Sakabe, N., Aneas, I., Knoblauch, N., Sobreira, D. R., Clark, N., Paz, C., et al. (2020). Transcriptome and regulatory maps of decidua-derived stromal cells inform gene discovery in preterm birth. *bioRxiv* [Preprint]. doi: 10.1101/2020.04.06.017079

Sasaki, K., Nakamura, T., Okamoto, I., Yabuta, Y., Iwatani, C., Tsuchiya, H., et al. (2016). The germ cell fate of cynomolgus monkeys is specified in the nascent amnion. *Dev. Cell* 39, 169–185. doi: 10.1016/j.devcel.2016.09.007

Sato, B. L., Collier, E. S., Vermudez, S. A., Junker, A. D., and Kendal-Wright, C. E. (2016). Human amnion mesenchymal cells are pro-inflammatory when activated by the Toll-like receptor 2/6 ligand, macrophage-activating lipoprotein-2. *Placenta* 44, 69–79. doi: 10.1016/j.placenta.2016.06.005

Schubeler, D. (2015). Function and information content of DNA methylation. *Nature* 517, 321–326. doi: 10.1038/nature14192

Serrano-Gomez, S. J., Maziveyi, M., and Alahari, S. K. (2016). Regulation of epithelial-mesenchymal transition through epigenetic and post-translational modifications. *Mol. Cancer* 15:18.

Seto, E., and Yoshida, M. (2014). Erasers of histone acetylation: the histone deacetylase enzymes. *Cold Spring Harb. Perspect. Biol.* 6:a018713. doi: 10.1101/cshperspect.a018713

Shen, C., and Zhong, N. (2015). Long non-coding RNAs: the epigenetic regulators involved in the pathogenesis of reproductive disorder. *Am. J. Reprod. Immunol.* 73, 95–108. doi: 10.1111/aji.12315

Siega-Riz, A. M., Promislow, J. H., Savitz, D. A., Thorp, J. M. Jr., and Mcdonald, T. (2003). Vitamin C intake and the risk of preterm delivery. *Am. J. Obstet. Gynecol.* 189, 519–525. doi: 10.1067/s0002-9378(03)00363-6

Silini, A., Parolini, O., Huppertz, B., and Lang, I. (2013). Soluble factors of amnion-derived cells in treatment of inflammatory and fibrotic pathologies. *Curr. Stem Cell Res. Ther.* 8, 6–14. doi: 10.2174/1574888x11308010003

Spruijt, C. G., Gnerlich, F., Smits, A. H., Pfaffeneder, T., Jansen, P. W. T. C., Bauer, C., et al. (2013). Dynamic readers for 5-(hydroxy) methylcytosine and its oxidized derivatives. *Cell* 152, 1146–1159. doi: 10.1016/j.cell.2013.02.004

Stephen, G. L., Lui, S., Hamilton, S. A., Tower, C. L., Harris, L. K., Stevens, A., et al. (2015). Transcriptomic profiling of human choriodecidua during term labor: inflammation as a key driver of labor. *Am. J. Reprod. Immunol.* 73, 36–55. doi: 10.1111/aji.12328

Suter, M. A., and Aagaard-Tillery, K. M. (2009). Environmental influences on epigenetic profiles. *Semin. Reprod. Med.* 27, 380–390. doi: 10.1055/s-0029-1237426

Suzuki, M., Maekawa, R., Patterson, N. E., Reynolds, D. M., Calder, B. R., Reznik, S. E., et al. (2016). Amnion as a surrogate tissue reporter of the effects of maternal preeclampsia on the fetus. *Clin. Epigenetics* 8:67.

Sykes, S. D., Mitchell, C., Pringle, K. G., Wang, Y., Zakar, T., and Lumbers, E. R. (2015). Methylation of promoter regions of genes of the human intrauterine renin angiotensin system and their expression. *Int. J. Endocrinol.* 2015:459818.

Tajima, S., Suetake, I., Takeshita, K., Nakagawa, A., and Kimura, H. (2016). Domain structure of the Dnmt1, Dnmt3a, and Dnmt3b DNA methyltransferases. *Adv. Exp. Med. Biol.* 945, 63–86. doi: 10.1007/978-3-319-43624-1_4

Tamura, I., Jozaki, K., Sato, S., Shirafuta, Y., Shinagawa, M., Maekawa, R., et al. (2018). The distal upstream region of insulin-like growth factor-binding protein-1 enhances its expression in endometrial stromal cells during decidualization. *J. Biol. Chem.* 293, 5270–5280. doi: 10.1074/jbc.ra117.000234

Tamura, I., Ohkawa, Y., Sato, T., Suyama, M., Jozaki, K., Okada, M., et al. (2014). Genome-wide analysis of histone modifications in human endometrial stromal cells. *Mol. Endocrinol.* 28, 1656–1669. doi: 10.1210/me.2014-1117

Tochigi, H., Kajihara, T., Mizuno, Y., Mizuno, Y., Tamaru, S., Kamei, Y., et al. (2017). Loss of miR-542-3p enhances IGFBP-1 expression in decidualizing human endometrial stromal cells. *Sci. Rep.* 7:40001.

Tong, J., Zhao, W., Lv, H., Li, W. P., Chen, Z. J., and Zhang, C. (2018). Transcriptomic profiling in human decidua of severe preeclampsia detected by RNA sequencing. *J. Cell. Biochem.* 119, 607–615. doi: 10.1002/jcb.26221

Vincent, Z. L., Farquhar, C. M., Mitchell, M. D., and Ponnampalam, A. P. (2011). Expression and regulation of DNA methyltransferases in human endometrium. *Fertil. Steril.* 95, 1522–1525.e1.

Vincent, Z. L., Mitchell, M. D., and Ponnampalam, A. P. (2015). Regulation of TIMP-1 in human placenta and fetal membranes by lipopolysaccharide and demethylating agent 5-aza-2'-deoxycytidine. *Reprod. Biol. Endocrinol.* 13:136.

Walsh, S. W., Chumble, A. A., Washington, S. L., Archer, K. J., Sahingur, S. E., and Strauss, J. F. III (2017). Increased expression of toll-like receptors 2 and 9 is associated with reduced DNA methylation in spontaneous preterm labor. *J. Reprod. Immunol.* 121, 35–41. doi: 10.1016/j.jri.2017.05.003

Wang, H., Ogawa, M., Wood, J. R., Bartolomei, M. S., Sammel, M. D., Kusanovic, J. P., et al. (2008). Genetic and epigenetic mechanisms combine to control MMP1 expression and its association with preterm premature rupture of membranes. *Hum. Mol. Genet.* 17, 1087–1096. doi: 10.1093/hmg/ddm381

Wang, Y., Lv, Y., Gao, S., Zhang, Y., Sun, J., Gong, C., et al. (2016). MicroRNA profiles in spontaneous decidualized menstrual endometrium and early pregnancy decidua with successfully implanted embryos. *PLoS One* 11:e0143116. doi: 10.1371/journal.pone.0143116

Wang, Y., Lv, Y., Wang, L., Gong, C., Sun, J., Chen, X., et al. (2015). MicroRNAome in decidua: a new approach to assess the maintenance of pregnancy. *Fertil. Steril.* 103, 980–989.e6.

Waterland, R. A., Kellermayer, R., Laritsky, E., Rayco-Solon, P., Harris, R. A., Travisano, M., et al. (2010). Season of conception in rural gambia affects DNA methylation at putative human metastable epialleles. *PLoS Genet.* 6:e1001252. doi: 10.1371/journal.pgen.1001252

Whittle, W. L., Gibb, W., and Challis, J. R. (2000). The characterization of human amnion epithelial and mesenchymal cells: the cellular expression, activity and glucocorticoid regulation of prostaglandin output. *Placenta* 21, 394–401. doi: 10.1053/plac.1999.0482

Wu, Q., Heidenreich, D., Zhou, S., Ackloo, S., Kramer, A., Nakka, K., et al. (2019). A chemical toolbox for the study of bromodomains and epigenetic signaling. *Nat. Commun.* 10:1915.

Yamagata, Y., Asada, H., Tamura, I., Lee, L., Maekawa, R., Taniguchi, K., et al. (2009). DNA methyltransferase expression in the human endometrium: down-regulation by progesterone and estrogen. *Hum. Reprod.* 24, 1126–1132. doi: 10.1093/humrep/dep015

Yao, Q., Chen, Y., and Zhou, X. (2019). The roles of microRNAs in epigenetic regulation. *Curr. Opin. Chem. Biol.* 51, 11–17. doi: 10.1016/j.cbpa.2019.01.024

Yoo, J. Y., You, Y. A., Kwon, E. J., Park, M. H., Shim, S., and Kim, Y. J. (2018). Differential expression and methylation of integrin subunit alpha 11 and thrombospondin in the amnion of preterm birth. *Obstet. Gynecol. Sci.* 61, 565–574. doi: 10.5468/ogs.2018.61.5.565

Yu, M., Hon, G. C., Szulwach, K. E., Song, C. X., Zhang, L., Kim, A., et al. (2012). Base-resolution analysis of 5-hydroxymethylcytosine in the mammalian genome. *Cell* 149, 1368–1380. doi: 10.1016/j.cell.2012.04.027

Zhang, G., Feenstra, B., Bacelis, J., Liu, X., Muglia, L. M., Juodakis, J., et al. (2017). Genetic associations with gestational duration and spontaneous preterm birth. *N. Engl. J. Med.* 377, 1156–1167.

Zhang, Q., Zhang, H., Jiang, Y., Xue, B., Diao, Z., Ding, L., et al. (2015). MicroRNA-181a is involved in the regulation of human endometrial stromal cell decidualization by inhibiting Kruppel-like factor 12. *Reprod. Biol. Endocrinol.* 13:23.

Zhang, X. H., Liang, X., Liang, X. H., Wang, T. S., Qi, Q. R., Deng, W. B., et al. (2013). The mesenchymal-epithelial transition during in vitro decidualization. *Reprod. Sci.* 20, 354–360. doi: 10.1177/1933719112472738

Zhao, G., Zhou, X., Chen, S., Miao, H., Fan, H., Wang, Z., et al. (2014). Differential expression of microRNAs in decidua-derived mesenchymal stem cells from patients with pre-eclampsia. *J. Biomed. Sci.* 21:81.

Zhao, L., Li, J., and Huang, S. (2018). Patients with unexplained recurrent spontaneous abortion show decreased levels of microRNA-146a-5p in the deciduae. *Ann. Clin. Lab. Sci.* 48, 177–182.

Zhu, H., Hou, C. C., Luo, L. F., Hu, Y. J., and Yang, W. X. (2014). Endometrial stromal cells and decidualized stromal cells: origins, transformation and functions. *Gene* 551, 1–14. doi: 10.1016/j.gene.2014.08.047

Cortisol Regeneration in the Fetal Membranes, A Coincidental or Requisite Event in Human Parturition?

Wang-Sheng Wang[1,2†], Chun-Ming Guo[3†] and Kang Sun[1,2]*

[1] *Center for Reproductive Medicine, Ren Ji Hospital, School of Medicine, Shanghai Jiao Tong University, Shanghai, China,* [2] *Shanghai Key Laboratory for Assisted Reproduction and Reproductive Genetics, Shanghai, China,* [3] *School of Life Sciences, Yunnan University, Kunming, China*

*Correspondence:
Kang Sun
sungangrenji@hotmail.com

†These authors have contributed equally to this work

The fetal membranes are equipped with high capacity of cortisol regeneration through the reductase activity of 11β-hydroxysteroid dehydrogenase 1 (11β-HSD1). The expression of 11β-HSD1 in the fetal membranes is under the feedforward induction by cortisol, which is potentiated by proinflammatory cytokines. As a result, the abundance of 11β-HSD1 increases with gestational age and furthermore at parturition with an escalation of cortisol concentration in the fetal membranes. Accumulated cortisol takes parts in a number of crucial events pertinent to the onset of labor in the fetal membranes, including extracellular matrix (ECM) remodeling and stimulation of prostaglandin output. Cortisol remodels the ECM through multiple approaches including induction of collagen I, III, and IV degradation, as well as inhibition of their cross-linking. These effects of cortisol are executed through activation of the autophagy, proteasome, and matrix metalloprotease 7 pathways, as well as inhibition of the expression of cross-linking enzyme lysyl oxidase in mesenchymal cells of the membranes. With regard to prostaglandin output, cortisol not only increases prostaglandin E2 and F2α syntheses through induction of their synthesizing enzymes such as cytosolic phospholipase A2, cyclooxygenase 2, and carbonyl reductase 1 in the amnion, but also decreases their degradation through inhibition of their metabolizing enzyme 15-hydroxyprostaglandin dehydrogenase in the chorion. Taking all together, data accumulated so far denote that the feedforward cortisol regeneration by 11β-HSD1 in the fetal membranes is a requisite event in the onset of parturition, and the effects of cortisol on prostaglandin synthesis and ECM remodeling may be enhanced by proinflammatory cytokines in chorioamnionitis.

Keywords: 11β-HSD1, collagen, prostaglandins, glucocorticoids, fetal membranes

INTRODUCTION

Glucocorticoids are essential for life, and it regulates a variety of important cardiovascular, metabolic, and immunologic functions in the maintenance of homeostasis (Schmid et al., 1995; Beato and Klug, 2000; Rhen and Cidlowski, 2005). Cortisol is the most important endogenous glucocorticoid in humans. The *de novo* synthesis of cortisol from cholesterol takes place primarily in the zona fasciculata of the adrenal cortex (Miller and Auchus, 2011). After secretion into the circulation, most of cortisol is bound by corticosteroid-binding protein (CBG) and to a lesser extent by albumin (Bae and Kratzsch, 2015; Meyer et al., 2016). There is approximately only 5 to 10% of cortisol that remains free in the circulation, which is important for the actions of cortisol as only the free fraction of cortisol is biologically active (Lewis et al., 2005). In compensation, glucocorticoid target organs develop a way to enhance cortisol concentrations within the cells through regeneration of cortisol by 11β-hydroxysteroid dehydrogenase 1 (11β-HSD1) (Chapman et al., 1997; Tomlinson et al., 2004; Chapman et al., 2013; Morgan et al., 2014). 11β-HSD1 is a microsomal reductase catalyzing the regeneration of cortisol from biologically inactive 17α-hydroxy-11-dehydrocorticosterone (cortisone), which derives mostly from the oxidase action of 11β-HSD2 in the mineralocorticoid target organs (**Figure 1**; Tannin et al., 1991; Albiston et al., 1994; Chapman et al., 2013). 11β-HSD2 is a counterpart enzyme of 11β-HSD1 and functions in an opposite way to 11β-HSD1 converting biologically active cortisol to inactive cortisone (**Figure 1**). Because 11β-HSD2 does not metabolize aldosterone, 11β-HSD2 is utilized by the mineralocorticoid target organs as a pre-receptor gate to ensure the indiscriminating mineralocorticoid receptor being occupied only by aldosterone but not by cortisol (White et al., 1997a,b,c). This differential expression pattern of 11β-HSD1 and 11β-HSD2 in glucocorticoid and mineralocorticoid target organs is developed perfectly to ensure the efficiency of cortisol's actions and the specificity of aldosterone's actions in their respective target organs.

In pregnancy, the placenta is responsible for nourishing and protecting the fetus as well as maintaining pregnancy by producing a plethora of hormones and immune factors. Attached to the edge of the discoid placenta is the atrophied chorionic villi, also known as the smooth chorion or chorion leave, which fuses with the amniotic membrane extended from the fetal surface of the placenta, and together they form the reflected fetal membranes (Leiser and Kaufmann, 1994; Ferner and Mess, 2011). The fetal membranes not only enclose the fetus bathed in the amniotic fluid but also become a source of initiating signals for parturition toward the end of gestation (Okazaki et al., 1981; Myatt and Sun, 2010; Menon, 2016; Wang et al., 2018; Menon and Moore, 2020). Like the specific distribution of 11β-HSD1 and 11β-HSD2 in glucocorticoid and mineralocorticoid target organs, the distribution of 11β-HSD1 and 11β-HSD2 in the placenta and fetal membranes also adopts a unique tissue-specific pattern (Sun et al., 1997; Yang et al., 2016). Although the placenta is not a typical mineralocorticoid target organ, it boasts abundant 11β-HSD2 but scarce 11β-HSD1 (Albiston et al., 1994; Sun et al., 1997; Yang et al., 2016). It is known that 11β-HSD2 in the placenta functions as a glucocorticoid barrier by inactivating maternal cortisol to cortisone so that the fetus can be protected from the growth-restricting effects of excessive maternal glucocorticoids (Osinski, 1960; Burton and Waddell, 1999; Drake et al., 2007). This function of 11β-HSD2 in the placenta is substantiated by its distinct distribution in the syncytiotrophoblast, the outmost layer of placental villi that immerse directly in the maternal blood (Krozowski et al., 1995; Ni et al., 2009; Li et al., 2011, 2013; Zhang et al., 2015; Zuo et al., 2017). In contrast to the placenta, the fetal membranes express abundant 11β-HSD1 with barely detectable 11β-HSD2 (Sun et al., 1997), which can utilize cortisone derived from both maternal mineralocorticoid organs and the placenta to regenerate cortisol (**Figure 1**; Murphy, 1977, 1979). The expression of 11β-HSD1 in the fetal membranes increases with gestational age and further increases in parturition with its abundance atop all fetal tissues by the end of gestation (Murphy, 1977, 1981; Alfaidy et al., 2003). This cortisol-regenerating capacity of the fetal membranes is even regarded as a supplemental extra-adrenal source of glucocorticoids in pregnancy (Murphy, 1977, 1981; Tanswell et al., 1977). Why should the fetal membranes be equipped with such a unique cortisol-regenerating capacity in pregnancy? Given that the smooth chorion is actually atrophied chorion villi, it is plausible to question whether this cortisol regeneration activity of the fetal membranes is merely an irrelevant by-product of pregnancy or a finely mapped-out event, which is absolutely required toward the end of gestation. In this review article, we will try to answer these questions by summarizing data from our laboratory as well as others.

FEEDFORWARD CORTISOL REGENERATION IN THE FETAL MEMBRANES

The fetal membrane components differ in different species (Mess et al., 2003). Human fetal membranes comprised the amnion and smooth chorion. The smooth chorion is the outer layer that connects the maternal decidua and can be subdivided into a trophoblast layer and a connective tissue layer adjacent to the amnion. The amnion is composed of a single layer of amnion epithelial cells sitting on a basement membrane and a tough compact layer that contains abundant interstitial fibers and fibroblasts (Bourne, 1960; Parry and Strauss, 3rd., 1998; Wang et al., 2018). Studies of 11β-HSD1 in the fetal membranes of other species are sparse. However, 11β-HSD1 has been localized to the placenta in a number of species including rat, sheep, and baboon (Burton and Waddell, 1994; Pepe et al., 1996; Yang et al., 1997). Immunohistochemical staining of human fetal membranes shows that 11β-HSD1 distributes in whole membrane layers (Sun et al., 1997; Wang et al., 2012; Liu et al., 2016a). In the amnion, 11β-HSD1 distributes in both epithelial and fibroblast cells, whereas in the smooth chorion, 11β-HSD1 is localized to trophoblasts, as well as fibroblasts (Sun et al., 1997; Wang et al., 2012; Liu et al., 2016a). Notably, in contrast to the expression of 11β-HSD2 in trophoblasts of human placenta chorionic villi, trophoblasts of the smooth chorion express mainly 11β-HSD1 rather than 11β-HSD2 (Sun et al., 1997). These discrepancies are suggestive of a unique role of 11β-HSD1 rather than a by-product of atrophied villi in the fetal membranes.

Intriguingly, cortisol, despite being a product of 11β-HSD1, induces rather than inhibits 11β-HSD1 expression in both smooth chorion trophoblasts and amnion fibroblasts (Sun et al., 2002; Sun and Myatt, 2003; Li et al., 2006; Yang et al., 2007), thus setting up a positive feedback loop between cortisol

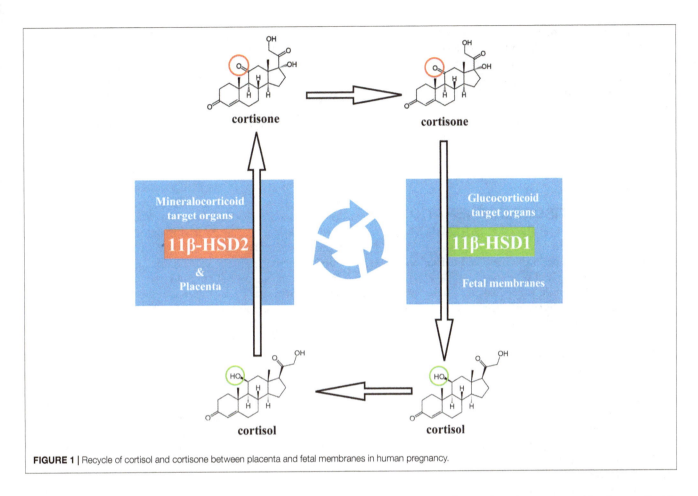

FIGURE 1 | Recycle of cortisol and cortisone between placenta and fetal membranes in human pregnancy.

regeneration and 11β-HSD1 expression in the fetal membranes. This feedforward expression pattern of 11β-HSD1 in the fetal membranes may account for its increasing expression with gestational age (Alfaidy et al., 2003) and its further increase at parturition (Liu et al., 2016a).

The actions of glucocorticoids and proinflammatory cytokines usually oppose each other at sites of inflammation. However, in the fetal membranes, proinflammatory cytokines induce the expression of 11β-HSD1 not only on their own, but also in synergy with glucocorticoids (Sun and Myatt, 2003; Li et al., 2006; Lu et al., 2019c). Given that inflammation is a common cause of both term and preterm birth, and overproduction of proinflammatory cytokines is a common feature of inflammation (Bollapragada et al., 2009; Menon et al., 2010; Romero et al., 2014; Singh et al., 2019), the synergy between glucocorticoids and proinflammatory cytokines in the induction of 11β-HSD1 expression is particularly noteworthy because this synergy is very likely to generate even more cortisol under conditions of chorioamnionitis. These distinct features of 11β-HSD1 expression in the fetal membranes denote again that the expression of 11β-HSD1 in the fetal membranes may be a requisite event in the end of normal gestation and may even be more intriguing in the condition of chorioamnionitis. In non-gestational tissues, proinflammatory cytokines have also been shown to induce 11β-HSD1 expression either on its own (Tomlinson et al., 2001; Yong et al., 2002; Ignatova et al., 2009; Esteves et al., 2014) or in synergy with glucocorticoids (Rae et al., 2004; Kaur et al., 2010), which is regarded as a self-restraining mechanism to avoid over immune responses in inflammation. Is cortisol regeneration by 11β-HSD1 in the fetal membranes simply a self-restraining mechanism to contain inflammation or does it mean more than an anti-inflammatory role in pregnancy? Convincing evidence has accumulated that glucocorticoids derived from fetal adrenal glands can trigger parturition in a number of animal species (Anderson et al., 1975; Flint et al., 1978; First and Bosc, 1979; Morrison et al., 1983; Fowden et al., 2008). However, adrenal glands of human fetus produce mainly dehydroepiandrosterone sulfate (DHEAS) rather than glucocorticoids (Mesiano and Jaffe, 1997; Ishimoto and Jaffe, 2011). This feature of human fetal adrenal glands may also explain why systemic administration of synthetic glucocorticoids such as betamethasone apparently does not induce labor (Craft et al., 1976). This is probably due to the strong negative feedback of synthetic glucocorticoids on the fetal hypothalamic–pituitary–adrenal axis, which may result in diminished production of both DHEAS and cortisol when synthetic glucocorticoids pass through the placenta and enter the fetal circulation. Because DHEAS is a precursor for estrogen synthesis in the placenta, diminished DHEAS will lead to reduced estrogen production (Ogueh et al., 1999), which is essential for preparation of the myometrium for contraction (Mesiano, 2001). Therefore, it is very likely that the feedforward cortisol regeneration by 11β-HSD1 in the fetal membranes is a compensatory mechanism in parturition for the insufficient cortisol synthesis by fetal adrenal glands in humans. In other words, local regeneration of cortisol in the fetal membranes is probably more important than cortisol derived from fetal adrenal glands in human parturition. This notion is endorsed by increased abundance of glucocorticoid receptor (GR) in the fetal membranes at parturition (Sun et al., 1996), suggesting that cortisol regenerated by 11β-HSD1 in the fetal membranes has enhanced local actions pertinent to human parturition.

ROLE OF CORTISOL REGENERATION IN THE RUPTURE OF FETAL MEMBRANES

During the gestational period, a tough and tensile amniotic sac is required for holding and protecting the fetus bathed in the amniotic fluid. The tensile strength of the fetal membranes is believed to derive mainly from the rich content of collagenous fibers in the compact layer of the amnion (Bourne, 1962; Parry and Strauss, 3rd., 1998; Oyen et al., 2006). Needless to say, the fetal membranes should break for the delivery of fetus at parturition, and rupture of membranes can, in turn, promote labor, suggesting that the fetal membranes are a source of labor initiating signals. As a matter of fact, the fetal membranes are indeed among the gestational tissues that give rise to signals leading to parturition (Parry and Strauss, 3rd., 1998; Menon, 2016; Menon et al., 2016). These multiple source signals may need to work in a coordinating manner to start labor at term. However, intensified signals from the fetal membranes as elicited by membrane rupture or infection can sometimes even start labor alone no matter at term and preterm, which highlights the importance of membrane rupture in parturition. In line with the rupture of membranes, the fetal membranes become increasingly weak toward the end of gestation. Our serial studies indicate that local regeneration of cortisol is an important attributor to membrane weakening and rupture (Liu et al., 2016a; Wang et al., 2016, 2019a; Mi et al., 2017, 2018).

The initial inspiration that has encouraged us to investigate whether cortisol regeneration is involved in membrane rupture comes from the side effects of clinical usage of glucocorticoids. Based on their potent anti-inflammatory properties, synthetic glucocorticoids are widely prescribed to treat a variety of acute and chronic inflammatory conditions (Rhen and Cidlowski, 2005). Among the side effects of glucocorticoids, skin atrophy is frequently encountered (Sterry and Asadullah, 2002; Schoepe et al., 2006). Fibroblasts have been shown to be the target cells of glucocorticoids for this side effect (Nuutinen et al., 2001; Oishi et al., 2002; Schoepe et al., 2006). It has been demonstrated that glucocorticoids reduce tensile strength and elasticity of the skin by decreasing the synthesis of extracellular matrix (ECM) proteins and increasing their turnover in fibroblasts (Cutroneo et al., 1975, 1981; Shull and Cutroneo, 1986; Nuutinen et al., 2001; Oishi et al., 2002; Boudon et al., 2017). For the same reason, glucocorticoids are being used topically to prevent excessive scar formation (Berliner et al., 1967; Jalali and Bayat, 2007). These clinical observations have prompted us to envisage that the feedforward cortisol regeneration in the fetal membranes may be related to ECM remodeling for membrane rupture.

It is now known that the tensile strength of the amnion is largely attributed to collagen I and III contents in the compact layer (Bourne, 1960; Malak et al., 1993; Bryant-Greenwood, 1998). Abundance of collagen I and III in the amnion decreases after the middle trimester to a nadir at term (Skinner et al., 1981; Casey and MacDonald, 1996; Hampson et al., 1997). In preterm premature rupture of membranes, a common cause of preterm labor, collagen content is further decreased (Skinner et al., 1981; Hampson et al., 1997; Stuart et al., 2005). These findings suggest that decreased collagen abundance characterizes the process of membrane rupture. We investigated whether cortisol regenerated in the fetal membranes is involved in the reduction of collagens in cultured primary human amnion fibroblasts, which are the major source of ECM proteins in the amnion compact layer (Casey and MacDonald, 1996). We have demonstrated that cortisol decreases the abundance of collagen I and III protein in a concentration-dependent manner with no effects on their mRNA abundance in amnion fibroblasts. Further mechanistic studies have revealed that cortisol decreases collagen I and III protein abundance by activating the autophagic and proteasome pathways, respectively (Mi et al., 2017, 2018). In addition to collagen I and III, collagen IV is essential for the maintenance of epithelial basal membrane as well as for the ECM structural protein assembling in the amnion (Malak et al., 1993; Bryant-Greenwood, 1998). For this reason, collagen IV is known as another crucial determinant of membrane integrity. By using human amnion fibroblasts, we have found that cortisol also causes the breakdown of collagen IV in a concentration-dependent manner through drastic induction of the expression of matrix metalloprotease 7 (MMP-7), also known as matrilysin, *via* activation of the AP-1 transcription factor (Wang et al., 2019a). These inhibitory effects of cortisol on collagen I, III, and IV have shown to be GR-mediated effects and have been confirmed in amnion tissue explant experiments. These findings are also substantiated by concurrent increases in cortisol, 11β-HSD1, MMP-7, and markers for autophagy and decreases in collagen I, III, and IV in the amnion tissue collected from spontaneous labor with membrane rupture (Liu et al., 2016a; Mi et al., 2017, 2018; Wang et al., 2019a,b).

The tensile strength of the amnion is determined not only by collagen abundance, but also by the degree of their cross-linking. Cross-linked collagens become tough and resistant to the breakdown by MMPs (Vater et al., 1979). It is now known that the cross-linking of collagens is catalyzed by lysyl oxidase (LOX), a copper-dependent amine oxidase (Kagan and Trackman, 1991). It has been shown that LOX protein and enzyme activity decrease dramatically in the amnion with advancing gestational age and further decrease in spontaneous labor with membrane rupture (Casey and MacDonald, 1997; Liu et al., 2016a,b). We have demonstrated that both cortisol and cortisone inhibit LOX expression in human amnion fibroblasts, and the effect of cortisone is abolished with inhibition of 11β-HSD1 (Liu et al., 2016a). Again, these effects have proved to be mediated by GR and have been replicated in amnion tissue explant experiments.

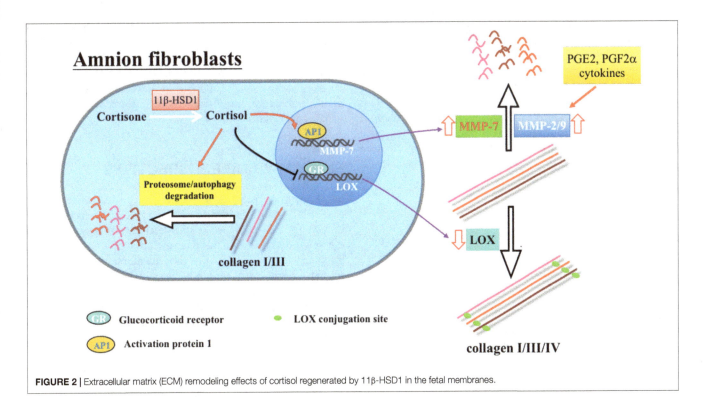

FIGURE 2 | Extracellular matrix (ECM) remodeling effects of cortisol regenerated by 11β-HSD1 in the fetal membranes.

In addition to the effects mediated directly by GR, an alternative mechanism is also present in ECM remodeling effects of cortisol. It has been shown that serum amyloid A1 (SAA1), an acute phase protein produced primarily by the liver, could be produced locally in the fetal membranes (Li et al., 2017), where SAA1 exerts extensive ECM remodeling effects including induction of MMP-1, MMP-2, MMP-8, MMP-9, and MMP-13; inhibition of LOX-like 1; and evoking collagen degradation (Wang et al., 2019b,c). Moreover, SAA1 can induce the expression of 11β-HSD1, and cortisol can in turn stimulate the expression of SAA1 (Lu et al., 2019b,c), thus formulating a mutual reinforcing mechanism in the production of SAA1 and cortisol in the fetal membranes. These findings are suggestive of existence of an alternative mechanism through induction of SAA1 to remodel the ECM structure by cortisol in the fetal membranes. Taken together, all these findings of cortisol's actions on collagens, LOX, and MMP-7 in human amnion fibroblasts are supportive of the view that cortisol regenerated by 11β-HSD1 plays an important role in the ECM remodeling for membrane rupture at parturition (**Figure 2**).

ROLE OF CORTISOL REGENERATION IN THE STIMULATION OF PROSTAGLANDIN E2 AND F2α OUTPUT IN THE FETAL MEMBRANES

Prostaglandins, particularly prostaglandin E2 (PGE2) and prostaglandin F2α (PGF2α), play crucial roles in human parturition (Challis et al., 1997; Romero et al., 2014). They increase myometrium contractility, ripen the cervix, and promote fetal membrane rupture (Challis et al., 1997; Romero et al., 2014). Although all gestational tissues including fetal membranes and maternal decidua/myometrium are virtually capable of PGE2 and PGF2α synthesis, the fetal amnion and maternal decidua/myometrium are recognized to synthesize the most PGE2 and PGF2α, respectively (Duchesne et al., 1978; Mitchell et al., 1978; Okazaki et al., 1981; Rehnstrom et al., 1983). In the amnion, the capacity of PGE2 synthesis in interstitial fibroblasts is approximately 5 times more than the capacity in epithelial cells (Sun et al., 2003). In addition, amnion fibroblasts are also capable of synthesizing PGF2α, although not as much as PGE2 (Guo et al., 2014). As narrated above, glucocorticoids are the most widely used class of anti-inflammatory drugs with prominent inhibitory effects on the synthesis of proinflammatory cytokines, as well as prostaglandins (Rhen and Cidlowski, 2005). These inhibitory effects of glucocorticoids on prostaglandin synthesis are known to be executed mostly through inhibition of cyclooxygenase 2 (COX-2) expression, the rate-limiting enzyme in prostaglandin synthesis (Goppelt-Struebe et al., 1989; Lasa et al., 2001; Lim et al., 2014). However, it has been noted for a long time that there are parallel increases in cortisol and prostaglandin levels in the maternal circulation toward the end of human gestation, and this apparent contradiction is described as a gestational paradox (Casey et al., 1985). Several groups have confirmed that this paradoxical phenomenon holds true in human amnion fibroblasts (Potestio et al., 1988; Zakar et al., 1995; Blumenstein et al., 2000; Sun et al., 2003, 2006). It has been shown that both cortisol and synthetic glucocorticoids stimulate rather than inhibit the expression of COX-2 in human amnion fibroblasts. Moreover, glucocorticoids also induce the expression of cytosolic phospholipase A2 (cPLA2) in human amnion fibroblasts (Sun et al., 2003; Guo et al., 2008, 2010). Cytosolic phospholipase A2 catalyzes the formation of arachidonic acid, a rate-limiting substrate in prostaglandin synthesis, from membrane phospholipids. The mechanism underlying the paradoxical induction of cPLA2 and COX-2 by glucocorticoids is fascinating because glucocorticoids inhibit the expression of proinflammatory cytokines in amnion fibroblasts at the same time. We set out to delineate this paradoxical mechanism and it turned out to be a very complicated mechanism. It is revealed that glucocorticoids induce cPLA2 and COX-2 expression through stimulation of the cAMP/PKA pathway with subsequent activation of multiple transcription factors including CREB and STAT3, and so on (Zhu et al., 2009; Guo et al., 2010; Wang et al., 2015; Lu et al., 2017, 2019a). Interestingly, the classical inflammatory transcription factor, nuclear factor κB, is nevertheless inhibited by glucocorticoids (Guo, 2010), which is responsible for the inhibition of proinflammatory cytokine expression in human amnion fibroblasts, a situation resembling most of non-gestational tissues.

As depicted above, the amnion is also capable of synthesizing PGF2α, although not as much as PGE2 (Guo et al., 2014). There are multiple pathways for PGF2α synthesis in amnion fibroblast. In addition to PGF synthase (PGFS)–catalyzed formation of PGF2α from PGH2, PGF2α can also be converted from PGE2 by the enzyme carbonyl reductase 1 (CBR1) (Ziboh et al., 1977). We have found that cortisol significantly induces the synthesis of PGF2α through induction of CBR1 but not PGFS in amnion fibroblasts (Sun et al., 2003; Guo et al., 2014). This induction of CBR1 by cortisol was revealed to be GR-mediated enhancement of CBR1 transcription (Guo et al., 2014).

During the gestational period, there is abundant expression of prostaglandin degrading enzyme 15-hydroxyprostaglandin dehydrogenase (PGDH) in trophoblasts of the smooth chorion, which is known as a prostaglandin barrier (Cheung et al., 1992; Johnson et al., 2004). PGDH catalyzes NAD^+-linked oxidation of 15 (S)-hydroxyl group of prostaglandins resulting in inactivation of their biological activities (Tai et al., 2002). Therefore, PGE2 and PGF2α synthesized in the amnion are mostly blocked from reaching the uterus by this barrier. Studies have shown that the abundant expression of PGDH in chorion trophoblasts is maintained mostly by progesterone (Challis et al., 1999; Patel and Challis, 2002). However, this maintenance is eventually undermined by increasing concentrations of cortisol derived from the feedforward regeneration through 11β-HSD1 (Patel et al., 1999a,b; Patel and Challis, 2002). The involvement of 11β-HSD1 is supported by findings that inhibition of PGDH by cortisone is reversed by 11β-HSD1 inhibitor (Patel et al., 1999b). It has been suggested that accumulating cortisol may compete with progesterone for progesterone receptor, thereby attenuating the maintaining effect of progesterone on PGDH expression and leading to progressively undermined prostaglandin barrier in the smooth chorion at term (Patel et al., 2003). Like the situation of cPLA2 and COX-2 induction by glucocorticoids, the inhibition of PGDH by glucocorticoids in the smooth chorion is also a kind of paradox, which is in marked contrast to the induction of PGDH expression by glucocorticoids in most of non-gestational tissues (Xun et al., 1991; Tong and Tai, 2005). All these findings of glucocorticoids on the induction of cPLA2/COX-2/CBR1 in amnion fibroblasts and inhibition of PGDH in chorion trophoblasts are supportive of a role of cortisol regeneration in the stimulation of PGE2 and PGF2α output either by induction of their synthesis or by inhibition of their degradation in the fetal membranes (**Figure 3**).

SUMMARY AND PERSPECTIVES

In pregnancy, there is increasing cortisol regeneration by 11β-HSD1 toward the end of gestation. 11β-HSD1 is expressed in virtually all cell types in the fetal membranes. Although the smooth chorion of the fetal membranes is considered as atrophied chorionic villi, the fetal membranes including the smooth chorion are endocrinologically active in pregnancy. Cortisol regeneration by 11β-HSD1 is one of such endocrine activities. Cortisol regenerated by 11β-HSD1 is involved not only in ECM remodeling for membrane rupture but also in the upregulation of PGE2 and PGF2α outputs. Both are requisite events for the onset of parturition. In addition to the actions described in this review, it remains to be uncovered whether cortisol regenerated by 11β-HSD1 in the fetal membranes possesses other unknown actions pertinent to the onset of labor. Another interesting issue remains to be clarified is the apparent contradictions between the concurrent induction of prostaglandins and inhibition of proinflammatory cytokines by glucocorticoids in the fetal membranes. Because

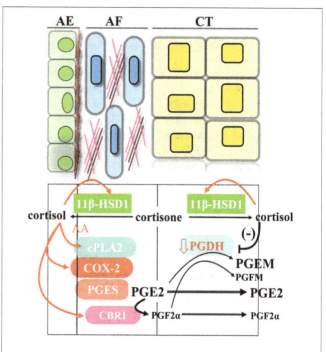

FIGURE 3 | Induction of PGE2 and PGF2α output by cortisol regenerated through 11β-HSD1 in human fetal membranes. AE, amnion epithelial cells; AF, amnion fibroblasts; CT, smooth chorion trophoblasts; AA, arachidonic acid.

both prostaglandins and proinflammatory cytokines are prolabor factors involved in ECM remodeling and uterine contractile activities (Keelan et al., 2003), it would be interesting to understand how these actions of cortisol on prostaglandins and proinflammatory cytokines are balanced in the fetal membrane at parturition, particularly in the situation of chorioamnionitis. Nevertheless, these effects of cortisol on ECM remodeling and prostaglandin output might be even enhanced in chorioamnionitis, given the potentiation of cortisol regeneration by proinflammatory cytokines. These apparent contradictions may represent a unique feature how glucocorticoids work locally in the fetal membranes in the promotion of labor. Simultaneous inhibition of proinflammatory cytokines and stimulation of prostaglandins by glucocorticoids may avoid deleterious effects of proinflammatory cytokines on the fetus on the one hand but save the labor promoting effects of prostaglandins on the other hand. Finally, it would be helpful to find a suitable animal model to replicate those findings in humans, such as the expression pattern of 11β-HSD1 across gestational age and those actions of glucocorticoids on ECM remodeling, prostaglandin synthesis, and degradation in the fetal membranes. What is more important is to test whether local artificial manipulation of 11β-HSD1 and GR expression in the fetal membranes can indeed change the course of gestation in the right animal model. Taking all together, we can conclude that cortisol regeneration in the fetal membranes is not a coincidental but a requisite event in parturition.

AUTHOR CONTRIBUTIONS

KS conceived the idea. KS, W-SW, and C-MG contributed to manuscript writing and figure preparation.

REFERENCES

Albiston, A. L., Obeyesekere, V. R., Smith, R. E., and Krozowski, Z. S. (1994). Cloning and tissue distribution of the human 11 beta-hydroxysteroid dehydrogenase type 2 enzyme. *Mol. Cell. Endocrinol.* 105, R11–R17. doi: 10.1016/0303-7207(94)90176-7

Alfaidy, N., Li, W., Macintosh, T., Yang, K., and Challis, J. (2003). Late gestation increase in 11beta-hydroxysteroid dehydrogenase 1 expression in human fetal membranes: a novel intrauterine source of cortisol. *J. Clin. Endocrinol. Metab.* 88, 5033–5038. doi: 10.1210/jc.2002-021915

Anderson, A. B., Flint, A. P., and Turnbull, A. C. (1975). Mechanism of action of glucocorticoids in induction of ovine parturition: effect on placental steroid metabolism. *J. Endocrinol.* 66, 61–70.

Bae, Y. J., and Kratzsch, J. (2015). Corticosteroid-binding globulin: modulating mechanisms of bioavailability of cortisol and its clinical implications. *Best Pract. Res. Clin. Endocrinol. Metab.* 29, 761–772. doi: 10.1016/j.beem.2015.09.001

Beato, M., and Klug, J. (2000). Steroid hormone receptors: an update. *Hum. Reprod. Update* 6, 225–236.

Berliner, D. L., Williams, R. J., Taylor, G. N., and Nabors, C. J. Jr. (1967). Decreased scar formation with topical corticosteroid treatment. *Surgery* 61, 619–625.

Blumenstein, M., Hansen, W. R., Deval, D., and Mitchell, M. D. (2000). Differential regulation in human amnion epithelial and fibroblast cells of prostaglandin E(2) production and prostaglandin H synthase-2 mRNA expression by dexamethasone but not tumour necrosis factor-alpha. *Placenta* 21, 210–217. doi: 10.1053/plac.1999.0473

Bollapragada, S., Youssef, R., Jordan, F., Greer, I., Norman, J., and Nelson, S. (2009). Term labor is associated with a core inflammatory response in human fetal membranes, myometrium, and cervix. *Am. J. Obstet. Gynecol.* 200, 104.e1-11. doi: 10.1016/j.ajog.2008.08.032

Boudon, S. M., Vuorinen, A., Geotti-Bianchini, P., Wandeler, E., Kratschmar, D. V., Heidl, M., et al. (2017). Novel 11beta-hydroxysteroid dehydrogenase 1 inhibitors reduce cortisol levels in keratinocytes and improve dermal collagen content in human ex vivo skin after exposure to cortisone and UV. *PLoS One* 12:e0171079. doi: 10.1371/journal.pone.0171079

Bourne, G. (1962). The foetal membranes. A review of the anatomy of normal amnion and chorion and some aspects of their function. *Postgrad. Med. J.* 38, 193–201. doi: 10.1136/pgmj.38.438.193

Bourne, G. L. (1960). The microscopic anatomy of the human amnion and chorion. *Am. J. Obstet. Gynecol.* 79, 1070–1073. doi: 10.1016/0002-9378(60)90512-3

Bryant-Greenwood, G. D. (1998). The extracellular matrix of the human fetal membranes: structure and function. *Placenta* 19, 1–11. doi: 10.1016/s0143-4004(98)90092-3

Burton, P. J., and Waddell, B. J. (1994). 11 beta-Hydroxysteroid dehydrogenase in the rat placenta: developmental changes and the effects of altered glucocorticoid exposure. *J. Endocrinol.* 143, 505–513. doi: 10.1677/joe.0.1430505

Burton, P. J., and Waddell, B. J. (1999). Dual function of 11beta-hydroxysteroid dehydrogenase in placenta: modulating placental glucocorticoid passage and local steroid action. *Biol. Reprod.* 60, 234–240. doi: 10.1095/biolreprod60.2.234

Casey, M. L., and MacDonald, P. C. (1996). Interstitial collagen synthesis and processing in human amnion: a property of the mesenchymal cells. *Biol. Reprod.* 55, 1253–1260. doi: 10.1095/biolreprod55.6.1253

Casey, M. L., and MacDonald, P. C. (1997). Lysyl oxidase (ras recision gene) expression in human amnion: ontogeny and cellular localization. *J. Clin. Endocrinol. Metab.* 82, 167–172. doi: 10.1210/jcem.82.1.3668

Casey, M. L., Macdonald, P. C., and Mitchell, M. D. (1985). Despite a massive increase in cortisol secretion in women during parturition, there is an equally massive increase in prostaglandin synthesis. A paradox? *J. Clin. Invest.* 75, 1852–1857. doi: 10.1172/JCI111899

Challis, J. R., Lye, S. J., and Gibb, W. (1997). Prostaglandins and parturition. *Ann. N. Y. Acad. Sci.* 828, 254–267.

Challis, J. R., Patel, F. A., and Pomini, F. (1999). Prostaglandin dehydrogenase and the initiation of labor. *J. Perinat. Med.* 27, 26–34.

Chapman, K., Holmes, M., and Seckl, J. (2013). 11beta-hydroxysteroid dehydrogenases: intracellular gate-keepers of tissue glucocorticoid action. *Physiol. Rev.* 93, 1139–1206. doi: 10.1152/physrev.00020.2012

Chapman, K. E., Kotelevtsev, Y. V., Jamieson, P. M., Williams, L. J., Mullins, J. J., and Seckl, J. R. (1997). Tissue-specific modulation of glucocorticoid action by the 11 beta-hydroxysteroid dehydrogenases. *Biochem. Soc. Trans.* 25, 583–587. doi: 10.1042/bst0250583

Cheung, P. Y., Walton, J. C., Tai, H. H., Riley, S. C., and Challis, J. R. (1992). Localization of 15-hydroxy prostaglandin dehydrogenase in human fetal membranes, decidua, and placenta during pregnancy. *Gynecol. Obstet. Invest.* 33, 142–146. doi: 10.1159/000294868

Craft, I., Brummer, V., Horwell, D., and Morgan, H. (1976). Betamethazone induction of labour. *Proc. R. Soc. Med.* 69, 827–828.

Cutroneo, K. R., Rokowski, R., and Counts, D. F. (1981). Glucocorticoids and collagen synthesis: comparison of in vivo and cell culture studies. *Coll. Relat. Res.* 1, 557–568. doi: 10.1016/s0174-173x(81)80037-4

Cutroneo, K. R., Stassen, F. L., and Cardinale, G. J. (1975). Anti-inflammatory steroids and collagen metabolism: glucocorticoid-mediated decrease of prolyl hydroxylase. *Mol. Pharmacol.* 11, 44–51.

Drake, A. J., Tang, J. I., and Nyirenda, M. J. (2007). Mechanisms underlying the role of glucocorticoids in the early life programming of adult disease. *Clin. Sci.* 113, 219–232. doi: 10.1042/CS20070107

Duchesne, M. J., Thaler-Dao, H., and De Paulet, A. C. (1978). Prostaglandin synthesis in human placenta and fetal membranes. *Prostaglandins* 15, 19–42.

Esteves, C. L., Kelly, V., Breton, A., Taylor, A. I., West, C. C., Donadeu, F. X., et al. (2014). Proinflammatory cytokine induction of 11beta-hydroxysteroid dehydrogenase type 1 (11beta-HSD1) in human adipocytes is mediated by MEK, C/EBPbeta, and NF-kappaB/RelA. *J. Clin. Endocrinol. Metab.* 99, E160–E168. doi: 10.1210/jc.2013-1708

Ferner, K., and Mess, A. (2011). Evolution and development of fetal membranes and placentation in amniote vertebrates. *Respir. Physiol. Neurobiol.* 178, 39–50. doi: 10.1016/j.resp.2011.03.029

First, N. L., and Bosc, M. J. (1979). Proposed mechanisms controlling parturition and the induction of parturition in swine. *J. Anim. Sci.* 48, 1407–1421. doi: 10.2527/jas1979.4861407x

Flint, A. P., Kingston, E. J., Robinson, J. S., and Thorburn, G. D. (1978). Initiation of parturition in the goat: evidence for control by foetal glucocorticoid through activation of placental C21-steroid 17alpha-hydroxylase. *J. Endocrinol.* 78, 367–378. doi: 10.1677/joe.0.0780367

Fowden, A. L., Forhead, A. J., and Ousey, J. C. (2008). The endocrinology of equine parturition. *Exp. Clin. Endocrinol. Diabetes* 116, 393–403. doi: 10.1055/s-2008-1042409

Goppelt-Struebe, M., Wolter, D., and Resch, K. (1989). Glucocorticoids inhibit prostaglandin synthesis not only at the level of phospholipase A2 but also at the level of cyclo-oxygenase/PGE isomerase. *Br. J. Pharmacol.* 98, 1287–1295. doi: 10.1111/j.1476-5381.1989.tb12676.x

Guo, C., Li, J., Myatt, L., Zhu, X., and Sun, K. (2010). Induction of Galphas contributes to the paradoxical stimulation of cytosolic phospholipase A2alpha expression by cortisol in human amnion fibroblasts. *Mol. Endocrinol.* 24, 1052–1061. doi: 10.1210/me.2009-0488

Guo, C., Wang, W., Liu, C., Myatt, L., and Sun, K. (2014). Induction of PGF2alpha synthesis by cortisol through GR dependent induction of CBR1 in human amnion fibroblasts. *Endocrinology* 155, 3017–3024. doi: 10.1210/en.2013-1848

Guo, C., Yang, Z., Li, W., Zhu, P., Myatt, L., and Sun, K. (2008). Paradox of glucocorticoid-induced cytosolic phospholipase A2 group IVA messenger RNA expression involves glucocorticoid receptor binding to the promoter in human amnion fibroblasts. *Biol. Reprod.* 78, 193–197. doi: 10.1095/biolreprod.107.063990

Guo, C. M. (2010). *Molecular Mechanism of the Paradoxical Induction of Cytosolic Phospholipase A2 by Glucocorticoids in Human Amnion Fibroblasts*. Doctoral thesis, Fudan University, Shanghai.

Hampson, V., Liu, D., Billett, E., and Kirk, S. (1997). Amniotic membrane collagen content and type distribution in women with preterm premature rupture of the membranes in pregnancy. *Br. J. Obstet. Gynaecol.* 104, 1087–1091. doi: 10.1111/j.1471-0528.1998.tb10107.x

Ignatova, I. D., Kostadinova, R. M., Goldring, C. E., Nawrocki, A. R., Frey, F. J., and Frey, B. M. (2009). Tumor necrosis factor-alpha upregulates 11beta-hydroxysteroid dehydrogenase type 1 expression by CCAAT/enhancer binding protein-beta in HepG2 cells. *Am. J. Physiol. Endocrinol. Metab.* 296, E367–E377. doi: 10.1152/ajpendo.90531.2008

Ishimoto, H., and Jaffe, R. B. (2011). Development and function of the human fetal adrenal cortex: a key component in the feto-placental unit. *Endocr. Rev.* 32, 317–355. doi: 10.1210/er.2010-0001

Jalali, M., and Bayat, A. (2007). Current use of steroids in management of abnormal raised skin scars. *Surgeon* 5, 175–180. doi: 10.1016/s1479-666x(07)80045-x

Johnson, R. F., Mitchell, C. M., Clifton, V., and Zakar, T. (2004). Regulation of 15-hydroxyprostaglandin dehydrogenase (PGDH) gene activity, messenger ribonucleic acid processing, and protein abundance in the human chorion in late gestation and labor. *J. Clin. Endocrinol. Metab.* 89, 5639–5648. doi: 10.1210/jc.2004-0540

Kagan, H. M., and Trackman, P. C. (1991). Properties and function of lysyl oxidase. *Am. J. Respir. Cell Mol. Biol.* 5, 206–210.

Kaur, K., Hardy, R., Ahasan, M. M., Eijken, M., Van Leeuwen, J. P., Filer, A., et al. (2010). Synergistic induction of local glucocorticoid generation by inflammatory cytokines and glucocorticoids: implications for inflammation associated bone loss. *Ann. Rheum. Dis.* 69, 1185–1190. doi: 10.1136/ard.2009.107466

Keelan, J. A., Blumenstein, M., Helliwell, R. J., Sato, T. A., Marvin, K. W., and Mitchell, M. D. (2003). Cytokines, prostaglandins and parturition–a review. *Placenta* 24 (Suppl A) S33–S46.

Krozowski, Z., Maguire, J. A., Stein-Oakley, A. N., Dowling, J., Smith, R. E., and Andrews, R. K. (1995). Immunohistochemical localization of the 11 beta-hydroxysteroid dehydrogenase type II enzyme in human kidney and placenta. *J. Clin. Endocrinol. Metab.* 80, 2203–2209. doi: 10.1210/jcem.80.7.7608280

Lasa, M., Brook, M., Saklatvala, J., and Clark, A. R. (2001). Dexamethasone destabilizes cyclooxygenase 2 mRNA by inhibiting mitogen-activated protein kinase p38. *Mol. Cell. Biol.* 21, 771–780. doi: 10.1128/MCB.21.3.771-780.2001

Leiser, R., and Kaufmann, P. (1994). Placental structure: in a comparative aspect. *Exp. Clin. Endocrinol.* 102, 122–134.

Lewis, J. G., Bagley, C. J., Elder, P. A., Bachmann, A. W., and Torpy, D. J. (2005). Plasma free cortisol fraction reflects levels of functioning corticosteroid-binding globulin. *Clin. Chim. Acta* 359, 189–194. doi: 10.1016/j.cccn.2005.03.044

Li, J., Wang, W., Liu, C., Wang, W., Li, W., Shu, Q., et al. (2013). Critical role of histone acetylation by p300 in human placental 11beta-HSD2 expression. *J. Clin. Endocrinol. Metab.* 98, E1189–E1197. doi: 10.1210/jc.2012-4291

Li, J. N., Ge, Y. C., Yang, Z., Guo, C. M., Duan, T., Myatt, L., et al. (2011). The Sp1 transcription factor is crucial for the expression of 11beta-hydroxysteroid dehydrogenase type 2 in human placental trophoblasts. *J. Clin. Endocrinol. Metab.* 96, E899–E907. doi: 10.1210/jc.2010-2852

Li, W., Gao, L., Wang, Y., Duan, T., Myatt, L., and Sun, K. (2006). Enhancement of cortisol-induced 11beta-hydroxysteroid dehydrogenase type 1 expression by interleukin 1beta in cultured human chorionic trophoblast cells. *Endocrinology* 147, 2490–2495. doi: 10.1210/en.2005-1626

Li, W., Wang, W., Zuo, R., Liu, C., Shu, Q., Ying, H., et al. (2017). Induction of pro-inflammatory genes by serum amyloid A1 in human amnion fibroblasts. *Sci. Rep.* 7:693. doi: 10.1038/s41598-017-00782-9

Lim, W., Park, C., Shim, M. K., Lee, Y. H., Lee, Y. M., and Lee, Y. (2014). Glucocorticoids suppress hypoxia-induced COX-2 and hypoxia inducible factor-1alpha expression through the induction of glucocorticoid-induced leucine zipper. *Br. J. Pharmacol.* 171, 735–745. doi: 10.1111/bph.12491

Liu, C., Guo, C., Wang, W., Zhu, P., Li, W., Mi, Y., et al. (2016a). Inhibition of lysyl oxidase by cortisol regeneration in human amnion: implications for rupture of fetal membranes. *Endocrinology* 157, 4055–4065. doi: 10.1210/en.2016-1406

Liu, C., Zhu, P., Wang, W., Li, W., Shu, Q., Chen, Z. J., et al. (2016b). Inhibition of lysyl oxidase by prostaglandin E2 via EP2/EP4 receptors in human amnion fibroblasts: implications for parturition. *Mol. Cell. Endocrinol.* 424, 118–127. doi: 10.1016/j.mce.2016.04.016

Lu, J., Wang, W., Mi, Y., Zhang, C., Ying, H., Wang, L., et al. (2017). AKAP95-mediated nuclear anchoring of PKA mediates cortisol-induced PTGS2 expression in human amnion fibroblasts. *Sci. Signal.* 10:eaac6160. doi: 10.1126/scisignal.aac6160

Lu, J. W., Wang, W. S., Zhou, Q., Gan, X. W., Myatt, L., and Sun, K. (2019a). Activation of prostaglandin EP4 receptor attenuates the induction of cyclooxygenase-2 expression by EP2 receptor activation in human amnion fibroblasts: implications for parturition. *FASEB J.* 33, 8148–8160. doi: 10.1096/fj.201802642R

Lu, Y., Wang, W. S., Lin, Y. K., Lu, J. W., Li, W. J., Zhang, C. Y., et al. (2019b). Enhancement of cortisol-induced SAA1 transcription by SAA1 in the human amnion. *J. Mol. Endocrinol.* 62, 149–158. doi: 10.1530/JME-18-0263

Lu, Y., Zhou, Q., Lu, J. W., Wang, W. S., and Sun, K. (2019c). Involvement of STAT3 in the synergistic induction of 11beta-HSD1 by SAA1 and cortisol in human amnion fibroblasts. *Am. J. Reprod. Immunol.* 82:e13150. doi: 10.1111/aji.13150

Malak, T. M., Ockleford, C. D., Bell, S. C., Dalgleish, R., Bright, N., and Macvicar, J. (1993). Confocal immunofluorescence localization of collagen types I, III, IV, V and VI and their ultrastructural organization in term human fetal membranes. *Placenta* 14, 385–406. doi: 10.1016/s0143-4004(05)80460-6

Menon, R. (2016). Human fetal membranes at term: dead tissue or signalers of parturition? *Placenta* 44, 1–5. doi: 10.1016/j.placenta.2016.05.013

Menon, R., Bonney, E. A., Condon, J., Mesiano, S., and Taylor, R. N. (2016). Novel concepts on pregnancy clocks and alarms: redundancy and synergy in human parturition. *Hum. Reprod. Update* 22, 535–560. doi: 10.1093/humupd/dmw022

Menon, R., and Moore, J. J. (2020). Fetal membranes, not a mere appendage of the placenta, but a critical part of the fetal-maternal interface controlling parturition. *Obstet. Gynecol. Clin. North Am.* 47, 147–162. doi: 10.1016/j.ogc.2019.10.004

Menon, R., Taylor, R. N., and Fortunato, S. J. (2010). Chorioamnionitis–a complex pathophysiologic syndrome. *Placenta* 31, 113–120. doi: 10.1016/j.placenta.2009.11.012

Mesiano, S. (2001). Roles of estrogen and progesterone in human parturition. *Front. Horm. Res.* 27, 86–104. doi: 10.1159/000061038

Mesiano, S., and Jaffe, R. B. (1997). Developmental and functional biology of the primate fetal adrenal cortex. *Endocr. Rev.* 18, 378–403. doi: 10.1210/edrv.18.3. 0304

Mess, A., Blackburn, D. G., and Zeller, U. (2003). Evolutionary transformations of fetal membranes and reproductive strategies. *J. Exp. Zool. A Comp. Exp. Biol.* 299, 3–12. doi: 10.1002/jez.a.10287

Meyer, E. J., Nenke, M. A., Rankin, W., Lewis, J. G., and Torpy, D. J. (2016). Corticosteroid-binding globulin: a review of basic and clinical advances. *Horm. Metab. Res.* 48, 359–371. doi: 10.1055/s-0042-108071

Mi, Y., Wang, W., Lu, J., Zhang, C., Wang, Y., Ying, H., et al. (2018). Proteasome-mediated degradation of collagen III by cortisol in amnion fibroblasts. *J. Mol. Endocrinol.* 60, 45–54. doi: 10.1530/JME-17-0215

Mi, Y., Wang, W., Zhang, C., Liu, C., Lu, J., Li, W., et al. (2017). Autophagic degradation of collagen 1A1 by cortisol in human amnion fibroblasts. *Endocrinology* 158, 1005–1014. doi: 10.1210/en.2016-1829

Miller, W. L., and Auchus, R. J. (2011). The molecular biology, biochemistry, and physiology of human steroidogenesis and its disorders. *Endocr. Rev.* 32, 81–151. doi: 10.1210/er.2010-0013

Mitchell, M. D., Bibby, J., Hicks, B. R., and Turnbull, A. C. (1978). Specific production of prostaglandin E by human amnion in vitro. *Prostaglandins* 15, 377–382. doi: 10.1016/0090-6980(78)90177-6

Morgan, S. A., Mccabe, E. L., Gathercole, L. L., Hassan-Smith, Z. K., Larner, D. P., Bujalska, I. J., et al. (2014). 11beta-HSD1 is the major regulator of the tissue-specific effects of circulating glucocorticoid excess. *Proc. Natl. Acad. Sci. U.S.A.* 111, E2482–E2491. doi: 10.1073/pnas.1323681111

Morrison, D. G., Humes, P. E., and Godke, R. A. (1983). The use of dimenhydrinate in conjunction with dexamethasone for induction of parturition in beef cattle. *Theriogenology* 19, 221–233. doi: 10.1016/0093-691x(83)90 008-0

Murphy, B. E. (1977). Chorionic membrane as an extra-adrenal source of foetal cortisol in human amniotic fluid. *Nature* 266, 179–181. doi: 10.1038/266179a0

Murphy, B. E. (1979). Cortisol and cortisone in human fetal development. *J. Steroid Biochem.* 11, 509–513.

Murphy, B. E. (1981). Ontogeny of cortisol-cortisone interconversion in human tissues: a role for cortisone in human fetal development. *J. Steroid Biochem.* 14, 811–817. doi: 10.1016/0022-4731(81)90226-0

Myatt, L., and Sun, K. (2010). Role of fetal membranes in signaling of fetal maturation and parturition. *Int. J. Dev. Biol.* 54, 545–553. doi: 10.1387/ijdb. 082771lm

Ni, X. T., Duan, T., Yang, Z., Guo, C. M., Li, J. N., and Sun, K. (2009). Role of human chorionic gonadotropin in maintaining 11beta-hydroxysteroid dehydrogenase type 2 expression in human placental syncytiotrophoblasts. *Placenta* 30, 1023–1028. doi: 10.1016/j.placenta.2009.10.005

Nuutinen, P., Autio, P., Hurskainen, T., and Oikarinen, A. (2001). Glucocorticoid action on skin collagen: overview on clinical significance and consequences. *J. Eur. Acad. Dermatol. Venereol.* 15, 361–362.

Ogueh, O., Jones, J., Mitchell, H., Alaghband-Zadeh, J., and Johnson, M. R. (1999). Effect of antenatal dexamethasone therapy on maternal plasma human chorionic gonadotrophin, oestradiol and progesterone. *Hum. Reprod.* 14, 303–306. doi: 10.1093/humrep/14.2.303

Oishi, Y., Fu, Z. W., Ohnuki, Y., Kato, H., and Noguchi, T. (2002). Molecular basis of the alteration in skin collagen metabolism in response to in vivo dexamethasone treatment: effects on the synthesis of collagen type I and III, collagenase, and tissue inhibitors of metalloproteinases. *Br. J. Dermatol.* 147, 859–868. doi: 10.1046/j.1365-2133.2002.04949.x

Okazaki, T., Casey, M. L., Okita, J. R., Macdonald, P. C., and Johnston, J. M. (1981). Initiation of human parturition. XII. Biosynthesis and metabolism of prostaglandins in human fetal membranes and uterine decidua. *Am. J. Obstet. Gynecol.* 139, 373–381.

Osinski, P. A. (1960). Steroid 11beta-ol dehydrogenase in human placenta. *Nature* 187:777.

Oyen, M. L., Calvin, S. E., and Landers, D. V. (2006). Premature rupture of the fetal membranes: is the amnion the major determinant? *Am. J. Obstet. Gynecol.* 195, 510–515. doi: 10.1016/j.ajog.2006.02.010

Parry, S., and Strauss, J. F, 3rd. (1998). Premature rupture of the fetal membranes. *N. Engl. J. Med.* 338, 663–670.

Patel, F. A., and Challis, J. R. (2002). Cortisol/progesterone antagonism in regulation of 15-hydroxysteroid dehydrogenase activity and mRNA levels in human chorion and placental trophoblast cells at term. *J. Clin. Endocrinol. Metab.* 87, 700–708. doi: 10.1210/jcem.87.2.8245

Patel, F. A., Clifton, V. L., Chwalisz, K., and Challis, J. R. (1999a). Steroid regulation of prostaglandin dehydrogenase activity and expression in human term placenta and chorio-decidua in relation to labor. *J. Clin. Endocrinol. Metab.* 84, 291–299. doi: 10.1210/jcem.84.1.5399

Patel, F. A., Sun, K., and Challis, J. R. (1999b). Local modulation by 11beta-hydroxysteroid dehydrogenase of glucocorticoid effects on the activity of 15-hydroxyprostaglandin dehydrogenase in human chorion and placental trophoblast cells. *J. Clin. Endocrinol. Metab.* 84, 395–400. doi: 10.1210/jcem. 84.2.5442

Patel, F. A., Funder, J. W., and Challis, J. R. (2003). Mechanism of cortisol/progesterone antagonism in the regulation of 15-hydroxyprostaglandin dehydrogenase activity and messenger ribonucleic acid levels in human chorion and placental trophoblast cells at term. *J. Clin. Endocrinol. Metab.* 88, 2922–2933. doi: 10.1210/jc.2002-021710

Pepe, G. J., Waddell, B. J., Burch, M. G., and Albrecht, E. D. (1996). Interconversion of cortisol and cortisone in the baboon placenta at midgestation: expression of 11beta-hydroxysteroid dehydrogenase type 1 messenger RNA. *J. Steroid Biochem. Mol. Biol.* 58, 403–410. doi: 10.1016/0960-0760(96)00049-0

Potestio, F. A., Zakar, T., and Olson, D. M. (1988). Glucocorticoids stimulate prostaglandin synthesis in human amnion cells by a receptor-mediated mechanism. *J. Clin. Endocrinol. Metab.* 67, 1205–1210. doi: 10.1210/jcem-67-6-1205

Rae, M. T., Niven, D., Critchley, H. O., Harlow, C. R., and Hillier, S. G. (2004). Antiinflammatory steroid action in human ovarian surface epithelial cells. *J. Clin. Endocrinol. Metab.* 89, 4538–4544. doi: 10.1210/jc.2003-032225

Rehnstrom, J., Ishikawa, M., Fuchs, F., and Fuchs, A. R. (1983). Stimulation of myometrial and decidual prostaglandin production by amniotic fluid from term, but not midtrimester pregnancies. *Prostaglandins* 26, 973–981. doi: 10. 1016/0090-6980(83)90158-2

Rhen, T., and Cidlowski, J. A. (2005). Antiinflammatory action of glucocorticoids-new mechanisms for old drugs. *N. Engl. J. Med.* 353, 1711–1723. doi: 10.1056/ NEJMra050541

Romero, R., Dey, S. K., and Fisher, S. J. (2014). Preterm labor: one syndrome, many causes. *Science* 345, 760–765. doi: 10.1126/science.1251816

Schmid, W., Cole, T. J., Blendy, J. A., and Schutz, G. (1995). Molecular genetic analysis of glucocorticoid signalling in development. *J. Steroid Biochem. Mol. Biol.* 53, 33–35. doi: 10.1016/0960-0760(95)00038-2

Schoepe, S., Schacke, H., May, E., and Asadullah, K. (2006). Glucocorticoid therapy-induced skin atrophy. *Exp. Dermatol.* 15, 406–420.

Shull, S., and Cutroneo, K. R. (1986). Glucocorticoids change the ratio of type III to type I procollagen extracellularly. *Coll. Relat. Res.* 6, 295–300. doi: 10.1016/ s0174-173x(86)80013-9

Singh, N., Herbert, B., Sooranna, G., Das, A., Sooranna, S. R., Yellon, S. M., et al. (2019). Distinct preterm labor phenotypes have unique inflammatory signatures and contraction associated protein profilesdagger. *Biol. Reprod.* 101, 1031–1045. doi: 10.1093/biolre/ioz144

Skinner, S. J., Campos, G. A., and Liggins, G. C. (1981). Collagen content of human amniotic membranes: effect of gestation length and premature rupture. *Obstet. Gynecol.* 57, 487–489.

Sterry, W., and Asadullah, K. (2002). "Topical glucocorticoid therapy in dermatology," in *Recent Advances in Glucocorticoid Receptor Action. Ernst Schering Research Foundation Workshop*, eds A. C. B Cato, H Schäcke, and K Asadullah, (Berlin: Springer) 39–54.

Stuart, E. L., Evans, G. S., Lin, Y. S., and Powers, H. J. (2005). Reduced collagen and ascorbic acid concentrations and increased proteolytic susceptibility with prelabor fetal membrane rupture in women. *Biol. Reprod.* 72, 230–235. doi: 10.1095/biolreprod.104.033381

Sun, K., He, P., and Yang, K. (2002). Intracrine induction of 11beta-hydroxysteroid dehydrogenase type 1 expression by glucocorticoid potentiates prostaglandin production in the human chorionic trophoblast. *Biol. Reprod.* 67, 1450–1455. doi: 10.1095/biolreprod.102.005892

Sun, K., Ma, R., Cui, X., Campos, B., Webster, R., Brockman, D., et al. (2003). Glucocorticoids induce cytosolic phospholipase A2 and prostaglandin H synthase type 2 but not microsomal prostaglandin E synthase (PGES) and cytosolic PGES expression in cultured primary human amnion cells. *J. Clin. Endocrinol. Metab.* 88, 5564–5571. doi: 10.1210/jc.2003-030875

Sun, K., and Myatt, L. (2003). Enhancement of glucocorticoid-induced 11beta-hydroxysteroid dehydrogenase type 1 expression by proinflammatory cytokines in cultured human amnion fibroblasts. *Endocrinology* 144, 5568–5577. doi: 10.1210/en.2003-0780

Sun, K., Qu, X., Gao, L., and Myatt, L. (2006). Dexamethasone fails to inhibit the induction of cytosolic phospholipase A(2) expression by interleukin-1beta in cultured primary human amnion fibroblasts. *Placenta* 27, 164–170. doi: 10.1016/j.placenta.2005.03.004

Sun, K., Yang, K., and Challis, J. R. (1997). Differential expression of 11 beta-hydroxysteroid dehydrogenase types 1 and 2 in human placenta and fetal membranes. *J. Clin. Endocrinol. Metab.* 82, 300–305. doi: 10.1210/jcem.82.1.3681

Sun, M., Ramirez, M., Challis, J. R., and Gibb, W. (1996). Immunohistochemical localization of the glucocorticoid receptor in human fetal membranes and decidua at term and preterm delivery. *J. Endocrinol.* 149, 243–248. doi: 10.1677/joe.0.1490243

Tai, H. H., Ensor, C. M., Tong, M., Zhou, H., and Yan, F. (2002). Prostaglandin catabolizing enzymes. *Prostaglandins Other Lipid Mediat.* 68–69, 483–493.

Tannin, G. M., Agarwal, A. K., Monder, C., New, M. I., and White, P. C. (1991). The human gene for 11 beta-hydroxysteroid dehydrogenase. Structure, tissue distribution, and chromosomal localization. *J. Biol. Chem.* 266, 16653–16658.

Tanswell, A. K., Worthington, D., and Smith, B. T. (1977). Human amniotic membrane corticosteroid 11-oxidoreductase activity. *J. Clin. Endocrinol. Metab.* 45, 721–725.

Tomlinson, J. W., Moore, J., Cooper, M. S., Bujalska, I., Shahmanesh, M., Burt, C., et al. (2001). Regulation of expression of 11beta-hydroxysteroid dehydrogenase type 1 in adipose tissue: tissue-specific induction by cytokines. *Endocrinology* 142, 1982–1989. doi: 10.1210/endo.142.5.8168

Tomlinson, J. W., Walker, E. A., Bujalska, I. J., Draper, N., Lavery, G. G., Cooper, M. S., et al. (2004). 11beta-hydroxysteroid dehydrogenase type 1: a tissue-specific regulator of glucocorticoid response. *Endocr. Rev.* 25, 831–866. doi: 10.1210/er.2003-0031

Tong, M., and Tai, H. H. (2005). 15-Hydroxyprostaglandin dehydrogenase can be induced by dexamethasone and other glucocorticoids at the therapeutic level in A549 human lung adenocarcinoma cells. *Arch. Biochem. Biophys.* 435, 50–55. doi: 10.1016/j.abb.2004.11.031

Vater, C. A., Harris, E. D. Jr., and Siegel, R. C. (1979). Native cross-links in collagen fibrils induce resistance to human synovial collagenase. *Biochem. J.* 181, 639–645. doi: 10.1042/bj1810639

Wang, L. Y., Wang, W. S., Wang, Y. W., Lu, J. W., Lu, Y., Zhang, C. Y., et al. (2019a). Drastic induction of MMP-7 by cortisol in the human amnion: implications for membrane rupture at parturition. *FASEB J.* 33, 2770–2781. doi: 10.1096/fj.201801216R

Wang, W. S., Li, W. J., Wang, Y. W., Wang, L. Y., Mi, Y. B., Lu, J. W., et al. (2019b). Involvement of serum amyloid A1 in the rupture of fetal membranes through induction of collagen I degradation. *Clin. Sci.* 133, 515–530. doi: 10.1042/CS20180950

Wang, Y. W., Wang, W. S., Wang, L. Y., Bao, Y. R., Lu, J. W., Lu, Y., et al. (2019c). Extracellular matrix remodeling effects of serum amyloid A1 in the human amnion: Implications for fetal membrane rupture. *Am. J. Reprod. Immunol.* 81:e13073. doi: 10.1111/aji.13073

Wang, W., Chen, Z. J., Myatt, L., and Sun, K. (2018). 11beta-HSD1 in human fetal membranes as a potential therapeutic target for preterm birth. *Endocr. Rev.* 39, 241–260. doi: 10.1210/er.2017-00188

Wang, W., Guo, C., Li, W., Li, J., Wang, W., Myatt, L., et al. (2012). Involvement of GR and p300 in the induction of H6PD by cortisol in human amnion fibroblasts. *Endocrinology* 153, 5993–6002. doi: 10.1210/en.2012-1531

Wang, W., Guo, C., Zhu, P., Lu, J., Li, W., Liu, C., et al. (2015). Phosphorylation of STAT3 mediates the induction of cyclooxygenase-2 by cortisol in the human amnion at parturition. *Sci. Signal.* 8:ra106. doi: 10.1126/scisignal.aac6151

Wang, W., Liu, C., and Sun, K. (2016). Induction of amnion epithelial apoptosis by cortisol via tPA/Plasmin system. *Endocrinology* 157, 4487–4498. doi: 10.1210/en.2016-1464

White, P. C., Mune, T., and Agarwal, A. K. (1997a). 11 beta-Hydroxysteroid dehydrogenase and the syndrome of apparent mineralocorticoid excess. *Endocr. Rev.* 18, 135–156. doi: 10.1210/edrv.18.1.0288

White, P. C., Mune, T., Rogerson, F. M., Kayes, K. M., and Agarwal, A. K. (1997b). 11 beta-Hydroxysteroid dehydrogenase and its role in the syndrome of apparent mineralocorticoid excess. *Pediatr. Res.* 41, 25–29.

White, P. C., Mune, T., Rogerson, F. M., Kayes, K. M., and Agarwal, A. K. (1997c). Molecular analysis of 11 beta-hydroxysteroid dehydrogenase and its role in the syndrome of apparent mineralocorticoid excess. *Steroids* 62, 83–88. doi: 10.1016/s0039-128x(96)00164-x

Xun, C. Q., Ensor, C. M., and Tai, H. H. (1991). Regulation of synthesis and activity of NAD(+)-dependent 15-hydroxy-prostaglandin dehydrogenase (15-PGDH) by dexamethasone and phorbol ester in human erythroleukemia (HEL) cells. *Biochem. Biophys. Res. Commun.* 177, 1258–1265. doi: 10.1016/0006-291x(91)90677-y

Yang, K., Langlois, D. A., Campbell, L. E., Challis, J. R., Krkosek, M., and Yu, M. (1997). Cellular localization and developmental regulation of 11 beta-hydroxysteroid dehydrogenase type 1 (11 beta-HSD1) gene expression in the ovine placenta. *Placenta* 18, 503–509. doi: 10.1016/0143-4004(77)90003-0

Yang, Q., Wang, W., Liu, C., Wang, Y., and Sun, K. (2016). Compartmentalized localization of 11beta-HSD 1 and 2 at the feto-maternal interface in the first trimester of human pregnancy. *Placenta* 46, 63–71. doi: 10.1016/j.placenta.2016.08.079

Yang, Z., Guo, C., Zhu, P., Li, W., Myatt, L., and Sun, K. (2007). Role of glucocorticoid receptor and CCAAT/enhancer-binding protein alpha in the feed-forward induction of 11beta-hydroxysteroid dehydrogenase type 1 expression by cortisol in human amnion fibroblasts. *J. Endocrinol.* 195, 241–253. doi: 10.1677/JOE-07-0303

Yong, P. Y., Harlow, C., Thong, K. J., and Hillier, S. G. (2002). Regulation of 11beta-hydroxysteroid dehydrogenase type 1 gene expression in human ovarian surface epithelial cells by interleukin-1. *Hum. Reprod.* 17, 2300–2306. doi: 10.1093/humrep/17.9.2300

Zakar, T., Hirst, J. J., Mijovic, J. E., and Olson, D. M. (1995). Glucocorticoids stimulate the expression of prostaglandin endoperoxide H synthase-2 in amnion cells. *Endocrinology* 136, 1610–1619. doi: 10.1210/endo.136.4.7895671

Zhang, N., Wang, W., Li, W., Liu, C., Chen, Y., Yang, Q., et al. (2015). Inhibition of 11beta-HSD2 expression by triclosan via induction of apoptosis in human placental syncytiotrophoblasts. *J. Clin. Endocrinol. Metab.* 100, E542–E549. doi: 10.1210/jc.2014-4376

Zhu, X. O., Yang, Z., Guo, C. M., Ni, X. T., Li, J. N., Ge, Y. C., et al. (2009). Paradoxical stimulation of cyclooxygenase-2 expression by glucocorticoids via a cyclic AMP response element in human amnion fibroblasts. *Mol. Endocrinol.* 23, 1839–1849. doi: 10.1210/me.2009-0201

Ziboh, V. A., Lord, J. T., and Penneys, N. S. (1977). Alterations of prostaglandin E2-9-ketoreductase activity in proliferating skin. *J. Lipid Res.* 18, 37–43.

Zuo, R., Liu, X., Wang, W., Li, W., Ying, H., and Sun, K. (2017). A repressive role of enhancer of zeste homolog 2 in 11beta-hydroxysteroid dehydrogenase type 2 expression in the human placenta. *J. Biol. Chem.* 292, 7578–7587. doi: 10.1074/jbc.M116.765800

Premature Rupture of Membranes and Severe Weather Systems

*Mackenzie L. Wheeler and Michelle L. Oyen**

Department of Engineering, East Carolina University, Greenville, NC, United States

**Correspondence:*
Michelle L. Oyen
oyenm18@ecu.edu

There has long been anecdotal evidence of early labor and delivery in severe weather events leading to preterm birth. In particular, significant barometric pressure changes are associated with hurricanes and bomb cyclones. Some authors have related these low pressure weather events to premature rupture of fetal membranes, hypothesizing that the membranes act as an inflated balloon and respond directly to pressure changes. In this article, the key literature including data supporting this hypothesis is reviewed. A simple numerical model, based on a competition between the driving and resisting forces for fetal membrane rupture, is presented. This model provides a quantitative mechanism for membrane failure in the context of storms with low atmospheric pressure. Other sequelae of severe storms that are unrelated to fetal membrane rupture are also discussed. Labor and delivery in the context of major weather events should be understood in a holistic framework that includes both exogenous and endogenous factors relevant to the pregnant patient.

Keywords: preterm, premature, PROM, chorioamnion, fetal, membranes, rupture, failure

1. INTRODUCTION

There have been many articles written in the popular press about a potential association between major weather events, such as hurricanes, and early childbirth (LaFrance, 2016; Blau, 2017; Bolluyt, 2018). There is some evidence in the scientific literature in support of such an association, particularly between low levels of barometric pressure and premature rupture of the fetal membranes (PROM) (Polansky et al., 1985; Akutagawa et al., 2007). In this context, "premature" refers not to the gestational age of the pregnancy (instead that is called "preterm") but the rupture of the membranes prior to the onset of labor. Other studies have found no association between barometric pressure and PROM (Marks et al., 1983). However, the methodology associated with many articles in this genre has been criticized for being insufficient in terms of patient numbers, weather-related data, inadequate control populations, or other deficiencies.

The current work aims to examine this hypothesis of preterm PROM associated with significant drops in barometric pressure associated with major weather events. A number of key studies in this area will be reviewed in the first section of this paper. The physical mechanics of PROM and barometric pressure change will be elucidated with an analytical model in the following section. This will be followed by discussion and conclusions, emphasizing the need for further study on the relationship between major weather events and late-gestation pregnant women, with a view toward potential intervention via evacuation or watchful and conservative medical management.

2. KEY LITERATURE

An early study completed at the University of Iowa Hospital and published in 1985 (Polansky et al., 1985) showed that PROM occurred more often when the barometric pressure decreased 3 h beforehand. The results of this study further showed that the onset of labor for matched control patients within the same geographical area were not associated with barometric pressure changes. If there was an increase in barometric pressure instead of a drop in pressure, PROM was not affected. This study noted that previous authors examining the issue of PROM and barometric pressure suffered methodological deficiencies in their studies, and that Polansky et al. had designed their study to avoid these flaws. The article postulated that barometric pressure could create a gradient across the chorioamniotic membranes to maintain in utero pressure, but suggested that prostaglandins or other biochemical mechanisms could also be responsible.

A 1997 study focussed on the onset of labor associated with significant decreases in barometric pressure (King et al., 1997). Although not focussed on PROM or membrane rupture, a significant increase in the onset of labor was found in the 24 h after a significant barometric pressure drop and not in the 24 h prior. This study in a journal aimed at nurse-midwives, recommended that low pressure weather systems should be monitored in the context of labor and delivery units and that this association should be mentioned to pregnant women in childbirth classes.

A landmark retrospective study covering 1997–2003 and published in 2007 (Akutagawa et al., 2007) demonstrated that deliveries increased on days with a larger change in barometric pressure in a statistically significant manner. Rupture of the membranes, including premature rupture, was associated with lower barometric pressures, in this study defined by a cut-off value of 758.1 mm Hg (1010.7 hPa in their manuscript). The authors note that labor pains bare associated with both hormones and the autonomic system, and that these both could be affected by local weather and by more general environmental changes. However, they clearly postulate that the membrane rupture and low barometric pressure are not just associated but causal, consistent with the model developed in the following section.

An extensive series of studies of the physical strength of the chorioamnion membrane was performed by Oyen et al. (2004), Oyen et al. (2006), Calvin and Oyen (2007), and Chua and Oyen (2009) showing the decrease in membrane strength with gestational age. These studies focussed on labored versus C-section deliveries and the effects of twin pregnancies, emphasizing endogenous effects. In addition, these authors developed a mechanics-based framework for prediction of preterm birth as a function of changes in pregnancy status, such as polyhydramnios (increased amniotic fluid pressure and volume) or infection within the chorioamnion membrane (Oyen et al., 2004). Here, that mechanics model is applied to consider exogenous factors, in particular the barometric pressure change associated with severe weather events, to test the hypothesis that hurricanes could cause PROM.

3. MODEL AND ANALYSIS

A simple model is constructed here for rupture of the fetal (chorioamnion) membrane as a function of substantial decreases in atmospheric pressure. Considerations of fetal membrane rupture will follow that of reference Oyen et al. (2004) where a similar model was examined for endogenous effects such as chorioamnionitis or polyhydramnios. The basis of the model is a competition between stress in and strength of the membrane. In this context, stress is a driving force for mechanical rupture of the membrane, deriving from exogenous causes. In contrast, strength is a resisting force for mechanical failure of the membrane, deriving from endogenous effects. Mechanical failure or rupture of the membrane occurs when the strength of the membrane is exceeded by the applied stress. It is assumed that membrane strength is a function of gestational age alone, and that there is no influence of weather systems on the material properties resisting rupture. In contrast, it is assumed here that the mechanical stress in the membrane is a function of barometric pressure and no consideration of endogenous physiological factors such as decreased membrane strength from infection or changes in other physiological processes is driving mechanical failure. It is entirely likely that the mechanical changes modeled here in isolation are combined with additional contributions to increase the likelihood of PROM in the difficult circumstances of a severe storm. We consider first the membrane strength values based on experimental measurements of puncture force.

Failure data for membranes were taken from the raw data from the study of puncture force F_{max} as a function of gestational age (GA, Oyen et al., 2006). The data were split into two GA groups, $GA \leq 29$ and $GA \geq 30$ weeks. The raw data were fit by linear regression for each GA range (**Figure 1**). These regression lines were used as the input force F_{max} as a function of gestational age for calculations of membrane strength, using the equation

$$\sigma_f = \frac{1}{h}\left(\frac{F_{max}Eh}{6\pi R}\right)^{1/2} \quad (1)$$

where h is the membrane thickness, E is the membrane elastic modulus, and $R = 1.6$ mm was the probe radius used in the puncture studies (Oyen et al., 2004, 2006). Here h was taken as 250 μm and E was taken as 5 MPa based on published data (Helmig et al., 1993). The failure strength σ_f shows an increase with GA up to 30 weeks and a decrease thereafter (solid line, **Figure 2**). We consider next the membrane stress and its changes with barometric pressure.

The membrane stress as a function of fluid pressure was computed according to Laplace's law, as utilized for this context in (Oyen et al., 2004):

$$\sigma = p\frac{r}{2h} \quad (2)$$

where r is the radius of the sac bounded by the membrane and h is again the membrane thickness. The same estimates were used as previously (Oyen et al., 2004) for the size of the sac, linearly

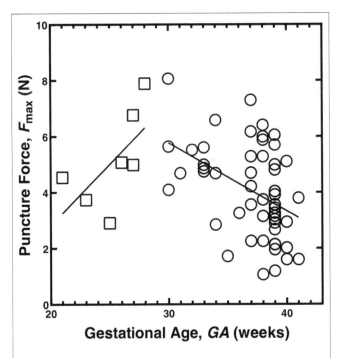

FIGURE 1 | Puncture force for the chorioamnion membrane as a function of gestational age, data from the studies (Oyen et al., 2004, 2006). The data have been split into two groups and fit with linear trend lines, $GA \leq 29$ weeks (open squares) and $GA \geq 30$ weeks (open circles).

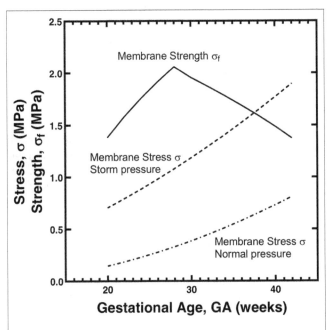

FIGURE 2 | Model for CA membrane stress σ and strength σ_f as a function of gestational age GA. The strength values are calculated from the data in **Figure 1** using Equation (1); the stress values for normal and storm atmospheric pressures are calculated from Equation (2) with parameter values as described in the text.

increasing from 7 cm at 20 weeks to 13 cm at 40 weeks GA. Amniotic fluid pressure was taken from Weiner et al. (1989) where the data were digitized and the best fit line was taken as $p = 0.661 * GA - 5.278$. This gives a fluid (gage) pressure of approximately 20 mm Hg above ambient (Faber et al., 1992) at full gestation of $GA = 40$ weeks (**Figure 2**, lower dashed line). This baseline was assumed to be for a normal atmospheric pressure of 760 mm Hg. For storm conditions, the atmospheric pressure was assumed to decrease to 730 mm Hg, and thus 30 mm Hg was added to each amniotic fluid pressure due to the change in computing the gage pressure (**Figure 2**, upper dashed line). It is critical to note that there are no free parameters in this modeling approach, nor are there any pre-factors that are adjusted without mechanism or associated literature data. The calculations of stress and strength are independent save for the shared parameter of membrane thickness (h).

The membrane stress is on the order of the membrane strength in the case of normal atmospheric pressure. The value of chorioamnion strength of about 1 MPa near term is consistent with a large review study that found a similar value across a large number of studies and measurement methods (Chua and Oyen, 2009). The stress and strength curves will be shifted slightly up or down depending on the choice of parameter values (p, E, r, h) used in the model and on the experimentally-measured force values used (F_{max}). However, the general trend is clear, that a 30 mm Hg drop in atmospheric pressure associated with a storm has the potential to raise the membrane stress significantly, and increase the likelihood that the membrane stress exceeds the membrane strength for a range of late-term gestational ages. Thus, a causal mechanism of membrane rupture due to pressure changes is numerically plausible.

4. DISCUSSION

A series of key studies over the course of the last 35 years have demonstrated that there is a clear association of birth with substantial drops in barometric pressure (King et al., 1997), and that this is in particular related to premature rupture of the fetal membranes (Polansky et al., 1985; Akutagawa et al., 2007). A simple model (Oyen et al., 2004) is adapted to consider this association, treating the membranes as a bubble and considering the trade-off between decreasing membrane strength as full term approaches, and increasing membrane stress associated with barometric pressure drops. It is found that a 30 mm Hg pressure drop, consistent with major hurricanes or bomb cyclones (which can occur in winter and not be tropical) is sufficient to provide a mechanistic association between membrane rupture and low atmospheric pressure (**Figure 2**).

The assumption in the model that atmospheric pressure could influence the stress in the chorioamnion does rely on the membrane being exposed to a pressure difference between the amniotic fluid and the surrounding ambient conditions. It seems more likely that this could be in the case in relatively late gestation when the cervical mucous plug has started to discharge or is missing entirely. This is particularly true if the cervix has also started to dilate, in which case the membranes begin to be directly exposed to ambient air via the vaginal canal.

The model here was plotted (**Figure 2**) for a pressure drop from a typical atmospheric pressure of 760 mm Hg to a representative storm pressure of 730 mm Hg. This pressure drop of 30 mm Hg in the model was associated with a prediction of membrane rupture at $GA = 37.5$ weeks at a stress value of 1.62

MPa. A pressure drop of 25 mm Hg, with all other parameters remaining unchanged, predicts rupture at GA = 39 weeks at a stress of 1.54 MPa, a drop of 35 mm Hg predicts rupture at GA = 36.1 weeks at a stress of 1.68 MPa, and a drop of 40 mm Hg predicts rupture at GA = 34.7 weeks at a stress of 1.75 MPa. Thus, a more severe storm in terms of decrease from baseline atmospheric pressure is associated with predictions of membrane rupture at younger gestational ages but greater stresses, since the membrane strength is assumed to decrease with GA (Oyen et al., 2006). These model predictions as noted assume all other model parameters are unchanged, and thus serve as a baseline indicator of the severity of storm pressure changing in isolation of all other potentially changing factors.

Membrane rupture due to low atmospheric pressure is not the only potential mechanism associated with early labor and delivery relative to weather events. Large increases in atmospheric pressure in a relatively short time have also been associated with premature delivery (Akutagawa et al., 2007) although the mechanism for that must be different than the one described herein, perhaps associated with other physiological changes in blood pressure or volume. Less extreme meteorological factors have been associated with both preterm delivery and PROM, including sharp changes in temperature and humidity and strong winds (Yackerson et al., 2008). Such weather conditions were also found to be associated with obstetrical complications such as placental abruption and pre-eclampsia (Yackerson et al., 2007).

There are many possible reasons as to why hurricanes can affect pregnancy, including complications in labor and delivery and subsequent morbidity in the neonate. For example, exposure to hurricanes during a pregnancy can increase the chance of a newborn having to rely on a ventilator (Currie and Rossin-Slater, 2013). The same authors found higher chances of an infant having aspirated meconium, a sign of fetal distress, and that hurricanes were generally associated with low birth weight. There was evidence in this study of significant sequelae in infants even when exposure to storms was early in the pregnancy, as in the first or second trimester (Currie and Rossin-Slater, 2013). Different potential explanations are discussed in this thorough work, including the effect of maternal stress, evacuation out of the path of the storm, and impact of the storm on delivery of medical services in the community. All of these results take on increased importance given our increasing awareness that abnormal conditions surrounding the newborn's arrival can cause poor outcomes for the child not just in the immediate aftermath of birth but also later in life.

One further issue thus far not addressed at all in the literature linking barometric pressure changes and pregnancy is race and ethnicity, and the corresponding health disparities that arise in preterm birth (Culhane and Goldenberg, 2011). The March of Dimes in the US rates states on maternal and infant health and in particular focuses on preterm birth (2019). Many of the states with the worst grades on the March of Dimes scale (2019) coincide with states that are also the most likely to be directly hit in a hurricane (Griggs, 2017). The lack of information linking these two topics presents an interesting opportunity for future research by an interdisciplinary team considering aspects from socioeconomics to biomechanics.

5. CONCLUSION

Labor and delivery in the context of major weather events should be understood in a holistic framework that includes both exogenous and endogenous factors. Management of pregnancies in the path of large storms with significantly low barometric pressures could include education of both health care practitioners and of expectant mothers about this phenomenon. It is entirely likely that evasive action such as evacuation could be warranted for some late-stage pregnancies directly in the path of significant barometric pressure drops on the basis of both the literature and on the basis of the numerical model presented herein. This study motivates further research on this subject, in the context of gathering far more detailed experimental data from regions with high risk for serious weather incidents to better inform expectant mothers and their health care providers. Such research will gain relevance as the occurrence of severe weather events increases due to climate change.

AUTHOR CONTRIBUTIONS

MW provided background research in the form of an annotated bibliography and participated in all aspects of writing and editing the manuscript. MO performed the analysis and created the figures in discussion with MW, and participated in all aspects of writing and editing the manuscript.

ACKNOWLEDGMENTS

The authors wish to acknowledge Dr. Steve Calvin for his past collaborations on this project and Robert F. Cook for reviewing an early version of this manuscript.

REFERENCES

(2019). *March of Dimes Report Card*. Available online at: https://www.marchofdimes.org/mission/reportcard.aspx (accessed April 18, 2020).

Akutagawa, O., Nishi, H., and Isaka, K. (2007). Spontaneous delivery is related to barometric pressure. *Arch. Gynecol. Obstet.* 275, 249–254. doi: 10.1007/s00404-006-0259-3

Blau, M. (2017). *Can a Hurricane Induce Labor? Women in the Path of Irma Are Worried*. Stat News. Available online at: https://www.statnews.com/2017/09/08/florida-hospitals-pregnant-women-hurricane-irma/ (accessed February 29, 2020).

Bolluyt, J. (2018). *Can a Hurricane Make Pregnant Women Go Into Labor? Why It's True*. The Showbiz CheatSheet. Available online at: https://www.cheatsheet.com/health-fitness/can-a-hurricane-induce-labor.html/ (accessed February 29, 2020).

Calvin, S. E., and Oyen, M. L. (2007). Microstructure and mechanics of the chorioamnion membrane with an emphasis on fracture properties. *Ann. N. Y. Acad. Sci.* 1101, 166–185. doi: 10.1196/annals.1389.009

Chua, W., and Oyen, M. L. (2009). Do we know the strength of the chorioamnion? A critical review and analysis. *Eur. J. Obstet. Gynecol. Reprod. Biol.* 144(Supp. 1), 128–133. doi: 10.1016/j.ejogrb.2009.02.029

Culhane, J. F., and Goldenberg, R. L. (2011). Racial disparities in preterm birth. *Semin. Perinatol.* 35, 234–9. doi: 10.1053/j.semperi.2011.02.020

Currie, J., and Rossin-Slater, M. (2013). Weathering the storm: hurricanes and birth outcomes. *J. Health Econ.* 32, 487–503. doi: 10.1053/j.semperi.2011.02.020

Faber, J. J., and Barbera, A. (1992). Convention for reporting amniotic fluid pressure. *Eur. J. Obstet. Gynecol. Reprod. Biol.* 47, 181–184. doi: 10.1016/0028-2243(92)90148-R

Griggs, B. (2017). *No Other State Gets Hit by Hurricanes as Often as Florida CNN.* Available online at: https://www.cnn.com/2017/09/11/us/hurricanes-landfall-by-state-trnd/index.html (accessed April 18, 2020).

Helmig, R., Oxlund, H., Petersen, L. K., and Uldbjerg, N. (1993). Different biomechanical properties of human fetal membranes obtained before and after delivery. *Eur. J. Obstet. Gynecol. Reprod. Biol.* 48, 183–189. doi: 10.1016/0028-2243(93)90086-R

King, E. A., Fleschler, R. G., and Cohen, S. M. (1997). Association between significant decrease in barometric pressure and onset of labor. *J. Nurse-Midwifery* 42, 32–34. doi: 10.1016/S0091-2182(96)00101-2

LaFrance, A. (2016). *Do Hurricanes Really Induce Labor?* The Atlantic. Available online at: https://www.theatlantic.com/health/archive/2016/10/do-hurricanes-really-induce-labor/503258/ (accessed February 17, 2020).

Marks, J., Church, C. K., and Benrubi, G. (1983). Effects of barometric pressure and lunar phases on premature rupture of the membranes. *J. Reprod. Med.* 28, 485–488.

Oyen, M. (2020). *Puncture Force vs GA. Mendeley Data,* V2. doi: 10.17632/cr9z9xd6g8.2

Oyen, M. L., Calvin, S. E., and Landers, D. V. (2006). Premature rupture of the fetal membranes: is the amnion the major determinant? *Am. J. Obstet. Gynecol.* 195, 510–515. doi: 10.1016/j.ajog.2006.02.010

Oyen, M. L., Cook, R. F., and Calvin, S. E. (2004). Mechanical failure of human fetal membrane tissues. *J. Mater. Sci. Mater. Med.* 15, 651–658. doi: 10.1023/B:JMSM.0000030205.62668.90

Polansky, G. H., Varner, M. W., and O'Gorman, T. (1985). Premature rupture of the membranes and barometric pressure changes. *J. Reprod. Med.* 30, 189–191.

Weiner, C. P., Heilskov, J., Pelzer, G., Grant, S., Wenstrom, K., and Williamson, R. A. (1989). Normal values for human umbilical venous and amniotic fluid pressures and their alteration by fetal disease. *Am. J. Obstet. Gynecol.* 161, 714–717. doi: 10.1016/0002-9378(89)90387-6

Yackerson, N., Piura, B., and Sheiner, E. (2008). The influence of meteorological factors on the emergence of preterm delivery and preterm premature rupture of membrane. *J. Perinatol.* 28, 707–711. doi: 10.1038/jp.2008.69

Yackerson, N. S., Piura, B., and Friger, M. (2007). The influence of weather state on the incidence of preeclampsia and placental abruption in semi-arid areas. *Clin. Exp. Obstet. Gynecol.* 34, 27–30. doi: 10.1016/j.jhealeco.2013.01.004

Toxicant Disruption of Immune Defenses: Potential Implications for Fetal Membranes and Pregnancy

Sean M. Harris[1†], Erica Boldenow[2*†], Steven E. Domino[3] and Rita Loch-Caruso[1]

[1] Department of Environmental Health Sciences, School of Public Health, University of Michigan, Ann Arbor, MI, United States, [2] Department of Biology, Calvin College, Grand Rapids, MI, United States, [3] Department of Obstetrics and Gynecology, University of Michigan Medical School, Ann Arbor, MI, United States

*Correspondence:
Erica Boldenow
ejb25@calvin.edu

†These authors have contributed equally to this work

In addition to providing a physical compartment for gestation, the fetal membranes (FM) are an active immunological barrier that provides defense against pathogenic microorganisms that ascend the gravid reproductive tract. Pathogenic infection of the gestational tissues (FM and placenta) is a leading known cause of preterm birth (PTB). Some environmental toxicants decrease the capacity for organisms to mount an immune defense against pathogens. For example, the immunosuppressive effects of the widespread environmental contaminant trichloroethylene (TCE) are documented for lung infection with *Streptococcus zooepidemicus*. Group B *Streptococcus* (GBS; *Streptococcus agalactiae*) is a bacterial pathogen that is frequently found in the female reproductive tract and can colonize the FM in pregnant women. Work in our laboratory has demonstrated that a bioactive TCE metabolite, S-(1, 2-dichlorovinyl)-L-cysteine (DCVC), potently inhibits innate immune responses to GBS in human FM in culture. Despite these provocative findings, little is known about how DCVC and other toxicants modify the risk for pathogenic infection of FM. Infection of the gestational tissues (FM and placenta) is a leading known cause of PTB, therefore toxicant compromise of FM ability to fight off infectious microorganisms could significantly contribute to PTB risk. This Perspective provides the current status of understanding of toxicant-pathogen interactions in FM, highlighting knowledge gaps, challenges, and opportunities for research that can advance protections for maternal and fetal health.

Keywords: fetal membranes, toxicant pathogen interactions, preterm birth (PTB), pregnancy, trichloroethylene (TCE)

INTRODUCTION

Preterm birth (PTB), or birth <37 weeks gestation, is a significant health problem with lasting consequences. Preterm birth affects more than 1 in 10 babies in the United States as well as globally (March of Dimes et al., 2012; Martin et al., 2019). Babies born preterm are at increased risk for numerous adverse health outcomes later in life, including neurological (Allin et al., 2006), lung (Pike and Lucas, 2015), and intestinal issues (Behrman et al., 2007). In a recent study, Grosse et al. (2017) estimated total medical costs associated with PTB in the United States to be between $6 and 14 billion per year. The fetal membranes (FM), which surround and protect the fetus during pregnancy, play a critical role in both term and preterm labor. In addition to providing a physical barrier, the FM are an important line of defense against pathogenic microorganisms that ascend the reproductive tract (Romero et al., 2007). Notably, pathogenic infection of the gestational tissues (FM and placenta) is a leading known cause of PTB (Goldenberg et al., 2000, 2008).

Epidemiology studies have identified a diverse array of factors associated with PTB (Goldenberg et al., 2008; Ferguson et al., 2013, 2019; Torchin and Ancel, 2016; Vogel et al., 2018). These include exposure to a range of toxic substances including air pollution (Liu et al., 2019), cigarette smoke (Soneji and Beltran-Sanchez, 2019), polyfluoroalkyl substances (Sagiv et al., 2018), polybrominated diphenyl ethers (PBDEs; Peltier et al., 2015), phthalate esters (Ferguson et al., 2014), lead (Taylor et al., 2015), and arsenic (Ahmad et al., 2001). Additional factors include infection with pathogenic bacteria (Bianchi-Jassir et al., 2017) and exposure to high outdoor air temperatures (Zhong et al., 2018; Gronlund et al., 2020). On a mechanistic basis, these exposures are thought to act by triggering oxidative stress and/or inflammatory pathways that are part of the normal labor process of weakening the membranes (Menon et al., 2011; Romero et al., 2014; Wallace et al., 2016; Ha et al., 2018). While biologically plausible, these mechanisms remain poorly understood.

Despite known examples of toxicant-induced immunosuppression occurring in organs such as the lung (Aranyi et al., 1986; Mitchell et al., 2009; Selgrade and Gilmour, 2010), toxicant mediation of immune responses to bacterial infection in FM is largely unexplored. This review focuses on our current understanding about environmental toxicants, pathogenic bacteria and interactions between the two in FM. Due to the potential lifelong health impacts of PTB (Allin et al., 2006; Behrman et al., 2007; Pike and Lucas, 2015) and the critical role that the membranes play in healthy pregnancy (Menon and Moore, 2020), a deeper understanding of these interactions has significant public health implications.

ANATOMY AND FUNCTION OF THE FETAL MEMBRANES

The FM are a heterogenous tissue with multiple cell types that make up two distinct layers, the inner amnion (surrounding the fetus) and the outer chorion (Strauss, 2013). The amnion layer is composed of a single amnion epithelial cell layer and dense layer of collagen fibrils synthesized by fibroblasts (Verbruggen et al., 2017). The chorion is composed of trophoblasts that are in close contact with maternally derived decidual cells (Wang et al., 2018; Menon and Moore, 2020). The FM also include a small number of resident innate immune cells (macrophages and monocytes) (Osman et al., 2003).

The culmination of a healthy pregnancy is marked with increased prostaglandin secretion, activation of matrix metalloproteinases, and recruitment of immune cells, leading to myometrial contractions, rupture of the membranes, and cervical ripening, respectively (Vadillo-Ortega et al., 1996; Hernandez-Guerrero et al., 2000; Challis et al., 2009; Yellon, 2019). Although our understanding of the role of FM in the initiation of labor remains incomplete, it is widely accepted that they contribute to the parturition pathway. As pregnancy progresses, the FM secrete increasingly more cytokines and chemokines, which leads to prostaglandin synthesis and release (Mesiano, 2007; Kota et al., 2013) as well as immune cell recruitment in the gestational compartment (Osman et al., 2003). Because the FM abut the uterine muscle (myometrium), they are important as a source of prostaglandins that stimulate uterine contractions in labor.

Furthermore, in normal pregnancies, FM undergo a process of weakening leading up to rupture soon after the start of uterine contractions (Menon, 2016; Menon et al., 2016). Molecular signaling pathways, such as oxidative stress and inflammation, as well as mechanical forces contribute to the weakening of the membranes near term, a process characterized by cellular senescence and aging of the membranes (Menon et al., 2016). Rupture usually occurs in a structurally weak region of the membranes with a thinner chorion that overlies the cervix, referred to as the zone of altered morphology (ZAM; McLaren et al., 1999; McParland et al., 2003; Marcellin et al., 2017).

Premature rupture of the FM, or PROM, is characterized by rupture of the FM more than one hour before the onset of labor. PROM occurring after 37 weeks of pregnancy typically presents relatively few complications. However, pPROM, or preterm premature rupture of the FM (i.e., PROM that occurs prior to 37 weeks of gestation) is associated with severe adverse pregnancy outcomes and is frequently associated with asymptomatic intrauterine infection (Mercer, 2004; Caughey et al., 2008; Huang et al., 2018). Examples of associated adverse neonatal outcomes include respiratory distress syndrome, pulmonary hypoplasia (Nourse and Steer, 1997; Linehan et al., 2016), and neurological outcomes (Manuck and Varner, 2014). pPROM affects around 1–3% of pregnancies (Huang et al., 2018).

FETAL MEMBRANES AS A TARGET OF BACTERIAL PATHOGENS

Intrauterine bacterial infection is well established as a cause of PTB (Romero et al., 2014). It is estimated that intrauterine infection accounts for at least 25–40% of PTBs (Goldenberg et al., 2008). Both placenta and FM from preterm and pPROM pregnancies have been shown to be more likely to contain bacterial DNA and a higher level of diversity in bacterial species compared to term pregnancies (Jones et al., 2009). Pathogenic bacteria associated with pPROM and PTB include species from genera such as *Staphylococcus, Escherichia, Mycoplasma, Ureaplasma,* and *Streptococcus* (Larsen and Hwang, 2010; Oh et al., 2010; Fortner et al., 2014; Zeng et al., 2014; Kong et al., 2019).

The predominant mechanism by which bacteria enter the gestational compartment causing intrauterine infection is through the ascending pathway by which bacteria first colonize the vagina and cervix, migrate to and then cross the FM, and then colonize the amniotic cavity and fetus (Goldenberg et al., 2000). Therefore, the FM play a critical role as a barrier to bacterial entry.

In addition to providing a physical barrier to protect against infection, the FM provide crucial immunological defense against pathogenic microorganisms that ascend the reproductive tract. The FM actively secrete antimicrobial peptides, such as human beta defensins, lactoferrin, and cathelicidin, to inhibit bacterial infection (Kjaergaard et al., 1999; King et al., 2007a,b; Boldenow et al., 2013). Furthermore, the choriodecidual cells as well as resident innate immune cells are capable of secreting proinflammatory cytokines such as IL-1β, IL-6, IL-8, and TNF-α, which help signal for additional immune cell recruitment (Challis et al., 2009; Yockey and Iwasaki, 2018). Proinflammatory cytokines can also potentially trigger increased release of prostaglandins and proteases, which are key molecular triggers of parturition (Norwitz et al., 1992; Mitchell et al., 1993; Brown et al., 1998; Young et al., 2002; Myatt and Sun, 2010; Romero et al., 2014). Even when bacteria do not infect the amniotic compartment, these proinflammatory responses to bacterial infection in the FM can lead to adverse pregnancy and neonatal outcomes (Adams Waldorf et al., 2011; Burd et al., 2012; Garcia-Flores et al., 2018).

Much of what is currently known about toxicant-bacteria interactions in FM comes from experiments using either *Streptococcus agalactiae*, commonly known as Group B *Streptococcus* (GBS). Group B *Streptococcus* infection in pregnant women is the leading cause of infectious neonatal morbidity and mortality in the United States (Verani et al., 2010). Group B *Streptococcus* induces preterm labor in non-human primates (Gravett et al., 1996; Boldenow et al., 2016). In women, GBS infection is associated with PTB at less than 32 weeks gestation (Hillier et al., 1991) and with chorioamnionitis, an inflammation of the chorion layer of the FM (Anderson et al., 2007). A recent publication from our laboratory showed that GBS inoculation caused a release of molecular effectors of parturition (matrix metalloproteinases and prostaglandin E2) from human FM explant punches *in vitro* (Park et al., 2018). In addition, pathway analysis of transcriptomic responses showed that pathways related to inflammation and PTB were activated by GBS inoculation (Park et al., 2018). Studies from our laboratory showed that a metabolite of trichloroethylene (TCE), a common environmental contaminant, modifies innate immune response to GBS in FM explants (Boldenow et al., 2015). Other groups have shown similar effects with other toxicant-bacteria combinations (e.g., carbon monoxide and *Escherichia coli* (Klimova et al., 2013). Although rarely explored, interactive effects between pathogens and toxicants in gestational tissues are plausible and have significant implications for maternal and fetal health.

FETAL MEMBRANES AS A TARGET OF ENVIRONMENTAL TOXICANTS

Pregnant women are exposed to a multitude of diverse environmental contaminants through drinking water, food packaging, air pollution workplace exposures, and other sources (Mitro et al., 2015). Ubiquitous environmental contaminants such as lead, cadmium, PBDEs, bisphenol A, and phthalates have been detected in human FM (Miller et al., 2009; Kot et al., 2019) and amniotic fluid (Miller et al., 2012; Geer et al., 2015), demonstrating that contaminants can come into contact with the FM either through blood flow to the decidua or via the amniotic fluid. Numerous epidemiology studies have found associations between exposures to environmental toxicants and increased risk of pPROM. These include toxic substances such as lead (Huang et al., 2018), ambient air pollution (Wang et al., 2019) and cigarette smoke (England et al., 2013). These epidemiology studies along with the detection of toxicants in human FM support the role of FM as a target of toxicant effects related to adverse pregnancy outcomes.

Toxicants Activate Pathways Involved in Fetal Membrane Rupture and PTB

Consideration of the FM as a mediator of toxicant effects is plausible based on their important role in membrane rupture and in the initiation of labor. As recently reviewed by Menon (2016), Menon et al. (2019), and Menon and Moore (2020), the FM contribute to the activation of labor and membrane rupture through a variety of molecular signaling pathways involving hormones, inflammatory cytokines, phosphorylated MAPK p38, reactive oxygen species and prostaglandins. Pro-inflammatory cytokines such as IL-1β, TNF-α, and IL-8 are secreted by the FM and promote the production of prostaglandins and proteases in the gestational compartment (Norwitz et al., 1992; Mitchell et al., 1993; Brown et al., 1998; Young et al., 2002; Myatt and Sun, 2010). Prostaglandins play a direct role in stimulating uterine contractions and cervical ripening, and proteases and ROS contribute to the weakening of the FM (Woods, 2001; Romero et al., 2014). The p38 MAPK pathway is critical for the initiation of cellular senescence and FM weakening, ultimately leading to membrane rupture (Menon et al., 2014). Increased generation of ROS in the gestational compartment is thought to activate the p38 pathway, leading to membrane senescence, damage to collagen, and weakening of the membranes in preparation for rupture in both term labor and pPROM (Woods, 2001).

Toxicants such as cigarette smoke extract and PBDEs activate one or more of these pathways in *in vitro* models of FM tissue or cells. For example, PBDEs induced oxidative stress, p38 MAPK activation and increased expression of cyclooxygenase-2 (a rate limiting enzyme of prostaglandin production) in human amnion epithelial cells (Behnia et al., 2015). Similarly, Menon et al. (2014) showed that cigarette smoke extract induced oxidative stress (assessed via formation of 3-nitrotyrosine staining) and activated the p38 MAPK pathway in FM explants *in vitro*. In addition, the environmental contaminant 2,3,7,8-tetrachlorodibenzo-p-dioxin (TCDD), often referred to as dioxin, increased expression of protease genes in human amnion epithelial cells (Abe et al., 2006) and increased a marker of senescence (β-galactosidase) in a FM "organ-on-chip" system consisting of primary human amnion epithelial cells co-cultured with decidual cells (Richardson et al., 2019). Thus, toxicology studies support molecular mechanisms that may explain epidemiological associations between toxicant exposures and adverse pregnancy outcomes mediated by the FM. However, several aspects of these phenomena, such as the thresholds of exposure and potential dimorphic responses based on fetal sex, remain largely unexplored.

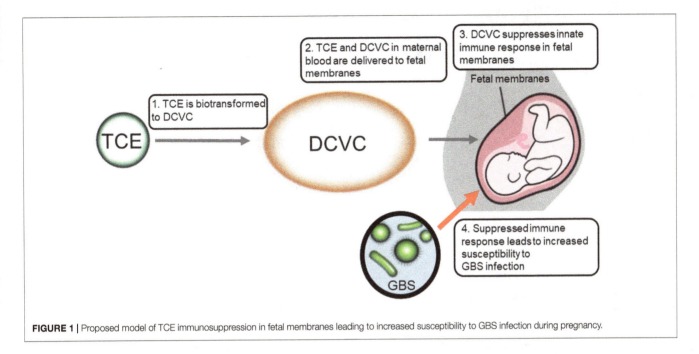

FIGURE 1 | Proposed model of TCE immunosuppression in fetal membranes leading to increased susceptibility to GBS infection during pregnancy.

TOXICANT-PATHOGEN INTERACTIONS: IMPACT ON FETAL MEMBRANES

Whereas several mechanisms have been identified which present plausible explanations for FM toxicity, immunomodulation in conjunction with bacterial infection remains an important but understudied phenomenon in gestational tissues. In a 2010 review, Feingold et al. (2010) highlighted the need for environmental toxicology research to incorporate interactions with infectious pathogens such as bacteria and viruses. Feingold et al. (2010) described four potential toxicant-pathogen interactions that could lead to disease: (1) toxicant and pathogen are both needed to cause disease; (2) pathogen and toxicant are individually capable of causing disease; (3) the chemical toxicant modifies the pathogen which leads to disease; and (4) the pathogen modifies the toxicant which leads to disease. In the same journal issue, Birnbaum and Jung (2010) called for increased attention to environmental health and infectious disease, noting that they can act concurrently, antagonistically, or synergistically. Despite this call to action, little research on toxicant-pathogen interactions during pregnancy has been conducted in the last decade.

Toxicant-Pathogen Co-treatment Leads to Enhanced Inflammation

Some toxicants have been shown to enhance pathogen-stimulated oxidative stress pathways and pro-inflammatory responses in gestational tissues. For example, some PBDEs increased *E. coli*-stimulated IL-1β and IL-6 secretion and COX-2 expression, as well as reduced *E. coli*-stimulated IL-10 release in human placental explants (Peltier et al., 2012; Arita et al., 2018c). Similarly, TCDD increased bacteria-stimulated PGE$_2$ and COX-2 gene expression and decreased IL-10 secretion (Peltier et al., 2013). Notably, the PBDE and TCDD effects were observed in the absence of impacts on explant viability and in placenta tissue obtained from both term (Arita et al., 2018c) and preterm (Peltier et al., 2012, 2013) stages of pregnancy, suggesting that immunomodulatory effects can occur throughout gestation. In addition, tributyltin enhanced *E. coli*-stimulated IL-6 release from placental explants (Arita et al., 2018a). Another study found that the flame retardant chemical tetrabromobisphenol A (TBBPA) increased the *E. coli*-induced release of IL-6 and TNF-α (Arita et al., 2018b). Research continues to be limited on how these toxicants modify bacterial host response in the FM and *in vivo*. Given the important nature of the FM in pPROM and PTB it is imperative that more research be conducted on toxicant-pathogen interactions in the FM.

Immunosupression as a Mechanism of Toxicity

Whereas some toxicants enhance inflammation and immune responses, others have demonstrated immunosuppressive effects (Selgrade, 2007). Examples of toxic substances that suppress immune responses include alcohol, cigarette smoke, and air pollution, all of which have been shown to inhibit macrophage phagocytosis (Karavitis and Kovacs, 2011). Epidemiology studies have found associations between decreased antibody responses to vaccinations in children exposed to perfluorinated compounds (Grandjean et al., 2012) and polychlorinated biphenyls (Heilmann et al., 2006). Immunosuppressive effects of toxicants have also been observed in gestational tissues. For example, TBBPA and tributyltin both inhibited bacteria-stimulated IL-1β secretion in placental explants (Arita et al., 2018a,b).

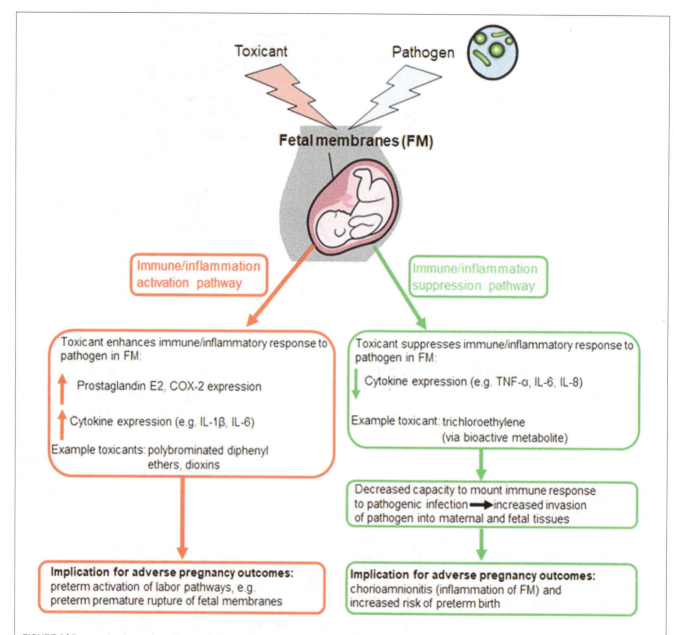

FIGURE 2 | Proposed pathways for toxicant activation or suppression of inflammation/immune responses in the fetal membranes with potential implications for pregnancy outcomes. Multiple environmental toxicants have been identified that either enhance or suppress immune responses in the fetal membranes, particularly in models of pathogenic infection. Both mechanisms of toxicity have potentially significant implications for adverse pregnancy outcomes, e.g., early activation of labor pathways (activation) or decreased capacity for membrane tissue to mount a defense against pathogens (suppression). These pathways may not be mutually exclusive.

Immunomodulatory Effects of Trichloroethylene

The common environmental contaminant TCE is a well-documented example of a compound with immunosuppressive effects. Trichloroethylene is a chlorinated volatile organic solvent commonly used as an industrial metal degreaser (Waters et al., 1977; Chiu et al., 2013). Trichloroethylene is ranked #16 on the U.S. Agency for Toxic Substances and Disease Registry's Priority List of Hazardous Substances and is a common environmental contaminant found in approximately 800 Environmental Protection Agency-designated Superfund sites (Wong, 2004; Chiu et al., 2013). Trichloroethylene is classified as a "known human carcinogen" (Guha et al., 2012) and is a renal and hepatic toxicant However, effects of TCE on gestational tissues have been minimally explored. Because of its continued industrial use and widespread persistent environmental contamination, TCE exposure continues to pose a threat to human health through ingestion of contaminated drinking water and inhalation of the volatilized chemical (Watson et al., 2006; Dumas et al., 2018). Trichloroethylene and its metabolites are detected in the blood of pregnant women exposed via inhalation and transfer across the placenta has been indicated by detection in the umbilical vein and artery (Beppu, 1968; Laham, 1970). Trichloroethylene and its metabolites are also found in the placenta and amniotic fluid of exposed pregnant mice (Ghantous et al., 1986). Thus, the effect of TCE and its downstream metabolites on gestational tissues in exposed women is of relevant concern.

The immunomodulatory effects of TCE are well documented in rodent and epidemiology studies. Mice co-treated with TCE and *Streptococcus zooepidemicus* showed increased mortality, decreased bacterial clearance from the lungs, and decreased alveolar phagocytosis (Aranyi et al., 1986; Selgrade and Gilmour, 2010). Trichloroethylene also suppressed activity of natural killer cells isolated from exposed rats (Wright et al., 1991). Immunosuppressive effects are observed in humans exposed to TCE. For example, lymphocyte counts as well as circulating levels of proinflammatory cytokines IL-6 and TNF-α were lower in exposed workers compared to controls (Hosgood et al., 2011; Xueqin et al., 2018). In a 2009 review, Cooper et al. (2009) concluded that "studies in mice and humans support an etiologic role of TCE in autoimmune disease." It appears that metabolism is required for at least some of TCE's immunotoxicity, because inhibition of the TCE metabolizing enzyme CYP2E1 mitigates some of these effects (Griffin et al., 2000). Despite these compelling findings, few researchers have investigated this phenomenon in gestational tissues such as the FM. Because the FM play a vital role in protecting the fetus and gestational compartment from pathogenic infection during pregnancy, an increased understanding of how environmental contaminant exposures modify FM responses to infection could greatly improve our ability to identify populations at risk for bacterial infection and associated adverse pregnancy outcomes.

TCE Metabolite Suppression of Immune Responses to Bacteria in Fetal Membranes

Work in our laboratory demonstrated that the bioactive TCE metabolite S-(1,2-dichlorovinyl)-L-cysteine (DCVC) inhibits innate immune responses to GBS. These findings were observed in FM tissue explants (tissue cultures established from FM obtained from planned caesarian deliveries). Explants co-treated with GBS and DCVC showed decreased expression of TNF-α, IL-1β, and IL-8 compared to those treated with GBS alone (Boldenow et al., 2015). Two other TCE metabolites (TCA and DCA) showed no effect (Boldenow et al., 2015). Importantly, the concentrations of DCVC used (5–10 μM) were within the range of metabolite blood concentrations in female volunteers exposed to airborne TCE at the current occupational exposure limit (Lash et al., 1999; Agency for Toxic Substances and Disease Registry, 2007). Moreover, the immunomodulatory effects of DCVC occurred in the absence of any effect on overall GBS viability. The cytokine suppression occurred not only in response to GBS, but also in response to lipoteichoic acid and lipopolysaccharide (virulence factors expressed by multiple species of bacteria) (Alexander and Rietschel, 2001; Ginsburg, 2002), suggesting that the observed effects were not pathogen specific.

Suppression of cytokine expression has important implications for innate immune responses in FM. Cytokines play important roles during bacterial infection, such as the recruitment of immune cells. Thus, suppression of these cytokine responses could lead to decreased recruitment of immune cells during bacterial infection, leading to prolonged or more severe pathogenic infections during pregnancy. Prolonged or more severe infections could in turn lead to pPROM, PTB or other adverse pregnancy outcomes such as neonatal sepsis.

Figure 1 summarizes the major events in the proposed mechanism by which TCE exposure could lead to increased susceptibility to GBS infection. Few epidemiology studies have assessed associations between TCE exposure and PTB. Studies thus far have found associations with small for gestational age, low birth weight and birth defects but not PTB (Bove et al., 2002; Forand et al., 2012; Ruckart et al., 2014). However, these studies did not report on presence or absence of maternal pathogenic infection as a variable and obtaining accurate assessments of TCE exposure is challenging (Bove et al., 2002). Future epidemiology studies focusing on potential toxicant-pathogen interactions could greatly improve our understanding of whether phenomena observed in FM models *in vitro* translate to *in vivo* human outcomes.

DISCUSSION

Despite intriguing findings, numerous aspects of toxicant-pathogen interactions in FM need to be clarified in order to reach conclusions about the implications for maternal or fetal health outcomes. Although DCVC suppression of innate immune responses could exacerbate GBS infection, proinflammatory pathways are also critical in the activation of parturition, meaning that DCVC could also suppress activation of labor processes (**Figure 1**). A better understanding of mechanisms underlying these phenomena would clarify the true level of risk for adverse pregnancy outcomes due to GBS infection combined with TCE exposure. In addition, findings thus far have only been observed in FM tissue *in vitro*. While useful, these models lack a number of tissue interactions between the decidua and the chorionic layer of the FM as well as maternal immune responses to infection. Validating these findings in pregnant animal models co-treated with GBS and TCE could provide important clarification in this area. Furthermore, clarification is needed on whether DCVC is the sole metabolite of TCE responsible for immunosuppressive effects or if downstream metabolites play a role. Improved understanding of virulence factors that allow bacteria such as GBS to evade the defenses of the FM and colonize the amniotic fluid and/or fetus would also represent a significant step forward. Fetal sex and gestational age are other potentially important variables that were not considered in prior studies of the FM. Finally, TCE is far from the only toxicant known to have immunosuppressive effects. For example, perfluorinated chemicals such as perfluorooctanoic acid have recently generated concern due to observed immunosuppressive effects (Shane et al., 2020) and therefore should be investigated for interactions with pathogens in the context of pregnancy. Other classes of chemicals that have demonstrated immunosuppressive effects include aromatic hydrocarbons, benzene and metals such as lead and arsenic (National Academy of Sciences, 1992).

Some studies have noted both immunosuppressive and immune activation effects for the same toxicant. For example, Arita, et al. observed an increase in E. coli-induced TNF-α in placental explants treated with TBBPA, whereas IL-1β secretion was reduced (Arita et al., 2018b). This is not surprising given the inherent complexity of immunological signaling pathways. For a given toxicant, it is possible that both immune activation and suppression could occur to differing degrees simultaneously or in sequence, which is especially important to recognize when utilizing *in vitro* models. For example, if cultured FM are exposed to the toxicant and pathogen simultaneously then the toxicant may not diffuse into the tissue before the pathogen stimulates the early TNF-α response, but the toxicant could still inhibit the later IL-1β response. Additionally, the toxicant may act to inhibit or activate different molecular pathways within the immune system. For example, the toxicant could be inhibiting caspase, which is needed for IL-1β secretion, while simultaneously activating TNF-α (Thornberry et al., 1992). If immune activation predominates, adverse pregnancy events may include preterm activation of labor pathways which could lead to premature rupture of the FM. If immune suppression is the dominant process, adverse events could include increased pathogenic infiltration into the gestational compartment due to inadequate FM immune response. The mechanisms determining whether suppression or activation predominate in the FM in response to toxicants are not currently well understood but are likely mediated by a number of factors including the dose of toxicant, stage of pregnancy, strain or species of pathogen or duration of toxicant exposure (e.g.,

chronic vs. acute exposure). For example, naturally occurring immunological changes occurring throughout pregnancy include a progressive increase in the number and responsiveness of circulating neutrophils (Aghaeepour et al., 2017). Therefore, being exposed to a toxicant and/or pathogen late in pregnancy may favor immune activation whereas a different response may be observed with exposure earlier in pregnancy. Whether toxicant immune activation, suppression or a more complex interaction between the two, is the most relevant to the FM for a given toxicant-pathogen interaction is difficult to predict, further highlighting the need for additional research on this topic.

In summary, limited studies have shown that toxicants can potentially modify immune responses in the FM through both "immune/inflammation activation" and "immune/inflammation suppression" pathways (see **Figure 2**). Because current research into these phenomena has relied mostly on *in vitro* models of gestational cells and tissues, further research is needed to determine whether effects observed *in vitro* are replicated in FM *in vivo*. *In vitro* models are necessarily removed from the inherent complexity of the *in vivo* immune system. Studies using animal models would improve our understanding of how toxicants affect immune responses in the FM in an intact organism. Further research could improve our understanding of toxicant-pathogen interactions during pregnancy and potentially identify populations at risk for adverse pregnancy outcomes.

AUTHOR CONTRIBUTIONS

EB, SH, and RL-C proposed the original idea for the manuscript. All authors wrote and edited the manuscript and have seen and approved the final version of the submitted manuscript.

REFERENCES

Agency for Toxic Substances and Disease Registry (2007) *Trryi Chloroethylene Toxicity: What Are the U.S. Standards for Trichloroethylene Exposure?* Available online at: https://www.atsdr.cdc.gov/csem/csem.asp?csem=15&po=8

Abe, Y., Sinozaki, H., Takagi, T., Minegishi, T., Kokame, K., Kangawa, K., et al. (2006). Identification of 2,3,7,8-tetrachlorodibenzo-p-dioxin (TCDD)-inducible genes in human amniotic epithelial cells. *Reprod Biol. Endocrinol.* 4:27.

Adams Waldorf, K. M., Gravett, M. G., McAdams, R. M., Paolella, L. J., Gough, G. M., Carl, D. J., et al. (2011). Choriodecidual group B streptococcal inoculation induces fetal lung injury without intra-amniotic infection and preterm labor in *Macaca nemestrina*. *PLoS One* 6:e28972. doi: 10.1371/journal.pone.0028972

Aghaeepour, N., Ganio, E. A., McIlwain, D., Tsai, A. S., Tingle, M., Van Gassen, S., et al. (2017). An immune clock of human pregnancy. *Sci. Immunol.* 2:eaan2946.

Ahmad, S. A., Sayed, M. H., Barua, S., Khan, M. H., Faruquee, M. H., Jalil, A., et al. (2001). Arsenic in drinking water and pregnancy outcomes. *Environ. Health Perspect.* 109, 629–631.

Alexander, C., and Rietschel, E. T. (2001). Bacterial lipopolysaccharides and innate immunity. *J. Endotoxin. Res.* 7, 167–202.

Allin, M., Rooney, M., Griffiths, T., Cuddy, M., Wyatt, J., Rifkin, L., et al. (2006). Neurological abnormalities in young adults born preterm. *J. Neurol. Neurosurg. Psychiatry* 77, 495–499.

Anderson, B. L., Simhan, H. N., Simons, K. M., and Wiesenfeld, H. C. (2007). Untreated asymptomatic group B streptococcal bacteriuria early in pregnancy and chorioamnionitis at delivery. *Am. J. Obstet. Gynecol.* 196:524.e1-5.

Aranyi, C., O'Shea, W. J., Graham, J. A., and Miller, F. J. (1986). The effects of inhalation of organic chemical air contaminants on murine lung host defenses. *Fundam Appl. Toxicol.* 6, 713–720.

Arita, Y., Kirk, M., Gupta, N., Menon, R., Getahun, D., and Peltier, M. R. (2018a). Effects of tributyltin on placental cytokine production. *J. Perinat. Med.* 46, 867–875. doi: 10.1515/jpm-2017-0336

Arita, Y., Pressman, M., Getahun, D., Menon, R., and Peltier, M. R. (2018b). Effect of Tetrabromobisphenol A on expression of biomarkers for inflammation and neurodevelopment by the placenta. *Placenta* 68, 33–39. doi: 10.1016/j.placenta.2018.06.306

Arita, Y., Yeh, C., Thoma, T., Getahun, D., Menon, R., and Peltier, M. R. (2018c). Effect of polybrominated diphenyl ether congeners on placental cytokine production. *J. Reprod. Immunol.* 125, 72–79. doi: 10.1016/j.jri.2017.12.002

Behnia, F., Peltier, M. R., Saade, G. R., and Menon, R. (2015). Environmental pollutant polybrominated diphenyl ether, a flame retardant. induces primary amnion cell senescence. *Am. J. Reprod. Immunol.* 74, 398–406.

Behrman, R. E., Butler, A. S., and Committee on Understanding Premature Birth and Assuring Healthy Outcomes, Board on Health Sciences Policy, Institute of Medicine (2007). *Preterm Birth: Causes, Consequences, and Prevention*, eds R. E. Behrman and A. S. Butler (Washington, DC: Board on Health Sciences Policy, Institute of Medicine).

Beppu, K. (1968). Transmission of the anesthetic agents through the placenta in painless delivery and their effects on newborn infants. *Keio J. Med.* 17, 81–107.

Bianchi-Jassir, F., Seale, A. C., Kohli-Lynch, M., Lawn, J. E., Baker, C. J., Bartlett, L., et al. (2017). Preterm Birth Associated With Group B Streptococcus Maternal Colonization Worldwide: Systematic Review and Meta-analyses. *Clin. Infect. Dis.* 65(Suppl._2), S133–S142. doi: 10.1093/cid/cix661

Birnbaum, L. S., and Jung, P. (2010). Evolution in environmental health: incorporating the infectious disease paradigm. *Environ. Health Perspect.* 118, a327–a328.

Boldenow, E., Gendrin, C., Ngo, L., Bierle, C., Vornhagen, J., Coleman, M., et al. (2016). Group B Streptococcus circumvents neutrophils and neutrophil extracellular traps during amniotic cavity invasion and preterm labor. *Sci. Immunol.* 1:aah4576. doi: 10.1126/sciimmunol.aah4576

Boldenow, E., Hassan, I., Chames, M. C., Xi, C., and Loch-Caruso, R. (2015). The trichloroethylene metabolite S-(1,2-dichlorovinyl)-l-cysteine but not trichloroacetate inhibits pathogen-stimulated TNF-alpha in human extraplacental membranes in vitro. *Reprod Toxicol.* 52, 1–6.

Boldenow, E., Jones, S., Lieberman, R. W., Chames, M. C., Aronoff, D. M., Xi, C., et al. (2013). Antimicrobial peptide response to group B Streptococcus in human extraplacental membranes in culture. *Placenta* 34, 480–485. doi: 10.1016/j.placenta.2013.02.010

Bove, F., Shim, Y., and Zeitz, P. (2002). Drinking water contaminants and adverse pregnancy outcomes: a review. *Environ. Health Perspect.* 110(Suppl. 1), 61–74.

Brown, N. L., Alvi, S. A., Elder, M. G., Bennett, P. R., and Sullivan, M. H. (1998). Regulation of prostaglandin production in intact fetal membranes by interleukin-1 and its receptor antagonist. *J. Endocrinol.* 159, 519–526.

Burd, I., Balakrishnan, B., and Kannan, S. (2012). Models of fetal brain injury, intrauterine inflammation, and preterm birth. *Am. J. Reprod. Immunol.* 67, 287–294. doi: 10.1111/j.1600-0897.2012.01110.x

Caughey, A. B., Robinson, J. N., and Norwitz, E. R. (2008). Contemporary diagnosis and management of preterm premature rupture of membranes. *Rev. Obstet. Gynecol.* 1, 11–22.

Challis, J. R., Lockwood, C. J., Myatt, L., Norman, J. E., Strauss, J. F. III, and Petraglia, F. (2009). Inflammation and pregnancy. *Reprod. Sci.* 16, 206–215.

Chiu, W. A., Jinot, J., Scott, C. S., Makris, S. L., Cooper, G. S., Dzubow, R. C., et al. (2013). Human health effects of trichloroethylene: key findings and scientific issues. *Environ. Health Perspect.* 121, 303–311. doi: 10.1289/ehp.1205879

Committee on Understanding Premature Birth and Assuring Healthy Outcomes, Board on Health Sciences Policy, Institute of Medicine (2007). *Preterm Birth: Causes, Consequences, and Prevention*, eds R. E. Behrman and A. S. Butler Washington, DC:Board on Health Sciences Policy, Institute of Medicine.

Cooper, G. S., Makris, S. L., Nietert, P. J., and Jinot, J. (2009). Evidence of autoimmune-related effects of trichloroethylene exposure from studies in mice and humans. *Environ. Health Perspect.* 117, 696–702. doi: 10.1289/ehp.11782

Dumas, O., Despreaux, T., Perros, F., Lau, E., Andujar, P., Humbert, M., et al. (2018). Respiratory effects of trichloroethylene. *Respir. Med.* 134, 47–53. doi: 10.1016/j.rmed.2017.11.021

England, M. C., Benjamin, A., and Abenhaim, H. A. (2013). Increased risk of preterm premature rupture of membranes at early gestational ages among maternal cigarette smokers. *Am. J. Perinatol.* 30, 821–826. doi: 10.1055/s-0032-1333408

Feingold, B. J., Vegosen, L., Davis, M., Leibler, J., Peterson, A., and Silbergeld, E. K. (2010). A niche for infectious disease in environmental health: rethinking the toxicological paradigm. *Environ. Health Perspect.* 118, 1165–1172. doi: 10.1289/ehp.0901866

Ferguson, K. K., McElrath, T. F., and Meeker, J. D. (2014). Environmental phthalate exposure and preterm birth. *JAMA Pediatr.* 168, 61–67. doi: 10.1001/jamapediatrics.2013.3699

Ferguson, K. K., O'Neill, M. S., and Meeker, J. D. (2013). Environmental contaminant exposures and preterm birth: a comprehensive review. *J. Toxicol. Environ. Health B Crit. Rev.* 16, 69–113. doi: 10.1080/10937404.2013.775048

Ferguson, K. K., Rosen, E. M., Barrett, E. S., Nguyen, R. H. N., Bush, N., McElrath, T. F., et al. (2019). Joint impact of phthalate exposure and stressful life events in pregnancy on preterm birth. *Environ. Int.* 133(Pt B), 105254. doi: 10.1016/j.envint.2019.105254

Forand, S. P., Lewis-Michl, E. L., and Gomez, M. I. (2012). Adverse birth outcomes and maternal exposure to trichloroethylene and tetrachloroethylene through soil vapor intrusion in New York State. *Environ. Health Perspect.* 120, 616–621. doi: 10.1289/ehp.1103884

Fortner, K. B., Grotegut, C. A., Ransom, C. E., Bentley, R. C., Feng, L., Lan, L., et al. (2014). Bacteria localization and chorion thinning among preterm premature rupture of membranes. *PLoS One* 9:e83338. doi: 10.1371/journal.pone.0083338

Garcia-Flores, V., Romero, R., Miller, D., Xu, Y., Done, B., Veerapaneni, C., et al. (2018). Inflammation-induced adverse pregnancy and neonatal outcomes can be improved by the immunomodulatory Peptide Exendin-4. *Front. Immunol.* 9:1291. doi: 10.3389/fimmu.2018.01291

Geer, L. A., Pycke, B. F., Sherer, D. M., Abulafia, O., and Halden, R. U. (2015). Use of amniotic fluid for determining pregnancies at risk of preterm birth and for studying diseases of potential environmental etiology. *Environ. Res.* 136, 470–481. doi: 10.1016/j.envres.2014.09.031

Ghantous, H., Danielsson, B. R., Dencker, L., Gorczak, J., and Vesterberg, O. (1986). Trichloroacetic acid accumulates in murine amniotic fluid after tri- and tetrachloroethylene inhalation. *Acta Pharmacol. Toxicol.* 58, 105–114.

Ginsburg, I. (2002). Role of lipoteichoic acid in infection and inflammation. *Lancet Infect. Dis.* 2, 171–179.

Goldenberg, R. L., Culhane, J. F., Iams, J. D., and Romero, R. (2008). Epidemiology and causes of preterm birth. *Lancet* 371, 75–84. doi: 10.1016/S0140-6736(08)60074-4

Goldenberg, R. L., Hauth, J. C., and Andrews, W. W. (2000). Intrauterine infection and preterm delivery. *N. Engl. J. Med.* 342, 1500–1507.

Grandjean, P., Andersen, E. W., Budtz-Jorgensen, E., Nielsen, F., Molbak, K., Weihe, P., et al. (2012). Serum vaccine antibody concentrations in children exposed to perfluorinated compounds. *JAMA* 307, 391–397. doi: 10.1001/jama.2011.2034

Gravett, M. G., Haluska, G. J., Cook, M. J., and Novy, M. J. (1996). Fetal and maternal endocrine responses to experimental intrauterine infection in rhesus monkeys. *Am. J. Obstet. Gynecol.* 174, 1725–1731.

Griffin, J. M., Gilbert, K. M., and Pumford, N. R. (2000). Inhibition of CYP2E1 reverses CD4+ T-cell alterations in trichloroethylene-treated MRL+/+ mice. *Toxicol. Sci.* 54, 384–389.

Gronlund, C. J., Yang, A. J., Conlon, K. C., Bergmans, R. S., Le, H. Q., Batterman, S. A., et al. (2020). Time series analysis of total and direct associations between high temperatures and preterm births in Detroit. Michigan. *BMJ Open* 10:e032476. doi: 10.1136/bmjopen-2019-032476

Grosse, S. D., Waitzman, N. J., Yang, N., Abe, K., and Barfield, W. D. (2017). Employer-sponsored plan expenditures for infants born preterm. *Pediatrics* 140, doi: 10.1542/peds.2017-1078

Guha, N., Loomis, D., Grosse, Y., Lauby-Secretan, B., El Ghissassi, F., Bouvard, V., et al. (2012). Carcinogenicity of trichloroethylene, tetrachloroethylene, some other chlorinated solvents, and their metabolites. *Lancet Oncol.* 13, 1192–1193.

Ha, S., Liu, D., Zhu, Y., Sherman, S., and Mendola, P. (2018). Acute associations between outdoor temperature and premature rupture of membranes. *Epidemiology* 29, 175–182. doi: 10.1097/EDE.0000000000000779

Heilmann, C., Grandjean, P., Weihe, P., Nielsen, F., and Budtz-Jorgensen, E. (2006). Reduced antibody responses to vaccinations in children exposed to polychlorinated biphenyls. *PLoS Med.* 3:e311. doi: 10.1371/journal.pmed.0030311

Hernandez-Guerrero, C., Tenorio-Ramos, J., Vadillo-Ortega, F., Arechavaleta-Velasco, F., Jimenez-Zamudio, L., Ahued-Ahued, J. R., et al. (2000). [Tumor necrosis factor-alpha and interleukin-1 beta in maternal, fetal and retroplacental intravascular compartments at term and preterm labor]. *Ginecol. Obstet. Mex* 68, 105–112.

Hillier, S. L., Krohn, M. A., Kiviat, N. B., Watts, D. H., and Eschenbach, D. A. (1991). Microbiologic causes and neonatal outcomes associated with chorioamnion infection. *Am. J. Obstet. Gynecol.* 165(4 Pt 1), 955–961.

Hosgood, H. D. III, Zhang, L., Tang, X., Vermeulen, R., Qiu, C., Shen, M., et al. (2011). Decreased Numbers of CD4(+) Naive and Effector Memory T Cells, and CD8(+) Naive T Cells, are associated with trichloroethylene exposure. *Front. Oncol.* 1:53. doi: 10.3389/fonc.2011.00053

Huang, S., Xia, W., Sheng, X., Qiu, L., Zhang, B., Chen, T., et al. (2018). Maternal lead exposure and premature rupture of membranes: a birth cohort study in China. *BMJ Open* 8:e021565. doi: 10.1136/bmjopen-2018-021565

Jones, H. E., Harris, K. A., Azizia, M., Bank, L., Carpenter, B., Hartley, J. C., et al. (2009). Differing prevalence and diversity of bacterial species in fetal membranes from very preterm and term labor. *PLoS One* 4:e8205. doi: 10.1371/journal.pone.0008205

Karavitis, J., and Kovacs, E. J. (2011). Macrophage phagocytosis: effects of environmental pollutants, alcohol, cigarette smoke, and other external factors. *J. Leukoc Biol.* 90, 1065–1078. doi: 10.1189/jlb.0311114

King, A. E., Kelly, R. W., Sallenave, J. M., Bocking, A. D., and Challis, J. R. (2007a). Innate immune defences in the human uterus during pregnancy. *Placenta* 28, 1099–1106.

King, A. E., Paltoo, A., Kelly, R. W., Sallenave, J. M., Bocking, A. D., and Challis, J. R. (2007b). Expression of natural antimicrobials by human placenta and fetal membranes. *Placenta* 28, 161–169.

Kjaergaard, N., Helmig, R. B., Schonheyder, H. C., Uldbjerg, N., Hansen, E. S., and Madsen, H. (1999). Chorioamniotic membranes constitute a competent barrier to group b streptococcus in vitro. *Eur. J. Obstet. Gynecol. Reprod. Biol.* 83, 165–169.

Klimova, N. G., Hanna, N., and Peltier, M. R. (2013). Does carbon monoxide inhibit proinflammatory cytokine production by fetal membranes? *J. Perinat. Med.* 41, 683–690. doi: 10.1515/jpm-2013-0016

Kong, Y., Yang, T., Yang, T., Ruan, Z., Song, T., Ding, H., et al. (2019). Correlation between Ureaplasma spp. sub-group 1 and preterm pre-labour rupture of membranes revealed by an eMLST scheme. *Infect. Genet. Evol.* 68, 172–176. doi: 10.1016/j.meegid.2018.12.025

Kot, K., Kosik-Bogacka, D., Lanocha-Arendarczyk, N., Malinowski, W., Szymanski, S., Mularczyk, M., et al. (2019). Interactions between 14 elements in the human placenta, fetal membrane and umbilical cord. *Int. J. Environ. Res. Public Health* 16:1615. doi: 10.3390/ijerph16091615

Kota, S. K., Gayatri, K., Jammula, S., Kota, S. K., Krishna, S. V., Meher, L. K., et al. (2013). Endocrinology of parturition. *Indian J. Endocrinol. Metab.* 17, 50–59.

Laham, S. (1970). Studies on placental transfer. Trichlorethylene. *IMS Ind. Med. Surg.* 39, 46–49.

Larsen, B., and Hwang, J. (2010). Mycoplasma, Ureaplasma, and adverse pregnancy outcomes: a fresh look. *Infect. Dis. Obstet. Gynecol* 2010:521921. doi: 10.1155/2010/521921

Lash, L. H., Putt, D. A., Brashear, W. T., Abbas, R., Parker, J. C., and Fisher, J. W. (1999). Identification of S-(1,2-dichlorovinyl)glutathione in the blood of human volunteers exposed to trichloroethylene. *J. Toxicol. Environ. Health A* 56, 1–21.

Linehan, L. A., Walsh, J., Morris, A., Kenny, L., O'Donoghue, K., Dempsey, E., et al. (2016). Neonatal and maternal outcomes following midtrimester preterm premature rupture of the membranes: a retrospective cohort study. *BMC Pregnancy Childbirth* 16:25. doi: 10.1186/s12884-016-0813-3

Liu, Y., Xu, J., Chen, D., Sun, P., and Ma, X. (2019). The association between air pollution and preterm birth and low birth weight in Guangdong, China. *BMC Public Health* 19:3. doi: 10.1186/s12889-018-6307-7

Manuck, T. A., and Varner, M. W. (2014). Neonatal and early childhood outcomes following early vs later preterm premature rupture of membranes. *Am. J. Obstet. Gynecol.* 211, 308.e1–308.e6. doi: 10.1016/j.ajog.2014.05.030

Marcellin, L., Schmitz, T., Messaoudene, M., Chader, D., Parizot, C., Jacques, S., et al. (2017). Immune modifications in fetal membranes overlying the cervix precede parturition in humans. *J. Immunol.* 198, 1345–1356. doi: 10.4049/jimmunol.1601482

March of Dimes, PMNCH, Save the Children, and WHO (2012). *Born Too Soon: The Global Action Report on Preterm Birth*, eds M. V. Kinney, C. P. Howson and J. E. Lawn (Geneva: World Health Organization).

Martin, J. A., Haa, B., and Osterman, M. J. K. (2019). *Births in the United States, Data Brief no. 436, National Center for Health Statistics*. Hyattsville, MA: National Center for Health Statistics.

McLaren, J., Malak, T. M., and Bell, S. C. (1999). Structural characteristics of term human fetal membranes prior to labour: identification of an area of altered morphology overlying the cervix. *Hum. Reprod.* 14, 237–241.

McParland, P. C., Taylor, D. J., and Bell, S. C. (2003). Mapping of zones of altered morphology and chorionic connective tissue cellular phenotype in human fetal membranes (amniochorion and decidua) overlying the lower uterine pole and cervix before labor at term. *Am. J. Obstet. Gynecol.* 189, 1481–1488.

Menon, R. (2016). Human fetal membranes at term: Dead tissue or signalers of parturition? *Placenta* 44, 1–5. doi: 10.1016/j.placenta.2016.05.013

Menon, R., Behnia, F., Polettini, J., Saade, G. R., Campisi, J., and Velarde, M. (2016). Placental membrane aging and HMGB1 signaling associated with human parturition. *Aging* 8, 216–230.

Menon, R., Boldogh, I., Hawkins, H. K., Woodson, M., Polettini, J., Syed, T. A., et al. (2014). Histological evidence of oxidative stress and premature senescence in preterm premature rupture of the human fetal membranes recapitulated in vitro. *Am. J. Pathol.* 184, 1740–1751. doi: 10.1016/j.ajpath.2014.02.011

Menon, R., Fortunato, S. J., Yu, J., Milne, G. L., Sanchez, S., Drobek, C. O., et al. (2011). Cigarette smoke induces oxidative stress and apoptosis in normal term fetal membranes. *Placenta* 32, 317–322. doi: 10.1016/j.placenta.2011.01.015

Menon, R., and Moore, J. J. (2020). Fetal Membranes, Not a Mere Appendage of the Placenta, but a Critical Part of the Fetal-Maternal Interface Controlling Parturition. *Obstet. Gynecol. Clin. North Am.* 47, 147–162.

Menon, R., Richardson, L. S., and Lappas, M. (2019). Fetal membrane architecture, aging and inflammation in pregnancy and parturition. *Placenta* 79, 40–45. doi: 10.1016/j.placenta.2018.11.003

Mercer, B. M. (2004). Preterm premature rupture of the membranes: diagnosis and management. *Clin. Perinatol.* 31, 765–782.

Mesiano, S. (2007). Myometrial progesterone responsiveness. *Semin. Reprod. Med.* 25, 5–13.

Miller, M. F., Chernyak, S. M., Batterman, S., and Loch-Caruso, R. (2009). Polybrominated diphenyl ethers in human gestational membranes from women in southeast Michigan. *Environ. Sci. Technol.* 43, 3042–3046.

Miller, M. F., Chernyak, S. M., Domino, S. E., Batterman, S. A., and Loch-Caruso, R. (2012). Concentrations and speciation of polybrominated diphenyl ethers in human amniotic fluid. *Sci. Total Environ.* 41, 294–298. doi: 10.1016/j.scitotenv.2011.11.088

Mitchell, L. A., Lauer, F. T., Burchiel, S. W., and McDonald, J. D. (2009). Mechanisms for how inhaled multiwalled carbon nanotubes suppress systemic immune function in mice. *Nat. Nanotechnol.* 4, 451–456. doi: 10.1038/nnano.2009.151

Mitchell, M. D., Edwin, S. S., Lundin-Schiller, S., Silver, R. M., Smotkin, D., and Trautman, M. S. (1993). Mechanism of interleukin-1 beta stimulation of human amnion prostaglandin biosynthesis: mediation via a novel inducible cyclooxygenase. *Placenta* 14, 615–625.

Mitro, S. D., Johnson, T., and Zota, A. R. (2015). Cumulative chemical exposures during pregnancy and early development. *Curr. Environ. Health Rep.* 2, 367–378.

Myatt, L., and Sun, K. (2010). Role of fetal membranes in signaling of fetal maturation and parturition. *Int. J. Dev. Biol.* 54, 545–553. doi: 10.1387/ijdb.082771lm

National Academy of Sciences (1992). *Chapter 5: The Capacity of Toxic Agents to Compromise the Immune System (Biologic Markers of Immunosuppression). Biologic Markers in Immunotoxicology. National Research Council (US) Subcommittee on Immunotoxicology*. Washington, DC: The National Academies Press.

Norwitz, E. R., Lopez Bernal, A., and Starkey, P. M. (1992). Tumor necrosis factor-alpha selectively stimulates prostaglandin F2 alpha production by macrophages in human term decidua. *Am. J. Obstet. Gynecol.* 167, 815–820.

Nourse, C. B., and Steer, P. A. (1997). Perinatal outcome following conservative management of mid-trimester pre-labour rupture of the membranes. *J. Paediatr. Child Health* 33, 125–130.

Oh, K. J., Lee, K. A., Sohn, Y. K., Park, C. W., Hong, J. S., Romero, R., et al. (2010). Intraamniotic infection with genital mycoplasmas exhibits a more intense inflammatory response than intraamniotic infection with other microorganisms in patients with preterm premature rupture of membranes. *Am. J. Obstet. Gynecol.* 203:211.e1-8. doi: 10.1016/j.ajog.2010.03.035

Osman, I., Young, A., Ledingham, M. A., Thomson, A. J., Jordan, F. I, Greer, A., et al. (2003). Leukocyte density and pro-inflammatory cytokine expression in human fetal membranes, decidua, cervix and myometrium before and during labour at term. *Mol. Hum. Reprod.* 9, 41–45.

Park, H. R., Harris, S. M., Boldenow, E., McEachin, R. C., Sartor, M., Chames, M., et al. (2018). Group B streptococcus activates transcriptomic pathways related to premature birth in human extraplacental membranes in vitro. *Biol. Reprod.* 98, 396–407. doi: 10.1093/biolre/iox147

Peltier, M. R., Arita, Y., Klimova, N. G., Gurzenda, E. M., Koo, H. C., Murthy, A., et al. (2013). 2,3,7,8-tetrachlorodibenzo-p-dioxin (TCDD) enhances placental inflammation. *J. Reprod. Immunol.* 98, 10–20. doi: 10.1016/j.jri.2013.02.005

Peltier, M. R., Klimova, N. G., Arita, Y., Gurzenda, E. M., Murthy, A., Chawala, K., et al. (2012). Polybrominated diphenyl ethers enhance the production of proinflammatory cytokines by the placenta. *Placenta* 33, 745–749. doi: 10.1016/j.placenta.2012.06.005

Peltier, M. R., Koo, H. C., Getahun, D., and Menon, R. (2015). Does exposure to flame retardants increase the risk for preterm birth? *J. Reprod. Immunol.* 107, 20–25. doi: 10.1016/j.jri.2014.11.002

Pike, K. C., and Lucas, J. S. (2015). Respiratory consequences of late preterm birth. *Paediatr. Respir. Rev.* 16, 182–188. doi: 10.1016/j.prrv.2014.12.001

Richardson, L., Gnecco, J., Ding, T., Osteen, K., Rogers, L. M., Aronoff, D. M., et al. (2019). Fetal membrane organ-on-chip: an innovative approach to study cellular interactions. *Reprod. Sci.* doi: 10.1177/1933719119828084 [Online ahead of print]

Romero, R., Dey, S. K., and Fisher, S. J. (2014). Preterm labor: one syndrome, many causes. *Science* 345, 760–765. doi: 10.1126/science.1251816

Romero, R., Espinoza, J., Goncalves, L. F., Kusanovic, J. P., Friel, L., and Hassan, S. (2007). The role of inflammation and infection in preterm birth. *Semin. Reprod. Med.* 25, 21–39.

Ruckart, P. Z., Bove, F. J., and Maslia, M. (2014). Evaluation of contaminated drinking water and preterm birth, small for gestational age, and birth weight at Marine Corps Base Camp Lejeune. North Carolina: a cross-sectional study. *Environ. Health* 13:99. doi: 10.1186/1476-069X-13-99

Sagiv, S. K., Rifas-Shiman, S. L., Fleisch, A. F., Webster, T. F., Calafat, A. M., Ye, X., et al. (2018). Early-Pregnancy Plasma Concentrations of Perfluoroalkyl Substances and Birth Outcomes in Project Viva: Confounded by Pregnancy Hemodynamics? *Am. J. Epidemiol.* 187, 793–802. doi: 10.1093/aje/kwx332

Selgrade, M. K. (2007). Immunotoxicity: the risk is real. *Toxicol. Sci.* 100, 328–332.

Selgrade, M. K., and Gilmour, M. I. (2010). Suppression of pulmonary host defenses and enhanced susceptibility to respiratory bacterial infection in mice following inhalation exposure to trichloroethylene and chloroform. *J. Immunotoxicol.* 7, 350–356. doi: 10.3109/1547691X.2010.520139

Shane, H. L., Baur, R., Lukomska, E., Weatherly, L., and Anderson, S. E. (2020). Immunotoxicity and allergenic potential induced by topical application of perfluorooctanoic acid (PFOA) in a murine model. *Food Chem. Toxicol.* 136, 111114.

Soneji, S., and Beltran-Sanchez, H. (2019). Association of maternal cigarette smoking and smoking cessation with preterm birth. *JAMA Netw Open* 2, e192514. doi: 10.1001/jamanetworkopen.2019.2514

Strauss, J. F. III (2013). Extracellular matrix dynamics and fetal membrane rupture. *Reprod. Sci.* 20, 140–153. doi: 10.1177/1933719111424454

Taylor, C. M., Golding, J., and Emond, A. M. (2015). Adverse effects of maternal lead levels on birth outcomes in the ALSPAC study: a prospective birth cohort study. *BJOG* 122, 322–328. doi: 10.1111/1471-0528.12756

Thornberry, N. A., Bull, H. G., Calaycay, J. R., Chapman, K. T., Howard, A. D., Kostura, M. J., et al. (1992). A novel heterodimeric cysteine protease is required for interleukin-1 beta processing in monocytes. *Nature* 356, 768–774.

Torchin, H., and Ancel, P. Y. (2016). [Epidemiology and risk factors of preterm birth]. *J. Gynecol. Obstet. Biol. Reprod.* 45, 1213–1230. doi: 10.1016/j.jgyn.2016.09.013

Vadillo-Ortega, F., Hernandez, A., Gonzalez-Avila, G., Bermejo, L., Iwata, K., and Strauss, J. F. III (1996). Increased matrix metalloproteinase activity and reduced tissue inhibitor of metalloproteinases-1 levels in amniotic fluids from pregnancies complicated by premature rupture of membranes. *Am. J. Obstet. Gynecol.* 174, 1371–1376.

Verani, J. R., McGee, L., Schrag, S. J., Division of Bacterial Diseases, N. C. F. I., and Respiratory Diseases and Prevention, C. F. D. C. (2010). Prevention of perinatal group B streptococcal disease–revised guidelines from CDC, 2010. *MMWR Recomm. Rep.* 59, 1–36.

Verbruggen, S. W., Oyen, M. L., Phillips, A. T., and Nowlan, N. C. (2017). Function and failure of the fetal membrane: Modelling the mechanics of the chorion and amnion. *PLoS One* 12:e0171588. doi: 10.1371/journal.pone.0171588

Vogel, J. P., Chawanpaiboon, S., Moller, A. B., Watananirun, K., Bonet, M., and Lumbiganon, P. (2018). The global epidemiology of preterm birth. *Best Pract. Res. Clin. Obstet. Gynaecol.* 52, 3–12. doi: 10.1016/j.bpobgyn.2018.04.003

Wallace, M. E., Grantz, K. L., Liu, D., Zhu, Y., Kim, S. S., and Mendola, P. (2016). Exposure to ambient air pollution and premature rupture of membranes. *Am. J. Epidemiol.* 183, 1114–1121. doi: 10.1093/aje/kwv284

Wang, K., Tian, Y., Zheng, H., Shan, S., Zhao, X., and Liu, C. (2019). Maternal exposure to ambient fine particulate matter and risk of premature rupture of membranes in Wuhan. Central China: a cohort study. *Environ. Health* 18:96. doi: 10.1186/s12940-019-0534-y

Wang, W., Chen, Z. J., Myatt, L., and Sun, K. (2018). 11beta-HSD1 in human fetal membranes as a potential therapeutic target for preterm birth. *Endocr. Rev.* 39, 241–260. doi: 10.1210/er.2017-00188

Waters, E. M., Gerstner, H. B., and Huff, J. E. (1977). Trichloroethylene. I. An overview. *J. Toxicol. Environ. Health* 2, 671–707.

Watson, R. E., Jacobson, C. F., Williams, A. L., Howard, W. B., and DeSesso, J. M. (2006). Trichloroethylene-contaminated drinking water and congenital heart defects: a critical analysis of the literature. *Reprod. Toxicol.* 21, 117–147.

Wong, O. (2004). Carcinogenicity of trichloroethylene: an epidemiologic assessment. *Clin. Occup. Environ. Med.* 4, 557–589.

Woods, J. R. Jr. (2001). Reactive oxygen species and preterm premature rupture of membranes-a review. *Placenta* 22(Suppl. A), S38–S44.

Wright, P. F., Thomas, W. D., and Stacey, N. H. (1991). Effects of trichloroethylene on hepatic and splenic lymphocytotoxic activities in rodents. *Toxicology* 70, 231–242.

Xueqin, Y., Wenxue, L., Peimao, L., Wen, Z., Xianqing, H., and Zhixiong, Z. (2018). Cytokine expression and cytokine-based T-cell profiling in occupational medicamentosa-like dermatitis due to trichloroethylene. *Toxicol. Lett.* 288, 129–135. doi: 10.1016/j.toxlet.2018.02.012

Yellon, S. M. (2019). Immunobiology of cervix ripening. *Front. Immunol.* 10:3156. doi: 10.3389/fimmu.2019.03156

Yockey, L. J., and Iwasaki, A. (2018). Interferons and proinflammatory cytokines in pregnancy and fetal development. *Immunity* 49, 397–412. doi: 10.1016/j.immuni.2018.07.017

Young, A., Thomson, A. J., Ledingham, M., Jordan, F. I, Greer, A., and Norman, J. E. (2002). Immunolocalization of proinflammatory cytokines in myometrium, cervix, and fetal membranes during human parturition at term. *Biol. Reprod.* 66, 445–449.

Zeng, L. N., Zhang, L. L., Shi, J., Gu, L. L., Grogan, W., Gargano, M. M., et al. (2014). The primary microbial pathogens associated with premature rupture of the membranes in China: a systematic review. *Taiwan J. Obstet. Gynecol.* 53, 443–451. doi: 10.1016/j.tjog.2014.02.003

Zhong, Q., Lu, C., Zhang, W., Zheng, X., and Deng, Q. (2018). Preterm birth and ambient temperature: Strong association during night-time and warm seasons. *J. Therm. Biol.* 78, 381–390. doi: 10.1016/j.jtherbio.2018.11.002

Innate Immune Mechanisms to Protect Against Infection at the Human Decidual-Placental Interface

Regina Hoo [1,2], Annettee Nakimuli [1,3] and Roser Vento-Tormo [1,2]*

[1] Wellcome Sanger Institute, Cambridge, United Kingdom, [2] Centre for Trophoblast Research, University of Cambridge, Cambridge, United Kingdom, [3] Department of Obstetrics and Gynecology, School of Medicine, Makerere University, Kampala, Uganda

*Correspondence:
Roser Vento-Tormo
rv4@sanger.ac.uk

During pregnancy, the placenta forms the anatomical barrier between the mother and developing fetus. Infectious agents can potentially breach the placental barrier resulting in pathogenic transmission from mother to fetus. Innate immune responses, orchestrated by maternal and fetal cells at the decidual-placental interface, are the first line of defense to avoid vertical transmission. Here, we outline the anatomy of the human placenta and uterine lining, the decidua, and discuss the potential capacity of pathogen pattern recognition and other host defense strategies present in the innate immune cells at the placental-decidual interface. We consider major congenital infections that access the placenta from hematogenous or decidual route. Finally, we highlight the challenges in studying human placental responses to pathogens and vertical transmission using current experimental models and identify gaps in knowledge that need to be addressed. We further propose novel experimental strategies to address such limitations.

Keywords: innate immunity, uterine-placental interface, trophoblast, decidua, vertical transmission

INTRODUCTION

The human placenta is the temporary extra-embryonic organ that is present only during pregnancy and is the anatomical boundary between the mother and fetus. It has a range of functions including transport of nutrients and gases, and hormonal production (1). The placenta forms a physical, selective barrier between the maternal and fetal circulations, preventing transfer of pathogens. The uterine mucosal lining, the endometrium, is transformed into the decidua during early pregnancy (2). A range of innate immune mechanisms can respond to pathogens in both the decidua and the placenta (3, 4). The maternal-fetal interface is a protective barrier against pathogens, but some pathogens can transfer from the mother to fetus by different routes and cause fetal infection (3, 4).

Vertical transmission during pregnancy can occur on distinct boundaries between the mother and the fetus: (i) the intervillous space (IVS), where placental villi is in direct contact with the maternal blood, (ii) the implantation site or decidua basalis, where maternal cells are in direct contact with the invading fetal trophoblast, and (iii) the fetal membranes, which are in direct contact with the uterine cavity (5). Defense mechanisms in the cervix, such as the production of mucus and antimicrobial peptides (AMP), limit ascending infection from pathogens present in the lower genital tract, that otherwise may access the uterine cavity (6). However, some pathogens can escape antimicrobial strategies at the cervix and ascend to the uterus, where they can bypass the fetal membranes and lead to the inflammation of the membranes- also known as chorioamnionitis- and infection of the amniotic fluid (7, 8). Pathologic and immune features of chorioamnionitis and intra-amniotic infection are generally associated with bacterial invasion and inflammation [refer to (8, 9) for a comprehensive review on these mechanisms]. Here, we focus on infections and innate immune mechanisms at the uterine-placental interface—cases (i) and (ii) (**Figure 1**).

Infections at the uterine-placental interface are commonly associated with viruses, parasites and few bacteria (**Table 1**). Viral pathogens such as human cytomegalovirus (HCMV), Zika (ZIKV), and rubella virus are the most common vertically transmitted pathogens through the decidual-placental interface (**Table 1**) (26, 27). Non-viral pathogens, such as *Toxoplasma gondii* and *Listeria monocytogenes*, can cross the placental barrier via cell-to-cell transmission (**Table 1**) (28, 29). Fetal infection can result in various forms of congenital anomalies in humans (**Table 1**). Understanding the pathogenic mechanisms used by infectious agents is central to preventing vertical transmission and controlling infection during pregnancy.

How the innate immune cells and mechanisms in the placenta and the uterus recognize and respond to protect both the fetus and mother remains controversial due to technical and ethical constraints. However, there are several different models currently used to interrogate the uterine-placental interface in pregnancy. Firstly, mice are frequently used as a pregnancy model for infection. Although the murine models have provided important insights into the pathogenesis of various infection agents in the context of pregnancy, there are still limitations with this approach. The anatomy of placentation, length of gestation, and use of inbred strains, make extrapolation to humans problematic (30, 31). Secondly, a range of human trophoblast and choriocarcinoma cell lines are used as *in vitro* models for infection with pathogens. In contrast to the first trimester trophoblast *in vivo*, these cell lines do not recapitulate normal human trophoblast characteristics such as expression of the human leukocyte antigen (HLA) class I and methylation of *ELF5* (32, 33). Thirdly, human primary placental explants are frequently used. The syncytium dies rapidly in these cultures and it is virtually impossible to standardize the types of villi sampled (30). Therefore, these *in vitro* experimental factors should be taken into careful consideration when interpreting studies of infection of trophoblast.

In this review, we cover the innate immune features of the decidual-placental interface throughout gestation. We identify the gaps in knowledge and highlight the limitations of current studies and experimental models. Finally, we discuss novel experimental strategies for understanding how infection affects pregnancy in humans.

Physiology of the Placenta Throughout Gestation

The trophoblasts of the placenta are the barrier between fetal and maternal tissues. They are derived from the trophectoderm, the outer layer of the blastocyst that forms an inner mononuclear layer with an outer primary syncytium following implantation (34). The trophoblast in contact with the maternal cells can be: (i) syncytiotrophoblast (SCT), a single layer multinucleated, syncytial layer formed by fusion of the underlying villous cytotrophoblast (VCT), and (ii) extravillous trophoblast (EVT), that invade from the cytotrophoblast shell and anchoring villi into the transformed maternal endometrium, the decidua (2).

The function of EVT is to transform the uterine spiral arteries so that maternal blood is delivered to the intervillous space at low pressure. The arteries are surrounded by interstitial EVT that destroys the smooth muscle cells of the arterial media, known as "fibrinoid" change (35, 36). Subsequently, endovascular EVT (eEVT) moves down the spiral arteries from the placenta-decidua boundary (35). These eEVT form a plug of cells, limiting surges of arterial blood from damaging the delicate villi. EVT invasion transforms the arteries to support optimal regulation of blood flow into the placenta during fetal development (36). The plugs dissipate between 8 and 10 weeks of gestation when the full hemochorial circulation is established (37). Maternal blood then flows into the IVS, and establishes direct contact with the SCT allowing for proper nutrient and gas exchange between the mother and the fetus.

HOFBAUER CELLS: THE TISSUE RESIDENT IMMUNE CELLS OF THE PLACENTA

Hofbauer (HB) cells are fetal macrophages of the human placenta (38). HB cells can be detected in the placental villous stroma as early as 3 weeks post-conception and are present throughout pregnancy (1, 39). They are likely to have a variety of functions including control of villous remodeling and differentiation, hormonal secretion, and trophoblast turnover (1, 40). Several lines of evidence have led to the postulation that HB cells may have a role in infection during pregnancy. HB cells with ZIKV viral particles detected intracellularly have been shown (41, 42). Human immunodeficiency virus 1 (HIV-1) has also been detected in HB cells from first trimester infected placenta (43). Whether the HB cells can serve as a reservoir or limit virus replication is still unknown. Isolated HB cells from healthy term placenta show elevation of pro-inflammatory cytokines such as IL-6, MCP-1, IP-10, and IFN-α upon *in vitro* infection with ZIKV (44). HB cells from the first trimester placenta are also permissive for ZIKV infection and replication (23). However, this must be interpreted with caution because *in vitro* culture of HB cells do not entirely recapitulate the complexity of villous stromal microenvironment, such as presence of hormone and growth factors, all of which will influence the function and activity of HB cells (45).

MATERNAL BLOOD AND SCT INTERFACE

The SCT is the barrier between maternal blood and the placental core as it separates the IVS from the underlying fetal villous stroma. Blood-borne pathogens such as viruses and parasites can potentially be transmitted through the SCT barrier (**Figure 1**).

How can pathogens cross the SCT barrier and the VCT to infect the villous stroma? Although the SCT is an efficient barrier due to its stiff, highly dense actin cytoskeleton network and continuous membrane (46), the syncytium undergoes

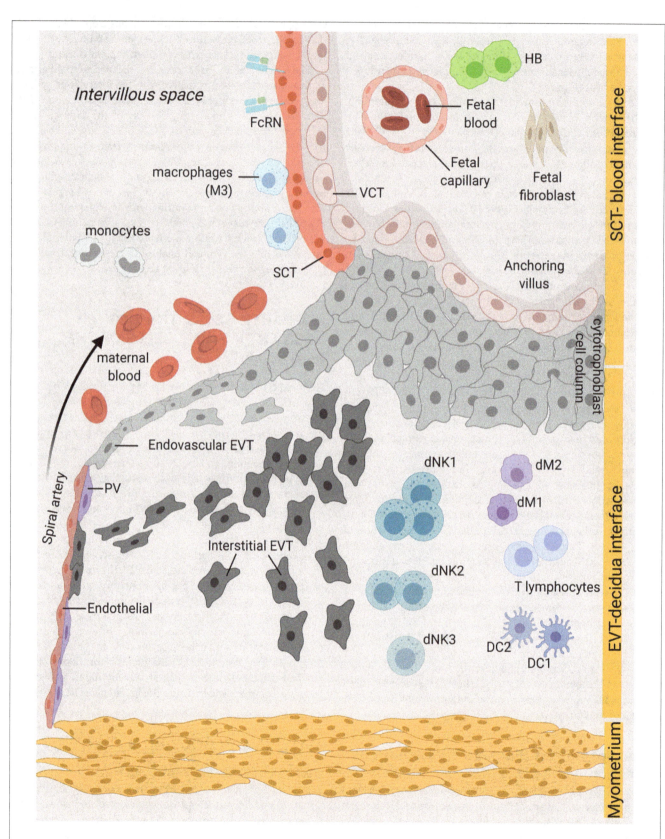

FIGURE 1 | Possible infection and vertical transmission route at the maternal-fetal interface. Illustration representing the anchoring placenta villi of early pregnancy, with onset of maternal blood circulation bathing the intervillous space. SCT-blood interface represents the SCT barrier exposed to maternal blood and immune cells. EVT-decidua interface represents the interface between EVT and maternal decidua cells. Major cell types of placenta trophoblast and decidua from Vento-Tormo et al. (10) are represented. SCT, syncytiotrophoblast; VCT, villous cytotrophoblast; EVT, extravillous trophoblast; DC, dendritic cell; dNK, decidua Natural killer cells; dM, decidua macrophages; HB, Hofbauer cell; PV, perivascular cells; FcRN, neonatal Fc receptor. Figure is created by BioRender.com.

TABLE 1 | Vertically transmitted pathogens with clinical evidence from natural human infection.

Species	Lifestyle	Life cycle and pathogenesis	Clinical manifestations	Evidence of cellular tropism in the human placenta or decidua by histology or PCR	References
Chlamydia trachomatis	Intracellular bacteria	Formation of reticulate body inside host cell allows for rapid replication. Conversion of reticulate body to elementary body inside host cell promotes the release of infectious bacteria to neighboring cell	Ectopic pregnancy, stillbirth, preterm labor, blinding corneal injury in neonates, neonatal pneumonia	Whole placenta, glandular epithelial cells, unidentified decidual cells	(11)
Group B Streptococcus (Streptococcus agalactiae)	Non-motile, extracellular bacteria	Beta-hemolytic. Strong adherence to epithelial layer. Able to form biofilm	Neonatal GBS (sepsis and meningitis), preterm birth	Amniotic epithelium, amniotic fluid, chorion, decidua	(12)
Listeria monocytogenes (Listeriosis)	Motile intracellular bacteria	Utilize two bacterial surface proteins (internalin A and B) to invade various non-phagocytic cell types. Able to escape phagosome-mediated lysis and multiply rapidly in host cytoplasm. Able to spread to adjacent cell through host cell actin polymerization	Spontaneous abortion, stillbirth, preterm labor	Placenta trophoblast	(13)
Coxiella burnetii (Q fever)	Intracellular bacteria	Able to escape phagosome-mediated lysis in macrophage	Spontaneous abortion, preterm delivery, fetal death	Placenta (unknown cell type)	(14)
Treponema pallidum	Motile spirochaete, extracellular bacteria	Able to transverse tight-junction between endothelial cells. Highly motile	Congenital syphilis	Placenta (unknown cell type)	(15, 16)
Toxoplasma gondii (Toxoplasmosis)	Intracellular parasite	Able to infect and replicate within various host cell types. Able to switch between non-motile (for replication) and motile state (for egress and invasion into new host cell)	Congenital toxoplasmosis, stillbirth	Placenta trophoblast	(17)
Trypanosoma cruzi (Chagas)	Intracellular and extracellular parasite	Able to propagate in various host cells and escape. Progeny released by host cells are motile, and able to infect distal tissue or organs	Stillbirth, preterm labor	SCT, villous stroma, placenta basal plate	(18)
Herpes simplex virus 1, 2 (HSV-1/2)	dsDNA virus	Able to cross through skin lesions and epithelial mucosal cells. Poor antibody neutralization to viral glycoprotein D (gD). Vertical transmission rate is very low	Spontaneous abortion, intrauterine growth restriction, preterm labor, neonatal herpes	Decidua	(11)
Human cytomegalovirus(HCMV)	dsDNA virus	Easily transmitted through bodily fluid. Poor antibody neutralization to viral glycoprotein B (gB). Can establish lifelong latency in myeloid cells	Variable; neonatal neurodevelopmental damage and hearing loss	VCT, decidua, amniotic membrane	(19)
Rubella	ssRNA virus	Able to enter the lymphatic system from the respiratory tract. Can lead to a systemic infection. Viral capsid can evade host immune recognition	Significant birth defects, neonatal deafness, miscarriage	Placenta basal plate and endothelial cells	(20)
Parvovirus B19	ssDNA virus	Spread through respiratory droplets. Preferential tropism for human erythroid progenitor	Fetus is usually unaffected, may result in severe fetal anemia	Whole placenta, placenta villi	(21)
Varicella zoster virus (Chicken pox)	ssDNA virus	Vertical transmission is very rare and only happens in primary infection	Congenital varicella syndrome, intrauterine growth restriction, low birth weight	No evidence, but chronic villitis has been described	(22)
ZIKA virus (ZIKV)	ssRNA virus	Mosquito borne infection transmitted from blood meal. Preferentially to invade blood monocytes	Congenital fetal anomalies (microcephaly), miscarriage, stillbirth	Whole placenta, amniotic epithelium, VCT, Hofbauer cells, decidual macrophages, decidual fibroblast	(23–25)

continuous breaks or gaps and dynamic repair processes (47). Breaks in the syncytium could potentially lead to transmission of pathogens into the underlying VCT. Our recent work showed that a novel population of maternal macrophages (M3) is associated with the SCT in early pregnancy and might be involved in repairing the breaks in the syncytium (10). It is intriguing that M3 macrophages infected with intracellular pathogens could possibly gain access to the underlying VCT via the syncytial breaks (**Figure 2**).

Only a few viral entry receptors on the SCT are described. Notably, the SCT lacks expression of ZIKV entry receptors, Axl, and Tyro3 (48) and the HCMV entry co-receptor integrin α/β (49). This is further supported by the transcriptomic expression of viral receptors in placental cells (10, 50, 51). Expression of surface receptors commonly used by ZIKV such as *AXL* and *HCMV* such as *NRP2* and *PDGFRA* are lowly expressed by the SCT (50). In addition, there is minimal co-expression of ACE2, the receptor gene for human severe acute respiratory syndrome coronavirus 2 (SARS-CoV-2), and TMPRSS2, the viral spike protein serine protease gene (50, 52). In line with this, there is no conclusive and direct evidence of vertical transmission of SARS-CoV-2 in a placenta from a healthy individual. There are some reports showing SARS-CoV-2 is predominantly localized at the SCT of the second trimester placenta (53, 54) and can lead to severe inflammatory infiltrate in the IVS (55). However, these findings are presented in a very small number of patients with severe disease or pre-existing pregnancy complications (54, 55).

Alternative transplacental mechanisms have been postulated at the syncytial barrier. Neonatal Fc receptor (FcRn) is expressed on the apical surface of the SCT and functions to selectively

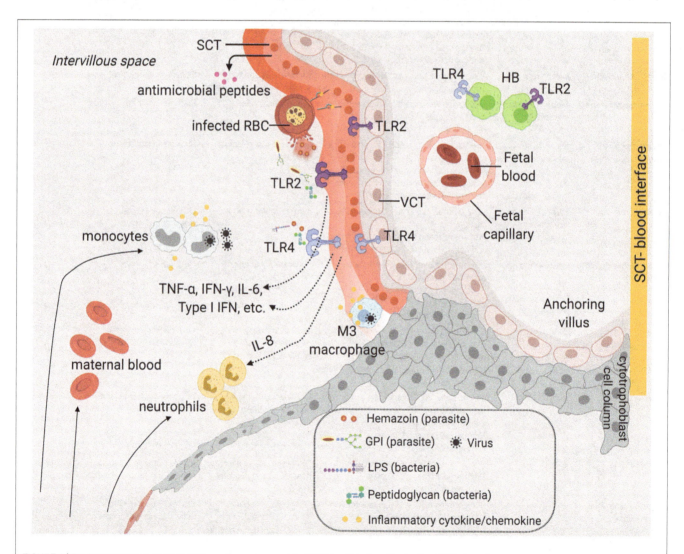

FIGURE 2 | Toll-like receptors and potential inflammatory response at the SCT-blood interface. Predominant TLRs found in the human placenta from early and term pregnancies. TLR2 and TLR4 are expressed in human placenta SCT, VCT, and in HB cells. Infiltration of infected maternal blood, infected immune cells, or release of pathogenic determinant such lipopolysaccharide (LPS), peptidoglycan, or parasite materials such as hemozoin or GPI (glycosylphosphatidylinositol) into the IVS will activate TLR-mediated signaling, leading to the production of a wide range of cytokines and chemokines. Severe infection is characterized by massive immune cell infiltration including monocytes and neutrophils from systemic circulation and overproduction of inflammatory cytokines upon TLR activation. This may lead to SCT inflammation and damage. SCT also secretes antimicrobial peptides as innate immune mechanisms. Figure is created by BioRender.com.

transport maternal IgG (56). FcRn could be exploited by certain viruses to enter the placenta including ZIKV, HIV-1, and HCMV (19, 57, 58). Transferrin receptor 1 (TfR1) is expressed on the apical end of the SCT, and functions as the primary iron transporter into the basal side of the SCT to provide sufficient iron stores into fetal circulation (59). TfR1 has been associated with viral entry into a broad host cell range, including Hepatitis C virus (60, 61) suggesting a possible mechanism of viral transport across the SCT barrier. Some pathogens, although unable to cross the SCT barrier, can still adhere to the syncytium and cause further pathology. For instance, *Plasmodium falciparum* infected red blood cells can bind with high affinity to chondroitin sulfate A expressed on the SCT, resulting in local inflammation, syncytial breaks, and damage (62–64).

Although the SCT is an effective barrier to most pathogens, local inflammation, tissue damage, and FcRN or TfR1-mediated viral entry at the SCT can potentially allow pathogen to breach the syncytial barrier, giving opportunity for transmission from maternal blood into placental villi (**Figure 2**).

MATERNAL DECIDUA AND EVT INTERFACE

During the first trimester of pregnancy, fetal EVT invades deeply into the uterus. The decidua basalis, the region located at the implantation site, is populated at this time by a distinctive subset of innate lymphocytes, decidual Natural Killer cells (dNK), which constitute up to 70% of leukocytes. We have identified three major populations of dNK by single-cell RNA-sequencing with unique phenotypes and functions in early pregnancy (10). In addition, there are populations of decidual macrophages (dMs) (~20%), conventional dendritic cells (DCs) and small proportions of T cells (~10–15%), whereas B cells, plasma cells, mast cells, and granulocytes are virtually absent (10) (**Figure 1**). The proportion of immune cells will vary throughout pregnancy, with an increase in the proportion of T cells at term (51).

Systemic infections will reach all organs including the decidua. Whether pathogens can also access the decidua via the cervix is still unclear. *Chlamydia trachomatis*, a common sexually-transmitted intracellular bacteria, was detected in glandular epithelial cells and unidentified decidual cells in decidual biopsies (11). This suggests the possibility of infections ascending and spreading from cell-to-cell from the lower genital tract into endometrial glands and vascular endothelium. The decidua basalis is in close contact with fetal cells and the maternal vasculature (**Figure 1**). First trimester dMs and decidual stromal cells are susceptible to ZIKV infection and replication *ex vivo* (23). Hence, infection could possibly spread from infected maternal immune and non-immune cells at the decidua, into uninfected VCT in the columns of the anchoring villi, and finally into the fetal compartment. However, this is likely to be limited to certain microorganisms which are capable of cell-to-cell spread, have an intracellular host niche, and are able to escape host innate defense mechanisms (**Table 1**).

HCMV, the most common cause of congenital infection, is mostly reported to infect from the decidua (11, 65). Women with primary HCMV infection and first pregnancy are more likely to transmit the virus to their fetus, compared to multiparous women with previous infection and demonstrable antibodies (66–68). Low affinity maternal antibodies against HCMV correlate with higher viral loads detected in the decidua, whereas patients with intermediate to high neutralizing antibodies have minimal viral replication (65), suggesting that maternal immunity against HCMV reduces risk of vertical transmission. HCMV protein was also detected in a range of cells within the decidua including endothelial, decidual stromal cells, DCs and macrophages (11, 65), suggesting that that infected maternal leukocytes could initiate transmission through contact and infection of endothelial cells that line decidual blood vessels.

Despite the evidence of decidual infection, the mechanism of vertical transmission for HCMV is still in debate. dNKs have been proposed to play a protective role against HCMV infection through several mechanisms including modulation of their cytotoxic effector function (69) and the interactions between the killer-cell immunoglobulin receptors (KIRs) expressed by dNK and HLA molecules expressed in the infected cells (70, 71). Activating KIR2DS1 by dNKs has been demonstrated to be more cytolytic against HLA-C2 HCMV-infected maternal decidual stromal cells (70). Similar cytotoxic response was also observed when peripheral blood NK cells expressing KIR2DS1 were exposed to HCMV-infected fibroblasts (71). Hence, this implies that in the decidua, dNKs are capable of eliminating harmful infection depending on the combination of KIR/HLA interactions between dNK and infected cells. dNKs are also able to control HIV-1 infection *in vitro* through production of IFN-γ (72). The role of dNK in controlling viral infection may protect against potential risk of vertical transmission from the decidua.

TRANSMEMBRANE PATTERN RECOGNITION RECEPTORS: TOLL-LIKE RECEPTORS

Pattern recognition receptors (PRR) are encoded in the germ-line and recognize specific, conserved pathogen-associated molecular patterns (PAMPs). These include Gram-negative bacteria lipopolysaccharide (LPS), Gram-positive bacteria lipoteichoic acids, lipoprotein, DNA, RNA, glucans, and peptidoglycans (73, 74). Pathogen recognition is not only an essential component of the innate immune response against infection, but also plays an important role in bridging the innate and adaptive systems by Toll-like receptors (TLR) activation of antigen presenting cells by up-regulation of major histocompatibility complex (MHC) and co-stimulatory molecules (75).

TLRs, the most studied family of PRR, are type I transmembrane proteins with large extracellular domains containing leucine-rich repeats that are expressed at the cell surface or intracellularly (76). Each TLR recognizes distinct PAMPs, leading to the activation of the transcription factor NF-κB and/or the interferon-regulatory factor (IRF) family, and the production of a wide range of cytokines and chemokines, including type I IFNs (76, 77). TLRs are expressed by immune cells (macrophages, DCs, and B cells) as well as non-immune cells (fibroblasts and epithelial cells) (74).

TLRs at the Human Uterine-Placental Interface

Expression of TLRs is dynamic and changes in response to different pathogens and cytokines (74). TLR2 (which recognizes bacterial proteoglycan) and TLR4 (which recognizes bacterial LPS) are the most well-studied, with immunohistochemical evidence of expression in healthy primary SCT at term (78–80). In contrast, in the first trimester, TLR2 and TLR4 proteins are expressed in VCT and EVT, but minimally in SCT (81, 82) (**Figure 3**). There is therefore variation in TLR2 and TLR4 expression in the different trophoblast lineages across pregnancy. Why and how such dynamic regulation of TLR expression occurs during gestation requires further investigation in a broader range of human placental samples (different donors, gestation stages, genetic background, sampling regions). It is likely that alteration in cytokines profiles in the microenvironment as pregnancy progresses (83) may result in the variation in the expression of TLRs in the placenta. Current evidence is only limited to *in vitro* TLR2/4 stimulation studies using placental explants and primary first trimester trophoblast cells, which drives the expression of

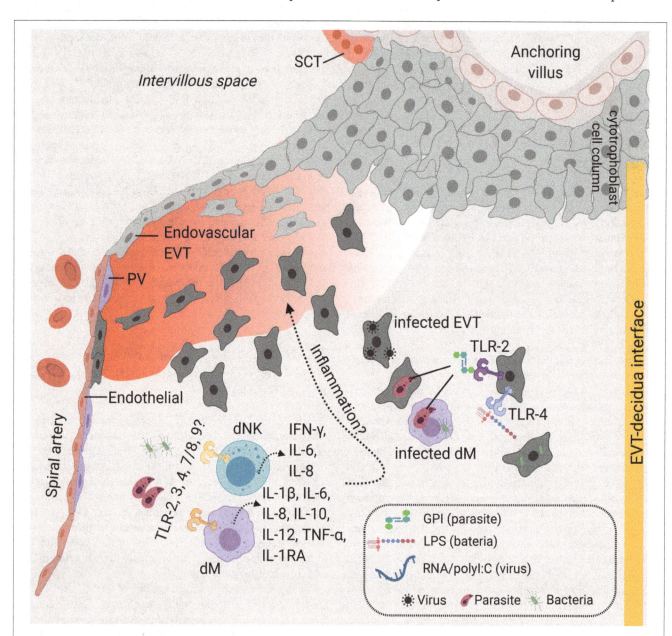

FIGURE 3 | Toll-like receptors and potential inflammatory response at the decidua. Predominant TLRs found in the human placenta from early and term pregnancies. TLR2 and TLR4 are expressed in EVT. dM and dNK also express a wide range of TLR families, where stimulation of TLR agonists lead to the production of a variety of cytokines and chemokines. Infiltration of infected cells and release of PAMPs in the decidua, which will activate TLR-mediated signaling. Overproduction of inflammatory cytokines at the decidua may lead to local inflammation. Figure is created by BioRender.com.

pro-inflammatory cytokines IL-6, IL-8, TNF-α, and IFN-γ (78, 80, 81).

TLR2 and TLR4 proteins are expressed in HB cells, confirmed by co-expression of CD68 in healthy term placentas (78). In early pregnancy, our findings indicate that only *TLR4* but not *TLR2* transcripts are expressed in steady-state HB cells (10) (**Figure 4**). Enhancement of IL-6 and IL-8 secretion upon stimulation of isolated first trimester HB cells with TLR4 agonist, LPS (84), does suggest a role for TLRs on HB cells in bacterial recognition and placental inflammation during early pregnancy. HB cells are postulated to have a role in viral replication (41, 42), however evidence on the expression and function of viral nucleic acid sensing receptors TLR3, TLR7, TLR8, and TLR9 in HB cells is lacking. Our findings show that *TLR7*, which recognizes viral single-strand RNA (ssRNA) (85) is expressed in steady-state HB cells (**Figure 4**) (10).

Other TLRs have also been shown to be expressed in decidua cells. dMs and dNKs isolated from first trimester pregnancies show steady state level expression of *TLR1-9* transcripts and respond to a broad range of PAMPs, including heat-killed bacteria, microbial membranes, and nucleic acids (86). Stimulating primary dMs with these PAMPs produces high levels of TNF-α, IL-1β, IL-6, IL-8, IL-12, IL-10, and IL-1RA, whereas dNKs secrete IL-6, IL-8, and IFN-γ (86). This study suggests that, in addition to the physiological roles of dMs and dNKs in accommodating the uterus for placentation, dMs and dNKs may play a role in pathogen recognition and antimicrobial response via activation of TLR signaling (**Figure 3**). The extent to which subsets of dMs or dNKs population (10) are critical for TLR-mediated response at the decidua is currently unknown.

In malaria endemic populations, single nucleotide polymorphisms (SNPs) within the TLR4 coding and TLR9 promoter regions are associated with variation in disease severity and parasitemia control (87, 88). In the case of pregnancy malaria, primiparous infected mothers with common TLR4 and TLR9 polymorphic variants are correlated with severe complications such as low birth weight and maternal anemia (89). This highlights the importance of studies involving large cohorts of individuals which include genotyping from pregnant mothers living in malaria endemic regions (see section on "Challenges and future perspective").

TLRs in Animal Models of Placental Parasite Infection

Animal models have also been used to study the functional role of TLR signaling, particularly for pathogens that are intracellular at some stage of their life cycle (**Table 1**). TLR4 and TLR9 are strongly activated by malaria parasite PAMPs such as glycosylphosphatidylinositol (GPI), DNA, and hemozoin (90, 91) (**Figure 2**). In a mouse model of placental malaria, TLR4, and Myd88 signaling activation resulted in placental expression of pro-inflammatory markers, such as IL-6 and TNF-α (92, 93). These studies also demonstrated that malaria parasite infection and inflammation in the mouse placenta lead to reduced fetus growth rate and disorganization of the vascular space in the placenta (92, 93). However, TLR-mediated inflammation and

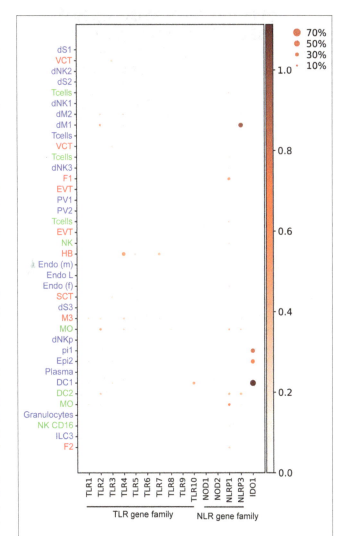

FIGURE 4 | Dotplot representing normalized and log transformed values expression of TLR (*TLR1-10*), NLR genes (*NOD1, NOD2, NLRP1, NLRP3*) and *IDO1* at steady state in early pregnancy from Vento-Tormo et al. (10). Origin of cell types from placenta (red), decidua (blue), and maternal blood (green) are labeled as differences in font color. Dot size represents the fraction of cells from a certain cluster expressing a gene and color scale represents normalized log transformed expression of the gene in that cluster. dS, decidua stroma; F, fibroblast; MO, monocyte; Endo, endothelial; Epi, epithelial; SCT, syncytiotrophoblast; VCT, villous cytotrophoblast; EVT, extravillous trophoblast; DC, dendritic cell; dNK, decidua Natural killer cells; dM, decidua macrophages; HB, Hofbauer cell; PV, perivascular cells. Figure is created by BioRender.com.

pathology in the human placenta upon malaria infection is unknown and remains to be further investigated.

Studies of congenital toxoplasmosis are also currently limited to animal models. TLR2 and TLR4 are associated with recognition of *T. gondii*'s infection in mice (94). Engagement of the *T. gondii* ligand by TLR2 and TLR4 at the SCT-blood or in the EVT-decidua compartments is plausible, although there is still no direct evidence for such host-parasite interaction in humans. TLR11 has a role in controlling *T. gondii* infection in mice (95, 96), however in humans TLR11 is a pseudogene and is not expressed (97).

CYTOSOLIC PATTERN RECOGNITION RECEPTORS: RIG-I, MDA5, AND NOD-LIKE RECEPTORS AT THE UTERINE-PLACENTAL INTERFACE

Cytosolic PRRs play an important role in fighting against viral infection by eliciting host type I interferons (IFN) antiviral response through recognition of single and double stranded RNA (ssRNA and dsRNA) (98, 99). Examples of PRRs are the cytosolic retinoic acid-inducible gene-I-like (RIG-I) and the melanoma differentiation-associated protein 5 (MDA5) receptors, both expressed in the SCT and VCT of term placenta (100). In the human placenta, there is limited information on the function of RIG-1 and MDA5, but they may play a crucial role in recognizing a variety of RNA viruses, including ZIKV and dengue virus (101).

The Nucleotide binding Oligomerization Domain-like receptors (NOD-like receptors; NLR) recognizes intracellular pathogen products which have entered into the host cytoplasmic compartment (74). Both NOD-1 and NOD-2 receptors, which are known to detect intracellular bacterial peptidoglycans (102), are expressed in the SCT in the first trimester and term placentas (103, 104). The NLR pyrin-containing 1 and 3 proteins (NLRP1 and NLRP3) form the major inflammasome complexes, which contribute to activation of inflammatory caspases and pathogen clearance (105, 106).

Activation of NLRP3 and AIM2 inflammasomes, together with high expression of IL-1R, IL-1β, and caspase-1 was recently shown in the placental tissue of mothers infected with *P. falciparum* with significant pathology (107). In a murine model of intra-amniotic inflammation induced by bacterial LPS, tissue sections from the decidua basalis region expressed high levels of NLRP3, but negligible caspase-1 activation suggesting a possible non-canonical activation of the NLRP3 inflammasome (108). Our analysis shows that decidual dM1 expresses high levels of *NLRP3* transcript at steady state compared to other cell types (10) (**Figure 4**), thus dM1 may play a role in NLRP3-mediated pathogen recognition during early pregnancy.

SECRETED HOST DEFENSES AT THE UTERINE-PLACENTAL INTERFACE

Antimicrobial Peptides

AMP secreted by epithelial and immune cells are small peptides that bind and destroy most groups of pathogens—bacteria, yeasts, fungi, and viruses (109). In addition to direct killing of pathogens, AMPs can rapidly modulate innate host immune responses by recruiting myeloid cells and lymphocytes to the site of infection and mediating activation of TLR (110, 111). The human placenta expresses high levels of β-defensins, a family of broad spectrum antimicrobial peptides which participate in direct bactericidal and anti-viral activity (112). Specific subtypes of β-defensins (HBD-1, 2, and 3) are expressed in SCTs (112), suggesting these AMPs can target potentially bacterial or viral infection from the maternal blood.

Antiviral Interferons

Recognition of PAMPs by PRRs during infection leads to production of pro-inflammatory cytokines that can aid in clearing the pathogen (74). Studies on the direct role of pro-inflammatory cytokines on the placenta in the case of infection is limited. Inflammatory mediators can directly influence infection outcome and fetal development, but they can also cause damage to the placenta if produced in excess (113). Amongst the proinflammatory cytokines associated with uterine-placental infection during pregnancy, the antiviral IFN are the most well-characterized.

IFNs are secreted by a variety of cell types as the first line of defense against viral infection (114). Type I IFNs, including IFN-α and IFN-β, are potent antiviral cytokines. IFN-α and IFN-β bind to the IFNAR1/2 receptor and lead to expression of IFN stimulated genes (ISGs), which control virus infection through a variety of mechanisms (114). Loss of IFNAR in the placenta leads to vertical transmission and fetal mortality in murine herpesvirus-68 (MHV68) infected mice (115). In the mouse model of ZIKV infection, type I IFN-mediated signaling is essential for the control of viral replication in the placenta, but can also lead to significant placental pathology and fetal mortality (116, 117). The mechanism of type I IFN-mediated placental pathology has been recently elucidated. IFN-induced transmembrane (IFITM) protein, which normally blocks viral entry into host cells, impairs syncytin-mediated fusion of VCT to form SCT, leading to aberrant placental development (118).

Type II IFN, IFNγ, predominantly produced by NK and CD4+ T cells is crucial in controlling parasitic infection, such as *T. gondii* in mice (94, 119). However, elevated levels of IFNγ in response to *T. gondii* infection can lead to pathological effects during pregnancy including fetal demise (119, 120). Severe placental pathology and fetal death have also been associated with elevation of IFNγ during pregnancy in a murine model of malaria (121). Hence, proper regulation of type I and II IFN-mediated signaling at the uterine-placental interface is crucial in limiting pathogen replication, whilst preserving a balanced environment for normal placental development (122). Type III IFN, IFNλ, are constitutively secreted by the human SCT, which presumably confers antiviral effects against ZIKV infection (123–125).

INTRACELLULAR HOST DEFENSES AT THE UTERINE-PLACENTAL INTERFACE

Tryptophan Metabolism by IDO

Indoleamine 2,3-dioxygenase (IDO) is a host intracellular enzyme which metabolizes the amino acid tryptophan (126). IDO has been associated with maternal immunoregulation during pregnancy (127). It also plays a key role in the control of bacterial and viral replication, through limiting the bioavailability of tryptophan (128). IDO also inhibits the replication of several parasitic pathogens including *T. gondii* in human fibroblasts (129) and *Leishmania spp* in human macrophages (130). Mouse infection with *L. monocytogenes* showed that IDO is elevated in an IFN-γ-dependent manner in stromal cells of the metrial gland and decidua basalis; a crucial process to resolve bacterial infection in the mouse placenta (131). Our findings also show *IDO1* expression is enriched in epithelial glandular and DC1 cell type in the first trimester decidua (10) (**Figure 4**). The presence of IDO in decidua suggests that the enzyme might have a central role in limiting parasitic, viral, and bacterial replication, thus preventing their spread to the fetus.

CHALLENGES AND FUTURE PERSPECTIVES

Research on how the human placenta safeguards itself against infections is challenging due to obvious logistical and ethical issues in obtaining tissue from early in gestation (**Box 1**). Although animal experimental models have provided important insights relating to the immune responses to pathogenic infection, major differences between human and animal placentas must be considered (30, 31). Likewise, differences between strains of pathogens adapted for mice compared with human clinical isolates should be taken into account as this may lead to variation in pathogenesis and cellular response. One such example is the use of mouse CMV, which is unable to cross the mouse placental barrier, unlike the HMVC counterpart which can be transmitted transplacentally in humans (132). Therefore, all data obtained from studies of infection in pregnant animals needs careful interpretation and consideration prior to translation to clinical infection in humans.

Inherent properties of trophoblast cell lines, primary cultures or explants vary between donors, and are likely to be confounded by the area of the placenta that is sampled and as well as stage of gestation (133). For instance, villous placental explants will vary depending on the types of villi sampled and the presence of attached decidual tissue (133). Caution is therefore needed when interpreting data using these experimental models.

To overcome such limitations, population-based cohort studies of women with infection during pregnancy with extensive tissue sampling should be performed. These need to include and focus on LMIC where infection is still a major cause of maternal and fetal mortality and morbidity. Cohort studies and epidemiological surveillance on maternal infections can offer significant insights into disease pathogenesis and accelerate clinical interventions (134). Collaborations between clinicians and researchers for population-based cohort collection and sample processing will be instrumental to achieving this goal. Biological samples such as blood or placenta collected from controls and infected pregnant individuals could be stored and cryopreserved retrospectively. To capture the overall heterogeneity of infected and non-infected placenta samples, sampling, and biobanking criteria of different regions of placenta should be considered (135). Protocols are now available to use frozen tissue processed for single-cell/nuclei and spatial genomics (136, 137). Hence, application of single-cell "omics" on infected vs. healthy human placental and decidual samples will enable us to evaluate cellular heterogeneity in response to infection.

The capacity to detect transcripts specific to host or pathogen mRNA from the same tissue using *in situ* nucleic acid hybridization methods will provide direct quantification of infection burden and identification of potential target host cells within the same tissue (138). Recent advances in spatial transcriptomics methods have also allowed gene expression signatures to be quantified and resolved from individual tissue sections (139). Combination of these emerging technologies with new methods to integrate single-cell and spatial data computationally (140) will provide an unbiased approach to characterize and profile the transcriptome of individual cells *in situ* from the placenta and decidua in response to infections. We anticipate that high-throughput datasets generated from cohort sampling studies will unravel novel cell states and tissue spatial localization associated with placental infections and inflammation. This will also allow us to better characterize not only the innate immune response or makers of infection, but also other adaptive immune states in the human placenta (**Box 1**).

The use of *in vitro* models will also further define host responses to infection. The recent generation of human trophoblast stem cells (hTSCs) (141) and three-dimensional (3D) trophoblast organoids (142, 143) offer a great opportunity to study infections in early pregnancy where the access to first trimester placental samples is a concern. More importantly, the hTSCs and trophoblast organoids fulfill the criteria characteristic of human first trimester trophoblast *in vivo* (32). Both hTSCs and trophoblast organoids can differentiate *in vitro* into SCT and EVT with appropriate media (142, 143) allowing infection experiments on both the major trophoblast subpopulations present at the two major sites of contact between maternal and

---

BOX 1 | Perspective of vertical transmission and innate immune function during pregnancy and infection.

A variety of maternal infections can lead to vertical transmission (**Table 1**). The exact mechanisms these pathogens use to escape host defense and cross the placental barrier into the fetal compartment are not entirely known. Experimental models that recapitulate infection of the human placenta and thus vertical transmission are challenging to set up. More data and representative experimental models are needed to answer these questions: (i) how do different pathogens escape or modulate the maternal-fetal host innate immune barrier (ii) why do some pathogens lead to congenital infection but not others? Studying infected human placentas will be essential in understanding this but access to these samples is difficult especially in low and middle-income countries (LMIC) where maternal infection is particularly prevalent (WHO, Maternal mortality index 2019). Despite evidence of expression in primary placental tissue, functional studies on important innate immune features such as TLRs, AMPs, RIG-I, MDA5, NLRs, and IDO during infection and pregnancy are lacking. Understanding how different cell types at the uterine-placental interface (HB cells, dNKs, and dMs) respond to pathogen challenge is essential, but remains under-researched. A critical obstacle is to also extrapolate the protective and pathological mechanisms of cytokines from mouse to human infection. Therefore, systematic comparison of the innate immune effector mechanisms across gestation, in the placenta and decidua from natural human infection vs. healthy pregnancy, will provide a more accurate representation in clinical settings.

fetal cells. Sequencing of both host and pathogen transcriptomes from infected trophoblast at single-cell resolution will also advance our understanding on host-pathogen interactions in placentas (144, 145).

Further refinement of the trophoblast organoid and hTSCs culture system is needed to address key biological questions unanswered by current models. These include studying the effect of infection on cellular crosstalk between trophoblast and other primary placental cells such as HB cells, or decidual cells in culture, such as dNK or decidual stromal cells. Adaptation of CRISPR/Cas9 genome editing technology for the trophoblast organoids or hTSCs will offer novel insights into essential host genes required for vertical transmission and placental defense mechanisms in humans.

CONCLUSION

Major maternal and fetal complications as a result of infection are still a concern, especially in LMIC with highest prevalence reported in countries of sub-Saharan Africa (WHO, Maternal mortality index 2019). Profound limitations on current study models and ethical regulations on studying human placenta have significantly delayed the development of therapies and vaccines for maternal-fetal infection. How vertical transmission occurs and how the uterine-placental innate immune system reacts to infection remain as major unresolved questions. Revolutionary advances in single-cell genomics, imaging, computational, and stem cell biology methods are currently underway to study the molecular and cellular mechanisms of human diseases. Therefore, it is now an exciting time to apply these transformative technologies to comprehensively address fundamental questions on host-pathogen interaction at the human uterine-placental interface.

AUTHOR CONTRIBUTIONS

RH, AN, and RV-T wrote and edited the manuscript. All authors contributed to the article and approved the submitted version.

ACKNOWLEDGMENTS

We would like to thank Ashely Moffett for the useful discussions and critical review of the manuscript. We are also very grateful to Sarah Aldridge, Loren Gibson, Damiana Alvarez, Carlos Talavera-Lopez, and Anna Arutyunyan for their insightful comments and corrections.

REFERENCES

Benirschke K, Kaufmann P, Baergen RN. *Pathology of the Human Placenta.* Berlin; Heidelberg: Springer (2006).

Schlafke S, Enders AC. Cellular basis of interaction between trophoblast and uterus at implantation. *Biol Reprod.* (1975) 12:41–65. doi: 10.1095/biolreprod12.1.41

PrabhuDas M, Bonney E, Caron K, Dey S, Erlebacher A, Fazleabas A, et al. Immune mechanisms at the maternal-fetal interface: perspectives and challenges. *Nat Immunol.* (2015) 16:328–34. doi: 10.1038/ni.3131

Ander SE, Diamond MS, Coyne CB. Immune responses at the maternal-fetal interface. *Sci Immunol.* (2019) 4:eaat6114. doi: 10.1126/sciimmunol.aat6114

Coyne CB, Lazear HM. Zika virus - reigniting the TORCH. *Nat Rev Microbiol.* (2016) 14:707–15. doi: 10.1038/nrmicro.2016.125

Yarbrough VL, Winkle S, Herbst-Kralovetz MM. Antimicrobial peptides in the female reproductive tract: a critical component of the mucosal immune barrier with physiological and clinical implications. *Hum Reprod Update.* (2015) 21:353–77. doi: 10.1093/humupd/dmu065

Romero R, Gomez-Lopez N, Winters AD, Jung E, Shaman M, Bieda J, et al. Evidence that intra-amniotic infections are often the result of an ascending invasion - a molecular microbiological study. *J Perinat Med.* (2019) 47:915–31. doi: 10.1515/jpm-2019-0297

Kim CJ, Romero R, Chaemsaithong P, Chaiyasit N, Yoon BH, Kim YM. Acute chorioamnionitis and funisitis: definition, pathologic features, and clinical significance. *Am J Obstet Gynecol.* (2015) 213:S29–52. doi: 10.1016/j.ajog.2015.08.040

Cappelletti M, Presicce P, Kallapur SG. Immunobiology of acute chorioamnionitis. *Front Immunol.* (2020) 11:649. doi: 10.3389/fimmu.2020.00649

Vento-Tormo R, Efremova M, Botting RA, Turco MY, Vento-Tormo M, Meyer KB, et al. Single-cell reconstruction of the early maternal-fetal interface in humans. *Nature.* (2018) 563:347–53. doi: 10.1038/s41586-018-0698-6

McDonagh S, Maidji E, Ma W, Chang H-T, Fisher S, Pereira L. Viral and bacterial pathogens at the maternal-fetal interface. *J Infect Dis.* (2004) 190:826–34. doi: 10.1086/422330

Vornhagen J, Adams Waldorf KM, Rajagopal L. Perinatal Group B streptococcal infections: virulence factors, immunity, and prevention strategies. *Trends Microbiol.* (2017) 25:919–31. doi: 10.1016/j.tim.2017.05.013

Hamon M, Bierne H, Cossart P. Listeria monocytogenes: a multifaceted model. *Nat Rev Microbiol.* (2006) 4:423–34. doi: 10.1038/nrmicro1413

Stein A, Raoult D. Q fever during pregnancy: a public health problem in southern France. *Clin Infect Dis.* (1998) 27:592–6. doi: 10.1086/514698

Thomas DD, Navab M, Haake DA, Fogelman AM, Miller JN, Lovett MA. Treponema pallidum invades intercellular junctions of endothelial cell monolayers. *Proc Natl Acad Sci USA.* (1988) 85:3608–12. doi: 10.1073/pnas.85.10.3608

Peeling RW, Mabey DCW. Syphilis. *Nat Rev Microbiol.* (2004) 2:448–9. doi: 10.1038/nrmicro914

Montoya JG, Liesenfeld O. Toxoplasmosis. *Lancet.* (2004) 363:1965–76. doi: 10.1016/S0140-6736(04)16412-X

Kemmerling U, Osuna A, Schijman AG, Truyens C. Congenital transmission of trypanosoma cruzi: a review about the interactions between the parasite, the placenta, the maternal and the fetal/neonatal immune responses. *Front Microbiol.* (2019) 10:1854. doi: 10.3389/fmicb.2019.01854

Maidji E, McDonagh S, Genbacev O, Tabata T, Pereira L. Maternal antibodies enhance or prevent cytomegalovirus infection in the placenta by neonatal Fc receptor-mediated transcytosis. *Am J Pathol.* (2006) 168:1210–26. doi: 10.2353/ajpath.2006.050482

Lazar M, Perelygina L, Martines R, Greer P, Paddock CD, Peltecu G, et al. Immunolocalization and distribution of rubella antigen in fatal congenital rubella syndrome. *EBioMedicine.* (2016) 3:86–92. doi: 10.1016/j.ebiom.2015.11.050

Ganaie SS, Qiu J. Recent advances in replication and infection of human parvovirus B19. *Front Cell Infect Microbiol.* (2018) 8:166. doi: 10.3389/fcimb.2018.00166

Enders G, Miller E, Cradock-Watson J, Bolley I, Ridehalgh M. Consequences of varicella and herpes zoster in pregnancy: prospective study of 1739 cases. *Lancet.* (1994) 343:1548–51. doi: 10.1016/S0140-6736(94)92943-2

El Costa H, Gouilly J, Mansuy J-M, Chen Q, Levy C, Cartron G, et al. ZIKA virus reveals broad tissue and cell tropism during the first trimester of pregnancy. *Sci Rep.* (2016) 6:35296. doi: 10.1038/srep35296

Foo S-S, Chen W, Chan Y, Bowman JW, Chang L-C, Choi Y, et al. Asian Zika virus strains target CD14+ blood monocytes and induce M2-skewed immunosuppression during pregnancy. *Nat Microbiol.* (2017) 2:1558–70. doi: 10.1038/s41564-017-0016-3

Michlmayr D, Andrade P, Gonzalez K, Balmaseda A, Harris E. CD14+CD16+ monocytes are the main target of Zika virus infection in peripheral blood mononuclear cells in a paediatric study in Nicaragua. *Nat Microbiol.* (2017) 2:1462–70. doi: 10.1038/s41564-017-0035-0

Delorme-Axford E, Sadovsky Y, Coyne CB. The placenta as a barrier to viral infections. *Annu Rev Virol.* (2014) 1:133–46. doi:10.1146/annurev-virology-031413-085524

Pereira L. Congenital viral infection: traversing the uterine-placental interface. *Annu Rev Virol.* (2018) 5:273–99. doi:10.1146/annurev-virology-092917-043236

Lecuit M. Understanding how listeria monocytogenes targets and crosses host barriers. *Clin Microbiol Infect.* (2005) 11:430–6. doi: 10.1111/j.1469-0691.2005.01146.x

Persson CM, Lambert H, Vutova PP, Dellacasa-Lindberg I, Nederby J, Yagita H, et al. Transmission of *Toxoplasma gondii* from infected dendritic cells to natural killer cells. *Infect Immun.* (2009) 77:970–6. doi: 10.1128/IAI.00833-08

Turco MY, Moffett A. Development of the human placenta. *Development.* (2019) 146:3613. doi: 10.1242/dev.163428

Carter AM. Animal models of human placentation - a review. *Placenta.* (2007) 28:S41–7. doi: 10.1016/j.placenta.2006.11.002

Lee CQE, Gardner L, Turco M, Zhao N, Murray MJ, Coleman N, et al. What is trophoblast? A combination of criteria define human first-trimester trophoblast. *Stem Cell Rep.* (2016) 6:257–72. doi: 10.1016/j.stemcr.2016.01.006

Hemberger M, Udayashankar R, Tesar P, Moore H, Burton GJ. ELF5- enforced transcriptional networks define an epigenetically regulated trophoblast stem cell compartment in the human placenta. *Hum Mol Genet.* (2010) 19:2456–67. doi: 10.1093/hmg/ddq128

Boyd JD, Hamilton WJ. *The Human Placenta.* London: Macmillan Press (1975).

Pijnenborg R, Bland JM, Robertson WB, Brosens I. Uteroplacental arterial changes related to interstitial trophoblast migration in early human pregnancy. *Placenta.* (1983) 4:397–413. doi: 10.1016/S0143-4004(83)80043-5

Pijnenborg R. Trophoblast invasion. *Reprod Med Rev.* (1994) 3:53–73. doi: 10.1017/S0962279900000776

Burton GJ, Jauniaux E, Watson AL. Maternal arterial connections to the placental intervillous space during the first trimester of human pregnancy: the Boyd collection revisited. *Am J Obstet Gynecol.* (1999) 181:718–24. doi: 10.1016/S0002-9378(99)70518-1

Enders AC, King BF. The cytology of Hofbauer cells. *Anat Rec.* (1970) 167:231–6. doi: 10.1002/ar.1091670211

Castellucci M, Zaccheo D, Pescetto G. A three-dimensional study of the normal human placental villous core. *Cell Tissue Res.* (1980) 210:235–47. doi: 10.1007/BF00237612

Wetzka B, Clark DE, Charnock-Jones DS, Zahradnik HP, Smith SK. Isolation of macrophages (Hofbauer cells) from human term placenta and their prostaglandin E2 and thromboxane production. *Hum Reprod.* (1997) 12:847–52. doi: 10.1093/humrep/12.4.847

de Noronha L, Zanluca C, Burger M, Suzukawa AA, Azevedo M, Rebutini PZ, et al. Zika virus infection at different pregnancy stages: anatomopathological findings, target cells and viral persistence in placental tissues. *Front Microbiol.* (2018) 9:2266. doi: 10.3389/fmicb.2018.02266

Bhatnagar J, Rabeneck DB, Martines RB, Reagan-Steiner S, Ermias Y, Estetter LBC, et al. Zika virus RNA replication and persistence in brain and placental tissue. *Emerg Infect Dis.* (2017) 23:405–14. doi: 10.3201/eid2303.161499

Lewis SH, Reynolds-Kohler C, Fox HE, Nelson JA. HIV-1 in trophoblastic and villous Hofbauer cells, and haematological precursors in eight-week fetuses. *Lancet.* (1990) 335:565–8. doi: 10.1016/0140-6736(90)90349-A

Quicke KM, Bowen JR, Johnson EL, McDonald CE, Ma H, O'Neal JT, et al. Zika virus infects human placental macrophages. *Cell Host Microbe.* (2016) 20:83–90. doi: 10.1016/j.chom.2016.05.015

Hunt JS, Pollard JW. Macrophages in the uterus and placenta. *Curr Top Microbiol Immunol.* (1992) 181:39–63. doi: 10.1007/978-3-642-77377-8_2

Zeldovich VB, Clausen CH, Bradford E, Fletcher DA, Maltepe E, Robbins JR, et al. Placental syncytium forms a biophysical barrier against pathogen invasion. *PLoS Pathogens.* (2013) 9:e1003821. doi: 10.1371/journal.ppat.1003821

Nelson DM. Apoptotic changes occur in syncytiotrophoblast of human placental villi where fibrin type fibrinoid is deposited at discontinuities in the villous trophoblast. *Placenta.* (1996) 17:387–91. doi: 10.1016/S0143-4004(96)90019-3

Tabata T, Petitt M, Puerta-Guardo H, Michlmayr D, Wang C, Fang-Hoover J, et al. Zika virus targets different primary human placental cells, suggesting two routes for vertical transmission. *Cell Host Microbe.* (2016) 20:155–66. doi: 10.1016/j.chom.2016.07.002

Maidji E, Genbacev O, Chang H-T, Pereira L. Developmental regulation of human cytomegalovirus receptors in cytotrophoblasts correlates with distinct replication sites in the placenta. *J Virol.* (2007) 81:4701–12. doi: 10.1128/JVI.02748-06

Pique-Regi R, Romero R, Tarca AL, Luca F, Xu Y, Alazizi A, et al. Does the human placenta express the canonical cell entry mediators for SARS-CoV-2? *Elife.* (2020) 9:e58716. doi: 10.7554/eLife.58716

Pique-Regi R, Romero R, Tarca AL, Sendler ED, Xu Y, Garcia-Flores V, et al. Single cell transcriptional signatures of the human placenta in term and preterm parturition. *Elife.* (2019) 8:e52004. doi: 10.7554/eLife.52004

Sungnak W, Huang N, Bécavin C, Berg M, Queen R, Litvinukova M, et al. SARS-CoV-2 entry factors are highly expressed in nasal epithelial cells together with innate immune genes. *Nat Med.* (2020) 681–7. doi: 10.1038/s41591-020-0868-6

Algarroba GN, Rekawek P, Vahanian SA, Khullar P, Palaia T, Peltier MR, et al. Visualization of SARS-CoV-2 virus invading the human placenta using electron microscopy. *Am J Obstet Gynecol.* (2020) 223:275–27. doi: 10.1016/j.ajog.2020.05.023

Hosier H, Farhadian SF, Morotti RA, Deshmukh U, Lu-Culligan A, Campbell KH, et al. SARS-CoV-2 infection of the placenta. *J Clin Invest.* (2020). doi: 10.1172/JCI139569. [Epub ahead of print].

Kirtsman M, Diambomba Y, Poutanen SM, Malinowski AK, Vlachodimitropoulou E, Parks WT, et al. Probable congenital SARS-CoV-2 infection in a neonate born to a woman with active SARS-CoV-2 infection. *CMAJ.* (2020) 192:E647–50. doi: 10.1503/cmaj.200821

Simister NE, Story CM, Chen HL, Hunt JS. An IgG-transporting Fc receptor expressed in the syncytiotrophoblast of human placenta. *Eur J Immunol.* (1996) 26:1527–31. doi: 10.1002/eji.1830260718

Rathore APS, Saron WAA, Lim T, Jahan N, St. John AL. Maternal immunity and antibodies to dengue virus promote infection and Zika virus–induced microcephaly in fetuses. *Sci Adv.* (2019) 5:eaav3208. doi: 10.1126/sciadv.aav3208

Gupta S, Gach JS, Becerra JC, Phan TB, Pudney J, Moldoveanu Z, et al. The Neonatal Fc receptor (FcRn) enhances human immunodeficiency virus type 1 (HIV-1) transcytosis across epithelial cells. *PLoS Pathog.* (2013) 9:e1003776. doi: 10.1371/journal.ppat.1003776

Georgieff MK, Wobken JK, Welle J, Burdo JR, Connor JR. Identification and localization of divalent metal transporter-1 (DMT-1) in term human placenta. *Placenta.* (2000) 21:799–804. doi: 10.1053/plac.2000.0566

Martin DN, Uprichard SL. Identification of transferrin receptor 1 as a hepatitis C virus entry factor. *Proc Natl Acad Sci USA.* (2013) 110:10777–782. doi: 10.1073/pnas.1301764110

Drakesmith H, Prentice A. Viral infection and iron metabolism. *Nat Rev Microbiol.* (2008) 6:541–52. doi: 10.1038/nrmicro1930

Rogerson SJ, Hviid L, Duffy PE, Leke RFG, Taylor DW. Malaria in pregnancy: pathogenesis and immunity. *Lancet Infect Dis.* (2007) 7:105–17. doi: 10.1016/S1473-3099(07)70022-1

Fried M, Duffy PE. Adherence of Plasmodium falciparum to chondroitin sulfate A in the human placenta. *Science.* (1996) 272:1502–4. doi: 10.1126/science.272.5267.1502

Crocker IP, Tanner OM, Myers JE, Bulmer JN, Walraven G, Baker PN. Syncytiotrophoblast degradation and the pathophysiology of the malaria-infected placenta. *Placenta.* (2004) 25:273–82. doi: 10.1016/j.placenta.2003.09.010

Pereira L, Maidji E, McDonagh S, Genbacev O, Fisher S. Human cytomegalovirus transmission from the uterus to the placenta correlates with the presence of pathogenic bacteria and maternal immunity. *J Virol.* (2003) 77:13301–14. doi: 10.1128/JVI.77.24.13301-13314.2003

Fowler KB, Stagno S, Pass RF. Interval between births and risk of congenital cytomegalovirus infection. *Clin Infect Dis.* (2004) 38:1035–7. doi: 10.1086/382533

Fowler KB, Stagno S, Pass RF. Maternal immunity and prevention of congenital cytomegalovirus infection. *JAMA.* (2003) 289:1008–11. doi: 10.1001/jama.289.8.1008

Parruti G, Polilli E, Ursini T, Tontodonati M. Properties and mechanisms of immunoglobulins for congenital cytomegalovirus disease. *Clin Infect Dis.* (2013) 57(Suppl. 4):S185–8. doi: 10.1093/cid/cit584

Siewiera J, El Costa H, Tabiasco J, Berrebi A, Cartron G, Le Bouteiller P, et al. Human cytomegalovirus infection elicits new decidual natural killer cell effector functions. *PLoS Pathog.* (2013) 9:e1003257. doi: 10.1371/journal.ppat.1003257

Crespo ÂC, Strominger JL, Tilburgs T. Expression of KIR2DS1 by decidual natural killer cells increases their ability to control placental HCMV infection. *Proc Natl Acad Sci USA.* (2016) 113:15072–7. doi: 10.1073/pnas.1617927114

van der Ploeg K, Chang C, Ivarsson MA, Moffett A, Wills MR, Trowsdale J. Modulation of human leukocyte Antigen-C by human cytomegalovirus stimulates KIR2DS1 recognition by natural killer cells. *Front Immunol.* (2017) 8:298. doi: 10.3389/fimmu.2017.00298

Quillay H, El Costa H, Duriez M, Marlin R, Cannou C, Madec Y, et al. NK cells control HIV-1 infection of macrophages through soluble factors and cellular contacts in the human decidua. *Retrovirology.* (2016) 13:39. doi: 10.1186/s12977-016-0271-z

Janeway CA Jr, Medzhitov R. Innate immune recognition. *Annu Rev Immunol.* (2002) 20:197–216. doi: 10.1146/annurev.immunol.20.083001.084359

Akira S, Uematsu S, Takeuchi O. Pathogen recognition and innate immunity. *Cell.* (2006) 124:783–801. doi: 10.1016/j.cell.2006.02.015

Banchereau J, Steinman RM. Dendritic cells and the control of immunity. *Nature.* (1998) 392:245–52. doi: 10.1038/32588

Kawasaki T, Kawai T. Toll-like receptor signaling pathways. *Front Immunol.* (2014) 5:461. doi: 10.3389/fimmu.2014.00461

Honda K, Taniguchi T. IRFs: master regulators of signalling by Toll-like receptors and cytosolic pattern-recognition receptors. *Nat Rev Immunol.* (2006) 6:644–58. doi: 10.1038/nri1900

Ma Y, Krikun G, Abrahams VM, Mor G, Guller S. Cell type-specific expression and function of toll-like receptors 2 and 4 in human placenta: implications in fetal infection. *Placenta.* (2007) 28:1024–31. doi: 10.1016/j.placenta.2007.05.003

Beijar ECE, Mallard C, Powell TL. Expression and subcellular localization of TLR-4 in term and first trimester human placenta. *Placenta.* (2006) 27:322–6. doi: 10.1016/j.placenta.2004.12.012

Holmlund U, Cebers G, Dahlfors AR, Sandstedt B, Bremme K, Ekström ES, et al. Expression and regulation of the pattern recognition receptors Toll-like receptor-2 and Toll-like receptor-4 in the human placenta. *Immunology.* (2002) 107:145–51. doi: 10.1046/j.1365-2567.2002.01491.x

Abrahams VM, Bole-Aldo P, Kim YM, Straszewski-Chavez SL, Chaiworapongsa T, Romero R, et al. Divergent trophoblast responses to bacterial products mediated by TLRs. *J Immunol.* (2004) 173:4286–96. doi: 10.4049/jimmunol.173.7.4286

Pudney J, He X, Masheeb Z, Kindelberger DW, Kuohung W, Ingalls RR. Differential expression of toll-like receptors in the human placenta across early gestation. *Placenta.* (2016) 46:1–10. doi: 10.1016/j.placenta.2016.07.005

Koga K, Aldo PB, Mor G. Toll-like receptors and pregnancy: trophoblast as modulators of the immune response. *J Obstet Gynaecol Res.* (2009) 35:191–202. doi: 10.1111/j.1447-0756.2008.00963.x

Young OM, Tang Z, Niven-Fairchild T, Tadesse S, Krikun G, Norwitz ER, et al. Toll-like receptor-mediated responses by placental Hofbauer Cells (HBCs): a potential pro-inflammatory role for Fetal M2 macrophages. *Am J Reprod Immunol.* (2015) 73:22–35. doi: 10.1111/aji.12336

Gantier MP, Tong S, Behlke MA, Xu D, Phipps S, Foster PS, et al. TLR7 is involved in sequence-specific sensing of single-stranded RNAs in human macrophages. *J Immunol.* (2008) 180:2117–24. doi: 10.4049/jimmunol.180.4.2117

Duriez M, Quillay H, Madec Y, El Costa H, Cannou C, Marlin R, et al. Human decidual macrophages and NK cells differentially express Toll-like receptors and display distinct cytokine profiles upon TLR stimulation. *Front Microbiol.* (2014) 5:316. doi: 10.3389/fmicb.2014.00316

Leoratti FMS, Farias L, Alves FP, Suarez-Mútis MC, Coura JR, Kalil J, et al. Variants in the toll-like receptor signaling pathway and clinical outcomes of malaria. *J Infect Dis.* (2008) 198:772–80. doi: 10.1086/590440

Mockenhaupt FP, Cramer JP, Hamann L, Stegemann MS, Eckert J, Oh N-R, et al. Toll-like receptor (TLR) polymorphisms in African children: common TLR-4 variants predispose to severe malaria. *Proc Natl Acad Sci USA.* (2006) 103:177–82. doi: 10.1073/pnas.0506803102

Mockenhaupt FP, Hamann L, von Gaertner C, Bedu-Addo G, von Kleinsorgen C, Schumann RR, et al. Common polymorphisms of toll-like receptors 4 and 9 are associated with the clinical manifestation of malaria during pregnancy. *J Infect Dis.* (2006) 194:184–8. doi: 10.1086/505152

Coban C, Ishii KJ, Kawai T, Hemmi H, Sato S, Uematsu S, et al. Toll-like receptor 9 mediates innate immune activation by the malaria pigment hemozoin. *J Exp Med.* (2005) 201:19–25. doi: 10.1084/jem.20041836

Krishnegowda G, Hajjar AM, Zhu J, Douglass EJ, Uematsu S, Akira S, et al. Induction of proinflammatory responses in macrophages by the glycosylphosphatidylinositols of plasmodium falciparum. *J Biol Chem.* (2005) 280:8606–16. doi: 10.1074/jbc.m413541200

Barboza R, Reis AS, da Silva LG, Hasenkamp L, Pereira KRB, Câmara NOS, et al. MyD88 signaling is directly involved in the development of murine placental malaria. *Infect Immun.* (2014) 82:830–8. doi: 10.1128/IAI.01288-13

Barboza R, Lima FA, Reis AS, Murillo OJ, Peixoto EPM, Bandeira CL, et al. TLR4-mediated placental pathology and pregnancy outcome in experimental malaria. *Sci Rep.* (2017) 7:8623. doi: 10.1038/s41598-017-08299-x

Yarovinsky F. Innate immunity to *Toxoplasma gondii* infection. *Nat Rev Immunol.* (2014) 14:109–21. doi: 10.1038/nri3598

Yarovinsky F, Zhang D, Andersen JF, Bannenberg GL, Serhan CN, Hayden MS, et al. TLR11 activation of dendritic cells by a protozoan profilin-like protein. *Science.* (2005) 308:1626–9. doi: 10.1126/science.1109893

Plattner F, Yarovinsky F, Romero S, Didry D, Carlier M-F, Sher A, et al. Toxoplasma profilin is essential for host cell invasion and TLR11-dependent induction of an interleukin-12 response. *Cell Host Microbe.* (2008) 3:77–87. doi: 10.1016/j.chom.2008.01.001

Zhang D, Zhang G, Hayden MS, Greenblatt MB, Bussey C, Flavell RA, et al. A toll-like receptor that prevents infection by uropathogenic bacteria. *Science.* (2004) 303:1522–6. doi: 10.1126/science.1094351

Yoneyama M, Onomoto K, Jogi M, Akaboshi T, Fujita T. Viral RNA detection by RIG-I-like receptors. *Curr Opin Immunol.* (2015) 32:48–53. doi: 10.1016/j.coi.2014.12.012

Kato H, Takeuchi O, Mikamo-Satoh E, Hirai R, Kawai T, Matsushita K, et al. Length-dependent recognition of double-stranded ribonucleic acids by retinoic acid-inducible gene-I and melanoma differentiation-associated gene 5. *J Exp Med.* (2008) 205:1601–10. doi: 10.1084/jem.20080091

Bryant AH, Menzies GE, Scott LM, Spencer-Harty S, Davies LB, Smith RA, et al. Human gestation-associated tissues express functional cytosolic nucleic acid sensing pattern recognition receptors. *Clin Exp Immunol.* (2017) 189:36–46. doi: 10.1111/cei.12960

Chazal M, Beauclair G, Gracias S, Najburg V, Simon-Lorière E, Tangy F, et al. RIG-I recognizes the 5 region of Dengue and Zika virus genomes. *Cell Rep.* (2018) 24:320–8. doi: 10.1016/j.celrep.2018.06.047

Girardin SE, Boneca IG, Carneiro LAM, Antignac A, Jéhanno M, Viala J, et al. Nod1 detects a unique muropeptide from gram-negative bacterial peptidoglycan. *Science.* (2003) 300:1584-7. doi: 10.1126/science.1084677

Bryant AH, Bevan RJ, Spencer-Harty S, Scott LM, Jones RH, Thornton CA. Expression and function of NOD-like receptors by human term gestation-associated tissues. *Placenta.* (2017) 58:25-32. doi: 10.1016/j.placenta.2017.07.017

Costello MJ, Joyce SK, Abrahams VM. NOD protein expression and function in first trimester trophoblast cells. *Am J Reprod Immunol.* (2007) 57:67- 80. doi: 10.1111/j.1600-0897.2006.00447.x

Martinon F, Burns K, Tschopp J. The inflammasome: a molecular platform triggering activation of inflammatory caspases and processing of proIL-beta. *Mol Cell.* (2002) 10:417-26. doi: 10.1016/S1097-2765(02)00599-3

Franchi L, Muñoz-Planillo R, Núñez G. Sensing and reacting to microbes through the inflammasomes. *Nat Immunol.* (2012) 13:325- 32. doi: 10.1038/ni.2231

Reis AS, Barboza R, Murillo O, Barateiro A, Peixoto EPM, Lima FA, et al. Inflammasome activation and IL-1 signaling during placental malaria induce poor pregnancy outcomes. *Sci Adv.* (2020) 6:eaax6346. doi: 10.1126/sciadv.aax6346

Faro J, Romero R, Schwenkel G, Garcia-Flores V, Arenas-Hernandez M, Leng Y, et al. Intra-amniotic inflammation induces preterm birth by activating the NLRP3 inflammasome†. *Biol Reprod.* (2019) 100:1290- 305. doi: 10.1093/biolre/ioy261

Hancock RE, Diamond G. The role of cationic antimicrobial peptides in innate host defences. *Trends Microbiol.* (2000) 8:402-10. doi: 10.1016/S0966-842X(00)01823-0

Yang D, Chertov O, Bykovskaia SN, Chen Q, Buffo MJ, Shogan J, et al. Beta-defensins: linking innate and adaptive immunity through dendritic and T cell CCR6. *Science.* (1999) 286:525-8. doi: 10.1126/science.286.5439.525

Lande R, Gregorio J, Facchinetti V, Chatterjee B, Wang Y-H, Homey B, et al. Plasmacytoid dendritic cells sense self-DNA coupled with antimicrobial peptide. *Nature.* (2007) 449:564-9. doi: 10.1038/nature06116

King AE, Paltoo A, Kelly RW, Sallenave J-M, Bocking AD, Challis JRG. Expression of natural antimicrobials by human placenta and fetal membranes. *Placenta.* (2007) 28:161-9. doi: 10.1016/j.placenta.2006.01.006

Yockey LJ, Iwasaki A. Interferons and proinflammatory cytokines in pregnancy and fetal development. *Immunity.* (2018) 49:397-412. doi: 10.1016/j.immuni.2018.07.017

Sadler AJ, Williams BRG. Interferon-inducible antiviral effectors. *Nat Rev Immunol.* (2008) 8:559-68. doi: 10.1038/nri2314

Racicot K, Aldo P, El-Guindy A, Kwon J-Y, Romero R, Mor G. Cutting edge: fetal/placental Type I IFN can affect maternal survival and fetal viral load during viral infection. *J Immunol.* (2017) 198:3029- 32. doi: 10.4049/jimmunol.1601824

Yockey LJ, Jurado KA, Arora N, Millet A, Rakib T, Milano KM, et al. Type I interferons instigate fetal demise after Zika virus infection. *Sci Immunol.* (2018) 3:eaao1680. doi: 10.1126/sciimmunol.aao1680

Miner JJ, Cao B, Govero J, Smith AM, Fernandez E, Cabrera OH, et al. Zika virus infection during pregnancy in mice causes placental damage and fetal demise. *Cell.* (2016) 165:1081-91. doi: 10.1016/j.cell.2016.05.008

Buchrieser J, Degrelle SA, Couderc T, Nevers Q, Disson O, Manet C, et al. IFITM proteins inhibit placental syncytiotrophoblast formation and promote fetal demise. *Science.* (2019) 365:176- 80. doi: 10.1126/science.aaw7733

Suzuki Y, Orellana MA, Schreiber RD, Remington JS. Interferon-gamma: the major mediator of resistance against *Toxoplasma gondii*. *Science.* (1988) 240:516-8. doi: 10.1126/science.3128869

Senegas A, Villard O, Neuville A, Marcellin L, Pfaff AW, Steinmetz T, et al. *Toxoplasma gondii*-induced foetal resorption in mice involves interferon-gamma-induced apoptosis and spiral artery dilation at the maternofoetal interface. *Int J Parasitol.* (2009) 39:481-7. doi: 10.1016/j.ijpara.2008.08.009

Niikura M, Inoue S-I, Mineo S, Asahi H, Kobayashi F. IFNGR1 signaling is associated with adverse pregnancy outcomes during infection with malaria parasites. *PLoS ONE.* (2017) 12:e0185392. doi: 10.1371/journal.pone.0185392

Yockey LJ, Lucas C, Iwasaki A. Contributions of maternal and fetal antiviral immunity in congenital disease. *Science.* (2020) 368:608-12. doi: 10.1126/science.aaz1960

Corry J, Arora N, Good CA, Sadovsky Y, Coyne CB. Organotypic models of type III interferon-mediated protection from Zika virus infections at the maternal-fetal interface. *Proc Natl Acad Sci USA.* (2017) 114:9433- 8. doi: 10.1073/pnas.1707513114

Bayer A, Lennemann NJ, Ouyang Y, Bramley JC, Morosky S, Marques ETDA Jr, et al. Type III interferons produced by human placental trophoblasts confer protection against Zika virus infection. *Cell Host Microbe.* (2016) 19:705-12. doi: 10.1016/j.chom.2016.03.008

Jagger BW, Miner JJ, Cao B, Arora N, Smith AM, Kovacs A, et al. Gestational stage and IFN-λ signaling regulate ZIKV infection *in utero*. *Cell Host Microbe.* (2017) 22:366-76.e3. doi: 10.1016/j.chom.2017.08.012

Munn DH, Mellor AL. Indoleamine 2,3 dioxygenase and metabolic control of immune responses. *Trends Immunol.* (2013) 34:137-43. doi: 10.1016/j.it.2012.10.001

Munn DH, Zhou M, Attwood JT, Bondarev I, Conway SJ, Marshall B, et al. Prevention of allogeneic fetal rejection by tryptophan catabolism. *Science.* (1998) 281:1191-3. doi: 10.1126/science.281.5380.1191

Schmidt SV, Schultze JL. New insights into IDO biology in bacterial and viral infections. *Front Immunol.* (2014) 5:384. doi: 10.3389/fimmu.2014.00384

Pfefferkorn ER. Interferon gamma blocks the growth of *Toxoplasma gondii* in human fibroblasts by inducing the host cells to degrade tryptophan. *Proc Natl Acad Sci USA.* (1984) 81:908-12. doi: 10.1073/pnas.81.3.908

Murray HW, Szuro-Sudol A, Wellner D, Oca MJ, Granger AM, Libby DM, et al. Role of tryptophan degradation in respiratory burst-independent antimicrobial activity of gamma interferon-stimulated human macrophages. *Infect Immun.* (1989) 57:845-9. doi: 10.1128/IAI.57.3.845-849.1989

Mackler AM, Barber EM, Takikawa O, Pollard JW. Indoleamine 2,3-dioxygenase is regulated by IFN-gamma in the mouse placenta during *Listeria monocytogenes* infection. *J Immunol.* (2003) 170:823-30. doi: 10.4049/jimmunol.170.2.823

Slavuljica I, Kveštak D, Huszthy PC, Kosmac K, Britt WJ, Jonjić S. Immunobiology of congenital cytomegalovirus infection of the central nervous system—the murine cytomegalovirus model. *Cell Mol Immunol.* (2015) 12:180-91. doi: 10.1038/cmi.2014.51

Heazlewood CF, Sherrell H, Ryan J, Atkinson K, Wells CA, Fisk NM. High incidence of contaminating maternal cell overgrowth in human placental mesenchymal stem/stromal cell cultures: a systematic review. *Stem Cells Transl Med.* (2014) 3:1305-11. doi: 10.5966/sctm.2014-0051

Bardají A, Steinhoff M, Macete E, Aguado T, Menéndez C. The burden of vaccine-preventable diseases in pregnancy in low-resource settings. *Lancet Glob Health.* (2016) 4:e152-3. doi: 10.1016/S2214-109X(16)0 0036-X

Burton GJ, Sebire NJ, Myatt L, Tannetta D, Wang Y-L, Sadovsky Y, et al. Optimising sample collection for placental research. *Placenta.* (2014) 35:9- 22. doi: 10.1016/j.placenta.2013.11.005

Slyper M, Porter CBM, Ashenberg O, Waldman J, Drokhlyansky E, Wakiro I, et al. A single-cell and single-nucleus RNA-Seq toolbox for fresh and frozen human tumors. *Nat Med.* (2019) 26:792-802. doi: 10.1038/s41591-020-0844-1

Amamoto R, Zuccaro E, Curry NC, Khurana S, Chen H-H, Cepko CL, et al. FIN-Seq: transcriptional profiling of specific cell types from frozen archived tissue of the human central nervous system. *Nucleic Acids Res.* (2020) 48:e4. doi: 10.1101/602847

Wang F, Flanagan J, Su N, Wang L-C, Bui S, Nielson A, et al. RNAscope: a novel in situ RNA analysis platform for formalin-fixed, paraffin-embedded tissues. *J Mol Diagn.* (2012) 14:22-9. doi: 10.1016/j.jmoldx.2011.08.002

Ståhl PL, Salmén F, Vickovic S, Lundmark A, Navarro JF, Magnusson J, et al. Visualization and analysis of gene expression in tissue sections by spatial transcriptomics. *Science.* (2016) 353:78-82. doi: 10.1126/science.aaf2403

Andersson A, Bergenstråhle J, Asp M, Bergenstråhle L, Jurek A, Navarro JF, et al. Spatial mapping of cell types by integration of transcriptomics data. *bioRxiv [Preprint].* (2019) 2019.12.13.874495. doi: 10.1101/2019.12.13.874495

Okae H, Toh H, Sato T, Hiura H, Takahashi S, Shirane K, et al. Derivation of human trophoblast stem cells. *Cell Stem Cell.* (2018) 22:50- 63.e6. doi: 10.1016/j.stem.2017.11.004

Turco MY, Gardner L, Kay RG, Hamilton RS, Prater M, Hollinshead MS, et al. Trophoblast organoids as a model for maternal–fetal interactions during human placentation. *Nature.* (2018) 564:263–7. doi: 10.1038/s41586-018-0753-3

Haider S, Meinhardt G, Saleh L, Kunihs V, Gamperl M, Kaindl U, et al. Self-renewing trophoblast organoids recapitulate the developmental program of the early human placenta. *Stem Cell Rep.* (2018) 11:537– 51. doi: 10.1016/j.stemcr.2018.07.004

Avraham R, Haseley N, Brown D, Penaranda C, Jijon HB, Trombetta JJ, et al. Pathogen cell-to-cell variability drives heterogeneity in host immune responses. *Cell.* (2015) 162:1309–21. doi: 10.1016/j.cell.2015.08.027

Avital G, Avraham R, Fan A, Hashimshony T, Hung DT, Yanai I. scDual-Seq: mapping the gene regulatory program of Salmonella infection by host and pathogen single-cell RNA-sequencing. *Genome Biol.* (2017) 18:200. doi: 10.1186/s13059-017-1340-x

CD206+ M2-Like Macrophages Are Essential for Successful Implantation

Yosuke Ono[1], Osamu Yoshino[2]*, Takehiro Hiraoka[2], Erina Sato[2], Yamato Fukui[3], Akemi Ushijima[4], Allah Nawaz[5], Yasushi Hirota[3], Shinichiro Wada[1], Kazuyuki Tobe[6], Akitoshi Nakashima[4], Yutaka Osuga[3] and Shigeru Saito[4]*

[1] Department of Obstetrics and Gynecology, Teine Keijinkai Hospital, Sapporo, Japan, [2] Department of Obstetrics and Gynecology, Kitasato University School Medicine, Tokyo, Japan, [3] Department of Obstetrics and Gynecology, Faculty of Medicine, University of Tokyo, Tokyo, Japan, [4] Department of Obstetrics and Gynecology, Faculty of Medicine, University of Toyama, Toyama, Japan, [5] Department of Molecular and Medical Pharmacology, Faculty of Medicine, University of Toyama, Toyama, Japan, [6] First Department of Internal Medicine, University of Toyama, Toyama, Japan

*Correspondence:
Osamu Yoshino
oyoshino624@gmail.com
Shigeru Saito
s30saito@med.u-toyama.ac.jp

Macrophages (MΦs) play important roles in implantation. Depletion of CD11b+ pan-MΦs in CD11b-diphtheria-toxin-receptor (DTR) mice is reported to cause implantation failure due to decreased progesterone production in the corpus luteum. However, of the M1 and M2, the type of MΦs that is important for implantation is unknown. In this study, we investigated the role of M2 MΦ in implantation using CD206-DTR mice. To deplete M2-MΦ, female CD206-DTR C57/BL6 mice were injected with DT before implantation. These M2-MΦ depleted mice (M2(-)) were naturally mated with Balb/C mice. As the control group, female C57/BL6 wild type (WT) mice injected with DT were mated with male Balb/C mice. The number of implantation sites and plasma progesterone levels at implantation were examined. Implantation-related molecule expression was determined using quantitative-PCR and immunohistochemistry of uterine tissues. The mRNA expression in the endometrial tissues of 38 patients with implantation failure was examined during the implantation window. In WT mice, CD206+M2-like MΦs accumulated in the endometrium at the implantation period, on embryonic (E) 4.5. In M2(-), the implantation number was significantly lower than that in control ($p < 0.001$, 7.8 ± 0.8 vs. 0.2 ± 0.4), although the plasma progesterone levels were not changed. Leukemia inhibitory factor (LIF) and CD206 mRNA expression was significantly reduced ($p < 0.01$), whereas the levels of TNFα were increased on E4.5 ($p < 0.05$). In M2(-), the number of Ki-67+ epithelial cells was higher than that in control at the pre-implantation period. Accelerated epithelial cell proliferation was confirmed by significantly upregulated uterine fibroblast growth factor (FGF)18 mRNA ($P < 0.05$), and strong FGF18 protein expression in M2(-) endometrial epithelial cells. Further, M2(-) showed upregulated uterine Wnt/β-catenin signals at the mRNA and protein levels. In the non-pregnant group, the proportion of M2-like MΦ to pan MΦ, CD206/CD68, was significantly reduced ($p < 0.05$) and the TNFα mRNA expression was significantly increased ($p < 0.05$) in the endometrial tissues compared to those in the pregnant group. CD206+ M2-like MΦs may be essential for embryo implantation through the regulation of endometrial proliferation via Wnt/β-catenin signaling.

Keywords: CD206, diphtheria-toxin receptor mouse, fibroblast growth factor, implantation, M2 macrophage, Wnt/β-catenin signal

INTRODUCTION

Macrophages (MΦ) are a crucial player in the generation and execution of immune responses through various functions, including phagocytosis, antigen presentation, and secretion of a variety of cytokines and growth factors (1–3). Recently, MΦs have been reported to play an essential role in tissue development and homeostasis through increased angiogenesis and vascular remodeling (1, 4, 5). MΦs also have attracted significant interest in human diseases as they play crucial roles in many diseases associated with chronic inflammation such as atherosclerosis, obesity, diabetes, cancer, skin diseases, and neurodegenerative diseases (6, 7). Implantation is a vital process of the first feto-maternal encounter in the uterus, leading to pregnancy. Good coordination between a blastocyst and receptive uterus is essential for successful implantation (8, 9). Although implantation is an important phenomenon in pregnancy, its precise mechanism is not fully understood due to its complexity involving multi-factors. Animal studies using different kinds of genetically altered mice have been undertaken to elucidate the mechanism of implantation (10–13). Although few studies have examined the relationship between MΦ and implantation, Care et al. first reported that MΦ plays an important role in the implantation process in CD11b-DTR mice (14). They showed that depletion of CD11b+ MΦs resulted in the implantation failure due to decreased progesterone production in the corpus luteum (14). MΦs are classified into two subtypes, M1 and M2 MΦs. M1 MΦs, or classically activated MΦs, are pro-inflammatory and play a central role in host defense against infection, whereas M2 MΦs, or alternatively activated MΦs, are associated with responses to anti-inflammatory reactions and tissue remodeling (15).

The precise role of MΦs in the uterus at the implantation period is unclear in implantation period.

MΦs demonstrate plasticity and polarize to the M1 or M2 type according to their surrounding microenvironment and stimuli (2, 16) and skewness to M1 or M2 MΦs has been reported in various diseases (4). But it is not clear which type of MΦs mostly contributes to the implantation. In the present study, we investigated the role of CD206+ M2-like MΦ in implantation using CD206-diphtheria-toxin (DT)-receptor transgenic mice (17–19), in which M2-like MΦs can be specifically depleted.

RESULTS

CD206+M2-Like MΦs Are Located in the Uterus at the Implantation Period

Most MΦs in non-pregnant mice are known to be present in the uterine stroma, but are reported to exist in the lumen and glands during the implantation period (20). To examine the localization of M2-like MΦs in the uterus at the implantation period on embryonic day 4.5 (E4.5), we performed CD206 immunohistochemistry in wild type (WT) mice. At the implantation period, we found that CD206+ M2-like MΦs were located in the uterine stromal region as well as close to the lumen and glands. Immunofluorescence analysis revealed that CD206+ cells were found in WT with DT and TG with PBS group, while these were completely depleted in TG with DT mice (**Figure 1A**-a). To examine the change of M2-like MΦs in the uterus at the implantation period, we compared CD206 mRNA expressions between non-pregnancy and implantation periods. The mRNA expressions of uterine CD206 was significantly increased during implantation period, peaking at embryonic (E) 3.5, compared to non-pregnancy (**Figure 1A**-b).

Implantation Was Impaired in the M2(-) Group

To investigate the role of CD206+ M2-like MΦ in implantation, we set the protocol of an implantation model using CD206 DTR mice (**Figure 1B**). We naturally mated C57/B6 female mice with Balb/c male mice as controls, or mated CD206 female DTR mice with Balb/c mice, defined as M2(-). DT was intraperitoneally administered to the control and M2(-) mice before the implantation period. The depletion of CD206+ M2-like MΦs was checked by qPCR. We compared the number of implantation sites between the two groups at E4.5 after in Chicago Blue dye administration. The implantation sites in M2(-) mice were significantly fewer compared to those in the control mice ($P < 0.001$, 7.8 ± 0.8 vs. 0.2 ± 0.4) (**Figures 2A,B**). As leukemia inhibitory factor (LIF)-Stat signaling is known to be essential for implantation (21), LIF mRNA expression was examined in the uterine tissues in M2(-) mice and was found to be significantly decreased compared to that in control ($p < 0.05$, **Figure 3A**). Immunostaining for phosphorylated Stat3 was also found in uterine epithelial cells of control mice but not in M2(-) mice (**Figure 3B**). The proportion of phosphorilated (p) STAT3-positive epithelial/total epithelial cells was significantly reduced in the M2(-) group compared to control (mean ± SD, $38.5 \pm 13.2\%$ vs. 0%; $p < 0.01$, **Figure 3C**).

The Accelerated Proliferation of Epithelial Cells Was Found in M2(-) Mice

We examined the morphological changes in the just after implantation period (E 5.5). In M2(-) mice, cell proliferation in the stromal region was impaired, and epithelial cells were proliferative compared to control (**Figure 4A**). We then examined the cell proliferation at pre-implantation period (E3.5). In M2(-) mice, the number of Ki-67-positive epithelial cells was higher compared to that in control at the pre-implantation period (E3.5). However, there were no histological differences in the corpus luteum and the plasma P4 concentration between both groups (**Figures 4B,C**). These suggest that endometrial epithelial cells had not transformed to become receptive to embryo implantation (**Figure 5**).

Uterine Wnt/β-Catenin Signaling Is Upregulated in M2(-) Mice at the Pre-implantation Period (E3.5)

Uterine Wnt/β-catenin signals regulate the production of fibroblast growth factor (FGF), and proper modification of these signals is essential for implantation (22). In M2(-) mice, at the implantation period, the mRNA expression of Wnt 4A, Wnt 7B, and β-catenin, was significantly increased ($p < 0.05$) compared

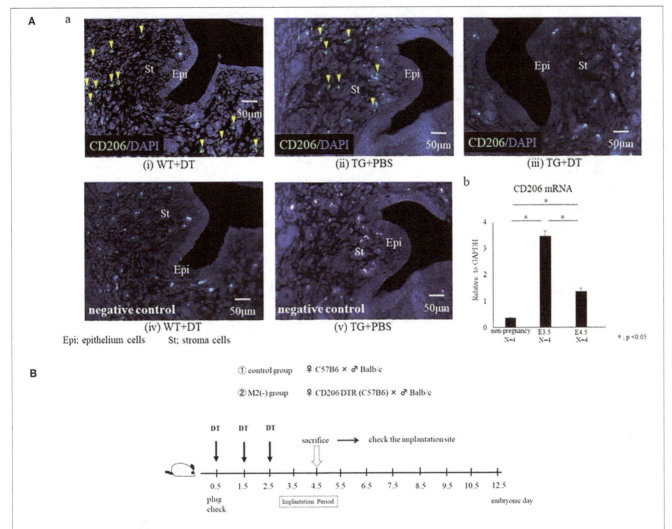

FIGURE 1 | (A) Localization of CD206+ M2-like macrophages (MΦ) in the uterus. Immunofluorescence for CD206 was performed for the uterus at embryonic day 4.5 (E4.5) in wild type (WT) and CD206 diphtheria toxin receptor transgenic mice (TG). The data of WT+DT(i), TG+PBS (ii), TG+DT (iii), WT+DT (iv), and TG+PBS(v) were shown. Anti- CD 206 antibody (i, ii, and iii) or control rabbit IgG (iv and v) were used for primary antibody. CD206-positive cells are in green, and nucleus were stained in blue. Yellow arrow heads show CD206+ M2-like MΦ. The uterine mRNA expression of CD206 at non pregnancy, E3.5 and E4.5 are shown in (b). Data were normalized to GAPDH mRNA levels to determine the relative abundance and are shown as the mean ± SEM. $*p < 0.05$. (B) Depletion protocol for CD206+ M2-like macrophages (MΦs) in the implantation model using CD206 DTR mouse. After checking the plug, diphtheria-toxin (DT) was intra-peritoneally injected prior to the implantation period (embryonic day; E0.5, E1.5, E2.5) in CD206-DTR female mice naturally mated with Balb/C male mice, defined as the M2(-) group. DT was also injected to C57/B6BL wild type (WT) female mice mated with Balb/C male mice, and were defined as the control group. The number of implantation sites and plasma progesterone levels at the implantation period (E4.5) were examined.

to the control, and endometrial epithelial cells exhibited strong staining for active β-catenin (**Figure 6A**). In detail, the basal site of uterine epithelial cells was strongly stained with β-catenin in M2(-) mice (**Figure 6B**). As expected, the mRNA expression of FGF18, downstream of the Wnt/β-catenin signal, was significantly upregulated ($P < 0.05$) compared to that in control; further, FGF18 protein was also strongly stained in the endometrial epithelial cells of M2(-) mice (**Figure 6C**).

Uterine Wnt/β-Catenin Signaling Was Enhanced by Inflammatory M1-Like MΦ

Wnt signaling is reported to be increased by TNFα in gastric tumor cells (23). We also found upregulated expression of TNFα, iNOS, and CD11c mRNAs produced by M1-like MΦs (4) in the uterus of M2(-) mice compared to control ($p < 0.05$) (**Figure 7**).

The Proportion of CD206+ M2-Like MΦs Among Total MΦs in Uterine Tissues Was Significantly Reduced in Patients With Infertility

We performed uterine endometrial biopsy in cohort of 38 infertility patients at the time of the implantation window. Implantation failure was diagnosed as the infertility factor for all these patients. After the endometrial biopsy, 19 patients got pregnant with assisted reproductive technology. The median age of the non-pregnant and the pregnant group was 40

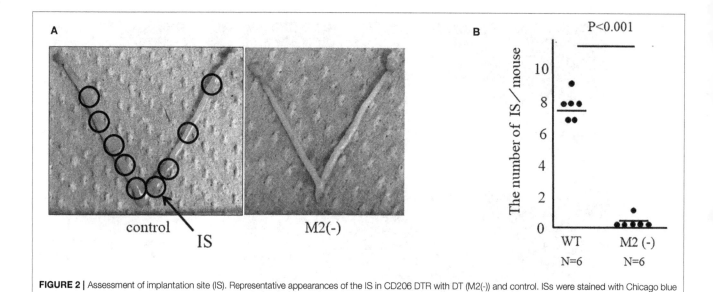

FIGURE 2 | Assessment of implantation site (IS). Representative appearances of the IS in CD206 DTR with DT (M2(-)) and control. ISs were stained with Chicago blue dye for facilitating their detection. ISs are shown (arrows) (A) and the number of ISs are shown as dots and the mean (B).

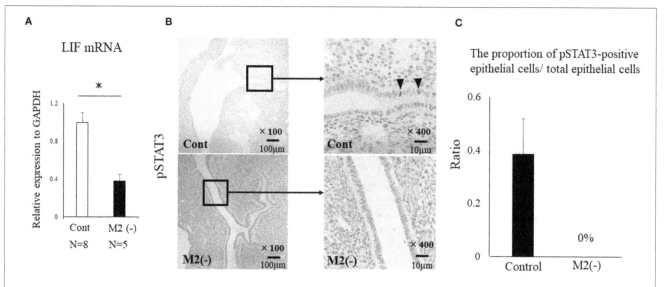

FIGURE 3 | LIF-STAT signal in the uterus at the implantation period. LIF mRNA expression in the uterus was examined. Data were normalized to GAPDH mRNA levels to determine the relative abundance and shown as (A). *$p < 0.05$. Immunohistochemistry was performed for phosphorylated (p) STAT3 in the control and M2(-) mice (B). We randomly selected six different sites on the section of immunostaining and counted the number of phosphorylation (p) STAT3-positive epithelial cells, which were divided by the total number of epithelial cells between both groups. The proportion of pSTAT3-positive epithelial cells/ total epithelial cells was examined (C).

(29–44) years and 37.5 (33–43) years old, respectively, which was comparable between two groups. We then compared the proportion of uterine CD206+ M2-like MΦs to pan MΦs at the mRNA levels of CD206/CD68, between pregnancy and non-pregnant groups. The relative ratio of M2-like MΦ to total MΦ was significantly reduced ($P < 0.05$) in non-pregnant group compared to that in the pregnant group, while upregulation of TNFα mRNA expression was observed in the non-pregnant group ($p < 0.05$) (Figure 8).

DISCUSSION

This is the first report investigating the role of M2 MΦs in the uterus at the implantation period in the mouse model. Previous reports showed that MΦs are important regulator of implantation and their depletion disrupts luteal vasculature resulting in reduced progesterone production from corpus luteum, which cause implantation failure (14, 24). These data suggest that depletion of pan MΦs during the implantation period causes implantation failure not owing to defects in the uterus but attributed to the ovary. Plaks et al. used the CD11c DTR mouse model to report that uterine dendric cells (DCs) are essential for embryonic implantation (25). However, as CD11c-positive cells include both MΦs and DCs, there was a limitation to determining the effect of each cell on implantation when CD11c cells were depleted. In the present study, we showed for the first time that CD206+ M2-like MΦs are essential to implantation by using CD206 DTR mice.

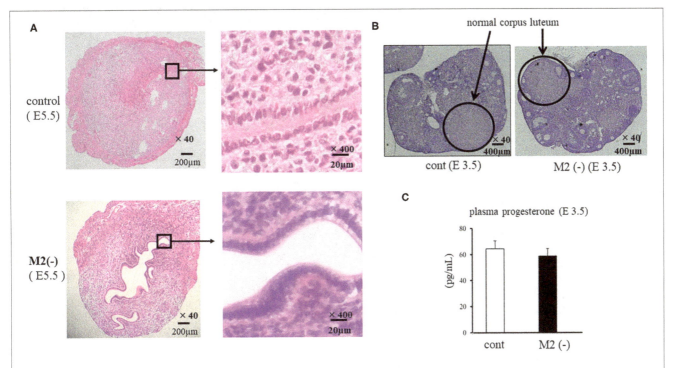

FIGURE 4 | Cross section of uterus and ovary. The cross sections of the implantation site (IS) are stained by hematoxylin and eosin (HE). The representative HE sections are shown at lower (x40) and higher (x400) magnification in the control and M2(-) at E5.5 **(A)**. The corpus luteum [**(B)**, hematoxylin and eosin stain] and the plasma progesterone levels **(C)** in control and M2(-) at E 3.5 are shown.

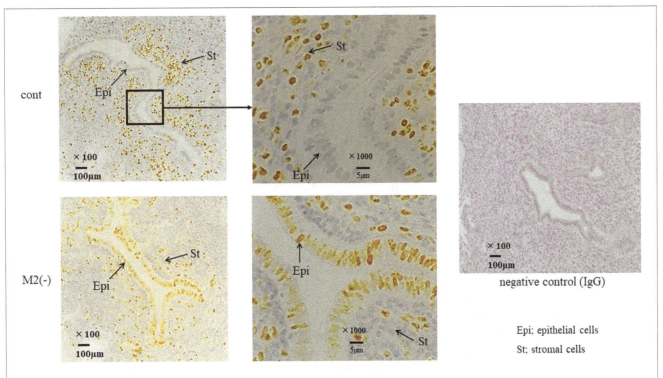

FIGURE 5 | Ki-67 immunostaining in the uterus at the pre-implantation period. Immunostaining for Ki-67, a proliferation marker, was performed in control and M2(-) mice. The arrows indicate the endometrial epithelial and stromal cells at E3.5. The representative sections are shown at lower (x100) and higher (x1000) magnification. Rabbit IgG was used for negative control.

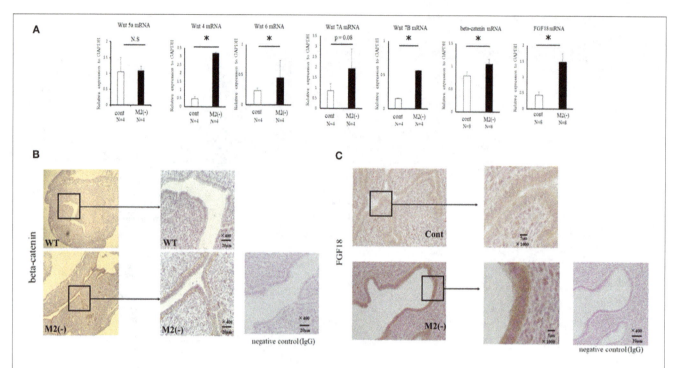

FIGURE 6 | Wnt/β-catenin signaling in the uterus at the pre-implantation period. The mRNA expression of Wnt4, Wnt5a, Wnt6, Wnt7A, Wnt7B, β-catenin, and FGF18 in the uterus at E 3.5 was examined by quantitative-PCR in the control and M2(-) mice **(A)**. Data were normalized to GAPDH mRNA levels to determine the relative abundance. The expression of β-catenin and FGF18 protein in the uterus at the pre-implantation period in control and M2(-) mice at E3.5 was examined by immunohistochemistry. Rabbit IgG was used for negative control **(B,C)**. Data are shown as the mean ± SEM. *$p < 0.05$.

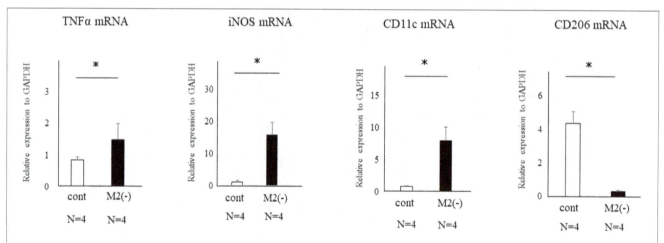

FIGURE 7 | Expression of TNFα, iNOS, CD11c, and CD206-mRNAs in the uterus of control and M2(-) mice at the pre-implantation period (E3.5). The mRNA expression of TNFα, iNOS, CD11c as the M1 MΦ marker, and CD206 in the uterus at the pre-implantation period in control and M2(-) mice was examined. Data were normalized to GAPDH mRNA levels to determine the relative abundance and are shown as the mean ± SEM. *$p < 0.05$.

In the CD206 DTR mouse model, implantation failure occurred exclusively by the depletion of CD206+ M2-like MΦs. As we have reported previously (19), we also found that the histological structure of the corpus luteum in M2(-) was not different from that of the control mice, and the plasma P4 levels were not changed, suggesting that the ovarian function at the implantation period was maintained in the absence of M2-like MΦs. Reduced plasma progesterone level by luteal dysfunction in depletion of pan MΦs mice model might be caused by the depletion of M1 MΦs. Therefore, the implantation failure may be attributed to the abnormal interaction between the embryo and uterus. In our previous study, we examined the effects of oocytes and embryos quality derived from M2MΦ depletion mouse on fertilization and implantation (19). In detail, after inducing superovulation in wild type (WT) and CD206+M2-like MΦ depleted mice, oocytes obtained from the fallopian tubes

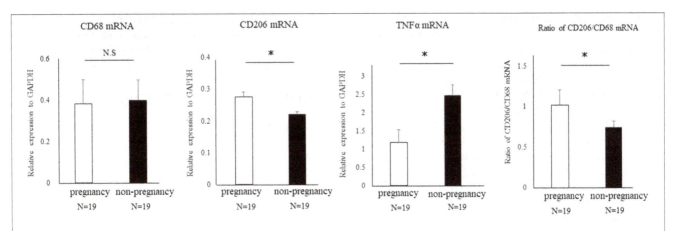

FIGURE 8 | The proportion of uterine CD206+ M2-like MΦ in human cases of pregnancy success and failure. A cohort of 38 patients with implantation failure were subjected to uterine endometrial biopsy at the timing of the implantation window. The mRNA expression of CD68 (pan-MΦ), CD206, and TNFα in uterus were examined between the pregnant and non-pregnant group after endometrial biopsy. Data were normalized to GAPDH mRNA levels to demonstrate the relative abundance. Also, the proportion of uterine CD206+ M2 MΦ to pan-MΦs at the mRNA level between two groups is shown. Data are shown as the mean ± SEM. *$p < 0.05$.

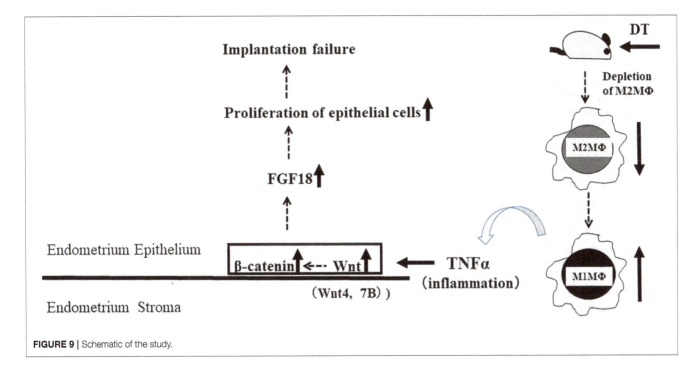

FIGURE 9 | Schematic of the study.

of these mice were *in vitro* fertilized, followed by transferring to pseudo pregnant WT mice. The fertilization rate, blastocyst formation rate, and pregnancy rate of CD206 DTR-mice derived oocytes were comparable to that of WT-mice derived oocytes, suggesting that oocytes derived from CD206+M2-like MΦ-depleted mice did not affect fertilization and implantation (19). In the present study, the structure of the corpus luteum and the plasma progesterone level was maintained during the implantation period. We detected morphological abnormality only in the uterus, so decreased uterine MΦs were considered the cause of implantation failure. In addition, at the pre-implantation period (E3.5), embryos obtained by flushing the uterine cavity with saline in both WT and CD206 DTR mice exhibited no morphological differences (data not shown). These data suggest that the depletion of M2MΦ *in vivo* did not affect the embryo quality and hormonal milieu. Therefore, the cause of implantation failure in M2(-) mice as observed in the present study, was the uterus and was not due to the abnormalities in the ovary or the embryo. Subsequently, we focused on the role of M2 MΦs in the endometrium during implantation. Elevated P4 concentrations after ovulation dramatically change the state of endometrial cell proliferation and render the uterus receptive to the embryo as a normal uterine morphological change that occurs during pre-implantation (26). In normal conditions, luminal epithelial cells are known to cease proliferation for implantation (26, 27); however, in M2(-) mice, the number of Ki-67-positive endometrial epithelial cells was higher compared to the control at the preimplantation period (E3.5), suggesting that the endometrial epithelial cells did not undergo the required change for receiving the embryo (**Figure 5**).

Nallasamy et al. have reported that targeted mutation of the homeobox transcription factors, Msx1 and Msx2, which control organogenesis and tissue interactions during embryonic development, in both the uterine epithelium and stroma, results in implantation failure. Based on gene expression profiling of the uterine epithelium and stroma from Msx1/2d/d mice, elevation of Wnt/β-catenin signaling leads to an increase in fibroblast growth factor (FGF) production in the uterine stroma (28). Moreover, upregulated FGFs act in a paracrine manner on the uterine epithelium to promote epithelial proliferation, which prevents endometrial differentiation and creates a non-receptive uterus for the embryo (28). This indicates that an excessive increase in Wnt/β-catenin signaling leads to an unreceptive uterus, which is refractory to implantation due to its inability to control epithelial proliferation, though moderately balanced uterine Wnt/β-catenin signaling is reported to be necessary for implantation (22). In the present study, the accelerated proliferation of epithelial cells in M2(-) mice might be due to a higher expression of FGF-18 in endometrial epithelial cells.

Aberrant expression of TNFα has been reported as one of the causes of enhanced Wnt/β-catenin signaling (23). In the present M2(-) mouse model, we found that the expression of TNFα and M1-like MΦ markers such as inducible nitric oxide synthase (iNOs) and CD11c (10), were significantly increased at the mRNA level ($P < 0.05$). This upregulation of M1-like MΦ related molecules might be due to a relative increase in M1-like MΦs owing to the depletion of CD206+ M2-like MΦs. Kambara et al. also reported that the expression of pro-inflammatory cytokines such as TNFα, IL-1β, IL-6, and MCP-1 were significantly upregulated in the lung tissues of CD206 DTR mice in response to DT treatment (17). Collectively, we hypothesized that upregulation of TNFα secreted by M1-like MΦs after depletion of CD206+ M2-like MΦ might accelerate the uterine Wnt/β-catenin signal in endometrial epithelial cells. Further, in epithelial cells, FGF18 expression was increased aberrantly, resulting in the proliferation of epithelial cells, which caused implantation failure (**Figure 9**). These results indicate that the balance of M1 and M2 MΦs may be critical for embryonic implantation. Additionally, LIF, essential for implantation, is also known to be produced by MΦ (29) and MΦ derived LIF is identified as a potential factor mediating MΦ-epithelial signaling (30). Therefore, the decrease in LIF expression (**Figure 3**) might be involved in the implantation failure. In our analysis of human samples, the proportion of uterine CD206+ M2-like MΦ, based on the CD206 mRNA expression compared to the total MΦ marker CD68, was significantly reduced ($P < 0.05$) in non-pregnant patients at the implantation period compared to that in the pregnant patients. And, in non-pregnant patients, the TNFα mRNA expression was significantly increased compared to that in the pregnant patients. Thus, dysregulation of M1/M2 MΦs may be one of the causes of implantation failure in humans.

In conclusion, we showed that the depletion of M2 MΦ led to implantation failure. Further studies are needed to clarify whether the mechanism of implantation failure is due to change in balance of M1/M2 MΦs, or decrease in number of M2 MΦs.

MATERIALS AND METHODS
Reagents and Materials
Roswell Park Memorial Institute (RPMI)-1640 medium and Diphtheria Toxin (DT) were purchased from Sigma-Aldrich (St. Louis, MO, USA). Fetal bovine serum (FBS) was purchased from Life Technologies (Minato-ku Tokyo, Japan). Antibiotics (a mixture of penicillin, streptomycin, and amphotericin B) were purchased from Wako Pure Chemical Industries (Chuo-ku, Osaka, Japan).

Immunohistochemistry
Paraffin-embedded tissues were cut into 5-μm-thick sections and mounted on slides. The mouse uterine and ovarian sections were deparaffinized in xylene, rehydrated through a graded series of ethanol, and washed in water. Antigen retrieval was performed in 10 mM sodium citrate buffer (pH 6.0) in a microwave for 10 min and then cooling to room temperature. Rabbit IgG was used as a negative control. Slide staining with the first and second antibodies was performed according to the manufacturer's instructions. Immunostaining was performed using antibodies specific to Ki-67 (Abcam, Tokyo, Japan, Cat# 15580, 1:100 dilution), β-catenin (Abcam, Tokyo, Japan, Cat# 138378, 1:100 dilution), phosphorilated-STAT3 (Cell Signaling Technology, Massachusetts, USA, Cat #9145, 1:100 dilution), and FGF18 (Abcam, Cat# ab169615, 1:100 dilution). An immunofluorescence analysis of implantation site (uterus) was performed using rabbit anti-mannose receptor (CD206) (Abcam, Cat# 64693, 1:100 dilution). And the primary antibody was incubated overnight at 4°C. As a second antibody, the rat anti-rabbit antibody was used. 4′,6-diamidino-2-phenylindole (DAPI; 1:500) was used to detect nuclei. Rabbit IgG were used instead of the primary antibody for negative control.

Mice and Diphtheria Toxin Administration
Female, CD206 DTR mice (17, 18), aged 12 to 20-weeks old were used. The mice were housed in a specific pathogen free (SPF) animal facility with a controlled environment of 22–24°C and 60–70% relative humidity, on a 12 h light/12 h dark cycle with food and water provided *ad libitum*. DT was diluted with sterile phosphate buffered saline (PBS) to the desired concentration and was intra-peritoneally injected to mice to deplete the CD206 positive cells. According to BioGPS, a complete resource for learning about gene and protein function (http://biogps.org/), CD206 seems to be expressed in mouse uterus more than other M2MΦ markers. In our preliminary experiment, in each organ, CD206 mRNA seemed to be more expressed than other M2MΦ markers (data not shown). Decidual MΦs are reported to be show higher expression of CD206 (31, 32). Wang et al. (33) reported that the CD206 expression in MΦs could be a marker for spontaneous abortion. From these results, CD206 is considered to be a valid marker for uterine M2 MΦ. The experiments

and procedures were performed at 48 h after the final DT administration, as previously reported by Nawaz et al. (18). The final DT injection was administered at E 2.5 before implantation. The depletion of CD206 positive cells was confirmed at mRNA levels by qPCR every experiment.

Assessment of the Implantation Site (IS)

We prepared control group by mating C57/B6 female WT mice with Balb/c male mice, and M2(-) group by mating CD206-DTR female mice with Balb/c mice (**Figure 1B**). To deplete M2-like MΦs at the implantation period, DT was administered to each mouse at a dose of 30 ng/gram body weight before implantation. We then checked the implantation sites between two groups. To identify implantation sites on embryonic day 4.5 (E4.5), mice were anesthetized using Avertin (2% tribromoethanol, 15 μl/g i.p.; Sigma-Aldrich), administered the Chicago blue dye solution (0.4% in PBS i.v.; Sigma-Aldrich) and then analyzed after 10 min. Uteri were dissected and assessed for clearly delineated blue bands as evidence of early implantation sites. In other mice, uterine paraffin sections from control and M2(-) mice were collected on E3.5 and E4.5 and stained with H&E to assess the implantation sites.

Patients With Implantation Failure

Uterine endometrial biopsy as performed at the time of the implantation window in 38 patients with implantation failure who visited the outpatient department of obstetrics and gynecology at the University of Tokyo. After the endometrial biopsy, we compared the proportion of uterine M2-like MΦ to the pan-MΦ based on the mRNA levels of CD206 and CD68 between the pregnancy and non-pregnant group.

Reverse Transcription (RT) and Quantitative Real-Time Polymerase Chain Reaction (PCR) Analysis

Total RNA was extracted from the mouse endometrial region from the peritoneal cavity, using the ISOGEN-II (NIPPON GENE, Tokyo, Japan). RT was performed using Rever Tra Ace qPCR RT Master Mix with gDNA Remover (TOYOBO, Tokyo, Japan). About 1.0 μg of total RNA was reverse-transcribed in a 20-μL volume. For the quantification of various mRNA levels, real-time PCR was performed using the Mx3000P Real-Time PCR System (Agilent Technologies, CA, USA) according to the manufacturer's instructions. The PCR primers used with the SYBR Green protocol were selected from different exons of the corresponding genes to discriminate the PCR products that might arise from possible chromosomal DNA contaminants. The SYBR Green thermal cycling conditions were as follows: 1 cycle of 95°C for 30 s, and cycles of 95°C for 10 s, 60°C for 10 s and 72°C for 10 s. The primer sequences used were as follows: 3-phosphate dehydrogenase (GAPDH, NM_002046: 628-648 and 1079-1060), mouse CD206 (NM_000710.3: 326-347 and 495-473), mouse TNFα (NM_000623.3: 432-453 and 605-584), mouse IL-10 (NM_010548.2: 390-412 and 464-443), mouse CD11c (NM_001363985.1: 82-103 and 194-175), mouse iNOS (NM_001313922.1: 2363-2382 and 2489-2470), β-catenin (NM_000623.3: 432-453 and 605-584), Fibroblast Growth Factor 18 (NM_000623.3: 432-453 and 605-584), Wnt 4 (NM_009523.2: 318-337 and 426-409), Wnt 5A (NM_009524.4: 565-583 and 668-650), Wnt 6 (XM_006495889.2: 670-688 and 796-779), Wnt 7A (NM_001363757.1: 501-518 and 578-558), and Wnt 7B (NM_009528.3: 421-440 and 492-472). The relative mRNA levels were calculated using the standard curve method and were normalized to the mRNA levels of GAPDH (forward, 5′-AATGTGTCCGTCGTGGATCTGA-3′ and reverse, 5′-GATGCCTGCTTCACCACCTTCT-3′) (**Supplementary Data 1**).

Measurement of Estradiol (E2) and Progesterone (P4) Levels

Mouse blood samples were collected during the analysis. Plasma levels of E2 and P4 were measured in duplicate using the specific EIA kits (Cayman, USA).

Statistical Analysis

Data were evaluated by Mann Whitney test using Jump version 10. $P < 0.05$ was accepted as statistically significant.

ETHICS STATEMENT

The studies involving human participants were reviewed and approved by the committee of the University of Tokyo (10991). The patients/participants provided their written informed consent to participate in this study. The animal study was reviewed and approved by the committee of University of Toyama (A 2015med-55).

AUTHOR CONTRIBUTIONS

SS, OY, KT, YH, and YOn: conception and design. YOn, ANak and AU: acquiring and processing samples. YOn, ANaw, YF, AU, OY, and ES: execution of the experiment. YOn and OY: analysis of data. SS, OY, ANaw, TH, ANak, and YOs: interpretation of data. YOn and OY: drafting the manuscript. SS, OY, YOn, and SW: revision of the manuscript for important intellectual content. All authors contributed to the article and approved the submitted version.

ACKNOWLEDGMENTS

The authors thank Mina Matsuo, Kaori Nomoto, and Hideki Hatta for their technical support and thank Editage (www.editage.com) for English language review.

REFERENCES

Gordon S. The macrophage: past, present and future. *Eur J Immunol.* (2007) 37:S9-17. doi: 10.1002/eji.200737638

Wynn TA, Chawla A, Pollard JW. Origins and hallmarks of macrophages: development, homeostasis, and disease. *Nature.* (2013) 496:445–55. doi: 10.1038/nature12034

Kebin H, Yang J, Zissis C, Xiaodong H, Hao L, Ling L. Macrophage functions and regulation: roles in diseases and implications in therapeutics. *J Immunol Res.* (2018) 2018:7590350. doi: 10.1155/2018/7590350

Yan CL, Xian BZ, Yan FC, Yong MY. Macrophage polarization in inflammatory diseases. *Int J Biol Sci.* (2014) 10:520–9. doi: 10.7150/ijbs.8879

Zhang L. Contribution of resident and recruited macrophages in vascular physiology and -athology. *Curr Opin Hematol.* (2018) 25:196–203. doi: 10.1097/MOH.0000000000000421

Schultze JL, Schmieder A, Goerdt S. Macrophage activation in human diseases. *Semin Immunol.* (2015) 27:249–56. doi: 10.1016/j.smim.2015.07.003

Decano JL, Aikawa M. Dynamic macrophages: understanding mechanisms of activation as guide to therapy for atherosclerotic vascular disease. *Front Cardiovasc Med.* (2018) 5:97. doi: 10.3389/fcvm.2018.00097

Egashira M, Hirota Y. Uterine receptivity and embryo–uterine interactions in embryo implantation: lessons from mice. *Reprod Med Biol.* (2013) 12:127–32. doi:10.1007/s12522-013-0153-1

Cha J, Sun X, Dey SK. Mechanisms of implantation: strategies for successful pregnancy. *Nat Med.* (2012) 18:1754–67. doi: 10.1038/nm.3012

Dey SK, Lim H, Das SK, Reese J, Paria BC, Daikoku T, et al. Molecular cues to implantation. *Endocr Rev.* (2004) 25:341–73. doi: 10.1210/er.2003-0020

Bilinski P, Roopenian D, Gossler A. Maternal IL-11r alpha function is required for normal decidua and fetoplacental development in mice. *Genes Dev.* (1998) 12:2234–43. doi: 10.1101/gad.12.14.2234

Daikoku T, Cha J, Sun X, Tranguch S, Xie H, Fujita T, et al. Conditional deletion of Msx homeobox genes in the uterus inhibits blastocyst implantation by altering uterine receptivity. *Dev Cell.* (2011) 21:1014–25. doi: 10.1016/j.devcel.2011.09.010

Sun X, Bartos A, Whitsett JA, Dey SK. Uterine deletion of Gp130 or Stat3 shows implantation failure with increased estrogenic responses. *Mol Endocrinol.* (2013) 27:1492–501. doi: 10.1210/me.2013-1086

Care AS, Diener KR, Jasper MJ, Brown HM, Ingman WV, Robertson SA. Macrophages regulate corpus luteum development during embryo implantation in mice. *J Clin Invest.* (2013) 123:3472–87. doi: 10.1172/JCI60561

Gordon S, Martinez FO. Alternative activation of macrophages: mechanism and functions. *Immunity.* (2010) 32:593–604. doi: 10.1016/j.immuni.2010.05.007

Martinez FO, Gordon S. The M1 and M2 paradigm of macrophage activation: time for reassessment. *F1000Prime Rep.* (2014) 6:13. doi: 10.12703/P6-13

Kambara K, Ohashi W, Tomita K, Takashina M, Fujisaka S, Hayashi R, et al. In vivo depletion of CD206+ M2 macrophages exaggerates lung injury in endotoxemic mice. *Am J Pathol.* (2015) 185:162–71. doi: 10.1016/j.ajpath.2014.09.005

Nawaz A, Aminuddin A, Kado T, Takikawa A, Yamamoto S, Tsuneyama K, et al. CD206+ M2-like macrophages regulate systemic glucose metabolism by inhibiting proliferation of adipocyte progenitors. *Nat Commun.* (2017) 8:286. doi: 10.1038/s41467-017-00231-1

Ono Y, Nagai M, Yoshino O, Koga K, Nawaz A, Hatta H, et al. CD11c+ M1-like macrophages (M<Is) but not CD206+ M2-like M<Is are involved in folliculogenesis in mice ovary. *Sci Rep.* (2018) 8:8171. doi: 10.1038/s41598-018-25837-3

Douglas NC, Zimmermann RC, Tan QK, Sullivan-Pyke CS, Sauer MV, Kitajewski JK, et al. VEGFR-1 blockade disrupts peri-implantation decidual angiogenesis and macrophage recruitment. *Vasc Cell.* (2014) 6:16. doi: 10.1186/2045-824X-6-16

Stewart CL, Kaspar P, Brunet LJ, Bhatt H, Gadi I, Köntgen F, et al. Blastocyst implantation depends on maternal expression of leukaemia inhibitory factor. *Nature.* (1992) 359:76–9. doi: 10.1038/359 076a0

Mohamed OA, Jonnaert M, Labelle-Dumais C, Kuroda K, Clarke HJ, Dufort D. Uterine Wnt/beta-catenin signaling is required for implantation. *Proc Natl Acad Sci USA.* (2005) 102:8579–84. doi: 10.1073/pnas.05006 12102

Oguma K, Oshima H, Aoki M, Uchio R, Naka K, Nakamura S, et al. Activated macrophages promote Wnt signalling through tumour necrosis factor-a in gastric tumour cells. *EMBO J.* (2008) 27:1671–81. doi: 10.1038/emboj.2008.105

Care AS, Ingman WV, Moldenhauer LM, Jasper MJ, Robertson SA. Ovarian steroid hormone-regulated uterine remodeling occurs independently of macrophages in mice. *Biol Reprod.* (2014) 91:60. doi: 10.1095/biolreprod.113.116509

Plaks V, Birnberg T, Berkutzki T, Sela S, BenYashar A, Kalchenko V, et al. Uterine DCs are crucial for decidua formation during embryo implantation in mice. *J Clin Invest.* (2008) 118:3954–65. doi: 10.1172/JCI 36682

Hirota Y. Progesterone governs endometrial proliferation differentiation switching and blastocyst implantation. *Endocr J.* (2019) 66:199–206. doi: 10.1507/endocrj.EJ18-0431

Haraguchi H, Saito-Fujita T, Hirota Y, Egashira M, Matsumoto L, Matsuo M, et al. MicroRNA-200a locally attenuates progesterone signaling in the cervix, preventing embryo implantation. *Mol Endocrinol.* (2014) 28:1108–17. doi: 10.1210/me.2014-1097

Nallasamy S, Li Q, Bagchi MK, Bagchi IC. Msx homeobox genes critically regulate embryo implantation by controlling paracrine signaling between uterine stroma and epithelium. *PLoS Genet.* (2012) 8:e1002500. doi:10.1371/journal.pgen.1002500

Nakamura H, Jasper MJ, Hull ML, Apilin JD, Robertson SA. Macrophages regulate expression of α1,2-fucosyltransferase genes in human endometrial epithelial cells. *Mol Hum Reprod.* (2011) 18:204–15. doi: 10.1093/molehr/gar070

Jasper MJ, Care AS, Sullivan B, Ingman WV, Aplin JD, Robertson SA. Macrophage-derived LIF and IL1B regulate alpha (1,2) fucosyltransferase 2 (Fut2) expression in mouse uterine epithelial cells during early pregnancy. *Biol Reprod.* (2011) 84:179–88. doi: 10.1095/biolreprod.110.085399

Laskarin G, Cupurdija K, Tokmadzic VS, Dorcic D, Dupor J, Juretic K, et al. The presence of functional mannose receptor on macrophages at the maternal-fetal interface. *Hum Reprod.* (2005) 20:1057–66. doi:10.1093/humrep/deh740

Svensson J, Jenmalm MC, Matussek A, Geffers R, Berg G, Ernerudh J. Macrophages at the fetal-maternal interface express markers of alternative activation and are induced by M-CSF and IL-10. *J Immunol.* (2011) 187:3671–82. doi: 10.4049/jimmunol.1100130

Wang WJ, Hao CF, Lin QD. Dysregulation of macrophage activation by decidual regulatory T cells in unexplained recurrent miscarriage patient. *J Reprod Immunol.* (2011) 92:97–102. doi: 10.1016/j.jri.2011.08.004

Progestins Inhibit Interleukin-1β-Induced Matrix Metalloproteinase 1 and Interleukin 8 Expression via the Glucocorticoid Receptor in Primary Human Amnion Mesenchymal Cells

William Marinello[1], Liping Feng[2] and Terrence K. Allen[1]*

[1] Department of Anesthesiology, Duke University Hospital, Durham, NC, United States,
[2] Department of Obstetrics and Gynecology, Duke University Hospital, Durham, NC, United States

*Correspondence:
Terrence K. Allen
terrence.allen@duke.edu

Preterm premature rupture of membranes is a leading cause of preterm births. Cytokine induced matrix metalloproteinase1 and interleukin 8 production from amnion mesenchymal cells may contribute to fetal membrane weakening and rupture. Progestins inhibit inflammation induced fetal membrane weakening but their effect on the inflammatory response of amnion mesenchymal cells is unknown. This study was designed to determine the role of progesterone receptor membrane component 1 and the glucocorticoid receptor in mediating the effects of progestins on interleukin-1β induced matrix metalloproteinase 1 and interleukin-8 expression in human amnion mesenchymal cells. Primary amnion mesenchymal cells harvested from human fetal membranes were passaged once and treated with vehicle, progesterone or medroxyprogesterone acetate at 10^{-6} M for 1 h followed by stimulation with interleukin-1β at 1 ng/ml for 24 h. Medroxyprogesterone acetate but not progesterone inhibited interleukin-1β-induced interleukin-8 and matrix metalloproteinase 1 mRNA expression. In subsequent dose response studies, medroxyprogesterone acetate, but not progesterone, at doses of 10^{-6}–10^{-8} M inhibited interleukin-1β induced interleukin-8 and matrix metalloproteinase 1 mRNA expression. We further demonstrated that inhibition of glucocorticoid receptor expression, but not progesterone receptor membrane component 1 knockdown with small interfering RNA transfection, resulted in a reversal in medroxyprogesterone acetate's (10^{-7} M) inhibition of interleukin-1β- induced matrix metalloproteinase 1 mRNA expression and interleukin-8 mRNA expression and protein expression. Our findings demonstrate that medroxyprogesterone acetate exerts its anti-inflammatory effect primarily through the glucocorticoid receptor in human amnion mesenchymal cells. Modulation of glucocorticoid receptor signaling pathways maybe a useful therapeutic strategy for preventing inflammation induced fetal membrane weakening leading to preterm premature rupture of membranes.

Keywords: progestins, preterm premature rupture of membranes, glucocorticoid receptor, progesterone receptor, interleukin-1 beta, Interleukin-8, matrix metalloproteinase 1

INTRODUCTION

Preterm birth (PTB) remains a major public health problem in the United States. Despite a slight decline in PTB rates from 2007 to 2014, rates have continued to increase in non-hispanic black women (Martin et al., 2017). Preterm births has multiple etiologies but the leading identifiable cause of preterm birth is preterm premature rupture of membranes (PPROM) (Parry and Strauss, 1998). Preterm premature rupture of membranes contributes significantly to perinatal morbidity and mortality, from adverse effects of prematurity and expectant management, increasing the risks of perinatal infections, placental abruption, umbilical cord prolapse, neonatal respiratory morbidity and adverse neurodevelopmental outcomes (Hadi et al., 1994; Lewis et al., 2007; Lee et al., 2010; Storness-Bliss et al., 2012; Korzeniewski et al., 2014; Ekin et al., 2015). Currently effective strategies for preventing PPROM are lacking.

The pathophysiology of PPROM involves the remodeling in fetal membranes of the extracellular matrix (ECM) in response to inflammation (Kumar et al., 2006). This inflammation induced ECM remodeling ultimately leads to fetal membrane weakening and rupture. *In vitro* biomechanical studies have also demonstrated that the amnion layer is the greatest contributor to the tensile strength of fetal membranes (Moore et al., 2006). The tensile strength of the amnion is due in part to the interstitial collagen type I and III in the compact layer of the amnion secreted by amnion mesenchymal cells in the fibroblast layer (Malak et al., 1993). Amnion mesenchymal cells are also a major source of matrix metalloproteinase 1 (MMP1) which initiates interstitial collagen degradation by cleaving the triple helix of the interstitial collagens (Mogami et al., 2013). Inflammatory cytokines induce MMP1 expression and activity in amnion mesenchymal cells which contributes to collagen degradation in the amnion ultimately leading to fetal membrane weakening and PPROM. Evidence suggesting that MMP1 plays a key role in PPROM include: elevated levels of MMP1 have been detected in the amniotic fluid of PPROM patients in both the presence and absence of infection (Maymon et al., 2000), a single nucleotide polymorphism in the promoter region of the MMP1 gene is associated with an increased risk of PPROM and changes in DNA methylation in the promotor region of the MMP1 gene have been associated with an increased risk of PPROM (Wang et al., 2008).

Our preliminary secretomic analysis of human amnion mesenchymal cells have demonstrated that amnion mesenchymal cells can release interleukin 8 (IL8) in response to interleukin-1 beta (IL1β) stimulation. interleukin 8 is a potent neutrophil chemoattractant and stimulator of neutrophil degranulation. Neutrophils in turn release MMP8 which cleaves the interstitial collagens. Neutrophil infiltration in fetal membranes has been associated with infection induced and abruption induced PPROM (Helmig et al., 2002; Lockwood et al., 2005). IL8 has also been implicated in epithelial to mesenchymal transition – a mechanism which has been implicated in the pathophysiology of PPROM (Radisky, 2005; Janzen et al., 2017). An increase in IL8 levels in amniotic fluid maybe associated with PPROM and predict the onset of preterm labor (Rizzo et al., 1997; Zhang et al., 2000; Jia, 2014). These findings collectively suggest that mesenchymal cells in response to inflammation play a role in the initiation of mechanism that lead to PPROM and PTB.

Progestins are used clinically for the prevention of PTB in women with a prior history of spontaneous PTB (Meis et al., 2003). *In vitro* studies have demonstrated that progestins are able to attenuate inflammation induced fetal membrane weakening (Kumar et al., 2015). The mechanisms by which progestins inhibit fetal membrane weakening still remains unclear. Given the role of the amnion mesenchymal cells in maintaining fetal membrane integrity, the effect of progestins on the inflammatory response of amnion mesenchymal cells may provide some insight into possible progestin-mediated mechanisms. Interestingly, fetal membranes do not express the classical nuclear progesterone receptors but still remain progesterone responsive and this progesterone responsiveness may be mediated through membrane-associated progesterone receptors (Merlino et al., 2009; Luo et al., 2010). For example, fetal membranes express progesterone receptor membrane component 1 (PGRMC1) whose role in fetal membranes remains to be elucidated (Feng et al., 2014, 2016; Allen et al., 2015). Furthermore, in fetal membranes, the amnion expresses higher levels of PGRMC1 when compared with the maternally derived decidual layer (Feng et al., 2014). We have previously demonstrated that PGRMC1 protein expression is diminished in PPROM patients when compared with term and preterm no labor patients highlighting the fact that PGRMC1 may play a role in molecular mechanisms that lead to fetal membrane rupture (Feng et al., 2014). Functionally we have shown that PGRMC1 partially mediates the inhibition of progestins on cytokine induced MMP9 activity in the HTR8 cytotrophoblast cell line and primary amnion epithelial cells (Allen et al., 2014, 2019). PGRMC1 may also play a role in oxidative stress induced senescence in fetal membranes (Feng et al., 2019). These findings demonstrate that PGRMC1 plays a role in maintaining fetal membrane integrity but its role in the amnion mesenchymal cells still remains unknown.

In the absence of the nuclear progesterone receptor, the glucocorticoid receptor (GR) may also explain some of the effects of progestins in fetal membranes. Glucocorticoids have been shown to inhibit lysyl oxidase (LOX) expression via the GR in amnion mesenchymal cells, a mechanism that may lead to fetal membrane rupture *in vivo* (Liu et al., 2016). Another study suggested that the inhibition of inflammation induced fetal membrane weakening *in vitro* by progestins could also be GR mediated (Kumar et al., 2015). Taken together our objectives were firstly to demonstrate that progestins inhibit IL1β-induced MMP1 and IL8 mRNA expression and secondly to determine if this mechanism is mediated through PGRMC1 or GR. Our primary hypothesis was that Progestins inhibit IL1β-induced MMP1 and IL8 mRNA expression primarily through PGRMC1.

MATERIALS AND METHODS

Isolation of Amnion Mesenchymal Cells

The collection of fetal membrane samples was approved by the Duke Medicine Institutional Review Board with a waiver of consent. As a result, fetal membrane samples were deidentified and there was no link to any clinical information. Fetal membrane samples were collected from term healthy patients at elective cesarean section without prior rupture of membranes or labor using a previously described protocol with modifications (Casey and MacDonald, 1996). Briefly, the amnion was separated from the choriodecidua and rinsed three times in Dulbecco modified Eagle medium: Nutrient Mixture F12 (DIMEM/F12) (Thermo Fisher Scientific) media with penicillin, streptomycin and amphotericin-B (Anti/Anti) (Thermo Fisher Scientific). Amnion epithelial cells were released from the amnion which was minced using scalpel blades and then digested with 1 g of 1:250 trypsin in DIMEM/F12 media with Anti/Anti for 30 min at 37°C. The remaining undigested amnion was collected and washed in DIMEM/F12 with Anti/Anti after filtering using a metal strainer. The process was repeated two more times. The undigested tissue fragments from three digestions were then pooled and incubated in DIMEM/F12 with Anti/Anti containing 0.75 mg/ml of Type I collagenase at 37°C for 30 min to release the amnion mesenchymal cells. The isolated cells were collected after filtration of the remaining undigested tissue through a 70 μm cell strainer. The filtrate was centrifuged at 1000 g for 5 min and the cell pellet was re-suspended in DMEM/F12 supplemented with 10% fetal bovine serum (FBS) (Thermo Fisher Scientific) and plated in 10 cm culture dishes. The cell cultures were incubated in humidified air and 5% CO2 for 5–7 days until they achieved confluence. Cells were passaged only once using 0.25% trypsin with EDTA and plated at approximately $0.2–0.5 \times 10^6$ cells/ml for all subsequent experiments.

Treatments

Amnion mesenchymal cells were plated at 0.5×10^6 cells/ml for 24 h. To determine the effect of progestin therapy on IL1β-induced MMP1 and IL8 mRNA expression the cell cultures were pre-treated with ethanol, medroxyprogesterone acetate (MPA), or progesterone (P4) (Millipore Sigma) at 10^{-6} M for 1 h followed by stimulation with IL1β at 1 ng/ml (RnD systems) for 24 h in DIMEM/F12 with Anti-Anti and 1% FBS. Subsequent dose response studies were performed using doses of MPA and P4 ranging from 10^{-6} to 10^{-8} M. At the end of the experimental incubation, cell culture media was harvested and centrifuged at 12,000 g for 5 min and the supernatant was collected, aliquoted and frozen at −80°C. Trizol® lysates were harvested and frozen at −80°C.

PGRMC1 and GR Depletion With siRNA

To determine the effect of PGRMC1 and GR on progestin mediated inhibition of IL1β-induced MMP1 and IL8 mRNA levels amnion mesenchymal cells were depleted of PGRMC1 or GR using siRNA. In a separate series of experiments amnion mesenchymal cells were initially plated at $0.2–0.5 \times 10^6$ cells/ml for 24 h in DIMEM F12 with 10%FBS. The cultures were then transfected using Lipofectamine RNAiMax and 10 nmol of PGRMC1 siRNA (ID: S21310), GR siRNA (ID: AM513311) or control siRNA (ID: AM4611) for 24 h in both serum and antibiotic free media. After 24 h transfection, the cultures were supplemented with 1 ml of DIMEM/F12 with 20% serum and incubated for an additional 48 h. At the end of the 72 h incubation the cells were then pre-treated with MPA or P4 for 1 h followed by stimulation with or without IL1β 1 ng/ml in DMEM/F12 with Anti/Anti and 1% FBS for an additional 24 h. We assessed the efficacy of PGRMC1 and GR knockdown with siRNA when compared with the control siRNA group using both real-time PCR and Western Blot.

Quantitation of IL8 and MMP1 Protein Concentrations by Magnetic Luminex Assay

Interleukin-8 and MMP1 levels in cell culture media were quantified simultaneously using the Human Magnetic Luminex assay (RnD systems) as directed by the manufacturer's protocol. The range of quantitation for MMP1 was 49.8–13,520 pg/ml. The range for quantitation of IL8 was 5.2–1227 pg/ml. Cell culture supernatant samples were diluted 1:10 due to the high concentration of IL8 in these samples to allow measurement within the range of the assay. When IL8 levels were below the lower limit of quantitation, we reported 1/2 of the lower limit of quantitation for IL8. In contrast, MMP1 levels were significantly lower in cell culture media and in the diluted samples they were below the level of quantitation of the assay and were not reported.

RNA Isolation and Real Time Quantitative PCR

Total RNA was extracted from amnion mesenchymal cells using Trizol, isolated using the RNeasy Mini-Kit and RNA concentrations were quantified using the NanoDrop® spectrophotometer. For each sample, 0.5–1.0 μg of RNA was reversed transcribed into cDNA using the Superscript III® first strand system (Thermo Fisher Scientific). Twenty-five to fifty nanograms of cDNA were used as the template for each real-time PCR reaction. Real-time PCR was performed using pre-validated Taqman probes directed against *MMP1* (assay ID: Hs00899658_m1) and GR (*NR3C1*) (Assay ID:Hs00353740_m1). Forward and reverse primers were used to detect PGRMC1, IL8 mRNA and the housekeeping gene *B2M* mRNA expression (**Table 1**). We performed Real-Time PCR using the following protocol: initial denaturation at 95°C for 3 min, followed by a 2-step amplification process of 95°C for 30 s and 60°C for 40 s for a total of 40 cycles.

TABLE 1 | Primer sequences used for real-time quantitative PCR.

Gene	Primer sequence
IL8	Forward 5′-ACT GAG AGT GAT TGA GAG TGG AC-3′
	Reverse 5′-AAC CCT CTG CAC CCA GTT TTC-3′
PGRMC1	Forward 5′-TGT GAC CAA AGG CCG CAA AT-3′
	Reverse 5′-TGC TTC CTT ATC CAG GCA AAA T 3′
B2M	Forward 5′-GAG GCT ATC CAG CGT ACT CCA-3′
	Reverse 5′-CGG CAG GCA TAC TCA TCT TTT-3′

Real-Time PCR was performed using the iCycler IQ™ Real-Time PCR detection system (Bio-Rad). All samples were run in duplicates with the mean cycle threshold C_t for the gene of interest normalized to the mean C_t value for the housekeeping gene *B2M*.

Western Blot

At the end of each experiment, cell culture media was removed, and the cells were washed with ice cold PBS and then lysed with radioimmunoprecipitation (RIPA) buffer containing the Complete Mini® protease inhibitor cocktail (Millipore Sigma). Total protein content for each sample was quantified using the Bradford protein assay. An equal amount of protein (10 μg) were separated on a 4–12% Bis–Tris gels (Thermo Fisher Scientific) at 125 V for 60 min and transferred onto a polyvinylidene fluoride (PVDF) membrane. The PVDF membranes were blocked with 5% milk in tris-buffered saline with 0.01% Tween for 1 h and then were incubated with polyclonal rabbit anti-human PGRMC1 (1:2000, catalog No. HPA08277, Millipore Sigma), polyclonal rabbit anti-human GR (1:1000 catalog No. 3660S, Cell Signaling) or monoclonal rabbit anti-human B2M (1:10,000, Catalog No. 12851S, Cell Signaling) antibodies overnight at 4°C. The membranes were then incubated with the appropriate secondary antibody (horseradish peroxidase-linked anti-rabbit or anti-mouse IgG at 1:1000 dilution, Cell Signaling) for 1 h at room temperature, after which they were incubated with the SuperSignal® West Pico Chemiluminescent Substrate (Thermo Fisher Scientific) and exposed on X-ray films. The band densities were quantified using ImageJ® and both PGRMC1 and GR were normalized to B2M.

Immunofluorescence

Primary amnion mesenchymal cells were plated on chamber slides at 1×10^4 cell/ml in DIMEM/F12 with antibiotics-antimycotics and 10% FBS for 48 h. Ice cold methanol was then used to fix the cells at −20°C for 10 min. The cells were then incubated for 30 min with Image – IT™ Signal Enhancer (Thermo Fisher Scientific) after which they were permeabilized and blocked with 5% goat serum and 0.1% Triton™ X for 1 h. To localize PGRMC1 or GR cells were incubated with rabbit anti-human polyclonal PGRMC1 antibody 1:100 (catalog No. HPA08277, Millipore Sigma) and/or mouse anti-human monoclonal GR antibody 1:250 (catalog no. SAB4800041, Millipore Sigma) overnight at 4°C in a humidified slide chamber. Cells incubated with a monoclonal anti-mouse (catalog no. MA5-14453, Thermo Fisher Scientific) and polyclonal anti-rabbit antibody (catalog no. ab27472, Abcam) were used as negative controls. To determine the homogeneity of the culture the cells were stained with the mesenchymal cell marker mouse anti-human monoclonal vimentin antibody (clone v9, catalog no. M0725, Agilent Dako) at 1:200 dilution. The cells were then incubated for 1 h with the Alexa Fluor™ 488 goat anti-mouse ReadyProbes™ (Thermo Fisher Scientific) and/or Alexa Fluor™ 594 goat anti-rabbit ReadyProbes™ (Thermo Fisher Scientific) diluted based on the manufacturer's specifications. The cells were then incubated with DAPI 1:1000 for 5 min.

ProLong™ Diamond Antifade (Thermo Fisher Scientific) was used as the mounting media and the cells were imaged with the Zeiss Axio Imager fluorescence microscope.

Statistical Analysis

All experimental groups were compared using one-way analysis of variance (ANOVA) with *post-hoc* pairwise comparisons using the Sidak test with each *P*-value was adjusted for multiple comparisons. A $p < 0.05$ was considered significant. Data were analyzed using GraphPad® Prism. Data are presented as mean ± standard error of the mean (sem).

RESULTS

Immunofluorescent staining demonstrated that PGRMC1 is localized to the nucleus, the perinuclear area, and the cytoplasm of amnion mesenchymal cells (**Figures 1B,E**). Interestingly, GR localized to the nucleus in some cells (**Figure 1A**) and in the cytoplasm in other cells (**Figure 1D**). When GR and PGRMC1 were both expressed in the nucleus they appeared to co-localize in the nucleus (**Figure 1C**). When GR was primarily expressed in the cytoplasm there was no evidence of co-localization with PGRMC1 (**Figure 1G**). The majority of the cells (>95%) stained positive for the mesenchymal cell marker vimentin (**Figure 1H**). Primary amnion mesenchymal cells were stained with DAPI to localize the nucleus (**Figure 1F**). The negative control demonstrated no evidence of non-specific staining (**Figure 1I**).

The Effect of Medroxyprogesterone Acetate and Progesterone on IL1β-Induced MMP1 and IL8 mRNA Expression in Amnion Mesenchymal Cells

Interleukin-1β significantly induced both *MMP1* and *IL8* mRNA levels in primary amnion mesenchymal cells when compared with the unstimulated (vehicle) control. In initial experiments MPA at a dose of 10^{-6} M significantly inhibited IL1β-induced *MMP1* and *IL8* mRNA expression when compared with the stimulated control (vehicle control plus IL1β) while P4 did not show any effects (**Figures 2A,B**). Both MPA and P4 did not suppress basal *MMP1* or *IL8* mRNA expression in amnion mesenchymal cells when compared with the unstimulated control.

In subsequent dose response studies pre-treatment with MPA at doses of 10^{-6}, 10^{-7}, and 10^{-8} M significantly inhibited IL1β-induced *MMP1* and *IL8* mRNA expression when compared with the stimulated controls (**Figures 2D,F**). Surprisingly, pre-treatment with P4 at doses of 10^{-7} and 10^{-8} M were associated with a significant increase in IL1β-induced *MMP1* mRNA expression when compared with the stimulated control (**Figure 2C**). Pre-treatment with all doses of P4 had no significant effect on IL1β-induced IL8 mRNA expression when compared with the stimulated control (**Figure 2E**). All doses of MPA and P4 tested had no effect on both basal *MMP1* and *IL8* mRNA expression when compared with the unstimulated control. In the

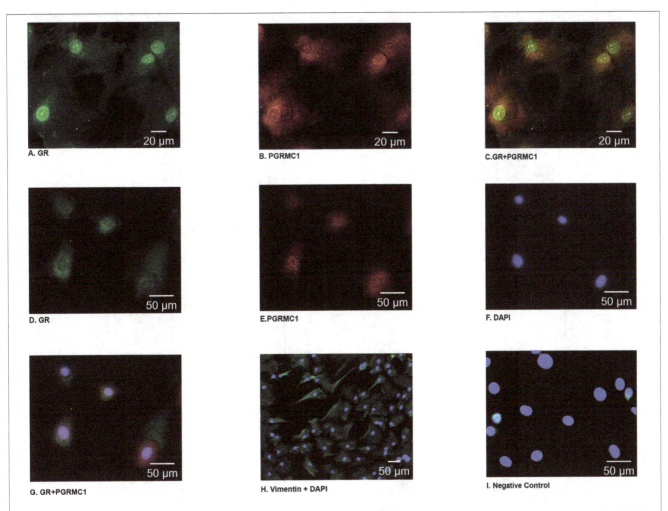

FIGURE 1 | In primary amnion mesenchymal cells GR was localized (green) primarily to the nucleus in some cells **(A)** and the cytoplasm in other cells **(D)**, PGRMC1 (red) localized to the nucleus and the perinuclear area of the cytoplasm **(B,E)**. Colocalization of GR and PGRMC1 in the nucleus when GR is expressed in the nucleus **(C)** vs. when GR is primarily expressed in the cytoplasm **(G)**. Primary mesenchymal cells stained with DAPI **(F)**, vimentin to identify primary mesenchymal cells **(H)**, and the negative control **(I)**. Images **(A–C)** were captured at 63× magnification **(D–G)**, **(I)** 40× magnification, and **(H)** at 20×.

subsequent siRNA experiments, we used MPA at a dose of 10^{-7} M and P4 at a dose of 10^{-6} M.

The Role of PGRMC1 and GR on Progestins Mediated Inhibition of IL1β-Induced MMP1 and IL8 Expression in Amnion Mesenchymal Cells

PGRMC1 siRNA significantly inhibited *PGRMC1* mRNA and protein expression in amnion mesenchymal cells but had no significant effect on GR mRNA and protein expression when compared with the control siRNA group (**Figure 3**). GR siRNA significantly inhibited GR mRNA and protein expression but had no significant effect on *PGRMC1* mRNA and protein expression when compared with the control siRNA group (**Figure 3**).

In the control siRNA group, the inhibition of IL1β-induced *MMP1* mRNA expression by MPA at 10^{-7} M when compared with the stimulated control was significantly attenuated by GR siRNA but was unaffected by PGRMC1 siRNA treatment (**Figure 4A**). As we had previously observed P4 at a dose of 10^{-6} M had no effect on IL1β-induced *MMP1* mRNA expression when compared with the stimulated control in the control siRNA group and this effect was unaffected by PGRMC1 or GR inhibition with siRNA. Furthermore, both MPA and P4 had no significant effect on basal MMP1 mRNA expression and this was unaffected by PGRMC1 and GR inhibition by siRNA.

In the control siRNA group, the inhibition of IL1β-induced *IL8* mRNA expression and IL8 protein levels in cell culture media by MPA at a dose of 10^{-7} M when compared with the stimulated control was significantly attenuated by GR inhibition with siRNA but was again unaffected by PGRMC1 inhibition with siRNA (**Figures 4B,C**). Progesterone at a dose of 10^{-6} M had no significant effect on both IL1β-induced IL8 mRNA expression and protein concentration when compared with the stimulated control in the control siRNA group and this lack of effect was unaffected by either PGRMC1 or GR inhibition. Both MPA and P4 had no significant effect on basal IL8 mRNA expression or protein concentration when compared with the

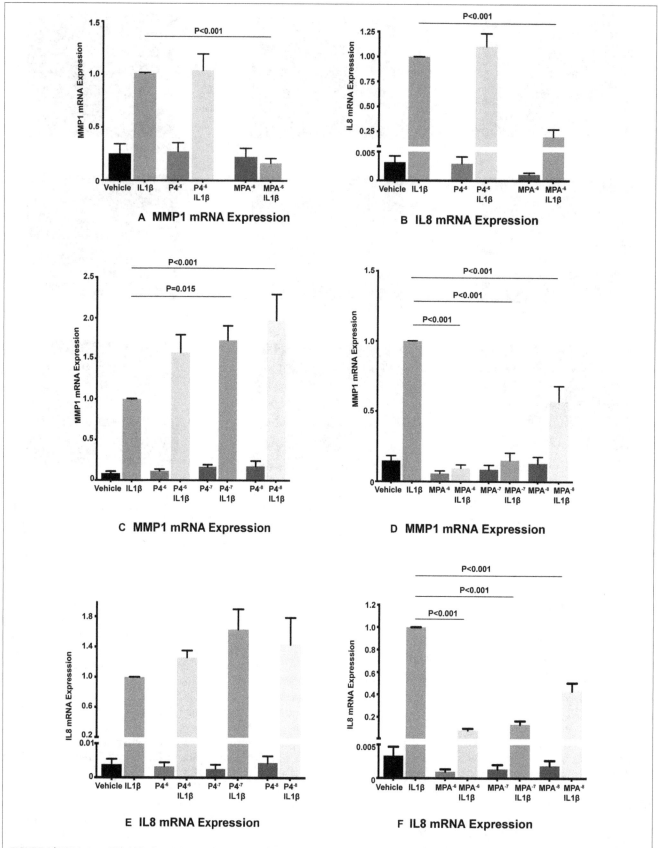

FIGURE 2 | MPA but not P4 inhibits IL1β-induced *MMP1* and *IL8* mRNA expression in primary amnion mesenchymal cells **(A,B)**. P4 dose response studies **(C,E)**, and MPA dose response studies **(D,F)** on IL1β-induced *MMP1* and *IL8* mRNA expression ($n = 6-7$ patients).

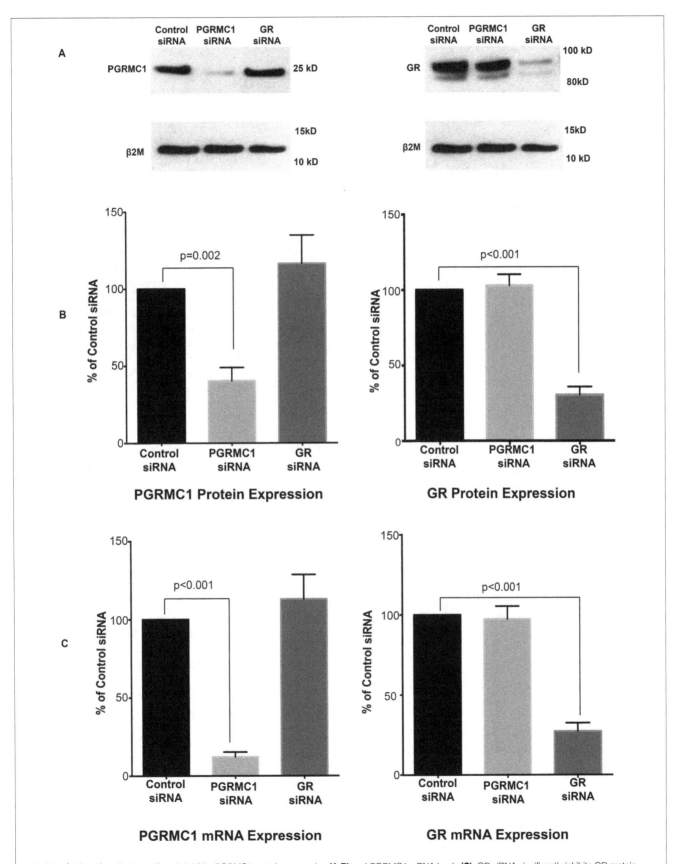

FIGURE 3 | PGRMC1 siRNA significantly inhibits PGRMC1 protein expression **(A,B)** and *PGRMC1* mRNA levels **(C)**. GR siRNA significantly inhibits GR protein expression **(A,B)** and GR mRNA levels **(C)** (n = 10 patients). For illustrative purposes the B2M image (top panel lower blot) was reused in both images.

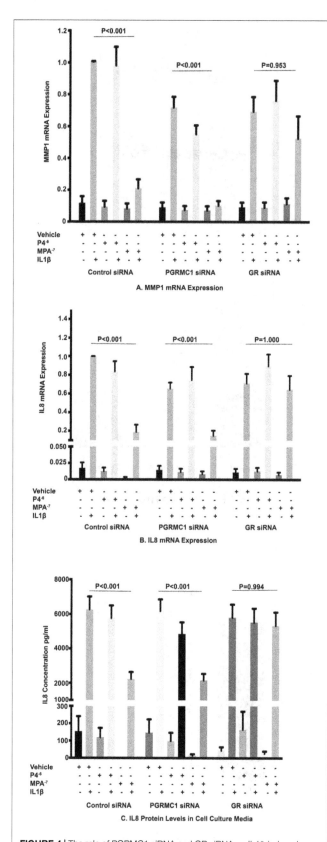

FIGURE 4 | The role of PGRMC1 siRNA and GR siRNA on IL1β-induced *MMP1* mRNA expression **(A)** and IL1β-induced *IL8* mRNA and protein levels **(B,C)** (n = 11 patients).

unstimulated control and this was unaffected by PGRMC1 and GR inhibition by siRNA.

DISCUSSION

Our findings demonstrate that MPA but not P4 inhibit IL1β-induced MMP1 mRNA expression and IL8 mRNA levels and secreted protein levels through GR and not through PGRMC1 in amnion mesenchymal cells. These findings are similar to our previous work in amnion epithelial cells which demonstrated that the inhibition of cytokine-induced MMP9 activity and mRNA levels in amnion epithelial cells was mediated through GR (Allen et al., 2019). Additionally, PGRMC1 localizes to the perinuclear area and the nucleus which is stark contrast to its expression pattern in amnion epithelial cells where it primarily localized to the cytoplasm and perinuclear area (Allen et al., 2019). GR in turn localizes to both the nucleus and cytoplasm as has been previously described (Wikström et al., 1987). Since in the inactive state, GR is localized to the cytoplasm as a part of a multiprotein complex with chaperone proteins and immunophilins, localization to the nucleus could represent activation by ligands present in cell culture media (Matthews et al., 2011). Alternatively the heterogeneity of GR localization in amnion mesenchymal cells could represent ligand independent trafficking of GR between the nucleus and cytoplasm which may occur normally during different phases of the cell cycle (Matthews et al., 2011). Both proteins appear to co-localize to the nucleus and even though the clinical relevance of this co-localization remains unclear, it could represent a functional interaction between both receptors in regulating genes involved in inflammation, cell cycle regulation and apoptosis in amnion mesenchymal cells and fetal membranes (Peluso et al., 2010; Allen et al., 2014, 2019; Sueldo et al., 2015).

This study provides further evidence that the anti-inflammatory effects of progestins, specifically MPA in the amnion are primarily mediated through GR and this is particularly important in fetally derived cells that lack the nuclear progesterone receptor (Merlino et al., 2009; Allen et al., 2014). The findings are even more important given the central role that amnion mesenchymal cells play in collagen turnover and immunomodulation in fetal membranes (Casey and MacDonald, 1996). The classic glucocorticoid receptor GRα, which is ubiquitously expressed, is known to mediate most of the known biological effects of glucocorticoids. However, there is still sparse data on the expression patterns of GR in fetal membranes in the preterm delivery phenotypes. This is further complicated by the fact that alternative mRNA splicing and translation initiation sites leads to the generation of multiple GR isoforms (Lu and Cidlowski, 2005; Lu et al., 2007; Turner et al., 2007). Currently, at least 8 GR isoforms have been identified in the placenta and are affected by gestational age and fetal sex and the roles of these isoforms still remain unclear (Saif et al., 2015). GRα-A is one of the isoforms involved in mediating glucocorticoid effects through its ability to transcriptionally activate and repress multiple gene targets. Interestingly the relative expression of GRα-A in the nucleus is less in preterm placentae than term placentae (Saif et al., 2015). The GR isoforms in the fetal membranes remain unknown, however, identification of the isoforms which mediate anti-inflammatory effects in fetal membranes could allow the development of safer glucocorticoids with reduced side effects.

Our findings in this study highlight the need for elucidating the underlying mechanism by which GR exerts these effects in fetal membranes. Recently it has been determined that distinct negative glucocorticoid response elements (nGRE) mediate the transcriptional repression effects of GR via an inverted quadrimetric palindrome separated by 0–2 nucleotide pairs (Surjit et al., 2011). Alternatively the protein-protein interaction between GR and specific transcription factors at promoters can result in inhibition (or stimulation) of target genes. These promoters either do not contain GRE (tethering) or have both GREs and responsive elements for the transcription factors that associate with GR (composite promoters) (Reichardt et al., 1998). Transcription factors that have been implicated in this protein-protein interaction include NF-κB, AP-1, and STATs (Heck et al., 1994; Stöcklin et al., 1996; De Bosscher et al., 1997). Interestingly NF-κB, AP-1 and STATs are some of the key transcription factors involved in the transcriptional regulation of MMP1 and IL8 gene expression (Chaudhary and Avioli, 1996; Overall and López-Otín, 2002; Fanjul-Fernández et al., 2010; Lin et al., 2016). Elucidating the anti-inflammatory mechanisms of GR in the amnion mesenchymal cells may allow the development of tissue specific GR modulators which inhibit inflammatory induced fetal membrane weakening and PPROM.

The role of PGRMC1 also remains unclear in fetal membranes. PGRMC1 did not mediate MPA's anti-inflammatory effect and we were also unable to demonstrate an anti-inflammatory effect of progesterone on IL1β-induced inflammation in amnion mesenchymal cells. However, emerging evidence demonstrates that PGRMC1's effects maybe cell type specific. In our previous work we demonstrated that PGRMC1 partially mediated the inhibition of TNFα-induced MMP9 activity by MPA in HTR8 cells, a cytotrophoblast cell line and to a lesser extent in primary human amnion epithelial cells (Allen et al., 2014, 2019). More recently we have demonstrated that PGRMC1 plays a role in mediating oxidative stress induced cellular aging through p38 MAPK and SIRT3 in primary human chorion cells (Feng et al., 2019). It has also been demonstrated that PGRMC1 may have anti-inflammatory effects by suppressing TNFα-induced gene expression independent of progesterone in N42 hypothalamic cells (Intlekofer et al., 2019). While in this study we were unable to demonstrate that PGRMC1 plays a role in IL1β-induced inflammation in amnion mesenchymal cells, it is likely that it may regulate other pathophysiological pathways that lead to PPROM and therefore warrants further investigation.

Interestingly in our *in vitro* study P4 was ineffective in preventing IL1β-induced MMP1 and IL8 expression and lower doses of P4 were associated with increased IL1β-induced MMP1 mRNA expression. In our prior work we have also been unable to demonstrate that P4 effectively prevents cytokine induced MMP9 activity and mRNA expression in primary amnion epithelial and chorion cells (Allen et al., 2015). The lack of effect of P4 and its augmentation of IL1β-induced MMP1 mRNA expression at lower doses could partly be explained by the lack of expression of the nuclear progesterone receptor in amnion mesenchymal cells and modulatory effects mediated via GR, respectively. The nuclear progesterone receptor isotypes PR-A and PR-B mediate most of the anti-inflammatory actions of P4 (Patel et al., 2014). In fact PR-A and PR-B null female mice demonstrate marked inflammatory changes in the endometrium (Lydon et al., 1995). Therefore in the absence of the nuclear progesterone receptor, P4's anti-inflammatory effects maybe significantly attenuated. However, P4 also binds GR but it does so with low relative affinity and it may also act as a weak partial agonist for GR-mediated transactivation and transreprepresion (Fuhrmann et al., 1996; Koubovec et al., 2005; Africander et al., 2011). Therefore the augmentation of IL1β-induced MMP1 mRNA expression could represent dose dependent conformational changes leading to GR-mediated transactivation and expression of proinflammatory genes. These anti and proinflammatory GR mediated effects highlight the complexity of GR signaling and the importance of finding the middle ground in maximizing GR-mediated therapeutic benefits.

Significant controversy surrounds the clinical use of progesterone for PTB prevention. Preclinical studies have demonstrated that progesterone promotes uterine quiescence by suppressing the expression of contraction associated proteins, inhibiting the expression of proinflammatory chemokines and cytokines and inhibiting immune cell infiltration and activation in the myometrium, potentially preventing mechanisms that may lead to PTB (Lei et al., 2015; Nadeem et al., 2016; Edey et al., 2017; Amini et al., 2019). In the cervix functional progesterone withdrawal is also associated with a local increase in proinflammatory mediators, matrix metalloproteinases and increased recruitment of immune cells that induces cervical remodeling that leads to PTB in human and animal models (Denison et al., 2000; Kuon et al., 2010; Kirby et al., 2016). While these findings suggest that progesterone supplementation maybe a useful therapeutic intervention for PTB prevention at least three large clinical trials have now demonstrated that vaginal progesterone does not significantly reduce preterm birth rates and in 2 of the studies, it did not reduce the rates of PPROM in subgroup analyses (O'Brien et al., 2007; Norman et al., 2016; Crowther et al., 2017; Norman and Bennett, 2017). The most recent PROLONG trial also demonstrated that another progestin 17αhydroxyprogesterone acetate did not significantly reduce recurrent spontaneous PTB (Blackwell et al., 2020). This has prompted some researchers to opine that it is now time to examine alternative therapies to progesterone for PTB prevention (Norman and Bennett, 2017). However, given the multiple mechanisms that may lead to PTB, research now needs to be focused on identifying the patient populations that may derive benefit from progesterone therapy.

Our study has several limitations. Firstly, we were unable to quantify MMP1 protein levels in part because the samples had to be diluted for IL8 level quantification using the magnetic Luminex assay. Another limitation of the study is that we only investigated inflammation induced molecular pathways, so our findings may not apply to other initiators of PPROM such as thrombin. Thrombin also induces *MMP1* mRNA expression, IL1β and IL8 protein levels in human amnion mesenchymal cells (Chigusa et al., 2016). In amnion mesenchymal cells this inflammatory response to thrombin can be inhibited by activators of nuclear factor erythroid 2- related factor 2 (NRF2) a transcription factor that mediates the expression of cell defense and antioxidant genes (Chigusa et al., 2016). Recently it has been demonstrated that GR signaling may also modulate NRF2 transcriptional activity, potentially highlighting the central role GR may play in pathways leading to PPROM and PTB (Alam et al., 2017).

In summary our findings provide additional evidence that the progestin MPA exerts its anti-inflammatory effects on molecular pathways implicated in PPROM through GR and not through PGRMC1 in fetal membranes. Identifying the downstream mechanisms by which GR exerts these effects could provide new insights into therapeutic interventions for PPROM prevention in at risk patients with the use of selective GR agonists and modulators.

ETHICS STATEMENT

Ethical review and approval was not required for the study on human participants in accordance with the local legislation and institutional requirements. Written informed consent for participation was not required for this study in accordance with the national legislation and the institutional requirements.

AUTHOR CONTRIBUTIONS

WM performed experiments, data analysis and interpretation, drafting of the manuscript, and approval of the final version of the manuscript. LF contributed to the study concept and design, drafting of the manuscript, and approval of the final version of the manuscript. TA contributed to the study concept and design, performed experiments, data analysis and interpretation, drafting of the manuscript, and approval of the final version of the manuscript. All authors contributed to the article and approved the submitted version.

ACKNOWLEDGMENTS

Biomarker profiling was performed under the management of Dr. Andrew N. Macintyre and direction of Dr. Gregory D. Sempowski in the Immunology Unit of the Duke Regional Biocontainment Laboratory (RBL), which received partial support for construction from the National Institutes of Health, National Institute of Allergy and Infectious Diseases (UC6-AI058607).

REFERENCES

Africander, D., Verhoog, N., and Hapgood, J. P. (2011). Molecular mechanisms of steroid receptor-mediated actions by synthetic progestins used in HRT and contraception. *Steroids* 76, 636–652. doi: 10.1016/j.steroids.2011.03.001

Alam, M. M., Okazaki, K., Nguyen, L. T. T., Ota, N., Kitamura, H., Murakami, S., et al. (2017). Glucocorticoid receptor signaling represses the antioxidant response by inhibiting histone acetylation mediated by the transcriptional activator NRF2. *J. Biol. Chem.* 292, 7519–7530. doi: 10.1074/jbc.m116.773960

Allen, T. K., Feng, L., Grotegut, C. A., and Murtha, A. P. (2014). Progesterone receptor membrane component 1 as the mediator of the inhibitory effect of progestins on cytokine-induced matrix metalloproteinase 9 activity in vitro. *Reprod. Sci.* 21, 260–268. doi: 10.1177/1933719113493514

Allen, T. K., Feng, L., Nazzal, M., Grotegut, C. A., Buhimschi, I. A., and Murtha, A. P. (2015). The effect of progestins on tumor necrosis factor α-induced matrix metalloproteinase-9 activity and gene expression in human primary amnion and chorion cells in vitro. *Anesth. Analg.* 120, 1085–1094. doi: 10.1213/ane.0000000000000708

Allen, T. K., Nazzal, M. N., Feng, L., Buhimschi, I. A., and Murtha, A. P. (2019). Progestins inhibit tumor necrosis factor α-induced matrix metalloproteinase 9 activity via the glucocorticoid receptor in primary amnion epithelial cells. *Reprod. Sci.* 26, 394–403.

Amini, P., Wilson, R., Wang, J., Tan, H., Yi, L., Koeblitz, W. K., et al. (2019). Progesterone and cAMP synergize to inhibit responsiveness of myometrial cells to pro-inflammatory/pro-labor stimuli. *Mol. Cell Endocrinol.* 479, 1–11. doi: 10.1016/j.mce.2018.08.005

Blackwell, S. C., Gyamfi-Bannerman, C., Biggio, J. R., Chauhan, S. P., Hughes, B. L., Louis, J. M., et al. (2020). 17-OHPC to prevent recurrent preterm birth in singleton gestations (PROLONG study): a multicenter, international, randomized double-blind trial. *Am. J. Perinatol.* 37, 127–136. doi: 10.1055/s-0039-3400227

Casey, M. L., and MacDonald, P. C. (1996). Interstitial collagen synthesis and processing in human amnion: a property of the mesenchymal cells. *Biol. Reprod.* 55, 1253–1260. doi: 10.1095/biolreprod55.6.1253

Chaudhary, L. R., and Avioli, L. V. (1996). Regulation of interleukin-8 gene expression by interleukin-1β, osteotropic hormones, and protein kinase inhibitors in normal human bone marrow stromal cells. *J. Biol. Chem.* 271, 16591–16596. doi: 10.1074/jbc.271.28.16591

Chigusa, Y., Kishore, A. H., Mogami, H., and Word, R. A. (2016). Nrf2 activation inhibits effects of thrombin in human amnion cells and thrombin-induced preterm birth in mice. *J. Clin. Endocrinol. Metab.* 101, 2612–2621. doi: 10.1210/jc.2016-1059

Crowther, C. A., Ashwood, P., McPhee, A. J., Flenady, V., Tran, T., Dodd, J. M., et al. (2017). Vaginal progesterone pessaries for pregnant women with a previous preterm birth to prevent neonatal respiratory distress syndrome (the PROGRESS study): a multicentre, randomised, placebo-controlled trial. *PLoS Med.* 14:e1002390. doi: 10.1371/journal.pone.01002390

De Bosscher, K., Schmitz, M. L., Vanden Berghe, W., Plaisance, S., Fiers, W., and Haegeman, G. (1997). Glucocorticoid-mediated repression of nuclear factor-κB dependent transcription involves direct interference with transactivation. *Proc. Natl. Acad. Sci. U.S.A.* 94, 13504–13509. doi: 10.1073/pnas.94.25.13504

Denison, F. C., Riley, S. C., Elliott, C. L., Kelly, R. W., Calder, A. A., and Critchley, H. O. (2000). The effect of mifepristone administration on leukocyte populations, matrix metalloproteinases and inflammatory mediators in the first trimester cervix. *Mol. Hum. Reprod.* 6, 541–548. doi: 10.1093/molehr/6.6.541

Edey, L. F., Georgiou, H., O'Dea, K. P., Mesiano, S., Herbert, B. R., Lei, K., et al. (2017). Progesterone, the maternal immune system and the onset of parturition in the mouse. *Biol. Reprod.* 98, 376–395. doi: 10.1093/biolre/iox146

Ekin, A., Gezer, C., Taner, C. E., and Ozeren, M. (2015). Perinatal outcomes in pregnancies with oligohydramnios after preterm premature rupture of membranes. *J. Matern. Fetal Neonatal Med.* 28, 1918–1922. doi: 10.3109/14767058.2014.972927

Fanjul-Fernández, M., Folgueras, A. R., Cabrera, S., and López-Otín, C. (2010). Matrix metalloproteinases: evolution, gene regulation and functional analysis in mouse models. *Biochim. Biophys. Acta* 1803, 3–19. doi: 10.1016/j.bbamcr.2009.07.004

Feng, L., Allen, T. K., Marinello, W. P., and Murtha, A. P. (2019). Roles of progesterone receptor membrane component 1 in oxidative stress-induced aging in chorion cells. *Reprod. Sci.* 26, 394–403. doi: 10.1177/1933719118776790

Feng, L., Antczak, B., Lan, L., Grotegut, C. A., Thompson, J. L., Allen, T. K., et al. (2014). Progesterone receptor membrane component 1 (PGRMC1) expression in fetal membranes among women with preterm premature rupture of the membranes (PPROM). *Placenta* 35, 331–333. doi: 10.1016/j.placenta.2014.03.008

Feng, L., Ransom, C. E., Nazzal, M. K., Allen, T. K., Li, Y.-J., Truong, T., et al. (2016). The role of progesterone and a novel progesterone receptor, progesterone receptor membrane component 1, in the inflammatory response of fetal membranes to *Ureaplasma parvum* infection. *PLoS One* 11:e0168102. doi: 10.1371/journal.pone.0168102

Fuhrmann, U., Krattenmacher, R., Slater, E. P., and Fritzemeier, K.-H. (1996). The novel progestin drospirenone and its natural counterpart progesterone: biochemical profile and antiandrogenic potential. *Contraception* 54, 243–251. doi: 10.1016/s0010-7824(96)00195-3

Hadi, H. A., Hodson, C. A., and Strickland, D. (1994). Premature rupture of the membranes between 20 and 25 weeks' gestation: role of amniotic fluid volume in perinatal outcome. *Am. J. Obstet. Gynecol.* 170, 1139–1144. doi: 10.1016/s0002-9378(94)70109-1

Heck, S., Kullmann, M., Gast, A., Ponta, H., Rahmsdorf, H. J., Herrlich, P., et al. (1994). A distinct modulating domain in glucocorticoid receptor monomers in the repression of activity of the transcription factor AP-1. *EMBO J.* 13, 4087–4095. doi: 10.1002/j.1460-2075.1994.tb06726.x

Helmig, B. R., Romero, R., Espinoza, J., Chaiworapongsa, T., Bujold, E., Gomez, R., et al. (2002). Neutrophil elastase and secretory leukocyte protease inhibitor in prelabor rupture of membranes, parturition and intra-amniotic infection. *J. Matern. Fetal Neonatal Med.* 12, 237–246. doi: 10.1080/jmf.12.4.237.246

Intlekofer, K. A., Clements, K., Woods, H., Adams, H., Suvorov, A., and Petersen, S. L. (2019). Progesterone receptor membrane component 1 inhibits tumor necrosis factor alpha induction of gene expression in neural cells. *PLoS One* 14:e0215389. doi: 10.1371/journal.pone.0215389

Janzen, C., Sen, S., Lei, M. Y. Y., Gagliardi de Assumpcao, M., Challis, J., and Chaudhuri, G. (2017). The role of epithelial to mesenchymal transition in human amniotic membrane rupture. *J. Clin. Endocrinol. Metab.* 102, 1261–1269.

Jia, X. (2014). Value of amniotic fluid IL-8 and annexin A2 in prediction of preterm delivery in preterm labor and preterm premature rupture of membranes. *J. Reprod. Med.* 59, 154–160.

Kirby, M. A., Heuerman, A. C., Custer, M., Dobyns, A. E., Strilaeff, R., Stutz, K. N., et al. (2016). Progesterone receptor-mediated actions regulate remodeling of the cervix in preparation for preterm parturition. *Reprod. Sci.* 23, 1473–1483. doi: 10.1177/1933719116650756

Korzeniewski, S. J., Romero, R., Cortez, J., Pappas, A., Schwartz, A. G., Kim, C. J., et al. (2014). A "multi-hit" model of neonatal white matter injury: cumulative contributions of chronic placental inflammation, acute fetal inflammation and postnatal inflammatory events. *J. Perinat. Med.* 42, 731–743.

Koubovec, D., Ronacher, K., Stubsrud, E., Louw, A., and Hapgood, J. P. (2005). Synthetic progestins used in HRT have different glucocorticoid agonist properties. *Mol. Cell Endocrinol.* 242, 23–32. doi: 10.1016/j.mce.2005.07.001

Kumar, D., Fung, W., Moore, R. M., Pandey, V., Fox, J., Stetzer, B., et al. (2006). Proinflammatory cytokines found in amniotic fluid induce collagen remodeling, apoptosis, and biophysical weakening of cultured human fetal membranes. *Biol. Reprod.* 74, 29–34. doi: 10.1095/biolreprod.105.045328

Kumar, D., Springel, E., Moore, R. M., Mercer, B. M., Philipson, E., Mansour, J. M., et al. (2015). Progesterone inhibits in vitro fetal membrane weakening. *Am. J. Obstet. Gynecol.* 213, 520.e521–520.e529.

Kuon, R. J., Shi, S. Q., Maul, H., Sohn, C., Balducci, J., Maner, W. L., et al. (2010). Pharmacologic actions of progestins to inhibit cervical ripening and prevent delivery depend on their properties, the route of administration, and the vehicle. *Am. J. Obstet. Gynecol.* 202, e451–e459.

Lee, S. E., Romero, R., Lee, S. M., and Yoon, B. H. (2010). Amniotic fluid volume in intra-amniotic inflammation with and without culture-proven amniotic fluid infection in preterm premature rupture of membranes. *J. Perinat. Med.* 38, 39–44.

Lei, K., Georgiou, E. X., Chen, L., Yulia, A., Sooranna, S. R., Brosens, J. J., et al. (2015). progesterone and the repression of myometrial inflammation: the roles of MKP-1 and the AP-1 system. *Mol. Endocrinol.* 29, 1454–1467. doi: 10.1210/me.2015-1122

Lewis, D. F., Robichaux, A. G., Jaekle, R. K., Salas, A., Canzoneri, B. J., Horton, K., et al. (2007). Expectant management of preterm premature rupture of membranes and nonvertex presentation: what are the risks? *Am. J. Obstet. Gynecol.* 196, 566–566.

Lin, C.-H., Wang, Y.-H., Chen, Y.-W., Lin, Y.-L., Chen, B.-C., and Chen, M.-C. (2016). Transcriptional and posttranscriptional regulation of CXCL8/IL-8 gene expression induced by connective tissue growth factor. *Immunol. Res.* 64, 369–384. doi: 10.1007/s12026-015-8670-0

Liu, C., Guo, C., Wang, W., Zhu, P., Li, W., Mi, Y., et al. (2016). Inhibition of lysyl oxidase by cortisol regeneration in human amnion: implications for rupture of fetal membranes. *Endocrinology* 157, 4055–4065. doi: 10.1210/en.2016-1406

Lockwood, C. J., Toti, P., Arcuri, F., Paidas, M., Buchwalder, L., Krikun, G., et al. (2005). Mechanisms of abruption-induced premature rupture of the fetal membranes. *Am. J. Pathol.* 167, 1443–1449. doi: 10.1016/s0002-9440(10)61230-8

Lu, N. Z., and Cidlowski, J. A. (2005). Translational regulatory mechanisms generate n-terminal glucocorticoid receptor isoforms with unique transcriptional target genes. *Mol. Cell* 18, 331–342. doi: 10.1016/j.molcel.2005.03.025

Lu, N. Z., Collins, J. B., Grissom, S. F., and Cidlowski, J. A. (2007). Selective regulation of bone cell apoptosis by translational isoforms of the glucocorticoid receptor. *Mol. Cell Biol.* 27, 7143–7160. doi: 10.1128/mcb.00253-07

Luo, G., Abrahams, V. M., Tadesse, S., Funai, E. F., Hodgson, E. J., Gao, J., et al. (2010). Progesterone inhibits basal and TNF(-induced apoptosis in fetal membranes: a novel mechanism to explain progesterone-mediated prevention of preterm birth. *Reprod. Sci.* 17, 532–539. doi: 10.1177/1933719110363618

Lydon, J. P., DeMayo, F. J., Funk, C. R., Mani, S. K., Hughes, A. R., Montgomery, C. A. Jr., et al. (1995). Mice lacking progesterone receptor exhibit pleiotropic reproductive abnormalities. *Genes Dev.* 9, 2266–2278. doi: 10.1101/gad.9.18.2266

Malak, T. M., Ockleford, C. D., Bell, S. C., Dalgleish, R., Bright, N., and Macvicar, J. (1993). Confocal immunofluorescence localization of collagen types I, III, IV, V and VI and their ultrastructural organization in term human fetal membranes. *Placenta* 14, 385–406. doi: 10.1016/s0143-4004(05)80460-6

Martin, J. A., Hamilton, B. E., Osterman, M. J., Driscoll, A. K., and Mathews, T. J. (2017). *Births: Final Data for 2015. National Vital Statistics Reports*. Hyattsville MD: National Center for Healthcare Statistics.

Matthews, L., Johnson, J., Berry, A., Trebble, P., Cookson, A., Spiller, D., et al. (2011). Cell cycle phase regulates glucocorticoid receptor function. *PLoS One* 6:e22289. doi: 10.1371/journal.pone.022289

Maymon, E., Romero, R., Pacora, P., Gervasi, M. T., Bianco, K., Ghezzi, F., et al. (2000). Evidence for the participation of interstitial collagenase (matrix metalloproteinase 1) in preterm premature rupture of membranes. *Am. J. Obstet. Gynecol.* 183, 914–920. doi: 10.1067/mob.2000.108879

Meis, P. J., Klebanoff, M., Thom, E., Dombrowski, M. P., Sibai, B., Moawad, A. H., et al. (2003). Prevention of recurrent preterm delivery by 17 alpha-hydroxyprogesterone caproate. *N. Eng. J. Med.* 348, 2379–2385.

Merlino, A., Welsh, T., Erdonmez, T., Madsen, G., Zakar, T., Smith, R., et al. (2009). Nuclear progesterone receptor expression in the human fetal membranes and decidua at term before and after labor. *Reprod. Sci.* 16, 357–363. doi: 10.1177/1933719108328616

Mogami, H., Kishore, A. H., Shi, H., Keller, P. W., Akgul, Y., and Word, R. A. (2013). Fetal fibronectin signaling induces matrix metalloproteases and cyclooxygenase-2 (COX-2) in amnion cells and preterm birth in mice. *J. Biol. Chem.* 288, 1953–1966. doi: 10.1074/jbc.m112.424366

Moore, R. M., Mansour, J. M., Redline, R. W., Mercer, B. M., and Moore, J. J. (2006). The physiology of fetal membrane rupture: insight gained from the determination of physical properties. *Placenta* 27, 1037–1051. doi: 10.1016/j.placenta.2006.01.002

Nadeem, L., Shynlova, O., Matysiak-Zablocki, E., Mesiano, S., Dong, X., and Lye, S. (2016). Molecular evidence of functional progesterone withdrawal in human myometrium. *Nat. Commun.* 7:11565.

Norman, J. E., and Bennett, P. (2017). Preterm birth prevention-time to PROGRESS beyond progesterone. *PLoS Med.* 14:e1002391. doi: 10.1371/journal.pone.01002391

Norman, J. E., Marlow, N., Messow, C.-M., Shennan, A., Bennett, P. R., Thornton, S., et al. (2016). Vaginal progesterone prophylaxis for preterm birth (the OPPTIMUM study): a multicentre, randomised, double-blind trial. *Lancet* 387, 2106–2116. doi: 10.1016/s0140-6736(16)00350-0

O'Brien, J. M., Adair, C. D., Lewis, D. F., Hall, D. R., Defranco, E. A., Fusey, S., et al. (2007). Progesterone vaginal gel for the reduction of recurrent preterm birth: primary results from a randomized, double-blind, placebo-controlled trial. *Ultrasound Obstet. Gynecol.* 30, 687–696. doi: 10.1002/uog.5158

Overall, C. M., and López-Otín, C. (2002). Strategies for MMP inhibition in cancer: innovations for the post-trial era. *Nat. Rev. Cancer* 2, 657–672. doi: 10.1038/nrc884

Parry, S., and Strauss, J. F. (1998). Premature rupture of the fetal membranes. *N. Eng. J. Med.* 338, 663–670.

Patel, B., Elguero, S., Thakore, S., Dahoud, W., Bedaiwy, M., and Mesiano, S. (2014). Role of nuclear progesterone receptor isoforms in uterine pathophysiology. *Hum. Reprod.* 21, 155–173. doi: 10.1093/humupd/dmu056

Peluso, J. J., Liu, X., Gawkowska, A., Lodde, V., and Wu, C. A. (2010). Progesterone inhibits apoptosis in part by PGRMC1-regulated gene expression. *Mol. Cell Endocrinol.* 320, 153–161. doi: 10.1016/j.mce.2010.02.005

Radisky, D. C. (2005). Epithelial-mesenchymal transition. *J. Cell Sci.* 118, 4325–4326.

Reichardt, H. M., Kaestner, K. H., Tuckermann, J., Kretz, O., Wessely, O., Bock, R., et al. (1998). DNA Binding of the glucocorticoid receptor is not essential for survival. *Cell* 93, 531–541.

Rizzo, G., Capponi, A., Vlachopoulou, A., Angelini, E., Grassi, C., and Romanini, C. (1997). The diagnostic value of interleukin-8 and fetal fibronectin concentrations in cervical secretions in patients with preterm labor and intact membranes. *J. Perinat. Med.* 25, 461–468. doi: 10.1515/jpme.1997.25.6.461

Saif, Z., Hodyl, N. A., Stark, M. J., Fuller, P. J., Cole, T., Lu, N., et al. (2015). Expression of eight glucocorticoid receptor isoforms in the human preterm placenta vary with fetal sex and birthweight. *Placenta* 36, 723–730. doi: 10.1016/j.placenta.2015.05.001

Stöcklin, E., Wissler, M., Gouilleux, F., and Groner, B. (1996). Functional interactions between Stat5 and the glucocorticoid receptor. *Nature* 383, 726–728. doi: 10.1038/383726a0

Storness-Bliss, C., Metcalfe, A., Simrose, R., Wilson, R. D., and Cooper, S. L. (2012). Correlation of residual amniotic fluid and perinatal outcomes in periviable preterm premature rupture of membranes. *J. Obstetr. Gynaecol. Can.* 34, 154–158. doi: 10.1016/s1701-2163(16)35158-1

Sueldo, C., Liu, X., and Peluso, J. J. (2015). Progestin and AdipoQ receptor 7, progesterone membrane receptor component 1 (PGRMC1), and PGRMC2 and their role in regulating progesterone's ability to suppress human granulosa/luteal cells from entering into the cell cycle. *Biol. Reprod.* 93:63.

Surjit, M., Ganti Krishna, P., Mukherji, A., Ye, T., Hua, G., Metzger, D., et al. (2011). Widespread negative response elements mediate direct repression by agonist-liganded glucocorticoid receptor. *Cell* 145, 224–241. doi: 10.1016/j.cell.2011.03.027

Turner, J. D., Schote, A. B., Keipes, M., and Muller, C. P. (2007). A new transcript splice variant of the human glucocorticoid receptor. *Ann. N. Y. Acad. Sci.* 1095, 334–341. doi: 10.1196/annals.1397.037

Wang, H., Ogawa, M., Wood, J. R., Bartolomei, M. S., Sammel, M. D., Kusanovic, J. P., et al. (2008). Genetic and epigenetic mechanisms combine to control MMP1 expression and its association with preterm premature rupture of membranes. *Hum. Mol. Genet.* 17, 1087–1096. doi: 10.1093/hmg/ddm381

Wikström, A.-C., Bakke, O., Okret, S., Brönnegård, M., and Gustafsson, J. -Å (1987). Intracellular localization of the glucocorticoid receptor: evidence for cytoplasmic and nuclear localization. *Endocrinology* 120, 1232–1242. doi: 10.1210/endo-120-4-1232

Zhang, W., Wang, L., Zhao, Y., and Kang, J. (2000). Changes in cytokine (IL-8, IL-6 and TNF-alpha) levels in the amniotic fluid and maternal serum in patients with premature rupture of the membranes. *Chin. Med. J.* 63, 311–315.

The Role(s) of Eicosanoids and Exosomes in Human Parturition

Eman Mosaad[1], Hassendrini N. Peiris[1], Olivia Holland[1,2], Isabella Morean Garcia[1] and Murray D. Mitchell[1]*

[1] School of Biomedical Science, Institute of Health and Biomedical Innovation – Centre for Children's Health Research, Faculty of Health, Queensland University of Technology, Brisbane, QLD, Australia, [2] School of Medical Science, Griffith University, Southport, QLD, Australia

***Correspondence:**
Murray D. Mitchell
murray.mitchell@qut.edu.au

The roles that eicosanoids play during pregnancy and parturition are crucial to a successful outcome. A better understanding of the regulation of eicosanoid production and the roles played by the various end products during pregnancy and parturition has led to our view that accurate measurements of a panel of those end products has exciting potential as diagnostics and prognostics of preterm labor and delivery. Exosomes and their contents represent an exciting new area for research of movement of key biological factors circulating between tissues and organs akin to a parallel endocrine system but involving key intracellular mediators. Eicosanoids and enzymes regulating their biosynthesis and metabolism as well as regulatory microRNAs have been identified within exosomes. In this review, the regulation of eicosanoid production, abundance and actions during pregnancy will be explored. Additionally, the functional significance of placental exosomes will be discussed.

Keywords: exosomes, eicosanoids, prostaglandins, pregnancy, parturition, gestation, preterm labor

INTRODUCTION

The fetal membranes perform unique functions to support fetal development and respond to signals for parturition. The correct timing for triggering this process is critical for the successful outcome of the pregnancy. The parturition process is mediated by a combination of signals from the fetus, placenta and mother. There are mainly two signallers of parturition that are interdependent and well reported, namely fetal endocrine signals and fetal growth-related signals (Challis et al., 2005; Menon, 2016; Mesiano, 2019). Both pathways directly and indirectly induce higher production of eicosanoids (particularly prostaglandins) which are important signaling molecules that affect the contractile activity of the myometrium leading to parturition (Challis et al., 2005; Reinl and England, 2015). Hence, administration of specific prostaglandins (E_2 or $F_{2\alpha}$) is proven to effectively induce labor and cervical ripening (E_2) in women. Additionally, a better understanding of the

Abbreviations: *5-LOX*, 5-lipoxygenase; *BLT1-2*, Leukotriene B4 receptor 1-2; *cAMP*, Cyclic AMP; *COX*, Cyclooxygenase; *CRH*, Corticotrophin-releasing hormone; *CysLT1-2*, Cysteinyl leukotriene receptor 1-2; *DP1-2*, Prostaglandin D_2 receptor 1-2; *EETs*, Epoxy-eicosatrienoic acids; *EP1-4*, Prostaglandin E_2 receptor 1-4; *ESCRT*, Endosomal Sorting Complexes for Transport; *EVs*, Extracellular vesicles; *FLAP*, Five-lipoxygenase activating protein; *FP*, Prostaglandin $F_{2\alpha}$ receptor; *GRO*α, Growth-related oncogene-α; *HETEs*, Hydroxy-eicosatetraenoic acids; *HPETE*, Hydroperoxyl eicosatetraenoic acid; *IL*, Interleukin; *ILVs*, Intraluminal vesicles; *IP*, Prostaglandin I_2 receptor; *LTA*$_4$, Leukotriene A_4; *LTB*$_4$, Leukotriene B_4; *LTC*$_4$, Leukotriene C_4; *LTD*$_4$, Leukotriene D_4; *LTs*, Leukotrienes; *MRPs*, Multidrug-resistance proteins; *MTOC*, Microtubule organization center; *MVB*, Multivesicular Bodies; *PG*, Prostaglandin; *PGD*$_2$, Prostaglandin D_2; *PGDH*, prostaglandin dehydrogenase; *PGE*$_2$, Prostaglandin E_2; *PGF*$_{2\alpha}$, Prostaglandin $F_{2\alpha}$; *PGH*$_2$, Prostaglandin H_2; *PGHS = PTGS-2*, prostaglandin endoperoxide synthase-2; *PGI*$_2$, Prostaglandin I_2; *TNF*α, Tumor necrosis factor-α; *TP*, Thromboxane receptor; *TXA*$_2$, Thromboxane A_2.

regulation of eicosanoid production and the roles played by the various end products during pregnancy and parturition has led to our view that accurate measurements of a panel of those end products has exciting potential as diagnostics and prognostics of preterm labor and delivery (Mitchell et al., 2015).

In this review, we explore the roles and distribution of eicosanoids in the human uterus and fetal membrane during parturition. We also describe exosome abundance during pregnancy and parturition. Finally, we discuss the potentially pivotal role of exosomes in distributing eicosanoids and the related diagnostic and therapeutic potential that this brings.

EICOSANOIDS

The term "eicosanoid" has evolved overtime as a definitive term for products of a family of polyunsaturated (C_{20}) fatty acids; including, but not limited to, lipoxins, leukotrienes, thromboxanes and prostaglandins. The biosynthesis of eicosanoids and their structural properties are well characterized in mammals (Smith, 1989). Eicosanoids are not stored, and their biosynthesis occurs in all mammalian tissues as a response to hormonal stimulation or mechanical trauma, acting as paracrine or autocrine modulators (Esser-von Bieren, 2017; Strauss and FitzGerald, 2019). Their actions are mediated by the activation of membrane receptors (Kim and Luster, 2007).

Eicosanoid Biosynthesis

A first essential and usually rate limiting step in eicosanoid biosynthesis is release of polyunsaturated (C_{20}) fatty acids from membrane phospholipid stores (Fitzpatrick and Soberman, 2001). Arachidonic acid is the major common precursor of eicosanoids and its release is precisely regulated by several types of phospholipase A_2 (Burke and Dennis, 2009) or phospholipase C and subsequent mono- and diacylglycerol lipases (Kano et al., 2009; Hanna and Hafez, 2018). Once released arachidonic acid is converted enzymatically to various eicosanoids via three main pathways (**Figure 1**): namely, the cyclooxygenase pathway, the lipoxygenase pathway, and the cytochrome P-450 epoxygenase pathway (Strauss and FitzGerald, 2019).

The major products of the cyclooxygenase (COX) pathway are prostanoids such as prostaglandins, thromboxanes and prostacyclin. There are two major COX enzymes that initiate the synthesis of prostaglandins, COX-1 is mainly expressed constitutively, and COX-2 is often induced via cytokines, growth factors and hormones (Herschman, 1996; Smith et al., 1996). Prostaglandin H_2 (PGH_2), a direct product of arachidonic acid release and reaction to COX enzymes, is converted to individual prostanoids that are tissue specific by the action of corresponding isomerases and synthases (Smith et al., 2000). For instance, thromboxane A_2 (TXA_2) synthase is expressed in platelets and macrophages; prostaglandin I_2 (PGI_2), also known as prostacyclin, synthase is expressed in endothelial cells and prostaglandin $F_{2\alpha}$ ($PGF_{2\alpha}$) synthase is abundant in the uterus (Ni et al., 2003; Ueno et al., 2005).

The lipoxygenase pathway produces leukotrienes (LTs). Products of this pathway in leukocytes are part of the LT family of lipid mediators, whose synthesis is mainly initiated by inflammatory cells. Formation of LTs is initiated via hydroperoxyl eicosatetraenoic acid (HPETE) formation from arachidonic acid by 5-lipoxygenase (5-LOX). 5-LOX in turn requires the cooperation of an accessory protein known as five-lipoxygenase activating protein (FLAP). Most HPETE molecules are converted to leukotriene A4 (LTA_4). LTA_4 can serve *in vitro* as a precursor for the transcellular biosynthesis of lipoxins and can undergo multiple routes of transformation (Bäck et al., 2011).

The cytochrome P450 epoxygenase pathway produces mainly epoxy-eicosatrienoic acids (EETs) via the catalysis of monooxygenation of arachidonic acid (Smith, 1989; Strauss and FitzGerald, 2019). However, hydroxygenases can also convert arachidonic acid to hydroxy-eicosatetraenoic acids (HETEs) (Strauss and FitzGerald, 2019).

Transport and Function

Despite the lipid nature of eicosanoids, they do not penetrate the cell membrane freely. Efflux transporters, such as multidrug-resistance proteins (MRPs), are necessary to transport newly synthesized eicosanoids outside the manufacturing cells. Additionally, the cellular uptake of eicosanoids is regulated by organic anion transporter proteins (Funk, 2001). The abundance of eicosanoid receptors and transporters is a limiting factor for their action. Therefore, they are believed to act as local or paracrine effectors initiating specific biochemical reactions in certain tissues.

Due to the different mechanisms that eicosanoids can induce on the cellular level, there are discrete receptor for each compound that mediate its action within the cell (Olson and Ammann, 2007). Thus far, there are 13 distinct cloned and characterized receptors for eicosanoids, including nine for cyclooxygenase-derived prostanoids and four for lipoxygenase-derived leukotrienes (Funk, 2001; Narumiya and Furuyashiki, 2011; Woodward et al., 2011). The nine prostanoid receptors mediate eicosanoid actions via cyclic AMP (cAMP), phosphatidylinositol turnover and Ca^{2+} shifts (**Table 1**).

Despite the short lifespan of eicosanoids, their biological effects are robust. Their biological properties have been studied in many contexts such as the cardiovascular system, immune system, nervous system and gastrointestinal tract as well as in inflammatory settings (Strauss and FitzGerald, 2019). The roles of eicosanoids in reproductive physiology are extensively studied in seminal fluid (Samuelsson, 1963; Alexandre et al., 2007; Remes Lenicov et al., 2012; Szczykutowicz et al., 2019), luteolytic actions (Vijayakumar and Walters, 1983; Bennegård et al., 1991; Miceli et al., 2001) and uterine physiology in pregnancy (Peiris et al., 2017); however, the roles of specific eicosanoids are still being elucidated. In the following sections, we will focus on the role of eicosanoids in uterine physiology during pregnancy and parturition.

Eicosanoids in Pregnancy and Parturition

The strong relationship between eicosanoids and pregnancy has been recognized for many years. Eicosanoids have various roles

The Role(s) of Eicosanoids and Exosomes in Human Parturition

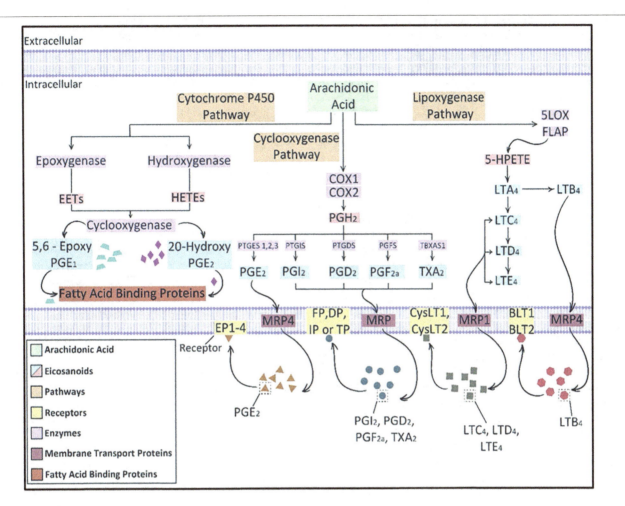

FIGURE 1 | Eicosanoid biosynthesis. The main three pathways involved in eicosanoids biosynthesis from the main precursor, arachidonic acid, are lipoxygenase, cyclooxygenase and cytochrome P450 pathways. The cytochrome P450 pathway produces epoxyeicosatrienoic acids (EETs) and hydroxyeicosatetraenoic acids (HETEs) from which some products can be further metabolized by cyclooxygenase. Cyclooxygenases (COX1 and 2) can act directly on arachidonic acid to produce the unstable intermediate prostaglandin (PG) H_2 (PGH_2) which then can produce various prostanoids such as PGE_2, PGI_2, PGD_2, and PGF_α and thromboxane A_2 (TXA_2). Lipoxygenase pathway yields leukotrienes (LTs), such as LTA_4 and LTB_4. Multidrug resistant proteins (MRPs) facilitate the transfer of eicosanoids through the cell membrane. Multiple cellular membrane receptors mediate the action of eicosanoids, such as EP1-4 for PGE_2 and BLT1-2 for LTB_4. [After (Funk, 2001; Strauss and FitzGerald, 2019)].

TABLE 1 | Eicosanoid receptors and their functional properties.

Eicosanoid category	Ligand	Receptor	Functional properties
Cyclooxygenase pathway (prostanoids)	TXA_2	TP	Increase intracellular calcium, Contractile
	PGI_2	IP	Increase intracellular cAMP, Relaxing
	$PGF_{2\alpha}$	FP	Increase intracellular calcium, Contractile
	PGD_2	DP1	Increase intracellular cAMP, Relaxing
		DP2	Induce intracellular calcium mobilization and chemoattractant
	PGE_2	EP1	Increase intracellular calcium, Contractile
		EP3	Inhibit cAMP production, Inhibitory
			Increase intracellular cAMP, Relaxing
Lipoxygenase pathway (leukotrienes)	LTB_4	BLT1 BLT2	Induce intracellular calcium mobilization and inhibit cAMP production
	LTD_4	CysLT1	Increase intracellular calcium
	LTC_4, LTD_4	CysLT2	Increase intracellular calcium

BLT1-2: Leukotriene B_4 receptor 1-2; cAMP: Cyclic AMP; CysLT1-2: Cysteinyl leukotriene receptor 1-2; DP1-2: Prostaglandin D_2 receptor 1-2; EP1-4: Prostaglandin E_2 receptor 1-4; FP: Prostaglandin $F_{2\alpha}$ receptor; IP: Prostaglandin I_2 receptor; LTB_4: Leukotriene B_4; LTC_4: Leukotriene C_4; LTD_4: Leukotriene D_4; PGD_2: Prostaglandin D_2; PGE_2: Prostaglandin E_2; $PGF_{2\alpha}$: Prostaglandin $F_{2\alpha}$; PGI_2: Prostaglandin I_2; TP: Thromboxane receptor; TXA_2: Thromboxane A_2.

in the reproduction process, including ovulation, corpus luteum function, luteolysis, fertilization and decidualisation as well as parturition as previously reviewed (Strauss and FitzGerald, 2019). COX-2-derived PGE_2 was found to play an important role in oocyte maturation and fertilization by affecting the activity of the cumulus cells surrounding the oocyte (McAdam et al., 1999). Defective embryo implantation and decidualisation were also observed in COX-2-deficient mice uteri, indicating the fundamental role of PGs in normal uterus physiology (Lim et al., 1999; McAdam et al., 1999).

The importance of eicosanoids in parturition has been subjected to detailed investigations using knockdown animal models. For example, parturition defects were observed in rodents deficient of COX enzymes and $PGF_{2\alpha}$ receptor. Mice with targeted disruption of COX-1 gene had delayed parturition, resulting in neonatal death (Gross et al., 1998; Yu et al., 2005). $PGF_{2\alpha}$ receptor-deficient mice, generated by gene knockdown, did not show the normal decline of serum levels of progesterone associated with parturition and consequentially were unable to deliver normal fetuses at term (Sugimoto et al., 1997). Additionally, many clinical observations have accumulated evidences that demonstrate the likely regulatory function of PGs on myometrial contractility and cervical softening. For instance, administration of PGs biosynthesis inhibitors such as aspirin or specific COX-2 (also known as prostaglandin endoperoxide synthase-2; PGHS or PTGS-2) inhibitors extend gestational length, however, does not prevent parturition (Lewis and Schulman, 1973; Collins and Turner, 1975; Khanprakob et al., 2012; Illanes et al., 2014; Triggs et al., 2020). Likewise, administration of PGE_2 and $PGF_{2\alpha}$ at any stage of gestation leads to increasing uterine contractile activity and cervical ripening (Embrey, 1971). Consequently, PGs are used clinically as a treatment to induce labor (Thomas et al., 2014). Furthermore, production of PGE_2 and $PGF_{2\alpha}$ increases during late stages of gestation and were found to be associated with the onset of parturition (Romero et al., 1994a, 1996; Slater et al., 1999). This confirms the notion that increased intrauterine PG biosynthesis is a cause rather than a result of the parturition process.

Term Labor and Intrauterine Prostaglandin Concentrations

During pregnancy, there are two main groups of regulatory factors that control the contractile activity of the uterus, uterotropins and uterotonins. Uterotropins and relaxatory uterotonins, such as progesterone and PGI, respectively, enhance myometrial relaxation and modulate uterine function and growth (Ilicic et al., 2020). Contrarily, stimulatory uterotonins, such as PGs, can induce contractions of the uteri. Before the parturition process starts, a relaxation state of the myometrium with minimum sensitivity to stimulatory uterotonins, such as PGs, is controlled by progesterone (Mesiano, 2004; Ilicic et al., 2020). Progesterone is a key player in the establishment and maintenance of pregnancy and its role and regulation have been extensively studied in human and experimental models (Arck et al., 2007; Forde et al., 2009; Solano and Arck, 2020). Progesterone withdrawal usually indicates the initiation of the parturition process with changes in the contractile activity of the myometrium. Human parturition is also associated with progesterone receptor subtypes changes (Merlino et al., 2007; Patel et al., 2015).

Although the required enzymes and receptors necessary for the synthesis and action of PGs are present in human myometrial tissue (Astle et al., 2007; Arulkumaran et al., 2012), their concentrations in the uterus may vary during various stages of gestation. During pregnancy, both maternal and fetal tissues produce PGE_2 and $PGF_{2\alpha}$. The increased intrauterine prostaglandin concentrations are key players in initiating and progressing labor and this occurs before the onset of labor (Romero et al., 1994a, 1996).

During the initial stage of the parturition process, myometrial cellular expression of PG-related genes is significantly increased: these genes include PG biosynthetic enzymes and PG receptors (Challis et al., 2002). The changed expression of these genes in turn increases the uterine tissue sensitivity to the elevated production of PGE_2 and $PGF_{2\alpha}$. This leads to greater contractile activity that leads to expulsion of the fetus and sequentially expulsion of the placenta (Challis, 2013).

The balance between PG biosynthesis and metabolizing activities in the fetal membranes plays an important role in the parturition process. Intrauterine PG biosynthesis via PGHS occurs in the amnion and to a lesser extent in the chorion, decidua and myometrium. Conversely, prostaglandin dehydrogenase (PGDH) enzyme, which controls the conversion of PGE_2 and $PGF_{2\alpha}$ to their inactive forms, is predominantly expressed in the chorion before the onset of labor. This leads to the prevention of active amnion-derived PGs reaching the myometrium due to the abundant presence of PGDH in the chorion which lies between the amnion and maternal tissues (Mesiano, 2019).

During parturition, expression of PGHS increases in the chorion, decidua and myometrium. In the meantime, expression of PGDH decreases in the chorion. This leads to greater abundance of active PGs in the chorion and permitting more PGE_2 and $PGF_{2\alpha}$ to reach and induce their contractile action on the myometrium leading to progression of labor.

Of note, progesterone stimulates PGDH and has been reported to inhibit PTGS2 in the relaxed state of the myometrium before the onset of the parturition process (Pomini et al., 2000; Patel et al., 2003). Conversely, placental cortisol and corticotrophin-releasing hormone (CRH) can stimulate PTGS2 and inhibit PGDH, causing increased access of active PGs to the myometrium (Olson and Ammann, 2007).

PG receptors also play a crucial role in regulating PG action during human parturition. Receptors for PGI_2, PGE_2, $PGF_{2\alpha}$ and thromboxane are expressed in the myometrium during pregnancy (Grigsby et al., 2006). $PGF_{2\alpha}$ receptor (FP) and thromboxane receptor (TP) enhance contractions by increasing the intracellular calcium (Ricciotti and FitzGerald, 2011). Both PGI_2 and PGE_2 have contrary contractile actions on the myometrium. PGI_2 receptor (IP) mediates elevated levels of cAMP which in turn leads to relaxation. However, PGI_2 has been found to play a role in increasing expression of contraction-associated proteins, such as PTGS2 and PG receptors. Interestingly, PGE_2 has four different receptors (EP1–4) with different physiologic actions. While contractile activity increases when PGE_2 interacts with EP1 and EP3, relaxation of the tissue can be mediated by PGE_2 interaction with EP2 and EP4 (Kotani et al., 1995). Therefore, PGE_2 can cause myometrial contraction or relaxation dependent upon the expression of receptor in different stages of pregnancy and during parturition.

A large literature illustrates the involvement of PGs in the five physiological events of human parturition: fetal membrane rupture via stimulating matrix mettaloproteinase activity and cell apoptosis (McLaren et al., 2000; Keelan et al., 2001), cervical ripening and dilation (Fletcher et al., 1993; Keirse, 1993; Steetskamp et al., 2020), myometrial contractility (Olson and Ammann, 2007), placental separation and uterine involution (Leung et al., 1987). This indicates the importance of further understanding the role of eicosanoids play in prognosis of pregnancy outcomes and their potential role as a diagnostic biomarker for fetus abnormalities and pregnancy complications, such as preeclampsia, gestational diabetes and preterm labor (Dalle Vedove et al., 2016; Hong et al., 2016; Aung et al., 2019; Welch et al., 2020).

Preterm Labor and Inflammatory Mechanisms

Labor that occurs before 37 completed weeks of gestation is considered as preterm, and preterm birth is the leading cause of perinatal mortality and morbidity (Goldenberg et al., 2008). The reasons behind the early onset of labor are not clearly identified (Green et al., 2005). Maternal infection is strongly correlated with preterm labor, such as intrauterine infection (Doi, 2020; Romero et al., 1994b). However, preterm delivery is associated with many other risk factors such as multifetal pregnancy, maternal obesity, maternal age, maternal nutrition and socioeconomic status (Johansson et al., 2014; Joseph et al., 2014; Koullali et al., 2016).

Inflammatory mechanisms are significantly involved in term and preterm labor (Christiaens et al., 2008; Peiris et al., 2019, 2020). Many studies focused on identifying labor-associated inflammatory genes profile, such as genes regulating cytokines, chemokines and related factors [reviewed in (Keelan et al., 2003)] which found to be upregulated in term deliveries and more apparently in preterm deliveries (Marvin et al., 2002; Mitchell, 2016). In term labor, infiltration of inflammatory cells increases in the cervix, myometrium, chorioamniotic membranes, and amniotic cavity. This is also found to be associated with increased expression and production of pro-inflammatory cytokines, such as interleukin (IL)-1β, IL-6 and tumor necrosis factor-α (TNFα), and chemokines, such as IL-8 and growth-related oncogene-α (GROα) (Keelan et al., 2003; Romero et al., 2006). Cytokine regulation of intrauterine prostaglandin production was found to be at the biosynthesis level and the catabolic inactivation level. For instance, IL-1β and TNF-α enhance upregulated expression of PGHS leading to increased biosynthesis of prostaglandins by gestational tissues (Hansen et al., 1999; Rauk and Chiao, 2000). Similarly, pro-inflammatory cytokines, IL-1β and TNFα may inhibit PGDH leading to decreased degradation of prostaglandins (Brown et al., 1998; Mitchell et al., 2000). The role of pro-inflammatory cytokines in regulating prostaglandin production is further evidence of the importance of inflammatory mechanisms in mediating parturition (Gross et al., 2000; Peiris et al., 2019, 2020).

Similarly, infection and non-infection-induced inflammation have been found to be associated with preterm labor (Yoon et al., 2001; Romero et al., 2014, 2015). There are many experimental and clinical evidences in support of the involvement of inflammation in preterm labor. For example, pregnant animal models with intrauterine infection or with exposure to microbial products can lead to preterm delivery [reviewed in (Elovitz and Mrinalini, 2004)]. Extrauterine and sub-clinical intrauterine maternal infections have been associated with premature parturition (Gomez et al., 1995; Romero et al., 2006). The production of pro-inflammatory cytokines such as IL-1β, IL-8, and IL-6 are usually increased in the amnion, decidua and myometrium in pregnancies with infection (Goldenberg et al., 2000). This confirms the notion that parturition is a consequence of failure of the maternal immune system to regulate inflammatory mechanisms (Romero et al., 2006).

Eicosanoid Distribution and Measurement

Due to the importance of eicosanoids in pregnancy and parturition, the accurate and specific measurement of eicosanoids is critical to our ability to enhance diagnostic and therapeutic strategies for preterm labor. However, the misidentification of PGs has been problematic with traditional methodologies such as immunoassays (Glass et al., 2005). Previously we reviewed the molecular resemblance between eicosanoids and associated compounds that may interfere and affect the specificity of immunoassays (Glass et al., 2005; Peiris et al., 2017). Thus, the gold standard of mass spectrometry that allows full identification of PGs is vital to any meaningful approach to this problem (Peiris et al., 2020).

Prostaglandins are produced by all tissues in the body. Hence measurements of circulating concentrations reflect overall changes in production and cannot be directly linked to a specific tissue or organ source. Moreover, due to rapid clearance of circulating eicosanoids by lungs and kidneys (Golub et al., 1975; Dunn and Hood, 1977; Peiris et al., 2017), we can only assess circulating metabolites of eicosanoids not the original compounds. Therefore, there is a strong argument for evaluating the utility of exosomes (which have a content that reflects the tissue/cellular source) as a stable biomarker for measuring and identifying eicosanoids from specific organs such as the uterus.

EXOSOMES

Exosome Morphology

Exosomes are a subtype of membrane bound extracellular vesicles (EVs); they are 30–120 nm in diameter and have a cup-shaped structure and a lipid bilayer which is similar in orientation of transmembrane constituents to that of the parental cells membrane (Record, 2014; Barile and Vassalli, 2017; Shao et al., 2018). Exosomes contain a diverse array of biologically active molecules such as proteins, lipids, RNA (mRNA, microRNA and noncoding RNA), DNA, protein mediators and eicosanoids (Pillay et al., 2017; Saez et al., 2018). Exosomal contents comprise specific proteins, lipids or genetic materials reflecting the source cell's physiological state, and can therefore serve as representative biomarkers (Menon et al., 2017).

Exosome Biogenesis

The biogenesis of exosomes involves the inward budding of the peripheral membrane and invagination of the late endosomes also known as Multivesicular Bodies (MVB) (Record, 2014); followed by the formation of intraluminal vesicles (ILVs) inside of the MVB's (Zhang et al., 2019). During the invagination process, proteins are incorporated into the membrane, leaving the cytosolic components to be engulfed into the ILVs (Zhang et al., 2019). MVBs are then fused with the plasma membrane of the cell releasing ILVs out into the extracellular space; once released ILVs are then referred to as exosomes (Kowal et al., 2014; Zhang et al., 2019; **Figure 2**). Exosomes biogenesis also requires; Endosomal Sorting Complexes for Transport (ESCRT) 0–III. This complex contains families of vacuolar sorting proteins, other associated proteins (e.g., Alix and tetraspanin) and lipids which also participate in protein sorting and ILV formation during biogenesis (Kowal et al., 2014). The selective packaging of molecules into exosomes occurs within the originating cell (Pillay et al., 2017); constituents within exosomes come from an array of cellular components such as the Golgi apparatus, endoplasmic reticulum, plasma membrane, nucleus and cytosol (Record, 2014), meaning that exosomes can represent many different parts of the cell. The few known selective mechanisms that regulate cargo sorting into exosomes have recently reviewed (Anand et al., 2019).

Exosome Secretion and Function

The exocytosis of exosomes is an active secretory process (Record, 2014). MVBs move along microtubules toward the cell's periphery fusing with the plasma membrane and causing the release of exosomes into the extracellular space (Zhang et al., 2019). Connection of the MVB and the microtubule organization center (MTOC) allows the sectorisation of exosome release, restricting the release of exosomes to non-random areas of the cell membrane (Record, 2014). Exosome release is also dependent on the cells and conditions of their surrounding environment (Kowal et al., 2014; Barile and Vassalli, 2017).

Once exosomes are released, they become involved in communication between cells through cargo delivery to the recipient cells. There are three main types signaling modes; autocrine affects the releasing cell, paracrine affects adjacent cells and endocrine is delivered to distal target cells via the circulation.

Exosomes are a device for both transportation and signaling; through their load of bioactive molecules, they have the innate ability to signal from inside a target cell; both from the periphery and intracellular compartments (Record, 2014).

The function of exosomes is to exchange information through the delivery of cargo to distal and adjacent target cells. In doing so, the interaction of target cells with exosomes results in reprogramming of their phenotype and regulation of their function; functions such as migration, proliferation, angiogenesis, translational activity, metabolism, and apoptosis (Ehrlich et al., 2016; Saez et al., 2018). This reprogramming and regulation consequently alters cellular physiology, and in some cases contributing to different pathological states (Pillay et al., 2017).

Exosomes in Pregnancy
Synthesis and Interactions With Surrounding Environment

Exosomes have been identified in the maternal circulation as early as 6 weeks into gestation (Salomon et al., 2014). As gestational age increases, there is an increase in circulating maternal exosome concentration (Pillay et al., 2017); with the increased exosome burden likely related to placental mass and derived primarily from placental mesenchymal stem cells.

First-trimester trophoblast cells act as environmental sensors, and these cells can respond to the changing environment via the synthesis and release of exosomes (Mitchell et al., 2015). For example, an increase of exosome numbers is observed when the *in vitro* environment has a low oxygen tension and is high in D-glucose concentration; these two factors synergistically interact to regulate the bioactivity and release of exosomes originating from first-trimester trophoblast cells.

The effect of environmental factors on the release of exosomes into the maternal circulation via endocrine communication is dependent on the integrity and stability of exosomes (Ehrlich et al., 2016). For example, increased release of exosomes from trophoblastic cells is seen as a response to challenging environmental conditions (e.g., elevated glucose concentrations and low oxygen tension) which might disrupt the balance of cytokines (Truong et al., 2017). Cytokines being a necessity for healthy implantation, placentation and successful pregnancy outcome (Mitchell et al., 2015).

Exchange, Mediatory Roles, and Other Functions

A function of placenta-derived exosomes is to be a mediator in the progression of pregnancy and cell fate. Exosomes are used in cell-to-cell communication between the placenta and maternal organs. This communication has many functions, one of which is the preparatory function of remote tissues for metabolic and placental changes during gestation (Greening et al., 2016; Jin and Menon, 2018).

Basic functions of exosomes in normal uncomplicated pregnancies are promotion of implantation and communication between endometrium and embryo (Jin and Menon, 2018). *In vitro* studies have also revealed the role of exosomes in differential endothelial cell migration and vascular tube formation. Additionally, exosomes have a pivotal immunoregulatory role via the initiation of activated maternal lymphocytes' local deletion and induction of maternal t-cell apoptosis, which prevents the degradation of invading trophoblastic cells (Greening et al., 2016; Pillay et al., 2017). Placenta-derived exosomes are also found to play a role in viral infection during pregnancy, where trophoblast cells can transfer the necessary capacity of resistance against viral infection to other nonplacental cells via exosomes (Mouillet et al., 2014).

Exosomes regulate all these functions through the transference of their content into target cells. This regulation of activity

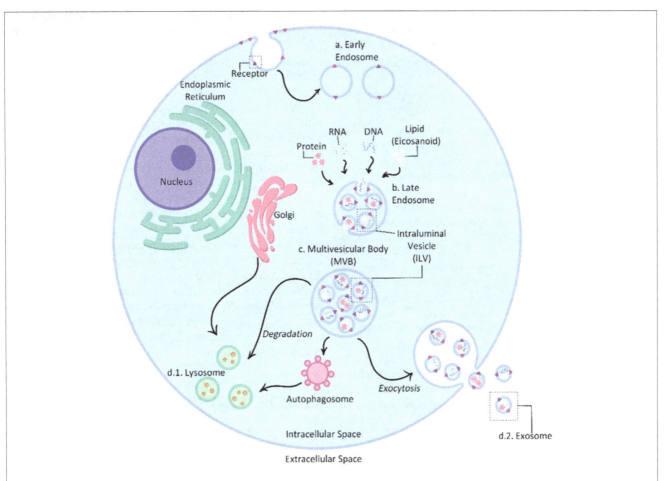

FIGURE 2 | Exosome biogenesis and secretion. The biogenesis of exosomes is initiated with the inward budding of the peripheral membrane into early endosomes **(a)**. Selective exosome packaging with molecules such as protein, RNA and DNA and lipids occurs within the originating cell and cellular compartments such as the Golgi apparatus, endoplasmic reticulum, plasma membrane, nucleus and cytosol. Invagination of the early endosomes into late endosomes **(b)** allows these diverse molecules to be taken up and individually packaged inside intraluminal vesicles (ILVs), turning the endosomes into multivesicular bodies (MVBs) **(c)**. During the invagination process, proteins are incorporated into the membrane, leaving the cytosolic components to be engulfed into the ILVs. Finally, MVBs either release ILVs intracellularly to be absorbed by lysosomes/autophagosomes **(d.1)** for degradation or fuse with the plasma membrane to secrete ILVs out into the extracellular space as exosomes **(d.2)**. [After (Kowal et al., 2014)].

can occur with either proximal or distal target cells via different interactions; this includes the modification of the extracellular milieu of the target cell, activation of cell membrane receptors, endocytosis by target cells in which the cell contents are released intracellularly and translational activity (e.g., angiogenesis, proliferation, metabolism and apoptosis). Exosomes can then modify the phenotype of these cells through maternal circulation.

The internalization of exosomes is also found to induce the release of pro-inflammatory cytokines (Greening et al., 2016). Exosomes released due to abnormal environmental factors lead to dysfunction of feto-placental endothelium and other various types of endothelial exosomes (Saez et al., 2018).

The involvement of exosomes in the transcellular metabolism of eicosanoids (and enzymes involved in substrate release for eicosanoids) has been described specifically and in terms of lipid mediators in a series of studies. In these studies exosomes from cells contained the full range of phospholipases and many free fatty acids (Subra et al., 2010; Record et al., 2014). The internalization of exosomes was described and the subsequent utilization of exosome cargo in cell metabolism (Subra et al., 2010) as well as involvement of this intercellular trafficking in pathophysiologies (Record et al., 2014). We have recently reviewed this in detail in an invited publication (Peiris et al., 2017).

Various studies have demonstrated the pivotal role of exosomes during human pregnancy and parturition (Sarker et al., 2014; Mitchell et al., 2015; Menon et al., 2017; Jin and Menon, 2018; Sheller-Miller and Menon, 2020). More interestingly, the potential role of exosomes in diagnosis/prognosis of pregnancy complications has gained a lot of attention in the scientific field in the last two decades. For example, preterm labor was one of the main topic that is under investigation (Cantonwine et al., 2016; Menon and Richardson, 2017; von Linsingen et al., 2017). Likewise, studies on gestational diabetes

(Powe, 2017; Liu et al., 2018; Saez et al., 2018) and preeclampsia (Pillay et al., 2016; Nielsen et al., 2017; Navajas et al., 2019) showed differential exosomal contents compared to that in uncomplicated pregnancies.

FINAL REMARKS

The intercellular communication mediated by exosomes has opened new era of research to study biological processes in healthy and pathophysiological conditions. From a clinical perspective, exosomes are mainly used in two applications: as biomarker detection and biologically active carriers. Exosomes are potential candidates as biomarkers detection tool circulating in blood. Enrichment of specific markers can be improved by exosome isolation and cargo identification (Record et al., 2018). Exosomes may transport proteins, lipids and nucleic acids that can be used as diagnostic or prognostic markers for specific clinical conditions. In this respect, several studies identified potential exosomal markers for early detection, diagnosis, and monitoring of cancer patients (Melo et al., 2015; Jalalian et al., 2019; Makler and Asghar, 2020). Similarly, exosomal contents are now gaining much attention in the field of pregnancy complications and fetal abnormalities (Yang et al., 2020). On the other hand, exosomes are now identified as potential platform for enhanced delivery of specific cargo in vivo, which can be biological compounds or therapeutic agents. The methods of loading exosomes with specific cargos of interest have been recently reviewed (Li et al., 2018; Donoso-Quezada et al., 2020; Mitchell et al., 2020). Exosomes have also inspired researchers to use cell-membrane-cloaked nanoparticles, also called synthetic exosome-mimics, as drug delivery platforms (Hu et al., 2011, 2015; Cao et al., 2016). These different applications of exosomes can provide hope to many patients including women with complicated pregnancies.

The relationship and importance of eicosanoids in pregnancy, labor and parturition are well established and have been an area of research for many decades. However, the limitations of immunoassays in the accurate measurement of specific eicosanoids have hampered research. The development of sensitive and specific mass spectrometry-based method to measure individual eicosanoids (e.g., prostaglandins and prostamides) via the monitoring of characteristic mass fragment pairs for each molecule at their distinct retention times has overcome these technical limitations and for the first time allowed accurate measurement of specific eicosanoids (Mitchell et al., 2016). A small but growing number of clinical studies have adopted mass spectrometric evaluations of these compounds, which has led to important new findings in the areas of labor and uterine infection (Maddipati et al., 2014, 2016; Peiris et al., 2020). The identification of the building blocks and enzymes needed for the synthesis of eicosanoids within exosomes is doubly exciting (Subra et al., 2010; Record et al., 2014). Firstly, the evaluation and quantitation of the cargo may provide a real-time snapshot of the cells' state. Secondly, exploration of the exosomes' abilities as vesicles of intercellular communication (i.e., to transport and deliver messages between cells) may further our understanding of the parturition process and provide opportunities to reconsider the mechanisms of pregnancy and parturition.

We postulate that together, understanding and quantitating eicosanoid biosynthesis, metabolism and actions in combination with exosome biology will enable the discovery of diagnostic and prognostic biomarkers for many pregnancy complications including preterm labor.

AUTHOR CONTRIBUTIONS

MM conceived the idea. EM and IMG prepared figures. EM, HP, OH, IMG, and MM contributed to manuscript writing. All authors contributed to the article and approved the submitted version.

ACKNOWLEDGMENTS

We thank our many colleagues who have assisted in the development of these studies over the years. We are also grateful to Queensland University of Technology for support and infrastructure. EM salary is supported by the Australian Research Council (Grant No: ARC LP160101854).

REFERENCES

Alexandre, B., Lemaire, A., Desvaux, P., and Amar, E. (2007). ORIGINAL RESEARCH—ED PHARMACOTHERAPY: intracavernous injections of prostaglandin E1 for erectile dysfunction: patient satisfaction and quality of sex life on long-term treatment. *J. Sex. Med.* 4, 426–431. doi: 10.1111/j.1743-6109.2006.00260.x

Anand, S., Samuel, M., Kumar, S., and Mathivanan, S. (2019). Ticket to a bubble ride: cargo sorting into exosomes and extracellular vesicles. *Biochim. Biophys. Acta Proteins Proteom.* 1867:140203. doi: 10.1016/j.bbapap.2019.02.005

Arck, P., Hansen, P. J., Mulac Jericevic, B., Piccinni, M.-P., and Szekeres-Bartho, J. (2007). Progesterone during pregnancy: endocrine–immune cross talk in mammalian species and the role of stress. *Am. J. Reprod. Immunol.* 58, 268–279. doi: 10.1111/j.1600-0897.2007.00512.x

Arulkumaran, S., Kandola, M. K., Hoffman, B., Hanyaloglu, A. C., Johnson, M. R., and Bennett, P. R. (2012). The roles of prostaglandin EP 1 and 3 receptors in the control of human myometrial contractility. *J. Clin. Endocrinol. Metab.* 97, 489–498. doi: 10.1210/jc.2011-1991

Astle, S., Newton, R., Thornton, S., Vatish, M., and Slater, D. M. (2007). Expression and regulation of prostaglandin E synthase isoforms in human myometrium with labour. *Mol. Hum. Reprod.* 13, 69–75. doi: 10.1093/molehr/gal093

Aung, M. T., Yu, Y., Ferguson, K. K., Cantonwine, D. E., Zeng, L., McElrath, T. F., et al. (2019). Prediction and associations of preterm birth and its subtypes with eicosanoid enzymatic pathways and inflammatory markers. *Sci. Rep.* 9, 1–17.

Bäck, M., Dahlén, S.-E., Drazen, J. M., Evans, J. F., Serhan, C. N., Shimizu, T., et al. (2011). International union of basic and clinical pharmacology. LXXXIV: leukotriene receptor nomenclature, distribution, and pathophysiological functions. *Pharmacol. Rev.* 63, 539–584.

Barile, L., and Vassalli, G. (2017). Exosomes: therapy delivery tools and biomarkers of diseases. *Pharmacol. Therap.* 174, 63–78. doi: 10.1016/j.pharmthera.2017.02.020

Bennegård, B., Hahlin, M., Wennberg, E., and Norém, H. (1991). Local luteolytic effect of prostaglandin F2α in the human corpus luteum. *Fertil. Steril.* 56, 1070–1076.

Brown, N. L., Alvi, S. A., Elder, M. G., Bennett, P. R., and Sullivan, M. H. (1998). Regulation of prostaglandin production in intact fetal membranes by interleukin-1 and its receptor antagonist. *J. Endocrinol.* 159, 519–526. doi: 10.1677/joe.0.1590519

Burke, J. E., and Dennis, E. A. (2009). Phospholipase A2 structure/function, mechanism, and signaling. *J. Lipid Res.* 50, S237–S242.

Cantonwine, D. E., Zhang, Z., Rosenblatt, K., Goudy, K. S., Doss, R. C., Ezrin, A. M., et al. (2016). Evaluation of proteomic biomarkers associated with circulating microparticles as an effective means to stratify the risk of spontaneous preterm birth. *Am. J. Obstetr. Gynecol.* 214:631.

Cao, H., Dan, Z., He, X., Zhang, Z., Yu, H., Yin, Q., et al. (2016). Liposomes coated with isolated macrophage membrane can target lung metastasis of breast cancer. *ACS Nano* 10, 7738–7748.

Challis, J. (2013). *Prostaglandins and Parturition. 51st Congress of the German Society for Gynecology and Obstetrics: Gynecology and Gynecological Oncology, Obstetrics, Perinatology and Prenatal Diagnostics, Gynecological Endocrinology and Reproductive Medicine.* Dresden: Springer-Verlag.

Challis, J. R. G., Bloomfield, F. H., Bocking, A. D., Casciani, V., Chisaka, H., Connor, K., et al. (2005). Fetal signals and parturition. *J. Obstetr. Gynaecol. Res.* 31, 492–499. doi: 10.1111/j.1447-0756.2005.00342.x

Challis, J. R. G., Sloboda, D. M., Alfaidy, N., Lye, S. J., Gibb, W., Patel, F. A., et al. (2002). Prostaglandins and mechanisms of preterm birth [Review]. *Reproduction* 124, 1–17. doi: 10.1530/rep.0.1240001

Christiaens, I., Zaragoza, D. B., Guilbert, L., Robertson, S. A., Mitchell, B. F., and Olson, D. M. (2008). Inflammatory processes in preterm and term parturition. *J. Reprod. Immunol.* 79, 50–57.

Collins, E., and Turner, G. (1975). Maternal effects of regular salicylate ingestion in pregnancy. *Lancet* 2, 335–338. doi: 10.1016/s0140-6736(75)92777-4

Dalle Vedove, F., Fava, C., Jiang, H., Zanconato, G., Quilley, J., Brunelli, M., et al. (2016). Increased epoxyeicosatrienoic acids and reduced soluble epoxide hydrolase expression in the preeclamptic placenta. *J. Hypertension* 34:1364.

Doi, K. (2020). "Multiple mechanisms of preterm labour other than intrauterine infection," in *Preterm Labour and Delivery*, ed. H. Sameshima (Singapore: Springer), 89–94.

Donoso-Quezada, J., Ayala-Mar, S., and González-Valdez, J. (2020). State-of-the-art exosome loading and functionalization techniques for enhanced therapeutics: a review. *Crit. Rev. Biotechnol.* 40, 804–820.

Dunn, M. J., and Hood, V. L. (1977). Prostaglandins and the kidney. *Am. J. Physiol. Renal Physiol.* 233, F169–F184.

Ehrlich, S., Lambers, D., Baccarelli, A., Khoury, J., Macaluso, M., and Ho, S. M. (2016). Endocrine disruptors: a potential risk factor for gestational diabetes mellitus. *Am. J. Perinatol.* 33, 1313–1318. doi: 10.1055/s-0036-1586500

Elovitz, M. A., and Mrinalini, C. (2004). Animal models of preterm birth. *Trends Endocrinol. Metab.* 15, 479–487. doi: 10.1016/j.tem.2004.10.009

Embrey, M. (1971). PGE compounds for induction of labour and abortion. *Ann. N. Y. Acad. Sci.* 180, 518–523. doi: 10.1111/j.1749-6632.1971.tb53219.x

Esser-von Bieren, J. (2017). Immune-regulation and-functions of eicosanoid lipid mediators. *Biol. Chem.* 398, 1177–1191.

Fitzpatrick, F., and Soberman, R. (2001). Regulated formation of eicosanoids. *J. Clin. Invest.* 107, 1347–1351.

Fletcher, H., Mitchell, S., Simeon, D., Frederick, J., and Brown, D. (1993). Intravaginal misoprostol as a cervical ripening agent. *Br. J. Obstet. Gynaecol.* 100, 641–644.

Forde, N., Carter, F., Fair, T., Crowe, M. A., Evans, A. C. O., Spencer, T. E., et al. (2009). Progesterone-regulated changes in endometrial gene expression contribute to advanced conceptus development in cattle1. *Biol. Reprod.* 81, 784–794. doi: 10.1095/biolreprod.108.074336

Funk, C. D. (2001). Prostaglandins and leukotrienes: advances in eicosanoid biology. *Science* 294, 1871–1875.

Glass, M., Hong, J., Sato, T. A., and Mitchell, M. D. (2005). Misidentification of prostamides as prostaglandins. *J. Lipid Res.* 46, 1364–1368.

Goldenberg, R. L., Culhane, J. F., Iams, J. D., and Romero, R. (2008). Epidemiology and causes of preterm birth. *Lancet* 371, 75–84.

Goldenberg, R. L., Hauth, J. C., and Andrews, W. W. (2000). Intrauterine infection and preterm delivery. *N. Engl. J. Med.* 342, 1500–1507. doi: 10.1056/nejm200005183422007

Golub, M., Zia, P., Matsuno, M., and Horton, R. (1975). Metabolism of prostaglandins A1 and E1 in man. *J. Clin. Invest.* 56, 1404–1410.

Gomez, R., Ghezzi, F., Romero, R., Muñoz, H., Tolosa, J. E., and Rojas, I. (1995). Premature labour and intra-amniotic infection: clinical aspects and role of the cytokines in diagnosis and pathophysiology. *Clin. Perinatol.* 22, 281–342. doi: 10.1016/S0095-5108(18)30286-0

Green, N. S., Damus, K., Simpson, J. L., Iams, J., Reece, E. A., Hobel, C. J., et al. (2005). Research agenda for preterm birth: recommendations from the March of Dimes. *Am. J. Obstet. Gynecol.* 193(Pt 1), 626–635. doi: 10.1016/j.ajog.2005.02.106

Greening, D. W., Nguyen, H. P., Elgass, K., Simpson, R. J., and Salamonsen, L. A. (2016). Human endometrial exosomes contain hormone-specific cargo modulating trophoblast adhesive capacity: insights into endometrial-embryo interactions. *Biol. Reprod.* 94:38.

Grigsby, P. L., Sooranna, S. R., Adu-Amankwa, B., Pitzer, B., Brockman, D. E., Johnson, M. R., et al. (2006). Regional expression of prostaglandin E2 and F2alpha receptors in human myometrium, amnion, and choriodecidua with advancing gestation and labour. *Biol. Reprod.* 75, 297–305. doi: 10.1095/biolreprod.106.051987

Gross, G., Imamura, T., Vogt, S. K., Wozniak, D. F., Nelson, D. M., Sadovsky, Y., et al. (2000). Inhibition of cyclooxygenase-2 prevents inflammation-mediated preterm labour in the mouse. *Am. J. Physiol. Regul. Integr. Comp. Physiol.* 278, R1415–R1423. doi: 10.1152/ajpregu.2000.278.6.R1415

Gross, G. A., Imamura, T., Luedke, C., Vogt, S. K., Olson, L. M., Nelson, D. M., et al. (1998). Opposing actions of prostaglandins and oxytocin determine the onset of murine labour. *Proc. Natl. Acad. Sci. U.S.A.* 95, 11875–11879. doi: 10.1073/pnas.95.20.11875

Hanna, V. S., and Hafez, E. A. A. (2018). Synopsis of arachidonic acid metabolism: a review. *J. Adv. Res.* 11, 23–32. doi: 10.1016/j.jare.2018.03.005

Hansen, W., Keelan, J., Skinner, S., and Mitchell, M. (1999). Key enzymes of prostaglandin biosynthesis and metabolism. Coordinate regulation of expression by cytokines in gestational tissues: a review. *Prostaglandins Other Lipid Mediat.* 57, 243–257.

Herschman, H. R. (1996). Prostaglandin synthase 2. *Biochim. Biophys. Acta* 1299, 125–140. doi: 10.1016/0005-2760(95)00194-8

Hong, J.-S., Romero, R., Lee, D.-C., Than, N. G., Yeo, L., Chaemsaithong, P., et al. (2016). Umbilical cord prostaglandins in term and preterm parturition. *J. Mater. Fetal Neonatal Med.* 29, 523–531.

Hu, C.-M. J., Fang, R. H., Wang, K.-C., Luk, B. T., Thamphiwatana, S., Dehaini, D., et al. (2015). Nanoparticle biointerfacing by platelet membrane cloaking. *Nature* 526, 118–121.

Hu, C.-M. J., Zhang, L., Aryal, S., Cheung, C., Fang, R. H., and Zhang, L. (2011). Erythrocyte membrane-camouflaged polymeric nanoparticles as a biomimetic delivery platform. *Proc. Natl. Acad. Sci. U.S.A.* 108, 10980–10985.

Ilicic, M., Zakar, T., and Paul, J. W. (2020). The regulation of uterine function during parturition: an update and recent advances. *Reprod. Sci.* 27, 3–28.

Illanes, S. E., Perez-Sepulveda, A., Rice, G. E., and Mitchell, M. D. (2014). Preterm labour: association between labour physiology, tocolysis and prevention. *Expert Opin. Invest. Drugs* 23, 759–771.

Jalalian, S. H., Ramezani, M., Jalalian, S. A., Abnous, K., and Taghdisi, S. M. (2019). Exosomes, new biomarkers in early cancer detection. *Anal. Biochem.* 571, 1–13.

Jin, J., and Menon, R. (2018). Placental exosomes: a proxy to understand pregnancy complications. *Am. J. Reprod. Immunol.* 79:e12788.

Johansson, S., Villamor, E., Altman, M., Bonamy, A. K., Granath, F., and Cnattingius, S. (2014). Maternal overweight and obesity in early pregnancy and risk of infant mortality: a population based cohort study in Sweden. *BMJ* 349:g6572. doi: 10.1136/bmj.g6572

Joseph, K. S., Fahey, J., Shankardass, K., Allen, V. M., O'Campo, P., Dodds, L., et al. (2014). Effects of socioeconomic position and clinical risk factors on spontaneous and iatrogenic preterm birth. *BMC Pregnancy Childbirth* 14:117. doi: 10.1186/1471-2393-14-117

Kano, M., Ohno-Shosaku, T., Hashimotodani, Y., Uchigashima, M., and Watanabe, M. (2009). Endocannabinoid-mediated control of synaptic transmission. *Physiol. Rev.* 89, 309–380.

Keelan, J. A., Blumenstein, M., Helliwell, R. J. A., Sato, T. A., Marvin, K. W., and Mitchell, M. D. (2003). Cytokines, prostaglandins and parturition-a review. *Placenta* 24, S33–S46. doi: 10.1053/plac.2002.0948

Keelan, J. A., Helliwell, R. J., Nijmeijer, B. E., Berry, E. B., Sato, T. A., Marvin, K. W., et al. (2001). 15-deoxy-Δ12, 14-prostaglandin J2-induced apoptosis in amnion-like WISH cells. *Prostaglandins Other Lipid Mediat.* 66, 265–282.

Keirse, M. (1993). Prostaglandins in preinduction cervical ripening. Meta-analysis of worldwide clinical experience. *J. Reprod. Med.* 38, 89–100.

Khanprakob, T., Laopaiboon, M., Lumbiganon, P., and Sangkomkamhang, U. S. (2012). Cyclo-oxygenase (COX) inhibitors for preventing preterm labour. *Cochrane Database Syst. Rev.* 10:CD007748.

Kim, N. D., and Luster, A. D. (2007). Regulation of immune cells by eicosanoid receptors. *ScientificWorldJournal* 7, 1307–1328.

Kotani, M., Tanaka, I., Ogawa, Y., Usui, T., Mori, K., Ichikawa, A., et al. (1995). Molecular cloning and expression of multiple isoforms of human prostaglandin E receptor EP3 subtype generated by alternative messenger RNA splicing: multiple second messenger systems and tissue-specific distributions. *Mol. Pharmacol.* 48, 869–879.

Koullali, B., Oudijk, M. A., Nijman, T. A., Mol, B. W., and Pajkrt, E. (2016). Risk assessment and management to prevent preterm birth. *Semin. Fetal Neonatal Med.* 21, 80–88. doi: 10.1016/j.siny.2016.01.005

Kowal, J., Tkach, M., and Théry, C. (2014). Biogenesis and secretion of exosomes. *Curr. Opin. Cell Biol.* 29, 116–125. doi: 10.1016/j.ceb.2014.05.004

Leung, A., Kwok, P., and Chang, A. (1987). Association between prostaglandin E2 and placental abruption. *Br. J. Obstetr. Gynaecol.* 94, 1001–1002.

Lewis, R. B., and Schulman, J. D. (1973). Influence of acetylsalicylic acid, an inhibitor of prostaglandin synthesis, on the duration of human gestation and labour. *Lancet* 2, 1159–1161. doi: 10.1016/s0140-6736(73)92934-6

Li, S.-P., Lin, Z.-X., Jiang, X.-Y., and Yu, X.-Y. (2018). Exosomal cargo-loading and synthetic exosome-mimics as potential therapeutic tools. *Acta Pharmacol. Sin.* 39, 542–551.

Lim, H., Gupta, R. A., Ma, W. G., Paria, B. C., Moller, D. E., Morrow, J. D., et al. (1999). Cyclo-oxygenase-2-derived prostacyclin mediates embryo implantation in the mouse via PPARdelta. *Genes Dev.* 13, 1561–1574. doi: 10.1101/gad.13.12.1561

Liu, J., Wang, S., Wang, Q., Du, J., and Wang, B. (2018). Gestational diabetes mellitus is associated with changes in the concentration and bioactivity of placental exosomes in the maternal circulation across gestation. *Eur. Rev. Med. Pharmacol. Sci.* 22, 2036–2043.

Maddipati, K. R., Romero, R., Chaiworapongsa, T., Chaemsaithong, P., Zhou, S. L., Xu, Z., et al. (2016). Lipidomic analysis of patients with microbial invasion of the amniotic cavity reveals up-regulation of leukotriene B4. *FASEB J.* 30, 3296–3307.

Maddipati, K. R., Romero, R., Chaiworapongsa, T., Zhou, S. L., Xu, Z., Tarca, A. L., et al. (2014). Eicosanomic profiling reveals dominance of the epoxygenase pathway in human amniotic fluid at term in spontaneous labour. *FASEB J.* 28, 4835–4846.

Makler, A., and Asghar, W. (2020). Exosomal biomarkers for cancer diagnosis and patient monitoring. *Expert Rev. Mol. Diagn.* 20, 387–400.

Marvin, K., Keelan, J., Eykholt, R., Sato, T., and Mitchell, M. (2002). Use of cDNA arrays to generate differential expression profiles for inflammatory genes in human gestational membranes delivered at term and preterm. *Mol. Hum. Reprod.* 8, 399–408.

McAdam, B. F., Catella-Lawson, F., Mardini, I. A., Kapoor, S., Lawson, J. A., and FitzGerald, G. A. (1999). Systemic biosynthesis of prostacyclin by cyclooxygenase (COX)-2: the human pharmacology of a selective inhibitor of COX-2. *Proc. Natl. Acad. Sci. U.S.A.* 96, 272–277. doi: 10.1073/pnas.96.1.272

McLaren, J., Taylor, D., and Bell, S. (2000). Prostaglandin E2-dependent production of latent matrix metalloproteinase-9 in cultures of human fetal membranes. *Mol. Hum. Reprod.* 6, 1033–1040.

Melo, S. A., Luecke, L. B., Kahlert, C., Fernandez, A. F., Gammon, S. T., Kaye, J., et al. (2015). Glypican-1 identifies cancer exosomes and detects early pancreatic cancer. *Nature* 523, 177–182.

Menon, R. (2016). Human fetal membranes at term: dead tissue or signalers of parturition? *Placenta* 44, 1–5. doi: 10.1016/j.placenta.2016.05.013

Menon, R., Mesiano, S., and Taylor, R. N. (2017). Programmed fetal membrane senescence and exosome-mediated signaling: a mechanism associated with timing of human parturition. *Front. Endocrinol.* 8:196. doi: 10.3389/fendo.2017.00196

Menon, R., and Richardson, L. S. (2017). Preterm prelabour rupture of the membranes: a disease of the fetal membranes. *Semin. Perinatol.* 41, 409–419.

Merlino, A. A., Welsh, T. N., Tan, H., Yi, L. J., Cannon, V., Mercer, B. M., et al. (2007). Nuclear progesterone receptors in the human pregnancy myometrium: evidence that parturition involves functional progesterone withdrawal mediated by increased expression of progesterone receptor-A. *J. Clin. Endocrinol. Metab.* 92, 1927–1933.

Mesiano, S. (2004). Myometrial progesterone responsiveness and the control of human parturition. *J. Soc. Gynecol. Invest.* 11, 193–202.

Mesiano, S. (2019). "Chapter 11 – endocrinology of human pregnancy and fetal-placental neuroendocrine development," in *Yen and Jaffe's Reproductive Endocrinology (Eighth Edition)*, eds J. F. Strauss and R. L. Barbieri (Amsterdam: Elsevier), 256–284e9. doi: 10.1016/B978-0-323-47912-7.00011-1

Miceli, F., Minici, F., Pardo, M. G., Navarra, P., Proto, C., Mancuso, S., et al. (2001). Endothelins enhance prostaglandin (PGE2 and PGF2α) biosynthesis and release by human luteal cells: evidence of a new paracrine/autocrine regulation of luteal function. *J. Clin. Endocrinol. Metab.* 86, 811–817. doi: 10.1210/jcem.86.2.7236

Mitchell, C. M. (2016). *Transcriptional and Epigenetic Regulation of Labour Associated Inflammatory Genes in the Amnion Faculty of Health*. Callaghan, NSW: The University of Newcastle.

Mitchell, M. D., Crookenden, M. A., Vaswani, K., Roche, J. R., and Peiris, H. N. (2020). The frontiers of biomedical science and its application to animal science in addressing the major challenges facing Australasian dairy farming. *Anim. Prod. Sci.* 60, 1–9. doi: 10.1071/AN18579

Mitchell, M. D., Goodwin, V., Mesnage, S., and Keelan, J. A. (2000). Cytokine-induced coordinate expression of enzymes of prostaglandin biosynthesis and metabolism: 15-hydroxyprostaglandin dehydrogenase. *Prostaglandins Leukot Essent Fatty Acids* 62, 1–5. doi: 10.1054/plef.1999.0117

Mitchell, M. D., Peiris, H. N., Kobayashi, M., Koh, Y. Q., Duncombe, G., Illanes, S. E., et al. (2015). Placental exosomes in normal and complicated pregnancy. *Am. J. Obstetr. Gynecol.* 213, S173–S181. doi: 10.1016/j.ajog.2015.07.001

Mitchell, M. D., Rice, G. E., Vaswani, K., Kvaskoff, D., and Peiris, H. N. (2016). Differential regulation of eicosanoid and endocannabinoid production by inflammatory mediators in human choriodecidua. *PLoS One* 11:e0148306. doi: 10.1371/journal.pone.0148306

Mouillet, J.-F., Ouyang, Y., Bayer, A., Coyne, C. B., and Sadovsky, Y. (2014). The role of trophoblastic microRNAs in placental viral infection. *Int. J. Dev. Biol.* 58, 281.

Narumiya, S., and Furuyashiki, T. (2011). Fever, inflammation, pain and beyond: prostanoid receptor research during these 25 years. *FASEB J.* 25, 813–818. doi: 10.1096/fj.11-0302ufm

Navajas, R., Corrales, F. J., and Paradela, A. (2019). Serum exosome isolation by size-exclusion chromatography for the discovery and validation of preeclampsia-associated biomarkers. *Methods Mol. Biol.* 1959, 39–50.

Ni, H., Sun, T., Ma, X.-H., and Yang, Z.-M. (2003). Expression and regulation of cytosolic prostaglandin E synthase in mouse uterus during the peri-implantation period. *Biol. Reprod.* 68, 744–750.

Nielsen, M. R., Frederiksen-Møller, B., Zachar, R., Jørgensen, J. S., Hansen, M. R., Ydegaard, R., et al. (2017). Urine exosomes from healthy and hypertensive pregnancies display elevated level of α-subunit and cleaved α-and γ-subunits of the epithelial sodium channel—ENaC. *Pflügers Arch.* 469, 1107–1119.

Olson, D. M., and Ammann, C. (2007). Role of the prostaglandins in labour and prostaglandin receptor inhibitors in the prevention of preterm labour. *Front. Biosci.* 12:1329–1343. doi: 10.2741/2151

Patel, B., Elguero, S., Thakore, S., Dahoud, W., Bedaiwy, M., and Mesiano, S. (2015). Role of nuclear progesterone receptor isoforms in uterine pathophysiology. *Hum. Reprod. Update* 21, 155–173.

Patel, F. A., Funder, J. W., and Challis, J. R. (2003). Mechanism of cortisol/progesterone antagonism in the regulation of 15-hydroxyprostaglandin dehydrogenase activity and messenger ribonucleic acid levels in human chorion and placental trophoblast cells at term. *J. Clin. Endocrinol. Metab.* 88, 2922–2933. doi: 10.1210/jc.2002-021710

Peiris, H. N., Romero, R., Vaswani, K., Reed, S., Gomez-Lopez, N., Tarca, A. L., et al. (2019). Preterm labour is characterized by a high abundance of amniotic fluid prostaglandins in patients with intra-amniotic infection or sterile intra-amniotic inflammation. *J. Matern. Fetal Neonatal Med.* doi: 10.1080/14767058.2019.1702953 [Epub ahead of print].

Peiris, H. N., Vaswani, K., Almughlliq, F., Koh, Y. Q., and Mitchell, M. D. (2017). Review: eicosanoids in preterm labour and delivery: Potential roles of exosomes in eicosanoid functions. *Placenta* 54, 95–103. doi: 10.1016/j.placenta.2016.12.013

Peiris, H. N., Vaswani, K., Holland, O., Koh, Y. Q., Almughlliq, F. B., Reed, S., et al. (2020). Altered productions of prostaglandins and prostamides by human amnion in response to infectious and inflammatory stimuli identified by mutliplex mass spectrometry. *Prostaglandins Leukot. Essential Fatty Acids* 154:102059.

Pillay, P., Maharaj, N., Moodley, J., and Mackraj, I. (2016). Placental exosomes and pre-eclampsia: maternal circulating levels in normal pregnancies and, early and late onset pre-eclamptic pregnancies. *Placenta* 46, 18–25.

Pillay, P., Moodley, K., Moodley, J., and Mackraj, I. (2017). Placenta-derived exosomes: potential biomarkers of preeclampsia. *Int. J. Nanomed.* 12, 8009–8023. doi: 10.2147/IJN.S142732

Pomini, F., Patel, F. A., Mancuso, S., and Challis, J. R. (2000). Activity and expression of 15-hydroxyprostaglandin dehydrogenase in cultured chorionic trophoblast and villous trophoblast cells and in chorionic explants at term with and without spontaneous labour. *Am. J. Obstet. Gynecol.* 182(Pt 1), 221–226. doi: 10.1016/s0002-9378(00)70516-3

Powe, C. E. (2017). Early pregnancy biochemical predictors of gestational diabetes mellitus. *Curr. Diabetes Rep.* 17:12.

Rauk, P. N., and Chiao, J. P. (2000). Interleukin−1 stimulates human uterine prostaglandin production through induction of cyclooxygenase−2 expression. *Am. J. Reprod. Immunol.* 43, 152–159.

Record, M. (2014). Intercellular communication by exosomes in placenta: a possible role in cell fusion? *Placenta* 35, 297–302. doi: 10.1016/j.placenta.2014.02.009

Record, M., Carayon, K., Poirot, M., and Silvente-Poirot, S. (2014). Exosomes as new vesicular lipid transporters involved in cell-cell communication and various pathophysiologies. *Biochim. Biophys. Acta* 1841, 108–120. doi: 10.1016/j.bbalip.2013.10.004

Record, M., Silvente-Poirot, S., Poirot, M., and Wakelam, M. J. (2018). Extracellular vesicles: lipids as key components of their biogenesis and functions. *J. Lipid Res.* 59, 1316–1324.

Reinl, E. L., and England, S. K. (2015). Fetal-to-maternal signaling to initiate parturition. *J. Clin. Invest.* 125, 2569–2571.

Remes Lenicov, F., Rodriguez Rodrigues, C., Sabatté, J., Cabrini, M., Jancic, C., Ostrowski, M., et al. (2012). Semen promotes the differentiation of tolerogenic dendritic cells. *J. Immunol.* 189:4777. doi: 10.4049/jimmunol.1202089

Ricciotti, E., and FitzGerald, G. A. (2011). Prostaglandins and inflammation. *Arterioscler. Thromb. Vasc. Biol.* 31, 986–1000.

Romero, R., Espinoza, J., Gonçalves, L. F., Kusanovic, J. P., Friel, L. A., and Nien, J. K. (2006). Inflammation in preterm and term labour and delivery. *Semin. Fetal Neonatal Med.* 11, 317–326. doi: 10.1016/j.siny.2006.05.001

Romero, R., Gonzalez, R., Baumann, P., Behnke, E., Rittenhouse, L., Barberio, D., et al. (1994a). Topographic differences in amniotic fluid concentrations of prostanoids in women in spontaneous labour at term. *Prostaglandins Leukot. Essential Fatty Acids* 50, 97–104.

Romero, R., Miranda, J., Chaemsaithong, P., Chaiworapongsa, T., Kusanovic, J. P., Dong, Z., et al. (2015). Sterile and microbial-associated intra-amniotic inflammation in preterm prelabour rupture of membranes. *J. Matern. Fetal Neonatal Med.* 28, 1394–1409. doi: 10.3109/14767058.2014.958463

Romero, R., Miranda, J., Chaiworapongsa, T., Korzeniewski, S. J., Chaemsaithong, P., Gotsch, F., et al. (2014). Prevalence and clinical significance of sterile intra-amniotic inflammation in patients with preterm labour and intact membranes. *Am. J. Reprod. Immunol.* 72, 458–474. doi: 10.1111/aji.12296

Romero, R., Munoz, H., Gomez, R., Galasso, M., Sherer, D. M., Cotton, D., et al. (1994b). Does infection cause premature labour and delivery? *Semin. Reprod. Endocrinol.* 17, 12–19.

Romero, R., Munoz, H., Gomez, R., Parra, M., Polanco, M., Valverde, V., et al. (1996). Increase in prostaglandin bioavailability precedes the onset of human parturition. *Prostaglandins Leukot. Essential Fatty Acids* 54, 187–191.

Saez, T., de Vos, P., Sobrevia, L., and Faas, M. M. (2018). Is there a role for exosomes in foetoplacental endothelial dysfunction in gestational diabetes mellitus? *Placenta* 61, 48–54. doi: 10.1016/j.placenta.2017.11.007

Salomon, C., Torres, M. J., Kobayashi, M., Scholz-Romero, K., Sobrevia, L., Dobierzewska, A., et al. (2014). A gestational profile of placental exosomes in maternal plasma and their effects on endothelial cell migration. *PLoS One* 9:e98667. doi: 10.1371/journal.pone.0098667

Samuelsson, B. (1963). Isolation and identification of prostaglandins from human seminal plasma 18. Prostaglandins and related factors. *J. Biol. Chem.* 238, 3229–3234.

Sarker, S., Scholz-Romero, K., Perez, A., Illanes, S. E., Mitchell, M. D., Rice, G. E., et al. (2014). Placenta-derived exosomes continuously increase in maternal circulation over the first trimester of pregnancy. *J. Transl. Med.* 12:204. doi: 10.1186/1479-5876-12-204

Shao, H., Im, H., Castro, C. M., Breakefield, X., Weissleder, R., and Lee, H. (2018). New technologies for analysis of extracellular vesicles. *Chem. Rev.* 118, 1917–1950. doi: 10.1021/acs.chemrev.7b00534

Sheller-Miller, S., and Menon, R. (2020). Isolation and characterization of human amniotic fluid-derived exosomes. *Methods Enzymol.* 645, 181–194.

Slater, D., Dennes, W., Sawdy, R., Allport, V., and Bennett, P. (1999). Expression of cyclo-oxygenase types-1 and -2 in human fetal membranes throughout pregnancy. *J. Mol. Endocrinol.* 22, 125–130. doi: 10.1677/jme.0.0220125

Smith, W. L. (1989). The eicosanoids and their biochemical mechanisms of action. *Biochem. J.* 259, 315–324. doi: 10.1042/bj2590315

Smith, W. L., DeWitt, D. L., and Garavito, R. M. (2000). Cyclooxygenases: structural, cellular, and molecular biology. *Annu. Rev. Biochem.* 69, 145–182.

Smith, W. L., Garavito, R. M., and DeWitt, D. L. (1996). Prostaglandin endoperoxide H synthases (cyclooxygenases)-1 and -2. *J. Biol. Chem.* 271, 33157–33160. doi: 10.1074/jbc.271.52.33157

Solano, M. E., and Arck, P. C. (2020). Steroids, pregnancy and fetal development [Review]. *Front. Immunol.* 10:3017. doi: 10.3389/fimmu.2019.03017

Steetskamp, J., Bachmann, E., Hasenburg, A., and Battista, M. J. (2020). Safety of misoprostol for near-term and term induction in small-for-gestational-age pregnancies compared to dinoprostone and primary cesarean section: results of a retrospective cohort study. *Arch. Gynecol. Obstet.* 302, 1369–1374.

Strauss, J. F., and FitzGerald, G. A. (2019). "Chapter 4 – steroid hormones and other lipid molecules involved in human reproduction," in *Yen and Jaffe's Reproductive Endocrinology (Eighth Edition)*, eds J. F. Strauss and R. L. Barbieri (Amsterdam: Elsevier), 75–114e117. doi: 10.1016/B978-0-323-47912-7.00004-4

Subra, C., Grand, D., Laulagnier, K., Stella, A., Lambeau, G., Paillasse, M., et al. (2010). Exosomes account for vesicle-mediated transcellular transport of activatable phospholipases and prostaglandins. *J. Lipid Res.* 51, 2105–2120.

Sugimoto, Y., Yamasaki, A., Segi, E., Tsuboi, K., Aze, Y., Nishimura, T., et al. (1997). Failure of parturition in mice lacking the prostaglandin F receptor. *Science* 277, 681–683. doi: 10.1126/science.277.5326.681

Szczykutowicz, J., Kałuża, A., Kaźmierowska-Niemczuk, M., and Ferens-Sieczkowska, M. (2019). The potential role of seminal plasma in the fertilization outcomes. *BioMed Res. Int.* 2019:5397804. doi: 10.1155/2019/5397804

Thomas, J., Fairclough, A., Kavanagh, J., and Kelly, A. J. (2014). Vaginal prostaglandin (PGE2 and PGF2a) for induction of labour at term. *Cochrane Database Syst. Rev.* 2014:Cd003101. doi: 10.1002/14651858.CD003101.pub3

Triggs, T., Kumar, S., and Mitchell, M. (2020). Experimental drugs for the inhibition of preterm labour. *Expert Opin. Invest. Drugs* 29, 507–523.

Truong, G., Guanzon, D., Kinhal, V., Elfeky, O., Lai, A., Longo, S., et al. (2017). Oxygen tension regulates the miRNA profile and bioactivity of exosomes released from extravillous trophoblast cells–liquid biopsies for monitoring complications of pregnancy. *PLoS One* 12:e0174514. doi: 10.1371/journal.pone.0174514

Ueno, N., Takegoshi, Y., Kamei, D., Kudo, I., and Murakami, M. (2005). Coupling between cyclooxygenases and terminal prostanoid synthases. *Biochem. Biophys. Res. Commun.* 338, 70–76. doi: 10.1016/j.bbrc.2005.08.152

Vijayakumar, R., and Walters, W. A. (1983). Human luteal tissue prostaglandins, 17β-estradiol, and progesterone in relation to the growth and senescence of the corpus luteum. *Fertil. Steril.* 39, 298–303.

von Linsingen, R., Bicalho, M. D. G., and de Carvalho, N. S. (2017). Baby born too soon: an overview and the impact beyond the infection. *J. Matern. Fetal Neonatal Med.* 30, 1238–1242. doi: 10.1080/14767058.2016.1209653

Welch, B. M., Keil, A. P., van 't Erve, T. J., Deterding, L. J., Williams, J. G., Lih, F. B., et al. (2020). Longitudinal profiles of plasma eicosanoids during pregnancy and size for gestational age at delivery: a nested case-control study. *PLoS Med.* 17:e1003271. doi: 10.1371/journal.pmed.1003271

Woodward, D. F., Jones, R. L., and Narumiya, S. (2011). International union of basic and clinical pharmacology. LXXXIII: classification of prostanoid receptors, updating 15 years of progress. *Pharmacol. Rev.* 63, 471–538. doi: 10.1124/pr.110.003517

Yang, H., Ma, Q., Wang, Y., and Tang, Z. (2020). Clinical application of exosomes and circulating microRNAs in the diagnosis of pregnancy complications and foetal abnormalities. *J. Transl. Med.* 18:32. doi: 10.1186/s12967-020-02227-w

Yoon, B. H., Romero, R., Moon, J. B., Shim, S. S., Kim, M., Kim, G., et al. (2001). Clinical significance of intra-amniotic inflammation in patients with preterm labour and intact membranes. *Am. J. Obstet. Gynecol.* 185, 1130–1136. doi: 10.1067/mob.2001.117680

Yu, Y., Cheng, Y., Fan, J., Chen, X.-S., Klein-Szanto, A., Fitzgerald, G. A., et al. (2005). Differential impact of prostaglandin H synthase 1 knockdown on platelets and parturition. *J. Clin. Invest.* 115, 986–995. doi: 10.1172/JCI23683

Zhang, Y., Liu, Y., Liu, H., and Tang, W. H. (2019). Exosomes: biogenesis, biologic function and clinical potential. *Cell Biosci.* 9:19. doi: 10.1186/s13578-019-0282-2

Mechanisms of Key Innate Immune Cells in Early- and Late-Onset Preeclampsia

Ingrid Aneman[1†], Dillan Pienaar[1†], Sonja Suvakov[2], Tatjana P. Simic[3,4], Vesna D. Garovic[2]* and Lana McClements[1]*

[1] Faculty of Science, School of Life Sciences, University of Technology Sydney, Sydney, NSW, Australia, [2] Division of Nephrology and Hypertension, Department of Internal Medicine, Mayo Clinic, Rochester, MN, United States, [3] Faculty of Medicine, Institute of Medical and Clinical Biochemistry, University of Belgrade, Belgrade, Serbia, [4] Department of Medical Sciences, Serbian Academy of Sciences and Arts, Belgrade, Serbia

*Correspondence:
Vesna D. Garovic
Garovic.Vesna@mayo.edu
Lana McClements
Lana.mcclements@uts.edu.au

[†] These authors have contributed equally to this work

Preeclampsia is a complex cardiovascular disorder of pregnancy with underlying multifactorial pathogeneses; however, its etiology is not fully understood. It is characterized by the new onset of maternal hypertension after 20 weeks of gestation, accompanied by proteinuria, maternal organ damage, and/or uteroplacental dysfunction. Preeclampsia can be subdivided into early- and late-onset phenotypes (EOPE and LOPE), diagnosed before 34 weeks or from 34 weeks of gestation, respectively. Impaired placental development in early pregnancy and subsequent growth restriction is often associated with EOPE, while LOPE is associated with maternal endothelial dysfunction. The innate immune system plays an essential role in normal progression of physiological pregnancy and fetal development. However, inappropriate or excessive activation of this system can lead to placental dysfunction or poor maternal vascular adaptation and contribute to the development of preeclampsia. This review aims to comprehensively outline the mechanisms of key innate immune cells including macrophages, neutrophils, natural killer (NK) cells, and innate B1 cells, in normal physiological pregnancy, EOPE and LOPE. The roles of the complement system, syncytiotrophoblast extracellular vesicles and mesenchymal stem cells (MSCs) are also discussed in the context of innate immune system regulation and preeclampsia. The outlined molecular mechanisms, which represent potential therapeutic targets, and associated emerging treatments, are evaluated as treatments for preeclampsia. Therefore, by addressing the current understanding of innate immunity in the pathogenesis of EOPE and LOPE, this review will contribute to the body of research that could lead to the development of better diagnosis, prevention, and treatment strategies. Importantly, it will delineate the differences in the mechanisms of the innate immune system in two different types of preeclampsia, which is necessary for a more personalized approach to the monitoring and treatment of affected women.

Keywords: immune cells, pregnancy, late-onset preeclampsia, early-onset preeclampsia, preeclampsia, inflammation, innate immunity

INTRODUCTION

Preeclampsia accounts for over 70,000 maternal and 500,000 fetal/neonatal deaths annually, with maternal deaths being highest in developing countries (1, 2). The exact etiology of preeclampsia is unknown, however, endothelial dysfunction, inappropriate angiogenesis, inadequate trophoblast invasion and spiral uterine artery remodeling, have all been identified as key contributors (3–6). Adequate remodeling of spiral uterine arteries into dilated, elastic, and low-resistance blood vessels enables unlimited supplies of oxygen and nutrients to the fetus. This requires appropriate invasion by extravillous trophoblasts and replacement of maternal endothelial cells (7). Inappropriate activation of the innate immune system and subsequent inflammation, however, can lead to placental dysfunction or poor maternal vascular adaptation and contribute to the development of preeclampsia (8). In this review, we will outline mechanisms of key innate immune cells implicated in the development of preeclampsia and differentiate how these mechanisms are affected in two phenotypes of preeclampsia, early-onset preeclampsia (EOPE) and late-onset preeclampsia (LOPE). The 2018 recommendations from The International Society for the Study of Hypertension in Pregnancy (ISSHP) define preeclampsia as *de-novo* hypertension (systolic blood pressure > 140 mmHg and diastolic blood pressure > 90 mmHg) after 20 weeks of gestation, accompanied by one or more of the following features: proteinuria (>300 mg/day), maternal organ dysfunction (including hepatic, renal, neurological), or hematological involvement such as thrombocytopenia, and/or uteroplacental dysfunction, such as fetal growth restriction and/or abnormal Doppler ultrasound findings of uteroplacental blood flow (1, 2, 9). Preeclampsia with severe features is defined as cases with blood pressure values ≥160/110 mmHg, accompanied by significant proteinuria (≥300 mg of protein/day), or pulmonary edema, cerebrovascular and/or liver function deterioration or thrombocytopenia (10). EOPE is diagnosed before 34 weeks of gestation whereas LOPE is diagnosed from 34 weeks of gestation (2).

INCIDENCE AND TREATMENT OF PREECLAMPSIA

A systematic review of the incidence of hypertensive disorders of pregnancy, including 39 million women from 40 countries, found that preeclampsia affects ~4.6% of all deliveries globally (11). Another review reported that preeclampsia complicates 2 to 8% of pregnancies (12). The reasons for differences in the incidence of preeclampsia among different countries, regions or hospitals include inconsistencies in the diagnostic criteria, difficulty in diagnosing preeclampsia, as well as differences in maternal age and nulliparity, access to prenatal care and education, and regional prevalence of other risk factors (2, 11, 13). Women who have chronic hypertension, autoimmune disorders, kidney disease, pre-gestational diabetes, maternal body mass index (BMI) > 30 kg/m^2 and a family or personal history of preeclampsia, are at higher risk of developing preeclampsia; older age (>40 years) is also associated with increased risk of preeclampsia (1). Treatment of preeclampsia can be divided into expectant care and interventionist care (14). Expectant care involves a balance of stabilizing the mother's condition and delaying delivery as far as the maternal condition allows, to reduce the mortality and morbidity associated with premature birth. Interventionist care involves early delivery to minimize serious maternal and fetal complications. Expectant care provides relief from symptoms, such as reducing blood pressure with antihypertensive therapy and the use of magnesium sulfate as anticonvulsant therapy (2, 15, 16). Evidence suggests that there is no clear difference between an expectant or interventionist care approach for preeclampsia with severe features (14). Without a clear contraindication, delaying delivery for as long as possible can improve outcomes for the fetus (17). Studies investigating the prophylactic use of aspirin in high-risk pregnancies have reported conflicting findings (9, 18). A meta-analysis including 18,907 women concluded that when taken before 16 weeks of gestation at a daily dose of ≥100 mg, aspirin could reduce the risk of preterm preeclampsia diagnosed before 37 weeks of gestation (19). As such, high-risk patients must be identified early in pregnancy for any beneficial effects to be observed (16). Calcium supplementation for women with low calcium diets may lead to a reduction in the severity of symptoms associated with preeclampsia and minimize the risk of preterm birth (2, 18). In the case of diabetic pregnancies, women who were given metformin with and without insulin treatment had a lower incidence of preeclampsia (20).

SIMILARITIES AND DIFFERENCES BETWEEN EARLY-ONSET AND LATE-ONSET PREECLAMPSIA

Gestational age has been identified as the most important clinical variable in predicting both maternal and perinatal outcomes (21). This led to stratification of preeclampsia into two phenotypes, EOPE and LOPE (1, 2, 22). LOPE accounts for the majority of preeclampsia cases, comprising ~80 to 95% of all preeclampsia cases worldwide (23). EOPE, although less common, is associated with higher rates of neonatal mortality and a greater degree of maternal morbidity compared to LOPE (3). As a result, EOPE has attracted greater interest and more studies have focused on elucidating the mechanisms underlying this disease phenotype (23), leading to implementation of preventative treatments (e.g., aspirin) and predictive biomarkers more suited for EOPE than LOPE. LOPE, nevertheless, is also a serious condition, associated with a high prevalence of eclampsia and HELLP (hemolysis, elevated liver enzymes, and low platelets) syndrome, which are two life-threatening complications (24). Further studies are needed to address this gap in research. Preeclampsia has been described as a two-stage disease, with initial deficient remodeling of the uterine spiral arteries leading to a stage of maternal systemic inflammation and vascular dysfunction (25). This model is more representative of EOPE. Impaired placental development in early pregnancy and subsequent growth restriction is often associated with EOPE, while LOPE is likely associated with maternal endothelial dysfunction (26). Both phenotypes exhibit an increased inflammatory response that leads to adverse maternal and fetal complications. Syncytiotrophoblast stress and placental hypoxia are implicated as the main cause of excessive systemic vascular inflammation. In EOPE, this is triggered by dysfunctional perfusion of the placenta. In the case of LOPE, syncytiotrophoblast stress likely occurs as a result of compression of placental terminal villi, as the placenta outgrows the space within the uterine cavity, which can also lead to uteroplacental malperfusion (24, 27).

Timely detection of preeclampsia is complicated by the fact that the disease is usually asymptomatic in its early stages (2). Close antenatal monitoring, especially during the third trimester, can be crucial in preventing maternal and fetal complications. Detection using angiogenesis-related biomarkers such as the ratio of soluble fms-like tyrosine kinase-1 (sFlt-1) and placental growth factor (PlGF), as well as Doppler ultrasound assessment, can be useful in detecting EOPE, and to a lesser extent LOPE. Recently, other angiogenesis-related biomarkers, FKBPL and CD44, were also implicated in prediction and diagnosis of preeclampsia, particularly LOPE (28). Further research is needed to elucidate the pathogenic mechanisms and develop diagnostic biomarkers for LOPE early in pregnancy, allowing interventions to begin before clinical features manifest.

COMPLICATIONS ASSOCIATED WITH PREECLAMPSIA

Women with a history of preeclampsia, in addition to short-term complications, have a higher risk of subsequent cardiovascular and metabolic disorders, especially following EOPE (29). A meta-analysis including datasets from 3,488,160 women found that women with previous preeclampsia were twice as likely to develop ischemic heart disease compared to normotensive pregnancies (30). It is not clear whether this increased risk of subsequent cardiovascular disease is caused by underlying maternal risk factors, which are exacerbated by preeclampsia, or if this increased risk is a consequence of preeclampsia (2). Potential overlapping mechanisms between preeclampsia and cardiovascular disease including hypertension and/or heart failure with preserved ejection fraction were recently identified using a bioinformatics "*in silico*" approach (31, 32).

Untreated preeclampsia, regardless of the phenotype, can result in severe complications including liver rupture, cerebral hemorrhage, myocardial infarction, stroke, acute respiratory distress syndrome, pulmonary edema, kidney failure, and abruptio placentae (1, 9, 16). Delivery of the baby, even if it is preterm, minimizes the risk of developing these maternal and fetal complications, including fetal growth restriction and fetal loss. Premature birth, nevertheless, is also associated with a number of neonatal complications such as respiratory distress syndrome, intraventricular hemorrhage, and necrotizing enterocolitis (14). While there are a multitude of factors that contribute to the pathogenesis and onset of preeclampsia, in recent years, it has been highlighted that an overactive maternal immune system can play a critical role in preeclampsia development.

INNATE IMMUNE SYSTEM IN HEALTHY PREGNANCY AND PREECLAMPSIA

The maternal innate immune system throughout the entire gestation period plays an important role in ensuring protection from pathogens, while concurrently inducing tolerance to the semi-allogeneic developing fetus and placental development. As outlined in **Figure 1**, this is achieved through a delicate balance of various cell functions and interactions between the innate immune system cells and other placental/uterine cells in a timely manner (33, 34). Unfortunately, this is not always the case and due to various factors, the aforementioned balance is disrupted by maladaptation of certain immune cells during gestation, which is demonstrated in **Figure 2**. In physiological pregnancies, decidual macrophages found in proximity to spiral uterine arteries help prepare these for remodeling via secretion of angiogenic molecules (35–37). Macrophages also phagocytize apoptotic cells during tissue remodeling, preventing the release of self-antigens or paternal alloantigens, which could trigger a maternal immunological response (38). There are two phenotypes of macrophages, M1 or classically activated macrophages, and M2 or alternatively activated macrophages. M1 macrophages are involved in phagocytosis, and are micro-biocidal and pro-inflammatory. M2 macrophages are immunomodulatory and responsible for inducing maternal tolerance, resolving inflammation, and are involved in tissue remodeling and cell proliferation (39, 40). Therefore, in normal physiological pregnancy, macrophages favor the M2 phenotype, whereas in preeclampsia, this balance is shifted toward the M1 phenotype (41). M1 cells secrete soluble fms-like tyrosine kinase-1 (sFlt-1), an anti-angiogenic molecule that is associated with impaired angiogenesis in preeclampsia (42). Consequently, the transition of macrophage phenotype from M2 to M1 is indicative of a pro-inflammatory response as observed in preeclampsia.

IMMUNOMODULATION BY INNATE IMMUNE CELLS

Innate immune cells, while assisting in the initial stages of pregnancy, also exhibit immunomodulatory characteristics targeted at immunological responses toward the fetus. Mast cells have demonstrated such characteristics through the release of histamine and stimulation of the G protein-coupled receptors ($H_{1-4}R$) (43). Activation of the H_4R appears to lead to proliferation of regulatory T cells (Tregs), and H_2R support angiogenesis at the fetal-maternal interface (43, 44). Tregs subsequently act to prevent lymphocytes from attacking the fetus. There is limited evidence regarding the behavior of mast cells during preeclampsia and their contribution to its onset. There are some reports that they accumulate at higher density adjacent to

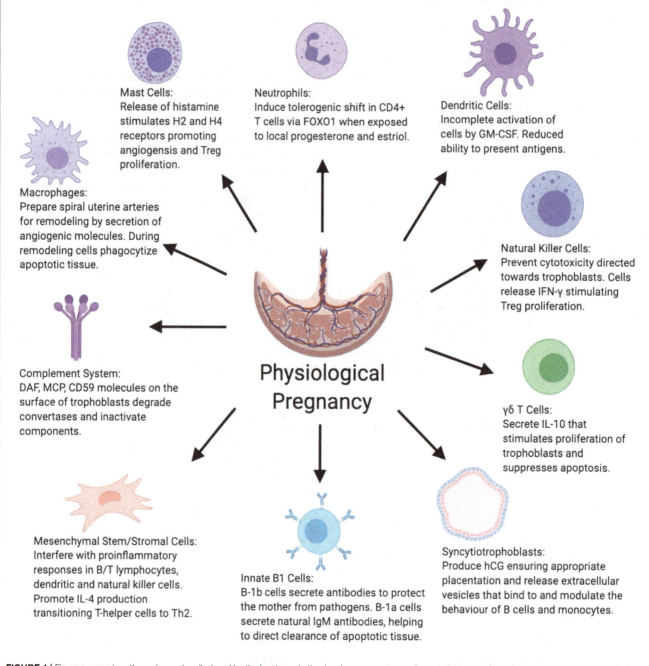

FIGURE 1 | Figure summarizes the various roles displayed by the innate and other key immune system cells as well as syncytiotrophoblasts and mesenchymal stem cells in normal physiological pregnancy. CD59+, Cluster of differentiation 59+; DAF, Decay-accelerating factor; FOXO1, Forkhead box protein-1; GM-CSF, Granulocyte-macrophage colony-stimulating factor; hCG, Human chorionic gonadotropin; IFN-γ, Interferon-gamma; IL-4, Interleukin-4; IL-10, Interleukin-10; MCP, Membrane cofactor protein.

spiral uterine arteries during preeclampsia and undergo intensive degranulation, leading to a release of large concentrations of histamines (45). The high histamine concentrations in the circulation stimulate pro-inflammatory responses from both the innate and adaptive immune system, leading to the secretion of pro-inflammatory cytokines and molecules, contributing to the increase in blood pressure, typical of preeclampsia (46).

THE ROLE OF NEUTROPHILS IN MATERNAL TOLERANCE DURING PREGNANCY

Neutrophils, also as part of a normal physiological pregnancy, are recruited to the developing placenta via the chemokine, IL-8 (47). Following the recruitment of circulating neutrophils

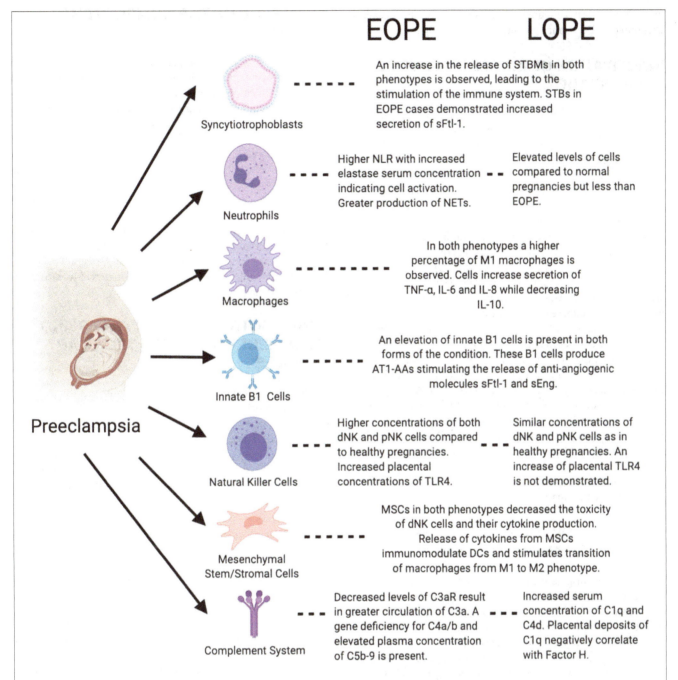

FIGURE 2 | Figure highlights the functions of both immune and placental cells in the context of preeclampsia and both of its phenotypes, EOPE and LOPE. AT1-AA, Angiotensin II type 1 receptor agonistic autoantibody; DC, Dendritic cell; dNK, Decidual natural killer; IL-6, Interleukin-6; IL-8, Interleukin-8; IL-10, Interleukin-10; MSC, Mesenchymal stem/stromal cell; NET, Neutrophil extracellular trap; pNK, Peripheral natural killer; NLR, Neutrophil to lymphocyte ratio; sEng, Soluble Endoglin; sFtl-1, Soluble fms-like tyrosine kinase-1; STB, Syncytiotrophoblast; STBM, syncytiotrophoblast micro-particles; TLR4, Toll-like receptor 4; TNF-α, Tumor necrosis factor-α.

to the placenta and under the influence of progesterone and estriol, CD4+ T cells undergo immunomodulation via transfer of the forkhead box protein 1 (FOXO1) from neutrophils (48). These neutrophil-induced T (niT) cells, in addition to establishing maternal tolerance of the fetus, secrete IL-10, IL-17, and vascular endothelial growth factor (VEGF) promoting angiogenic processes (48). Also in normal physiological pregnancy, the natural cytotoxicity receptors (NCRs) on maternal decidual natural killer (NK) cells are inactivated to ensure maternal tolerance. This is not the case in preeclampsia due to abnormalities in the NCR structure, which increases their synthesis and expression on NK cells, thus affecting maternal tolerance to the fetus (49). Overactivation of NCRs on NK cells leads to discharge of pro-inflammatory cytokines, thus contributing to weakened immunological tolerance potentially endangering the fetus (50).

INACTIVATION OF INNATE IMMUNE CELLS IN PREGNANCY

Whereas the aforementioned cells either assist in required gestational processes or exhibit immunoregulatory roles, other innate immune cells become partially or fully inactivated during pregnancy. NK cells within the uterus and decidua, for example, maintain their immunological function against infections without compromising the fetus. This is achieved by inhibiting NK cell-mediated cytotoxicity toward trophoblasts by interfering with their degranulation process (51). NK cells additionally release IFN-γ, which stimulates decidual $CD14^+$ myelomonocytic cells to induce Treg proliferation via transforming growth factor-beta (TGF-β) (52). The incomplete activation of DCs by granulocyte-macrophage colony-stimulating factor (GM-CSF) similarly leads to a reduction in the capacity of these cells to adequately present antigens (53). This effect consequently limits the development and activation of T cells, increasing maternal tolerance toward the fetus (54). DCs located proximally to the placenta remain inactivated or immature during normal pregnancy; however, these cells become inappropriately stimulated during preeclampsia. Although GM-CSF initially acts as a regulator of DCs, in higher concentrations, GM-CSF along with lnc-DC (long non-coding RNA expressed in DCs), induces DC maturation (55, 56). Once mature, DCs can more efficiently present antigens leading to an increase in the proliferation of Th1/Th17 cells (56, 57). The Th1/Th17 cells consequently stimulate pro-inflammatory responses, which significantly reduce maternal tolerance.

B1 CELL ACTIVATION IN HEALTHY PREGNANCY AND PREECLAMPSIA

B1 cells, despite originating from the lymphoid group of immune cells, also belong to the innate immune system and are important in the initiation and maintenance of a healthy pregnancy. The B1 cell population is subdivided into two groups, B-1a and B-1b, each exhibiting unique roles throughout gestation (58). B-1b cells produce typical antibodies in response to antigen identification, providing protection against invading pathogens (58). On the other hand, B-1a cells secrete "natural IgM antibodies" with low-affinity, poly-reactivity, and self-reactivity, regardless of antigenic stimuli (58, 59). These natural antibodies assist in the clearance of apoptotic tissue cell bodies, affecting the immune response during tissue remodeling (59). B1 innate cells, similar to other immune cells, are irregularly activated in preeclampsia. Notably, B-1a cells are stimulated to produce angiotensin II type 1 receptor agonist autoantibodies (AT1-AA) in preeclampsia, which does not occur in normal physiological pregnancies (60). These antibodies, as the name suggests, act as agonists and induce signaling pathways, leading to the vasoconstriction of blood vessels and the secretion of aldosterone, which stimulates the renin-angiotensin system and increases blood pressure (61).

INFLUENCE OF THE COMPLEMENT SYSTEM

The capacity of the complement system during healthy physiological pregnancy is also modulated to prevent its activation, which could endanger the fetus. Regulatory proteins including decay-accelerating factor (DAF), membrane cofactor protein (MCP), and CD59, found on the surface membrane of trophoblasts, help to degrade convertases within the complement system inducing components of this system into their inactive forms by way of cleavage (62). Due to the widespread dysregulation of the maternal immune system during preeclampsia, the complement system becomes overstimulated as part of a compensatory mechanism. Over-activation of both the classical and lectin complement pathways leads to greater terminal activation, causing inflammation and the recruitment of large numbers of phagocytes to the origin of the stimuli (63). This subsequently contributes to the onset of maternal hypertension and organ damage (63).

SYNCYTIOTROPHOBLAST CELLS AND THEIR SECRETED EXTRACELLULAR VESICLES

The blastocyst, in anticipation of implantation, initiates secretion of human chorionic gonadotropin (hCG) before its synthesis is superseded by syncytiotrophoblast cells (STBs) (7). The continued secretion of hCG by STBs ensures appropriate invasion of trophoblast cells into the endometrium. Upon shedding of the STB layer, extracellular vesicles (EVs) are released from apoptotic STBs, which bind to monocytes and B cells (64). EVs encompass three main vesicle types: exosomes, micro-particles/micro-vesicles and apoptotic bodies (65–67). These EVs, upon binding, induce a shift in the cytokine secretion profile of the neighboring cells, causing the release of anti-inflammatory cytokines (64). On the other hand, in preeclampsia when placental ischemia and hypoxia are present, a greater number of the STB cells undergo apoptosis (68). There is subsequently an increase in secreted EVs into the maternal circulation, overwhelming the body's ability to adequately scavenge and clear them effectively (68, 69). These vesicles then act as antigenic stimuli for components of the immune system leading to unintended endothelial injury, inflammation, and hyper-coagulation (68).

IMMUNOMODULATION BY MESENCHYMAL STEM/STROMAL CELLS

Emerging evidence suggest that mesenchymal stem/stromal cells (MSCs) also have important immunomodulatory roles in pregnancy. Facilitated by paracrine signaling, MSCs target B/T lymphocytes, DCs, and NK cells and interfere with their pro-inflammatory responses. Simultaneously, MSCs stimulate the shift of T-helper cells from a Th1 to Th2 phenotype by promoting IL-4 production and inhibiting IFN-γ production, thus heightening maternal immunological tolerance of the fetus.

Furthermore, MSCs have also been shown to have a key pro-angiogenic role in pregnancy (70). In preeclampsia, the function of MSCs is likely impaired due to exposure to increased numbers of reactive oxygen species (ROS) (70, 71). The presence of aldehyde dehydrogenases (ALDH) during normal pregnancy assists in detoxification from ROS, thus providing a degree of protection against oxidative damage (71). However, due to an unknown mechanism, levels of ALDH in preeclampsia are decreased, exposing the MSCs to oxidative stress with resulting damage and reduced functional ability to modulate other immune cells (71).

In summary, immune cells are critical in the progression of normal physiological pregnancy, both in terms of maternal tolerance and placental development; the roles of key innate and other immunogenic cells in normal physiological pregnancy are depicted in **Figure 1**. The vast majority of immune cells and other associated placental/uterine cells become over-activated or dysregulated in preeclampsia, contributing to the overall symptoms and features of the condition, including hypertension and organ damage.

MACROPHAGE PHENOTYPE PLASTICITY IN PREECLAMPSIA

Macrophages can alter their phenotypic profiles in response to a variety of environmental factors (39). M1 macrophages develop in response to exposure to Th1 cytokines such as IFN-γ, tumor necrosis factor (TNF)-α and lipopolysaccharide (LPS) (72, 73). The development of M2 macrophages is favored in the presence of TGF-β, IL-4, IL-10, and IL-13. Inflammatory cytokines, TNF-α, IL-6, and IL-8, are significantly increased in preeclampsia, and IL-10 is significantly decreased compared to normal pregnancy, therefore promoting the M1 phenotype (74, 75). Decidual macrophages comprise 20% of the immune cells present within the placenta (76). Placental decidual macrophages in normal pregnancy are mainly of the M2 subset and can be found near spiral uterine arteries (40). They have an important role in preparing spiral uterine arteries for remodeling by trophoblasts, as well as phagocytozing pro-inflammatory substances formed during the process of remodeling. The predominance of the M1 decidual macrophage phenotype is conducive to the release of substances such as TNF-α, IFN-γ and nitric oxide (NO), which inhibit trophoblast invasion and spiral uterine artery remodeling (39, 72, 76). Various studies have reported increased levels of decidual macrophages in preeclampsia (55, 77, 78). Other studies have reported a reduction in macrophages in the placental decidua in preeclampsia, possibly due to reduced monocyte migration to the decidua or lack of differentiation into macrophages (79, 80). Chitinase-3-like protein 1 (CHI3L1), also known as YKL-40, is indicative of the number of macrophages, and it has been shown to be present in significantly lower levels in women who developed EOPE compared to normal pregnancy (81). These conflicting findings may be a result of different macrophage cell markers, methods employed, use of tissue samples from different preeclampsia phenotypes and different sections of the placenta being studied, considering that decidual macrophages reside predominantly around spiral uterine arteries (82).

MARKERS OF SYSTEMIC INFLAMMATION: NEUTROPHIL EXTRACELLULAR TRAPS AND THE NEUTROPHIL-LYMPHOCYTE RATIO

Neutrophils are likely the main class of leukocytes that cause the majority of vascular cell dysfunction in women with preeclampsia (83). Neutrophil activation may occur from exposure to oxidized lipids secreted by the placenta as a consequence of placental damage. Activated neutrophils infiltrate the maternal systemic vasculature and release substances such as ROS, TNF-α and myeloperoxidase (MPO), causing endothelial dysfunction (74, 83). MPO has been associated with hypertension, and elevation in TNF-α is recognized as a driving inflammatory mechanisms to preeclampsia (84, 85).

Neutrophil numbers in the maternal systemic circulation and within the decidua steadily increase in pregnancy throughout gestation, yet this increase is further amplified in preeclampsia (4, 74, 86–88). Elevation in neutrophil count has been noted in both EOPE and LOPE compared to normal pregnancy, with a greater elevation present in EOPE (26). This surge in neutrophils may be an adverse reaction to the interaction between the maternal immune system and micro-debris originating from the placenta (89). Although the number of neutrophil granulocytes increases, the phagocytic function of these cells reportedly decreases in pregnancy, particularly in preeclampsia (88). Plasma elastase, a marker of neutrophil activation, has been noted to be elevated in preeclampsia when compared to normal pregnancy (90). A small sample cohort study reported a significant increase in plasma elastase in EOPE compared to normotensive controls (3). Neutrophil extracellular traps (NETs) have been found in the intervillous spaces of placentae in women with preeclampsia (25). The formation of these web-like chromatin structures is induced by STB microparticles (STBMs) released from the placenta and ROS (91). Neutrophils, in addition to causing inflammation, represent the first wave of leukocytes responding to inflammation (5, 83). NETs are abundant within sites of inflammation causing endothelial damage as demonstrated in cases of sepsis, and may also cause damage to villous trophoblast cells in preeclampsia (92, 93). The presence of NETs in the maternal circulation during pregnancy can contribute to thrombotic events, inflammation, and ultimately, fetal death (94). The neutrophil-to-lymphocyte ratio (NLR), is a measure of systemic inflammation, and has demonstrated prognostic value in several cardiovascular diseases, including preeclampsia (4). Both normal pregnancy and preeclampsia present with an increased NLR compared to non-pregnant controls (95). Several studies, however, have reported the NLR to be significantly higher in women with preeclampsia compared to normotensive controls (6, 16, 96, 97). A retrospective case-control study conducted with 186 patients found the NLR to be highest in EOPE, and LOPE demonstrating higher NLRs compared to normotensive controls (26). A change in the NLR can be noted at 16–18 weeks of gestation, and thus has a potential as an inexpensive biomarker for the early detection, monitoring and prompt intervention particularly for EOPE (97).

NATURAL KILLER CELLS IN PREECLAMPSIA

As discussed previously, in normal pregnancy the appropriate remodeling of spiral uterine arteries into low resistance and high capacity vessels coordinated with appropriate trophoblast invasion is pivotal. When these two processes are not well-coordinated, the consequent insufficient blood flow leads to a series of events, which ultimately result in the development of preeclampsia. This suggests that interactions at the maternal-fetal interface in early gestation are important for determining the course of pregnancy. In order to preserve an adequate immuno-tolerant environment, DCs and T-lymphocytes have limited access to the decidua during pregnancy (98). NK cells, in fact, represent 70% of the immune cells in the decidua (99, 100). These decidual NK (dNK) cells are a distinct population from peripheral NK (pNK), both phenotypically and functionally. Unlike pNK, the dNK subpopulation has a $CD56^+/CD16^-$ phenotype (101) and demonstrates a lower cytotoxic potential and higher cytokine secretory profile (102). Decidual NK cells, by secreting VEGF and PlGF, stimulate spiral uterine artery remodeling, a process crucial for successful establishment of the placenta and the feto-maternal interface in pregnancy (103, 104). The lack of dNK cells has been shown to lead to lower fertility and higher fetal resorption (105). NK cells, on the other hand, are recruited by the innate immune system in response to inadequate trophoblast invasion or insufficient spiral uterine artery remodeling, processes observed in preeclampsia. There are some inconsistencies among studies, however, with respect to the number of these cells present in preeclampsia compared to normotensive pregnancy. While some studies have reported significantly lower numbers of NK $CD56^+$ cells within the decidua in preeclampsia (77, 106), other reports have indicated the opposite trend (107, 108). The heterogeneity among studies and the differences in patient characteristics offer possible explanations for these discrepancies. A recent study demonstrated that the increases in both dNK and pNK cells were higher in EOPE compared to LOPE (108).

TOLL-LIKE RECEPTORS IN PREECLAMPSIA

Toll-like receptors (TLRs) represent a family of transmembrane signaling receptors found on all innate immune cells. Ten different TLRs have been identified in humans based on their cellular localization and respective ligands (109). All 10 TLRs activate nuclear factor κB- (NF-κB) dependent and NF-κB-independent pathways to generate cytokines and chemokines (109). TLR expressions vary throughout pregnancy. Trophoblast expression of TLRs changes throughout gestation, with TLR2-4 being highly expressed during the first trimester and TLR1-10 in the third trimester (110–114). TLRs activate inflammatory responses by recognizing damage-associated molecular patterns (DAMPs) released following tissue injury, as well as pathogen-associated molecular patterns (PAMPs) specific to microbial components (115–117). Continuous signaling from DAMPs due to persistent cell death and remodeling of spiral uterine arteries leads to over-activation of TLRs. Excessive TLR activity may contribute to the pro-inflammatory effects and hypertension observed in preeclampsia. Studies report that overstimulation of these receptors due to either viral or bacterial infections may lead to adverse pregnancy outcomes including preeclampsia (114, 118). Upon trophoblast TLR-3 and TLR-4 activation by microbial byproducts, chemokine secretion initiates the innate immune response and the decidua becomes infiltrated with pNK cells and macrophages (113). TLR4 activation by bacterial LPS, in addition, inhibits trophoblast migration (119), while TLR3 activation by poly I:C, a double-stranded RNA (dsRNA) viral mimetic, increases inflammation and results in the development of preeclampsia-like symptoms in pregnant rats (120). Increased immunoreactivity of the TLR4 protein in placentae from complicated pregnancies suggests that their role in the activation of the innate immune system is in response to the presence of infectious agents (112). It has been recently shown that the expression of TLR4 in placentae from women with EOPE was higher than TLR4 expression in women with LOPE (121). It is possible that this upregulation is part of a compensatory mechanism in preeclampsia, given that higher expression of TLR4 has been described in human term placentae compared to first trimester (122). Activation of TLR3 in pregnant mice increased systolic blood pressure and endothelial damage, both of which were further exacerbated in the absence of IL-10 (123). Moreover, dsRNA and single-stranded RNA (ssRNA) were shown to upregulate expressions of TLR3, TLR7, and TLR8 in mouse placentae. This caused pregnancy-dependent hypertension, endothelial dysfunction, and placental inflammation (124). Women with preeclampsia displayed activation of the aforementioned TLRs; however the association between severity of the disease and activation of TLRs was not confirmed (124). Increased expression of TLR9 in the placentae and peripheral blood mononuclear cells from women with preeclampsia compared to normotensive controls has also been described (125, 126). A study by He et al. showed that when mice were treated with a TLR9 agonist, they developed preeclampsia-like symptoms. This preeclampsia murine model also showed that with exogenous overexpression of TLR9, the levels of sFlt-1 increased while VEGF was downregulated. This suggests that TLR9 is capable of suppressing angiogenesis (127) and that aberrantly activated ligand binding to different TLRs may significantly influence pregnancy outcomes. In a relatively recent study, it was demonstrated that inhibition of TLR activation and thus inhibition of downstream signaling, could not prevent embryo resorption in the absence of dNK cells (105, 128). Differential expressions of TLRs throughout pregnancy and in preeclampsia, suggest that these receptors might represent potential therapeutic targets.

THE ROLE OF INNATE B1 CELLS IN PREECLAMPSIA

As indicated above, there are two different subsets of B1 cells. B1a cells are $CD5^+$ and produce "natural antibodies," which are polyreactive, low-affinity and self-reactive antibodies. On the other hand, B1b cells are $CD5^-$ and produce adaptive antibodies when exposed to antigens (58). It is, however, the role of B1a cells that is more closely associated with adverse pregnancy outcomes. Namely, the proportion of B1a cells decreases throughout gestation likely as a protective mechanism against poly-reactive antibodies produced by B1 these cells, which recognize and target a variety of antigens including fetal antigens (129). Their role in preeclampsia has not fully been investigated. However, there are studies emerging regarding their association with hypertensive disorders in pregnancy. The number of peripheral blood B1a cells in women with preeclampsia is significantly increased compared to normal pregnant women (60), however no difference in their number between severe and mild preeclampsia has been observed (130). In addition to the well-established Th1/Th2/Th17-Treg paradigm of the pathogenesis of preeclampsia [as reviewed in (131)], the role of B1 cells is likely linked to stimulation of $CD4^+$ T cells and their differentiation into Th17 effector cells (132). It has also been demonstrated that B1a cells can produce agonistic autoantibodies to AT1-AA in pregnancy, which can lead to the development of preeclampsia (133). High affinity binding of AT1-AA to receptors within the placenta leads to increased secretion of anti-angiogenic factors (sFlt-1 and Endoglin), both of which are associated with the onset of preeclampsia (134-136). These autoantibodies appear to correlate with severity of preeclampsia (137). The depletion of B-cells in an animal model of preeclampsia resulted in a decrease in the level of AT1-AA and a reduction in preeclampsia symptoms (138). Natural antibodies secreted by B1a cells are mostly IgM antibodies and are important in clearing and neutralizing pro-inflammatory targets (139). Although the specific roles of B1 cells have not been elucidated yet, their numbers were not significantly increased following placental ischemia (140). Substantial depletion of B cells by the monoclonal anti-human CD20 antibody, rituximab, interestingly did not have a significant effect on the hypertensive response in the RUPP model (140).

In summary, only a limited number of studies have assessed the role of innate B1 cells in preeclampsia. Further research is needed to evaluate the association of innate B1 cells with hypertensive disorders in pregnancy, as well as their role and pathogenic mechanisms in EOPE vs. LOPE.

EMERGING ROLE OF γδ T CELLS IN PREECLAMPSIA

Within the decidua, γδ T cells despite originating from the lymphoid lineage facilitate proliferation of trophoblast cells while concurrently suppressing their apoptosis through the secretion of IL-10 (141, 142). This ensures adequate migration and invasion of trophoblast cells leading to appropriate placental development. The role of γδ T cells has not yet been determined in preeclampsia, but increases in the production of pro-inflammatory stimuli, interferon (IFN)-γ & IL-17, by γδ T cells have been reported in women with idiopathic recurrent pregnancy loss (143). Furthermore, in mice, a competitive antagonist binding of the histocompatibility complex (MHC) class II found on the surface of γδ T cells, resulted in the reduction of their immunological capabilities (144). The γδ T cell "knockout mice" displayed a resistance to developing preeclampsia-like features, implying that these cells could have a role in the pathogenesis of the condition (144). In the same study, preeclamptic placentae demonstrated significantly increased levels of γδ T cells (144).

THE DYSREGULATION AND OVER-ACTIVATION OF THE COMPLEMENT SYSTEM DURING PREECLAMPSIA

The distribution and activity of the complement system's components vary between EOPE and LOPE, likely stemming from their different underlying pathogeneses. Dysfunction related to the complement system in EOPE has been correlated with single nucleotide polymorphisms (SNPs) as demonstrated by Wu et al. (145). More specifically, C6 (rs7444800, rs4957381) and MASP1 (rs1108450, rs3774282, rs698106) polymorphisms were shown to correspond independently to a risk of EOPE and severe preeclampsia (145). Another modification to the complement system that is unique to EOPE is the reduction in the placental concentrations of complement 3a receptor (C3aR) mRNA and protein (146). These reductions lead to an increase in the plasma concentration of C3a, the ligand for this receptor (146). Lokki et al. expanded upon these findings and compared the activation of the complement pathways in EOPE vs. normal pregnancies. In their cohort study of 22 women, those with EOPE displayed higher placental deposition of C1q, specifically proximal to areas of fibrinoid necrosis (147). They demonstrated that 43% of EOPE cases had a gene deficiency for C4a/b, a deficiency known to also be implicated in certain autoimmune disorders (147). Finally, Lokki et al. noted that areas of C3b deposition were positively correlated with C1q and negatively with Factor H, a regulatory factor of the alternative pathway (147). The over-activation of the complement system in EOPE is reinforced by the rise in the plasma concentration of C5b-9, which is indicative of terminal activation (148). C-reactive proteins of the system, specifically, C3a, have also been found circulating in high concentration within the amniotic fluid in EOPE (149).

LOPE shares many characteristics with EOPE in dysregulation of the complement system, with some key distinctions. As in EOPE, the MASP1 gene has been shown to display SNPs, however, in LOPE the variants indicated are rs1357134 and rs698090 (145). The aforementioned variations in the genes are completely different from the ones detected in EOPE cases and are specifically correlated with LOPE (145). Examining the sera of both EOPE and LOPE, severe preeclampsia cases revealed some degree of activation of the complement system, as demonstrated by Jia et al. (150). Serum levels of C1q, Factor H, C3 and C4 significantly decreased, while the Bb concentration increased in the presence of either EOPE or LOPE compared to their respective controls (150). Despite this, the concentrations of the C-reactive proteins observed in LOPE were not significantly different than in the EOPE cohort (150). Nevertheless, another recent study by He et al. using similar sample size, characterized the components of the complement system using plasma samples from 30 EOPE and 30 LOPE patients with severe preeclampsia. The results obtained contradicted Jia's investigation, showing elevated Bb, C3a, C5a, and MAC in both EOPE and LOPE, whereas LOPE was specifically associated with elevated C1q and C4d compared to normotensive controls (151). Lokki et al. built upon this data, by inspecting the dissimilarities of C1q deposition in the STB layer of the placenta of LOPE patients. This investigation revealed that the C1q deposits negatively correlated with Factor H, characterizing a shift toward activation within the complement system (147).

SYNCYTIOTROPHOBLASTS PLAY IMPORTANT ROLE IN PREECLAMPSIA

STBs form the feto-maternal placental barrier, which separates the fetal and maternal circulations (65). The STB-containing layer, as described above, is shed into the maternal circulation by the placenta during normal pregnancy, releasing STBMs (152, 153). STBMs levels were increased in EOPE compared to matched normal pregnancies, whereas no change was observed between LOPE and normal pregnancy samples (154). This increase in STMBs potentially contributes to endothelial dysfunction and systemic inflammation (155). Another study confirmed no significant difference between levels of EVs from various cells including STBs, in normal pregnancy compared to LOPE (156). Further studies are needed to determine whether this shedding is potentially more prominent in EOPE compared to LOPE. STBM shedding has been linked to increased levels of active tissue factor, leading to enhanced aggregation of platelets (157). This is evident in EOPE with severe features, but not observed in LOPE, which supports evidence suggesting two distinct phenotypic pathogeneses. Further studies are needed to explore if higher levels of STBMs in EOPE are due to their prevalence being greater in early gestation, independent of the presence of preeclampsia (153). STBMs act as ligands for receptors, growth and coagulation factors, and RNA molecules, and have an important role in cell-cell communication (65). STBMs bind TLRs and activate monocytes, DCs, NK cells, and neutrophils. The subsequent release of various inflammatory cytokines and superoxide radicals contributes to the systemic inflammation associated with preeclampsia (74, 88, 94, 158).

The release of sFlt-1 from STBs exerts indirect anti-angiogenic effects by competitively blocking binding of VEGF and PlGF to their respective receptors (158, 159). Levels of sFlt-1 are increased in preeclampsia and can be used as a biomarker of STB stress associated with EOPE (67, 158). LOPE does not present with this early pathology, with studies reporting changes in angiogenic biomarkers near term, observing similar plasma concentrations in both normal pregnancies and LOPE, thus not providing reliable detection of LOPE (160). Contrary to findings describing the prominent role of STBMs, it has been suggested that soluble factors directly released from STBs mediate endothelial dysfunction in preeclampsia rather than EVs (161).

MSC REGULATION OF INNATE IMMUNE SYSTEM RESPONSE IS IMPAIRED IN PREECLAMPSIA

Increased attention has been directed toward investigating the role of MSCs and their immunomodulatory capacity during pregnancy and its complications. As their potential therapeutic role in preeclampsia has been discussed elsewhere (70, 162, 163), here we discuss their contribution to irregular innate immune system signaling in preeclampsia. MSCs are found in many tissues, such as bone marrow, and adipose, decidual and fetal tissue (164–166). Adipose-derived MSCs have demonstrated impaired function associated with senescence in women with preeclampsia (167). Decidual MSCs mediate appropriate placentation and ensure immune tolerance to the semi-allograft fetus (168, 169). These decidual MSCs have the ability to decrease NK cell cytotoxicity and cytokine production (170). This may potentiate the transition of peripheral into decidual NK cells, a process critical for adequate decidual function. Decidual MSCs in addition regulate dNK through their intracellular cytokine expression profile, including TNF-α and IL-4 and via the interaction between collagen and LAIR-1 (171). Bone marrow-derived MSCs are also capable of modulating NK cells by inhibiting their proliferation, cytokine secretion, and cytotoxicity against HLA-class I- expressing targets, either via soluble factors or via cell-to-cell specific interactions (172, 173). A study by Aggarwal and Pittenger showed that immunosuppressive MSC features are associated with the inhibition of TNF-α and IFN-γ, and the secretion of prostaglandin E_2 (PGE2) (174, 175). Notably, it has been previously suggested that the lack of this prostaglandin in preeclampsia leads to a decrease in both renal blood flow and sodium excretion (176). The immunomodulatory interactions between MSCs and NK cells, along with existing studies, provide promising results that strengthen the potential immunomodulatory effects of MSCs. Although MSC are considered privileged immune cells, they can be recognized and eliminated by activated NK cells (172).

Human placental MSCs also have an immunoregulatory effect on macrophage differentiation, favoring the expression of the M2-immunosuppressive phenotype (177). This immunoregulatory effect may be mediated by soluble molecules acting partially via glucocorticoid and progesterone receptors. MSC treatment decreases IL-6 and TNF-α, while increasing anti-inflammatory cytokine, IL-10 (178). A previous study has suggested that PGE2 plays an important role in the immunoregulatory effects of MSC, indicating that M2 macrophage polarization is initiated via the COX-2-PGE2 pathway (178, 179). MSCs are the most widely used stem cell-based therapies due to their beneficial immunomodulation, anti-oxidant, pro-angiogenic, and regenerative therapeutic effects. Their therapeutic potential for the prevention and treatment of

TABLE 1 | Therapeutic strategies targeting aberrant innate immune system mechanisms implicated in preeclampsia.

Innate immunity target	Treatment	Mechanism	Safety in pregnancy	References
Macrophages	Salidroside (SLDS) is a phenylpropanoid glycoside extracted from the root of *Rhodiola rosea* L	Reduction in M1 macrophage/microglia polarization and an increase in M2 macrophage/microglia polarization in mice	Unknown	(73, 181)
Macrophages	Macrophages transplantation	Increase in M2-polarized macrophages	Risk for fetal and maternal micro-chimerism	(182)
Neutrophils	Maternal corticosteroid administration- Betamethasone	Reversal of delayed neutrophil apoptosis (returning the normal rate of spontaneous neutrophil apoptosis)	Betamethasone acetate Category C (TGA) Betamethasone dipropionate Category B1 (TGA)	(90)
STBM	Neprilysin (NEP) inhibitors Racecadotril (Hidrasec®)	Inhibition of STBM released, promoting vasodilatation, and natriuresis	Category B1 (FASS)	(183, 184)
Maternal microbiome	Probiotic-rich food Milk-based probiotics e.g., *Lactobacillus acidophilus* and *Lactobacillus rhamnosus*	Consumption of probiotic-rich food during pregnancy has been associated with lower rates of preterm birth and preeclampsia Probiotics have been implicated in the modification of placental trophoblast inflammation, systemic inflammation, and blood pressure, all features of preeclampsia *Lactobacillus* could be associated with lower risk of preeclampsia in primiparous women Overstimulation of the innate immune system due to dysbiosis of the maternal microbiome has been linked to preeclampsia	Generally recognized as safe (GRAS) by FDA	(185-188)
IL-10	Recombinant Human Interleukin-10	Increased anti-inflammatory capacity	Recombinant IL-10 reverses hypoxia-induced effects in pregnant mice No significant effect on fetal development in mice	(189-191)
TNFα	Infliximab	TNFα antagonist Anti-inflammatory effects	Category B (FDA) No increases in miscarriage, structural neonatal malformations or prematurity were observed compared with non-exposed pregnancies	(85, 192)
Complement system	Ravulizumab (Ultomiris®)	Inhibit cleavage of C5 into C5a and C5b	Category B2 (FASS)	(193)
TLR9	TLR9 antagonist Low-dose naltrexone (LDN)	Reduced inflammatory activity (studied in Crohn's disease)	Category B3 (FASS)	(194-196)
TLR2 & TLR4	Sparstolonin B (SsnB) derived from the Chinese herb *Spaganium stoloniferum*	Blocks TLR2- and TLR4-mediated NFκB activation in mouse macrophages induced by LPS and Pam3CSK4	Anti-angiogenic and anti-estrogen toxicity effects in pregnant rodents	(197)
TLR4	Ibudilast	Upregulation of anti-inflammatory cytokines (IL-10, IL-4) Antagonism of TLR4	Not tested in pregnant women	(198) www.clinicaltrials.gov (NCT01389193)
TLR9	TLR9 inhibitory oligodinucleotide (ODN2088)	Antagonism of TLR9 associated with reduction in systolic blood pressure	No adverse effects were observed in mice receiving this treatment in a model of type 1 diabetes mellitus ODN2088-treated mice gave birth to healthy pups	(199-201)
TLR4	Berberine- isoquinoline alkaloid mainly extracted from *Rhizoma Coptidis*	LPS antagonist Inhibition of LPS/TLR4 signaling	Berberine can cause or worsen jaundice in newborn infants and could lead to kernicterus	(202-206)
TLR4/NF-κB pathway	Parthenolide- Feverfew (*Tanacetum parthenium* L.)	Inhibition of the TLR4/NF-κB pathway	Not safe in pregnancy Feverfew (Tanacetum parthenium L.) shows potential emmenagogue activity and induces abortion	(202, 207, 208)

(Continued)

TABLE 1 | Continued

Innate immunity target	Treatment	Mechanism	Safety in pregnancy	References
IL-1 beta	Canakinumab	Antibody targeting IL-1β. Suppression of the innate immune response and systemic anti-inflammatory effects	Category B1 (FASS)	(209)
MSC	MSC-derived EVs	MSC-derived EVs containing molecular cargo and functional mitochondria metabolically reprogram macrophages M1 pro-inflammatory phenotype toward M2 anti-inflammatory phenotype	Unknown/no major adverse effects were reported in preclinical studies with pregnant rodents	(210) (Reviewed in (70))
MSC	PLacental eXpanded (PLX-PAD) cells	Suppress TLR-induced inflammation. Release anti-inflammatory cytokines (IL-15 & GM-CSF) and growth factors (EGF & VEGF-A)	No detrimental effects on fetal development of mice pups	(162)

The Swedish classification system (Farmaceutiska Specialiteter i Sverige (FASS), American Food and Drug Administration (FDA) and Australian Therapeutic Goods Administration (TGA) were used to determine the safety profile of drugs used during pregnancy. FASS reports on medications on the European market and reflects international text book recommendations (211).
Category A—safe in pregnancy; Category B1, B2, B3—unknown risk in pregnancy or based on animal studies/Categories B (C and D)—unsafe in pregnancy; Category C—possible harmful effects on the human fetus or neonate without causing malformations. The "probably safe" group include FASS and Australian categories A, B1, and B2 and FDA categories A and B; the "potentially risky" group include FASS and Australian categories B3, C, and D, Australian category X, and FDA categories C, D, and X.

preeclampsia is emerging from a number of pre-clinical studies, which show the ability of MSCs and their associated EVs to abrogate symptoms and features of preeclampsia (reviewed in (70). Their relevance specifically to EOPE and LOPE needs to be elucidated further.

THERAPEUTIC STRATEGIES FOR TARGETING INNATE IMMUNE SYSTEM ABERRANT MECHANISMS AS POTENTIAL TREATMENTS FOR PREECLAMPSIA

Finding potential novel treatments for preeclampsia is an area of unmet clinical need and is inherently challenging. Significant knowledge gaps exist surrounding the safety, effectiveness and long-term effects of drugs for the use in pregnancy (180). Clinical trials investigating therapeutics that could be potentially repurposed for preeclampsia often have pregnancy as an exclusion criterion because of possible teratogenic risks or other harmful effects to the fetus (**Table 1**). Consequently, phase 2 or 3 trial data in pregnancy are generally lacking, making it difficult to inform novel treatment strategies. Physiological changes occur in nearly all organs during pregnancy and the pharmacokinetics and pharmacodynamics of drugs are often significantly altered, although the specific changes are mostly undetermined (212). New micro-physiological systems technology such as "Organ on a chip" models may in the future be used to help fill these gaps in knowledge (213).

Dysregulation of TLRs and detection of host-derived DAMPs contribute to the pathogenesis of preeclampsia, as described above (214). Novel TLR antagonists, especially inhibitors of TLR4 and TLR9, have potential as exciting new therapeutic agents for inflammatory disorders. The anti-inflammatory properties of TLR antagonists have been explored in numerous clinical trials for diseases such as systemic lupus erythematosus, infection-associated sepsis and vascular disorders such as hypertension (194), yet it is unknown if these agents are safe to use in pregnancy. This is a research area that therefore warrants further investigation perhaps in pre-clinical models of preeclampsia. Many of the aforementioned immune cells have similar unexplored potential and are presented in **Table 1**. The understanding of the role of the innate immune system in the multifactorial pathogenesis of preeclampsia has been significantly advanced. This progress makes novel therapeutic strategies for targeting aberrant mechanisms within the innate immune system possible as potential treatments for preeclampsia. To support this advancement, greater research capacity and robust and safe clinical trials with pregnant women are needed, with particular focus on delineating differences in EOPE and LOPE management. Anti-inflammatory and immunomodulatory drugs used for other diseases may not be appropriate and safe to use in preeclampsia. It is important to rule out drugs that are not suitable for repurposing in order to streamline future research strategies to focus on more viable alternatives.

DISCUSSION

There is a plethora of evidence supporting the role of the maternal innate immune system in the pathogenesis of preeclampsia. Mechanisms of irregular signaling and function of the innate immune cells could be explored as potential biomarkers or therapeutic targets in preeclampsia. Moreover, these cells appear to play different roles in the two phenotypes of preeclampsia, EOPE and LOPE, which could lead to better risk stratification and personalized management of preeclampsia. Developing reliable predictive and diagnostic biomarkers especially for LOPE has been challenging given that preeclampsia is a multifactorial disease with a poorly understood pathogenesis (215). As depicted in this review, there are a number of different cell types, both from the innate immune system and other supportive systems such as MSCs and STBs, which if exhibiting irregular signaling, can lead to the development of EOPE or LOPE, or both (**Figure 2**).

While in some cases quantifying a particular cell types could be utilized as a biomarker of the disease, such as the number of innate B1 cells or NK cells (both pNK and dNK), the mechanisms involved are often diverse and therefore a panel of biomarkers would be necessary to accurately predict or diagnose preeclampsia. Given that the two phenotypes of preeclampsia are often not considered and distinguished in research, it is encouraging that in terms of the innate immune system, there is important evidence emerging regarding the influence of the innate immune system in both EOPE and LOPE. For example, both dNK and pNK cells, as well as TLR4, are likely increased in EOPE, whereas in LOPE there does not appear to be a difference in these factors compared to healthy pregnancy. Another frequently observed difference between EOPE and LOPE is the proliferation of neutrophils and neutrophil associated processes, with increases in NLR, elastase and NETs being much higher in EOPE than in LOPE. Macrophages and innate B1 cells, on the other hand, do not seem to be dysregulated differently between EOPE and LOPE.

Despite the emergence of novel research highlighting the differences in the behavior of certain innate immune cells in terms of the pathogenesis of EOPE and LOPE, it is important to acknowledge that given the complexity of this condition, there are often inter-personal variations in both the mechanisms and symptoms of the disease. Consequently, these factors impose further difficulties in monitoring, diagnosis, and treatment of preeclampsia. In light of this, it is not surprising that there is a lack of effective treatment strategies for this devastating pregnancy condition. A holistic approach to disease monitoring is necessary to identify women at high risk of developing preeclampsia in conjunction with determining a panel of biomarkers representative of the multifactorial nature and different phenotypes of this disease.

Our evaluation of the existing literature describing interactions between maternal innate immune cells and cells of placental/uterine origin identified a number of limitations in the field. As the heterogeneous nature of preeclampsia has only been recently classified, there is a delay in current research, with a limited number of studies fully examining the interplay among innate immune cells and components of the placenta in the context of both EOPE and LOPE. Certain cell types, nevertheless, have been well-characterized for these two phenotypes of preeclampsia. Evidence is lacking, however, for other cell types of the innate immune system regarding their involvement in the pathogenesis of preeclampsia regardless of the phenotype. These include eosinophils, basophils, mast cells, DCs, and Langerhans cells. It is possible that some of these do not play an important role in the development of preeclampsia. However, given the key roles of mast cells and DCs in pregnancy (**Figure 1**) and some evidence of their roles in the placental bed in preeclampsia, albeit with conflicting results (40), it is likely that these cells could influence preeclampsia monitoring and treatment in the future. A portion of the reviewed literature did examine the various cell types discussed above, however, evidence was provided regarding their behavior in cases of mild and severe preeclampsia, rather than EOPE and LOPE. As a consequence, while there is currently some literature reporting on the behavior of innate immune cell types in preeclampsia, more substantial evidence is required to accurately distinguish immune cell behaviors in both phenotypes of the condition.

Carrying out research with vulnerable groups such as pregnant women is inherently challenging and results in certain limitations. Adherence to stringent ethical considerations and difficulty in obtaining early placental tissue reduces the ability of an investigation to fully elucidate the roles that the immune cells may play in the pathogenesis of preeclampsia. Recent developments in a number of microfluidics or 3D multicellular platforms may greatly increase our understanding of the cellular and molecular mechanisms of the innate immune system associated with inadequate remodeling of spiral uterine arteries or placental development/growth relevant to preeclampsia. The DAX-1™ chip manufactured by AIM Biotechnology has been demonstrated to successfully and accurately recapitulate human tumor immune microenvironments (216). Utilizing this microfluidics platform, investigators were able to examine cell type dependent interactions and provide a novel insight into the tumor immune responses (216). Utilization of these or similar platforms might be able to reproduce the multicellular autocrine and paracrine conditions of preeclampsia, and the behavior of innate immune cells within the microenvironment could be further studied. Thus, researchers can circumnavigate the hurdles of collecting early pregnancy placental tissue while still producing accurate and relevant data. Replicating an EOPE or LOPE environment will be challenging given the distinct and overlapping features of these two phenotypes of preeclampsia. Nevertheless, additional benefits of the microfluidics platforms include the ability to track molecular changes in real-time and the potential to test emerging drug treatments.

CONCLUSION

Components of the innate immune system are fully or partially inactivated, or experience a tolerogenic shift in their immunological function throughout gestation. This, in conjunction with the ability of certain placental cells to modulate the immune system, confers a level of protection to the developing fetus against detrimental immunological responses. This delicate balance is disrupted in preeclampsia, leading to the inappropriate over-activation of these immune cells, causing disruption of appropriate placentation and contributing to the development of this hypertensive condition with end-organ damage. Although the dysfunction of these cells is observed in LOPE, the imbalance appears to be most pronounced in EOPE. While existing literature provides some evidence regarding the roles of the innate immune cells, including NK cells and neutrophils in EOPE and LOPE, further investigation specifically in the context of both phenotypes of preeclampsia, is required to address knowledge gaps. This could lead to the identification of specific disease mechanisms, which could be explored as new diagnostic biomarkers or treatment targets, hence improving the management of preeclampsia and identifying potential emerging treatments for both EOPE and LOPE.

AUTHOR CONTRIBUTIONS

IA, SS, and DP carried out literature search and created a draft of the manuscript. LM, VG, and TS conceptualized the topic, supervised, and revised the draft. All authors approved the manuscript.

REFERENCES

Brown MA, Magee LA, Kenny LC, Karumanchi SA, McCarthy FP, Saito S, et al. Hypertensive disorders of pregnancy: ISSHP classification, diagnosis, and management recommendations for international practice. *Hypertension.* (2018) 72:24–43. doi: 10.1161/HYPERTENSIONAHA.117.10803

Burton GJ, Redman CW, Roberts JM, Moffett A. Pre-eclampsia: pathophysiology and clinical implications. *BMJ.* (2019) 366:l2381. doi: 10.1136/bmj.l2381

Gupta AK, Gebhardt S, Hillermann R, Holzgreve W, Hahn S. Analysis of plasma elastase levels in early and late onset preeclampsia. *Arch Gynecol Obstet.* (2006) 273:239–42. doi: 10.1007/s00404-005-0093-z

Oylumlu M, Ozler A, Yildiz A, Oylumlu M, Acet H, Polat N, et al. New inflammatory markers in pre-eclampsia: echocardiographic epicardial fat thickness and neutrophil to lymphocyte ratio. *Clin Exp Hypertens.* (2014) 36:503–7. doi: 10.3109/10641963.2013.863324

Gezer C, Ekin A, Ertas IE, Ozeren M, Solmaz U, Mat E, et al. High first-trimester neutrophil-to-lymphocyte and platelet-to-lymphocyte ratios are indicators for early diagnosis of preeclampsia. *Ginekol Pol.* (2016) 87:431–5. doi: 10.5603/GP.2016.0021

Gogoi P, Sinha P, Gupta B, Firmal P, Rajaram S. Neutrophil-to-lymphocyte ratio and platelet indices in pre-eclampsia. *Int J Gynaecol Obstet.* (2019) 144:16–20. doi: 10.1002/ijgo.12701

McNally R, Alqudah A, Obradovic D, McClements L. Elucidating the pathogenesis of pre-eclampsia using *in vitro* models of spiral uterine artery remodelling. *Curr Hypertens Rep.* (2017) 19:93. doi: 10.1007/s11906-017-0786-2

Pierik E, Prins JR, van Goor H, Dekker GA, Daha MR, Seelen MAJ, et al. Dysregulation of complement activation and placental dysfunction: a potential target to treat preeclampsia? *Front Immunol.* (2019) 10:3098. doi: 10.3389/fimmu.2019.03098

Mol BWJ, Roberts CT, Thangaratinam S, Magee LA, de Groot CJM, Hofmeyr GJ. Pre-eclampsia. *Lancet.* (2016) 387:999–1011. doi: 10.1016/S0140-6736(15)00070-7

Mihu D, Razvan C, Malutan A, Mihaela C. Evaluation of maternal systemic inflammatory response in preeclampsia. *Taiwan J Obstet Gynecol.* (2015) 54:160–6. doi: 10.1016/j.tjog.2014.03.006

Abalos E, Cuesta C, Grosso AL, Chou D, Say L. Global and regional estimates of preeclampsia and eclampsia: a systematic review. *Eur J Obstet Gynecol Reprod Biol.* (2013) 170:1–7. doi: 10.1016/j.ejogrb.2013.05.005

Duley L. The global impact of pre-eclampsia and eclampsia. *Semin Perinatol.* (2009) 33:130–7. doi: 10.1053/j.semperi.2009.02.010

Schindler AE. New data about preeclampsia: some possibilities of prevention. *Gynecol Endocrinol.* (2018) 34:636–7. doi: 10.1080/09513590.2018.1441401

Churchill D, Duley L, Thornton JG, Moussa M, Ali HS, Walker KF. Interventionist versus expectant care for severe pre-eclampsia between 24 and 34 weeks' gestation. *Cochrane Database Syst Rev.* (2018) 10:CD003106. doi: 10.1002/14651858.CD003106.pub3

Heil SG, Herzog EM, Griffioen PH, van Zelst B, Willemsen SP, de Rijke YB, et al. Lower S-adenosylmethionine levels and DNA hypomethylation of placental growth factor (PlGF) in placental tissue of early-onset preeclampsia-complicated pregnancies. *PLoS ONE.* (2019) 14:e0226969. doi: 10.1371/journal.pone.0226969

Mannaerts D, Heyvaert S, De Cordt C, Macken C, Loos C, Jacquemyn Y. Are neutrophil/lymphocyte ratio (NLR), platelet/lymphocyte ratio (PLR), and/or mean platelet volume (MPV) clinically useful as predictive parameters for preeclampsia? *J Matern Fetal Neonatal Med.* (2019) 32:1412– 9. doi: 10.1080/14767058.2017.1410701

Sato Y, Moriuchi K, Sakae-Matsumoto C, Ueda M, Fujita K. Factors contributing to favourable neonatal outcomes in early-onset severe preeclampsia. *J Obstet Gynaecol.* (2020) 1–6. doi: 10.1080/01443615.2019.1706160

Tskhay V, Schindler A, Shestakova M, Klimova O, Narkevich Capital AC The role of progestogen supplementation (dydrogesterone) in the prevention of preeclampsia. *Gynecol Endocrinol.* (2019) 36:698–701. doi: 10.1080/09513590.2019.1706085

Roberge S, Bujold E, Nicolaides KH. Aspirin for the prevention of preterm and term preeclampsia: systematic review and meta-analysis. *Am J Obstet Gynecol.* (2018) 218:287–93 e281. doi: 10.1016/j.ajog.2017.11.561

Alqudah A, McKinley MC, McNally R, Graham U, Watson CJ, Lyons TJ, et al. Risk of pre-eclampsia in women taking metformin: a systematic review and meta-analysis. *Diabet Med.* (2018) 35:160–72. doi: 10.1111/dme.13523

Von Dadelszen P, Magee LA, Roberts JM. Subclassification of preeclampsia. *Hypertens Pregnancy.* (2003) 22:143–8. doi: 10.1081/PRG-120021060

Bouter AR, Duvekot JJ. Evaluation of the clinical impact of the revised ISSHP and ACOG definitions on preeclampsia. *Pregnancy Hypertens.* (2020) 19:206–11. doi: 10.1016/j.preghy.2019.11.011

Huppertz B. The critical role of abnormal trophoblast development in the etiology of preeclampsia. *Curr Pharm Biotechnol.* (2018) 19:771–80. doi: 10.2174/1389201019666180427110547

Staff AC. The two-stage placental model of preeclampsia: an update. *J Reprod Immunol.* (2019) 134–5:1–10. doi: 10.1016/j.jri.2019.07.004

Gardiner C, Vatish M. Impact of haemostatic mechanisms on pathophysiology of preeclampsia. *Thromb Res.* (2017) 151(Suppl. 1):S48–52. doi: 10.1016/S0049-3848(17)30067-1

Orgul G, Aydin Hakli D, Ozten G, Fadiloglu E, Tanacan A, Beksac MS. First trimester complete blood cell indices in early and late onset preeclampsia. *Turk J Obstet Gynecol.* (2019) 16:112–7. doi: 10.4274/tjod.galenos.2019. 93708

Redman CW, Sargent IL, Staff AC. IFPA Senior Award Lecture: making sense of pre-eclampsia - two placental causes of preeclampsia? *Placenta.* (2014) 35(Suppl.):S20–5. doi: 10.1016/j.placenta.2013.12.008

Todd N, McNally R, Alqudah A, Jerotic DJ, Suvakov S, Obradovic D, et al. Role of a novel angiogenesis FKBPL-CD44 pathway in preeclampsia risk stratification and mesenchymal stem cell treatment. *JCEM.* (2020). doi: 10.1210/clinem/dgaa403. [Epub ahead of print].

Phipps E, Prasanna D, Brima W, Jim B. Preeclampsia: updates in pathogenesis, definitions, and guidelines. *Clin J Am Soc Nephrol.* (2016) 11:1102–13. doi: 10.2215/CJN.12081115

Bellamy L, Casas JP, Hingorani AD, Williams DJ. Pre-eclampsia and risk of cardiovascular disease and cancer in later life: systematic review and meta-analysis. *BMJ.* (2007) 335:974. doi: 10.1136/bmj.39335.385301.BE

Suvakov S, Bonner E, Nikolic V, Jerotic DJ, Simic TP, Garovic VD, et al. Overlapping pathogenic signalling pathways and biomarkers in preeclampsia and cardiovascular disease. *Pregnancy Hypertens.* (2020) 20:131–6. doi: 10.1016/j.preghy.2020.03.011.263-5

Lopez-Campos G, Bonner E, McClements L. An integrative biomedical informatics approach to elucidate the similarities between pre- eclampsia and hypertension. *Stud Health Technol Inform.* (2019) 264:988–92. doi: 10.3233/SHTI190372

Mor G, and Cardenas I. The immune system in pregnancy: a unique complexity. *Am J Reprod Immunol.* (2010) 63:425–33. doi:10.1111/j.1600-0897.2010.00836.x

Bonney EA. Immune regulation in pregnancy: a matter of perspective? *Obstetr Gynecol Clin.* (2016) 43:679–98. doi: 10.1016/j.ogc.2016.07.004

Al-khafaji LA, Al-Yawer MA. Localization and counting of CD68-labelled macrophages in placentas of normal and preeclamptic women. In: *AIP Conference Proceedings.* Erbil: AIP Publishing LLC (2017). p. 020012.

Owen JL, Mohamadzadeh M. Macrophages and chemokines as mediators of angiogenesis. *Front Physiol.* (2013) 4:159. doi: 10.3389/fphys.2013.00159

Faas MM, De Vos P. Uterine NK cells and macrophages in pregnancy. *Placenta.* (2017) 56:44–52. doi: 10.1016/j.placenta.2017.03.001

Abrahams VM, Kim YM, Straszewski SL, Romero R, Mor G. Macrophages and apoptotic cell clearance during pregnancy. *Am J Reprod Immunol.* (2004) 51:275–82. doi:10.1111/j.1600-0897.2004.00156.x

Ning F, Liu H, Lash GE. The role of decidual macrophages during normal and pathological pregnancy. *Am J Reprod Immunol.* (2016) 75:298–309. doi: 10.1111/aji.12477

Faas MM, De Vos P. Innate immune cells in the placental bed in healthy pregnancy and preeclampsia. *Placenta.* (2018) 69:125–33. doi: 10.1016/j.placenta.2018.04.012

Faas MM, Spaans F, De Vos P. Monocytes and macrophages in pregnancy and pre-eclampsia. *Front Immunol.* (2014) 5:298. doi: 10.3389/fimmu.2014.00298

Schonkeren D, van der Hoorn M-L, Khedoe P, Swings G, van Beelen E, Claas F, et al. Differential distribution and phenotype of decidual macrophages in preeclamptic versus control pregnancies. *Am J Pathol.* (2011) 178:709–17. doi: 10.1016/j.ajpath.2010.10.011

Del Rio R, Noubade R, Saligrama N, Wall EH, Krementsov DN, Poynter ME, et al. Histamine H4 receptor optimizes T regulatory cell frequency and facilitates anti-inflammatory responses within the central nervous system. *J Immunol.* (2012) 188:541–7. doi: 10.4049/jimmunol.1101498

Woidacki K, Meyer N, Schumacher A, Goldschmidt A, Maurer M, Zenclussen AC. Transfer of regulatory T cells into abortion-prone mice promotes the expansion of uterine mast cells and normalizes early pregnancy angiogenesis. *Sci Rep.* (2015) 5:1–10. doi: 10.1038/srep13938

Szewczyk G, Pyzlak M, Klimkiewicz J, Smiertka W, Miedzinska-Maciejewska M, Szukiewicz D. Mast cells and histamine: do they influence placental vascular network and development in preeclampsia? *Mediators Inflamm.* (2012) 2012:307189. doi: 10.1155/2012/307189

O'Mahony L, Akdis M, Akdis CA. Regulation of the immune response and inflammation by histamine and histamine receptors. *J Allergy Clin Immunol.* (2011) 128:1153–62. doi: 10.1016/j.jaci.2011.06.051

Cemgil Arikan D, Aral M, Coskun A, Ozer A. Plasma IL-4, IL-8, IL- 12, interferon-γ and CRP levels in pregnant women with preeclampsia, and their relation with severity of disease and fetal birth weight. *J Matern Fetal Neonat Med.* (2012) 25:1569–73. doi: 10.3109/14767058.2011. 648233

Nadkarni S, Smith J, Sferruzzi-Perri AN, Ledwozyw A, Kishore M, Haas R, et al. Neutrophils induce proangiogenic T cells with a regulatory phenotype in pregnancy. *Proc Natl Acad Sci USA.* (2016) 113:E8415–24. doi: 10.1073/pnas.1611944114

Fukui A, Funamizu A, Yokota M, Yamada K, Nakamua R, Fukuhara R, et al. Uterine and circulating natural killer cells and their roles in women with recurrent pregnancy loss, implantation failure and preeclampsia. *J Reprod Immunol.* (2011) 90:105–10. doi: 10.1016/j.jri.2011.04.006

Hashemi V, Dolati S, Hosseini A, Gharibi T, Danaii S, Yousefi M. Natural killer T cells in Preeclampsia: an updated review. *Biomed Pharmacother.* (2017) 95:412–8. doi: 10.1016/j.biopha.2017.08.077

Sun J, Yang M, Ban Y, Gao W, Song B, Wang Y, et al. Tim-3 is upregulated in NK cells during early pregnancy and inhibits NK cytotoxicity toward trophoblast in galectin-9 dependent pathway. *PLoS ONE.* (2016) 11:e0147186. doi: 10.1371/journal.pone.0147186

Vacca P, Moretta L, Moretta A, Mingari MC. Origin, phenotype and function of human natural killer cells in pregnancy. *Trends Immunol.* (2011) 32:517– 23. doi: 10.1016/j.it.2011.06.013

Moldenhauer LM, Keenihan SN, Hayball JD, Robertson SA. GM-CSF is an essential regulator of T cell activation competence in uterine dendritic cells during early pregnancy in mice. *J Immunol.* (2010) 185:7085–96. doi:10.4049/jimmunol.1001374

Della Bella S, Giannelli S, Cozzi V, Signorelli V, Cappelletti M, Cetin I, et al. Incomplete activation of peripheral blood dendritic cells during healthy human pregnancy. *Clin Exp Immunol.* (2011) 164:180–92. doi:10.1111/j.1365-2249.2011.04330.x

Huang SJ, Zenclussen AC, Chen C-P, Basar M, Yang H, Arcuri F, et al. The implication of aberrant GM-CSF expression in decidual cells in the pathogenesis of preeclampsia. *Am J Pathol.* (2010) 177:2472–82. doi:10.2353/ajpath.2010.091247

Zhang W, Zhou Y, Ding Y. Lnc-DC mediates the over-maturation of decidual dendritic cells and induces the increase in Th1 cells in preeclampsia. *Am J Reprod Immunol.* (2017) 77:e12647. doi: 10.1111/aji.12647

Wang J, Tao Y-M, Cheng X-Y, Zhu T-F, Chen Z-F, Yao H, et al. Dendritic cells derived from preeclampsia patients influence Th1/Th17 cell differentiation in vitro. *Int J Clin Exp Med.* (2014) 7:5303–9.

Muzzio D, Zenclussen AC, Jensen F. The role of B cells in pregnancy: the good and the bad. *Am J Reprod Immunol.* (2013) 69:408–12. doi:10.1111/aji.12079

Nguyen T, Ward C, Morris J. To B or not to B cells-mediate a healthy start to life. *Clin Exp Immunol.* (2013) 171:124–34. doi: 10.1111/cei.12001

Jensen F, Wallukat G, Herse F, Budner O, El-Mousleh T, Costa S-D, et al. CD19+ CD5+ cells as indicators of preeclampsia. *Hypertension.* (2012) 59:861–8.doi: 10.1161/HYPERTENSIONAHA.111.188276

Cornelius DC, Cottrell J, Amaral LM, LaMarca B. Inflammatory mediators: a causal link to hypertension during preeclampsia. *Br J Pharmacol.* (2019) 176:1914–21. doi: 10.1111/bph.14466

Denny KJ, Woodruff TM, Taylor SM, Callaway LK. Complement in pregnancy: a delicate balance. *Am J Reprod Immunol.* (2013) 69:3–11. doi: 10.1111/aji.12000

Derzsy Z, Prohászka Z, Rigó Jr J, Füst G, Molvarec A. Activation of the complement system in normal pregnancy and preeclampsia. *Mol Immunol.* (2010) 47:1500–6. doi: 10.1016/j.molimm.2010.01.021

Southcombe J, Tannetta D, Redman C, Sargent I. The immunomodulatory role of syncytiotrophoblast microvesicles. *PLoS ONE.* (2011) 6:e20245. doi:10.1371/journal.pone.0020245

Familari M, Cronqvist T, Masoumi Z, Hansson SR. Placenta-derived extracellular vesicles: their cargo and possible functions. *Reprod Fertil Dev.* (2017) 29:433–47. doi: 10.1071/RD15143

Tannetta D, Masliukaite I, Vatish M, Redman C, Sargent I. Update of syncytiotrophoblast derived extracellular vesicles in normal pregnancy and preeclampsia. *J Reprod Immunol.* (2017) 119:98–106. doi: 10.1016/j.jri.2016.08.008

Göhner C, Plosch T, Faas MM. Immune-modulatory effects of syncytiotrophoblast extracellular vesicles in pregnancy and preeclampsia. *Placenta.* (2017) 60(Suppl. 1):S41–51. doi: 10.1016/j.placenta.2017.06.004

Han C, Han L, Huang P, Chen Y, Wang Y, Xue F. Syncytiotrophoblast-derived extracellular vesicles in pathophysiology of preeclampsia. *Front Physiol.* (2019) 10:1236. doi: 10.3389/fphys.2019.01236

Kaminska A, Enguita FJ, Stepien EŁ. Lactadherin: an unappreciated haemostasis regulator and potential therapeutic agent. *Vasc Pharmacol.* (2018) 101:21–8. doi: 10.1016/j.vph.2017.11.006

Suvakov S, Richards C, Nikolic V, Simic T, McGrath K, Krasnodembskaya A, et al. Emerging therapeutic potential of mesenchymal stem/stromal cells in preeclampsia. *Curr Hypertens Rep.* (2020) 22:37–37. doi: 10.1007/s11906-020-1034-8

Kusuma GD, Abumaree MH, Perkins AV, Brennecke SP, Kalionis B. Reduced aldehyde dehydrogenase expression in preeclamptic decidual mesenchymal stem/stromal cells is restored by aldehyde dehydrogenase agonists. *Sci Rep.* (2017) 7:42397. doi: 10.1038/srep42397

Wheeler KC, Jena MK, Pradhan BS, Nayak N, Das S, Hsu CD, et al. VEGF may contribute to macrophage recruitment and M2 polarization in the decidua. *PLoS ONE.* (2018) 13:e0191040. doi: 10.1371/journal.pone.0191040

Wang Y, Smith W, Hao D, He B, Kong L. M1 and M2 macrophage polarization and potentially therapeutic naturally occurring compounds. *Int Immunopharmacol.* (2019) 70:459–66. doi: 10.1016/j.intimp.2019.02.050

Laresgoiti-Servitje E. A leading role for the immune system in the pathophysiology of preeclampsia. *J Leukoc Biol.* (2013) 94:247–57. doi:10.1189/jlb.1112603

Sharma A, Satyam A, Sharma JB. Leptin, IL-10 and inflammatory markers (TNF-alpha, IL-6 and IL-8) in pre-eclamptic, normotensive pregnant and healthy non-pregnant women. *Am J Reprod Immunol.* (2007) 58:21–30. doi: 10.1111/j.1600-0897.2007.00486.x

Li ZH, Wang LL, Liu H, Muyayalo KP, Huang XB, Mor G, et al. Galectin-9 alleviates LPS-induced preeclampsia-like impairment in rats via switching decidual macrophage polarization to M2 subtype. *Front Immunol.* (2018) 9:3142. doi: 10.3389/fimmu.2018.03142

Milosevic-Stevanovic J, Krstic M, Radovic-Janosevic D, Popovic J, Tasic M, Stojnev S. Number of decidual natural killer cells & macrophages in pre-eclampsia. *Indian J Med Res.* (2016) 144:823–30. doi: 10.4103/ijmr.IJMR_776_15

Li M, Piao L, Chen CP, Wu X, Yeh CC, Masch R, et al. Modulation of decidual macrophage polarization by macrophage colony-stimulating factor derived from first-trimester decidual cells: implication in preeclampsia. *Am J Pathol.* (2016) 186:1258–66. doi: 10.1016/j.ajpath.2015.12.021

Bürk MR, Troeger C, Brinkhaus R, Holzgreve W, Hahn S. Severely reduced presence of tissue macrophages in the basal plate of pre-eclamptic placentae. *Placenta.* (2001) 22:309–16. doi: 10.1053/plac.2001.0624

Jena MK, Nayak N, Chen K, Nayak NR. Role of macrophages in pregnancy and related complications. *Arch Immunol Ther Exp.* (2019) 67:295–309. doi: 10.1007/s00005-019-00552-7

Kucur M, Tuten A, Oncul M, Acikgoz AS, Yuksel MA, Imamoglu M, et al. Maternal serum apelin and YKL-40 levels in early and late-onset pre-eclampsia. *Hypertens Pregnancy.* (2014) 33:467–75. doi: 10.3109/10641955.2014.944709

Yao Y, Xu XH, Jin L. Macrophage polarization in physiological and pathological pregnancy. *Front Immunol.* (2019) 10:792. doi: 10.3389/fimmu.2019.00792

Cadden KA, Walsh SW. Neutrophils, but not lymphocytes or monocytes, infiltrate maternal systemic vasculature in women with preeclampsia. *Hypertens Pregnancy.* (2008) 27:396–405. doi: 10.1080/10641950801958067

Shukla J, Walsh SW. Neutrophil release of myeloperoxidase in systemic vasculature of obese women may put them at risk for preeclampsia. *Reprod Sci.* (2015) 22:300–7. doi: 10.1177/1933719114557899

Alijotas-Reig J, Esteve-Valverde E, Ferrer-Oliveras R, Llurba E, Gris JM. Tumor necrosis factor-alpha and pregnancy: focus on biologics. An updated and comprehensive review. *Clin Rev Allergy Immunol.* (2017) 53:40–53. doi: 10.1007/s12016-016-8596-x

Lurie S, Frenkel E, Tuvbin Y. Comparison of the differential distribution of leukocytes in preeclampsia versus uncomplicated pregnancy. *Gynecol Obstet Invest.* (1998) 45:229–31. doi: 10.1159/000009973

Regal JF, Lillegard KE, Bauer AJ, Elmquist BJ, Loeks-Johnson AC, Gilbert JS. Neutrophil depletion attenuates placental ischemia-induced hypertension in the rat. *PLoS ONE.* (2015) 10:e0132063. doi: 10.1371/journal.pone.0132063

Lampe R, Kover A, Szucs S, Pal L, Arnyas E, Poka R. The effect of healthy pregnant plasma and preeclamptic plasma on the phagocytosis index of neutrophil granulocytes and monocytes of nonpregnant women. *Hypertens Pregnancy.* (2017) 36:59–63. doi: 10.1080/10641955.2016.1237644

Hahn S, Giaglis S, Hoesli I, Hasler P. Neutrophil NETs in reproduction: from infertility to preeclampsia and the possibility of fetal loss. *Front Immunol.* (2012) 3:362. doi: 10.3389/fimmu.2012.00362

Fuchisawa A, van Eeden S, Magee LA, Whalen B, Leung PC, Russell JA, et al. Neutrophil apoptosis in preeclampsia, do steroids confound the relationship? *J Obstet Gynaecol Res.* (2004) 30:342–8. doi: 10.1111/j.1447-0756.2004.00209.x

Konecna B, Laukova L, Vlkova B. Immune activation by nucleic acids: a role in pregnancy complications. *Scand J Immunol.* (2018) 87:e12651. doi: 10.1111/sji.12651

Brinkmann V, Reichard U, Goosmann C, Fauler B, Uhlemann Y, Weiss DS, et al. Neutrophil extracellular traps kill bacteria. *Science.* (2004) 303:1532–5. doi: 10.1126/science.1092385

Gupta AK, Joshi MB, Philippova M, Erne P, Hasler P, Hahn S, et al. Activated endothelial cells induce neutrophil extracellular traps and are susceptible to NETosis-mediated cell death. *FEBS Lett.* (2010) 584:3193–7. doi: 10.1016/j.febslet.2010.06.006

Giaglis S, Stoikou M, Grimolizzi F, Subramanian BY, van Breda SV, Hoesli I, et al. Neutrophil migration into the placenta: good, bad or deadly? *Cell Adh Migr.* (2016) 10:208–25. doi: 10.1080/19336918.2016.1148866

Mannaerts D, Faes E, Goovaerts I, Stoop T, Cornette J, Gyselaers W, et al. Flow-mediated dilation and peripheral arterial tonometry are disturbed in preeclampsia and reflect different aspects of endothelial function. *Am J Physiol Regul Integr Comp Physiol.* (2017) 313:R518–R525. doi: 10.1152/ajpregu.00514.2016

Serin S, Avci F, Ercan O, Kostu B, Bakacak M, Kiran H. Is neutrophil/lymphocyte ratio a useful marker to predict the severity of pre-eclampsia? *Pregnancy Hypertens.* (2016) 6:22–5. doi: 10.1016/j.preghy.2016.01.005

Panwar M, Kumari A, Hp A, Arora R, Singh V, Bansiwal R. Raised neutrophil lymphocyte ratio and serum beta hCG level in early second trimester of pregnancy as predictors for development and severity of preeclampsia. *Drug Discov Ther.* (2019) 13:34–7. doi: 10.5582/ddt.2019.01006

Nancy P, Erlebacher A. T cell behavior at the maternal-fetal interface. *Int J Dev Biol.* (2014) 58:189–98. doi: 10.1387/ijdb.140054ae

King A. Uterine leukocytes and decidualization. *Hum Reprod Update.* (2000) 6:28–36. doi: 10.1093/humupd/6.1.28

Bulmer JN, Morrison L, Longfellow M, Ritson A, Pace D. Granulated lymphocytes in human endometrium: histochemical and immunohistochemical studies. *Hum Reprod.* (1991) 6:791–8. doi: 10.1093/oxfordjournals.humrep.a137430

Lanier LL, Le AM, Civin CI, Loken MR, Phillips JH. The relationship of CD16 (Leu-11) and Leu-19 (NKH-1) antigen expression on human peripheral blood NK cells and cytotoxic T lymphocytes. *J Immunol.* (1986) 136:4480–6.

Laskarin G, Tokmadzic VS, Strbo N, Bogovic T, Szekeres-Bartho J, Randic L, et al. Progesterone induced blocking factor (PIBF) mediates progesterone induced suppression of decidual lymphocyte cytotoxicity. *Am J Reprod Immunol.* (2002) 48:201–9. doi: 10.1034/j.1600-0897.2002.01133.x

Lash GE, Schiessl B, Kirkley M, Innes BA, Cooper A, Searle RF, et al. Expression of angiogenic growth factors by uterine natural killer cells during early pregnancy. *J Leukoc Biol.* (2006) 80:572–80. doi: 10.1189/jlb. 0406250

Gibson DA, Greaves E, Critchley HO, Saunders PT. Estrogen-dependent regulation of human uterine natural killer cells promotes vascular remodelling via secretion of CCL2. *Hum Reprod.* (2015) 30:1290–301. doi: 10.1093/humrep/dev067

Wang W, Lin Y, Zeng S, Li D-J. Improvement of fertility with adoptive CD25+ natural killer cell transfer in subfertile non-obese diabetic mice. *Reprod Biomed Online.* (2009) 18:95–103. doi: 10.1016/S1472-6483(10)60430-0

Williams PJ, Bulmer JN, Searle RF, Innes BA, Robson SC. Altered decidual leucocyte populations in the placental bed in pre-eclampsia and foetal growth restriction: a comparison with late normal pregnancy. *Reproduction.* (2009) 138:177–84. doi: 10.1530/REP-09-0007

Bachmayer N, Rafik Hamad R, Liszka L, Bremme K, Sverremark-Ekstrom E. Aberrant uterine natural killer (NK)-cell expression and altered placental and serum levels of the NK-cell promoting cytokine interleukin-12 in pre-eclampsia. *Am J Reprod Immunol.* (2006) 56:292–301. doi: 10.1111/j.1600-0897.2006.00429.x

Du M, Wang W, Huang L, Guan X, Lin W, Yao J, et al. Natural killer cells in the pathogenesis of preeclampsia: a double-edged sword. *J Matern Fetal Neonatal Med.* (2020) 1–8. doi: 10.1080/14767058.2020.1740675

Takeda K, Kaisho T, Akira S. Toll-like receptors. *Annu Rev Immunol.* (2003) 21:335–76. doi: 10.1146/annurev.immunol.21.120601.141126

Holmlund U, Cebers G, Dahlfors AR, Sandstedt B, Bremme K, Ekstrom ES, et al. Expression and regulation of the pattern recognition receptors Toll-like receptor-2 and Toll-like receptor-4 in the human placenta. *Immunology.* (2002) 107:145–51. doi: 10.1046/j.1365-2567.2002.01491.x

Zarember KA, Godowski PJ. Tissue expression of human toll-like receptors and differential regulation of toll-like receptor mRNAs in leukocytes in response to microbes, their products, and cytokines. *J Immunol.* (2002) 168:554–51. doi: 10.4049/jimmunol.168.2.554

Kumazaki K, Nakayama M, Yanagihara I, Suehara N, Wada Y. Immunohistochemical distribution of Toll-like receptor 4 in term and preterm human placentas from normal and complicated pregnancy including chorioamnionitis. *Hum Pathol.* (2004) 35:47–54. doi: 10.1016/j.humpath.2003.08.027

Abrahams VM, Visintin I, Aldo PB, Guller S, Romero R, Mor G. A role for TLRs in the regulation of immune cell migration by first trimester trophoblast cells. *J Immunol.* (2005) 175:8096–104. doi:10.4049/jimmunol.175.12.8096

Abrahams VM, Bole-Aldo P, Kim YM, Straszewski-Chavez SL, Chaiworapongsa T, Romero R, et al. Divergent trophoblast responses to bacterial products mediated by TLRs. *J Immunol.* (2004) 173:4286–96. doi: 10.4049/jimmunol.173.7.4286

Ann-Charlotte I. Inflammatory mechanisms in preeclampsia. *Pregnancy Hypertens.* (2013) 3:58. doi: 10.1016/j.preghy.2013.04.005

McCarthy CG, Goulopoulou S, Wenceslau CF, Spitler K, Matsumoto T, Webb RC. Toll-like receptors and damage-associated molecular patterns: novel links between inflammation and hypertension. *Am J Physiol Heart Circ Physiol.* (2014) 306:H184–96. doi: 10.1152/ajpheart.00328.2013

Takeda K, Akira S. Toll-like receptors. *Curr Protoc Immunol.* (2015) 109:14 12 11-14 12 10. doi: 10.1002/0471142735.im1412s109

Romero R, Chaiworapongsa T, Espinoza J. Micronutrients and intrauterine infection, preterm birth and the fetal inflammatory response syndrome. *J Nutr.* (2003) 133(5 Suppl. 2):1668S–73S. doi: 10.1093/jn/133.5.1668S

Chaiworapongsa T, Romero R, Espinoza J, Kim YM, Edwin S, Bujold E, et al. Macrophage migration inhibitory factor in patients with preterm parturition and microbial invasion of the amniotic cavity. *J Matern Fetal Neonatal Med.* (2005) 18:405–16. doi: 10.1080/14767050500361703

Tinsley JH, Chiasson VL, Mahajan A, Young KJ, Mitchell BM. Toll-like receptor 3 activation during pregnancy elicits preeclampsia-like symptoms in rats. *Am J Hypertens.* (2009) 22:1314–9. doi: 10.1038/ajh.2009.185

Nizyaeva N, Kulikova G, Nagovitsyna M, Shchegolev A. Peculiarities of the expression of TLR4 and inhibitor of TLR-cascade tollip in the placenta in early and late-onset preeclampsia. *Bull Exp Biol Med.*(2019) 166:507–11. doi: 10.1007/s10517-019-04383-6

Beijar EC, Mallard C, Powell TL. Expression and subcellular localization of TLR-4 in term and first trimester human placenta. *Placenta.* (2006) 27:322– 6.doi: 10.1016/j.placenta.2004.12.012

Chatterjee P, Chiasson VL, Kopriva SE, Young KJ, Chatterjee V, Jones KA, et al. Interleukin 10 deficiency exacerbates toll-like receptor 3-induced preeclampsia-like symptoms in mice. *Hypertension.* (2011) 58:489–96. doi: 10.1161/HYPERTENSIONAHA.111.172114

Chatterjee P, Weaver LE, Doersch KM, Kopriva SE, Chiasson VL, Allen SJ, et al. Placental Toll-like receptor 3 and Toll-like receptor 7/8 activation contributes to preeclampsia in humans and mice. *PLoS ONE.* (2012) 7:e41884. doi: 10.1371/journal.pone.0041884

Pineda A, Verdin-Terán SL, Camacho A, Moreno-Fierros L. Expression of toll-like receptor TLR-2, TLR-3, TLR-4 and TLR-9 is increased in placentas from patients with preeclampsia. *Arch Med Res.* (2011) 42:382–91. doi:10.1016/j.arcmed.2011.08.003

Panda B, Panda A, Ueda I, Abrahams VM, Norwitz ER, Stanic AK, et al. Dendritic cells in the circulation of women with preeclampsia demonstrate a pro-inflammatory bias secondary to dysregulation of TLR receptors. *J Reprod Immunol.* (2012) 94:210–5. doi: 10.1016/j.jri.2012.01.008

He B, Yang X, Li Y, Huang D, Xu X, Yang W, et al. TLR9 (Toll-Like Receptor 9) agonist suppresses angiogenesis by differentially regulating VEGFA (Vascular Endothelial Growth Factor A) and sFLT1 (Soluble Vascular Endothelial Growth Factor Receptor 1) in preeclampsia. *Hypertension.* (2018) 71:671–80. doi:10.1161/HYPERTENSIONAHA.117.10510

Wang J, Wu F, Xie Q, Liu X, Tian F, Xu W, et al. Anakinra and etanercept prevent embryo loss in pregnant nonobese diabetic mice. *Reproduction.* (2015) 149:84. doi: 10.1530/REP-14-0614

Bhat NM, Mithal A, Bieber MM, Herzenberg LA, Teng NN. Human CD5+ B lymphocytes (B-1 cells) decrease in peripheral blood during pregnancy. *J Reprod Immunol.* (1995) 28:53–60. doi: 10.1016/0165-0378 (94)00907-o

Eledel RH, Bassuoni MA, Radwan WM, Masoud A, Eldeeb SM. CD19+ CD5+ B-cell expansion and risk of pre-eclampsia. *Menoufia Med J.* (2016) 29:319. doi: 10.4103/1110-2098.192433

Saito S, Nakashima A, Shima T, Ito M. Th1/Th2/Th17 and regulatory T- cell paradigm in pregnancy. *Am J Reprod Immunol.* (2010) 63:601–10. doi: 10.1111/j.1600-0897.2010.00852.x

Zhong X, Gao W, Degauque N, Bai C, Lu Y, Kenny J, et al. Reciprocal generation of Th1/Th17 and Treg cells by B1 and B2 B cells. *Eur J Immunol.* (2007) 37:2400–4. doi: 10.1002/eji.200737296

Lamarca B, Parrish MR, Wallace K. Agonistic autoantibodies to the angiotensin II type i receptor cause pathophysiologic characteristics of preeclampsia. *Gender Med.* (2012) 9:139–46. doi: 10.1016/j.genm.2012.03.001

Robinson CJ, Johnson DD, Chang EY, Armstrong DM, Wang W. Evaluation of placenta growth factor and soluble Fms-like tyrosine kinase 1 receptor levels in mild and severe preeclampsia. *Am J Obstet Gynecol.* (2006) 195:255– 9. doi: 10.1016/j.ajog.2005.12.049

Erez O, Romero R, Espinoza J, Fu W, Todem D, Kusanovic JP, et al. The change in concentrations of angiogenic and anti-angiogenic factors in maternal plasma between the first and second trimesters in risk assessment for the subsequent development of preeclampsia and small- for-gestational age. *J Matern Fetal Neonatal Med.* (2008) 21:279–87. doi: 10.1080/14767050802034545

Wang W, Irani RA, Zhang Y, Ramin SM, Blackwell SC, Tao L, et al. Autoantibody-mediated complement C3a receptor activation contributes to the pathogenesis of preeclampsia. *Hypertension.* (2012) 60:712–21. doi: 10.1161/HYPERTENSIONAHA.112.191817

Siddiqui AH, Irani RA, Blackwell SC, Ramin SM, Kellems RE, Xia Y. Angiotensin receptor agonistic autoantibody is highly prevalent in preeclampsia: correlation with disease severity. *Hypertension.* (2010) 55:386– 93. doi:10.1161/HYPERTENSIONAHA.109.140061

LaMarca B, Wallace K, Herse F, Wallukat G, Martin JNJr, Weimer A, et al. Hypertension in response to placental ischemia during pregnancy: role of B lymphocytes. *Hypertension.* (2011) 57:865–71. doi: 10.1161/HYPERTENSIONAHA.110.167569

Binder CJ. Natural IgM antibodies against oxidation-specific epitopes. *J Clin Immunol.* (2010) 30:56–60. doi: 10.1007/s10875-010-9396-3

Laule CF, Odean EJ, Wing CR, Root RM, Towner KJ, Hamm CM, et al. Role of B1 and B2 lymphocytes in placental ischemia-induced hypertension. *Am J Physiol Heart Circ Physiol.* (2019) 317:H732–H742. doi: 10.1152/ajpheart.00132.2019

Fox A, Maddox JF, de Veer MJ, Meeusen EN. γδTCR+ cells of the pregnant ovine uterus express variable T cell receptors and contain granulysin. *J Reprod Immunol.* (2010) 84:52–6. doi: 10.1016/j.jri.2009.10.003

Fan D-X, Duan J, Li M-Q, Xu B, Li D-J, Jin L-P. The decidual gamma- delta T cells up-regulate the biological functions of trophoblasts via IL- 10 secretion in early human pregnancy. *Clin Immunol.* (2011) 141:284–92. doi: 10.1016/j.clim.2011.07.008

Talukdar A, Rai R, Sharma KA, Rao D, Sharma A. Peripheral Gamma Delta T cells secrete inflammatory cytokines in women with idiopathic recurrent pregnancy loss. *Cytokine.* (2018) 102:117–22. doi: 10.1016/j.cyto.2017.07.018

Chatterjee P, Chiasson VL, Seerangan G, De Guzman E, Milad M, Bounds KR, et al. Depletion of MHC class II invariant chain peptide or γ-δ T- cells ameliorates experimental preeclampsia. *Clin Sci.* (2017) 131:2047–58. doi: 10.1042/CS20171008

Wu W, Yang H, Feng Y, Zhang P, Li S, Wang X, et al. Polymorphisms in complement genes and risk of preeclampsia in Taiyuan, China. *Inflamm Res.* (2016) 65:837–45. doi: 10.1007/s00011-016-0968-4

Lim R, Lappas M. Decreased expression of complement 3a receptor (C3aR) in human placentas from severe preeclamptic pregnancies. *Eur J Obstetr Gynecol Reprod Biol.* (2012) 165:194–8. doi: 10.1016/j.ejogrb.2012. 08.003

Lokki AI, Heikkinen-Eloranta J, Jarva H, Saisto T, Lokki M-L, Laivuori H, et al. Complement activation and regulation in preeclamptic placenta. *Front Immunol.* (2014) 5:312. doi: 10.3389/fimmu.2014.00312

Burwick RM, Velásquez JA, Valencia CM, Gutiérrez-Marín J, Edna-Estrada F, Silva JL, et al. Terminal complement activation in preeclampsia. *Obstet Gynecol.* (2018) 132:1477–85. doi: 10.1097/AOG.0000000000002980

Banadakoppa M, Vidaeff AC, Yallampalli U, Ramin SM, Belfort MA, Yallampalli C. Complement split products in amniotic fluid in pregnancies subsequently developing early-onset preeclampsia. *Dis Markers.* (2015) 2015. doi: 10.1155/2015/263109

Jia K, Ma L, Wu S, Yan W. Serum levels of complement factors C1q, Bb, and H in normal pregnancy and severe pre-eclampsia. *Med Sci Monit.* (2019) 25:7087. doi: 10.12659/MSM.915777

He Y, Xu B, Song D, Yu F, Chen Q, Zhao M. Expression of the complement system's activation factors in plasma of patients with early/late- onset severe pre-eclampsia. *Am J Reprod Immunol.* (2016) 76:205–11. doi: 10.1111/aji.12541

Guller S, Tang Z, Ma YY, Di Santo S, Sager R, Schneider H. Protein composition of microparticles shed from human placenta during placental perfusion: Potential role in angiogenesis and fibrinolysis in preeclampsia. *Placenta.* (2011) 32:63–9. doi: 10.1016/j.placenta.2010.10.011

Chen Y, Huang Y, Jiang R, Teng Y. Syncytiotrophoblast-derived microparticle shedding in early-onset and late-onset severe pre-eclampsia. *Int J Gynaecol Obstet.* (2012) 119:234–8. doi: 10.1016/j.ijgo.2012.07.010

Goswami D, Tannetta DS, Magee LA, Fuchisawa A, Redman CW, Sargent IL, et al. Excess syncytiotrophoblast microparticle shedding is a feature of early- onset pre-eclampsia, but not normotensive intrauterine growth restriction. *Placenta.* (2006) 27:56–61. doi: 10.1016/j.placenta.2004.11.007

Gilani SI, Weissgerber TL, Garovic VD, Jayachandran M. Preeclampsia and extracellular vesicles. *Curr Hypertens Rep.* (2016) 18:68. doi:10.1007/s11906-016-0678-x

Dragovic RA, Southcombe JH, Tannetta DS, Redman CW, Sargent IL. Multicolor flow cytometry and nanoparticle tracking analysis of extracellular vesicles in the plasma of normal pregnant and pre-eclamptic women. *Biol Reprod.* (2013) 89:151. doi: 10.1095/biolreprod.113.113266

Gardiner C, Tannetta DS, Simms CA, Harrison P, Redman CW, Sargent IL. Syncytiotrophoblast microvesicles released from pre-eclampsia placentae exhibit increased tissue factor activity. *PLoS ONE.* (2011) 6:e26313. doi: 10.1371/journal.pone.0026313

Redman CW, Staff AC. Preeclampsia, biomarkers, syncytiotrophoblast stress, and placental capacity. *Am J Obstet Gynecol.* (2015) 213(4 Suppl.):S9 e1–11. doi: 10.1016/j.ajog.2015.08.003

Yonekura Collier AR, Zsengeller Z, Pernicone E, Salahuddin S, Khankin EV,

Karumanchi SA. Placental sFLT1 is associated with complement activation and syncytiotrophoblast damage in preeclampsia. *Hypertens Pregnancy.* (2019) 38:193–9. doi: 10.1080/10641955.2019.1640725

Flint EJ, Cerdeira AS, Redman CW, Vatish M. The role of angiogenic factors in the management of preeclampsia. *Acta Obstet Gynecol Scand.* (2019) 98:700–7. doi: 10.1111/aogs.13540

O'Brien M, Baczyk D, Kingdom JC. Endothelial dysfunction in severe preeclampsia is mediated by soluble factors, rather than extracellular vesicles. *Sci Rep.* (2017) 7:5887. doi: 10.1038/s41598-017-06178-z

Chatterjee P, Chiasson VL, Pinzur L, Raveh S, Abraham E, Jones KA, et al. Human placenta-derived stromal cells decrease inflammation, placental injury and blood pressure in hypertensive pregnant mice. *Clin Sci.* (2016) 130:513–23. doi: 10.1042/CS20150555

Wang M, Yuan Q, Xie L. Mesenchymal stem cell-based immunomodulation: properties and clinical application. *Stem Cells Int.* (2018) 2018:3057624. doi: 10.1155/2018/3057624

Huang P, Lin LM, Wu XY, Tang QL, Feng XY, Lin GY, et al. Differentiation of human umbilical cord Wharton's jelly-derived mesenchymal stem cells into germ-like cells in vitro. *J Cell Biochem.* (2010) 109:747–54. doi: 10.1002/jcb.22453

Pelekanos RA, Sardesai VS, Futrega K, Lott WB, Kuhn M, Doran MR. Isolation and expansion of mesenchymal stem/stromal cells derived from human placenta tissue. *JoVE.* (2016) 112:e54204. doi: 10.3791/54204

Ayenehdeh JM, Niknam B, Rasouli S, Hashemi SM, Rahavi H, Rezaei N, et al. Immunomodulatory and protective effects of adipose tissue-derived mesenchymal stem cells in an allograft islet composite transplantation for experimental autoimmune type 1 diabetes. *Immunol Lett.* (2017) 188:21–31. doi: 10.1016/j.imlet.2017.05.006

Suvakov S, Cubro H, White WM, Butler Tobah YS, Weissgerber TL, Jordan KL, et al. Targeting senescence improves angiogenic potential of adipose-derived mesenchymal stem cells in patients with preeclampsia. *Biol Sex Differ.* (2019) 10:49. doi: 10.1186/s13293-019-0

Dimitrov R, Kyurkchiev D, Timeva T, Yunakova M, Stamenova M, Shterev A, et al. First-trimester human decidua contains a population of mesenchymal stem cells. *Fertil Steril.* (2010) 93:210–9. doi: 10.1016/j.fertnstert.2008.09.061

Nakashima A, Shima T, Inada K, Ito M, Saito S. The balance of the immune system between T cells and NK cells in miscarriage. *Am J Reprod Immunol.* (2012) 67:304–10. doi: 10.1111/j.1600-0897.2012.01115.x

Croxatto D, Vacca P, Canegallo F, Conte R, Venturini PL, Moretta L, et al. Stromal cells from human decidua exert a strong inhibitory effect on NK cell function and dendritic cell differentiation. *PLoS ONE.* (2014) 9:e89006. doi: 10.1371/journal.pone.0089006

Fu Q, Man X, Yu M, Chu Y, Luan X, Piao H, et al. Human decidua mesenchymal stem cells regulate decidual natural killer cell function via interactions between collagen and leukocyte associated immunoglobulin like receptor 1. *Mol Med Rep.* (2017) 16:2791–8. doi: 10.3892/mmr.2017.6921

Sotiropoulou PA, Perez SA, Gritzapis AD, Baxevanis CN, Papamichail M. Interactions between human mesenchymal stem cells and natural killer cells. *Stem Cells.* (2006) 24:74–85. doi: 10.1634/stemcells.2004-0359

Michelo CM, Fasse E, van Cranenbroek B, Linda K, van der Meer A, Abdelrazik H, et al. Added effects of dexamethasone and mesenchymal stem cells on early Natural Killer cell activation. *Transpl Immunol.* (2016) 37:1–9. doi: 10.1016/j.trim.2016.04.008

Harris SG, Padilla J, Koumas L, Ray D, Phipps RP. Prostaglandins as modulators of immunity. *Trends Immunol.* (2002) 23:144–50. doi: 10.1016/s1471-4906(01)02154-8

Aggarwal S, Pittenger MF. Human mesenchymal stem cells modulate allogeneic immune cell responses. *Blood.* (2005) 105:1815–22. doi: 10.1182/blood-2004-04-1559

Pedersen EB, Christensen NJ, Christensen P, Johannesen P, Kornerup HJ, Kristensen S, et al. Preeclampsia – a state of prostaglandin deficiency? Urinary prostaglandin excretion, the renin-aldosterone system, and circulating catecholamines in preeclampsia. *Hypertension.* (1983) 5:105–11. doi: 10.1161/01.hyp.5.1.105

Abumaree MH, Al Jumah MA, Kalionis B, Jawdat D, Al Khaldi A, Abomaray FM, et al. Human placental mesenchymal stem cells (pMSCs) play a role as immune suppressive cells by shifting macrophage differentiation from inflammatory M1 to anti-inflammatory M2 macrophages. *Stem Cell Rev Rep.* (2013) 9:620–41. doi: 10.1007/s12015-013-9455-2

Jin L, Deng Z, Zhang J, Yang C, Liu J, Han W, et al. Mesenchymal stem cells promote type 2 macrophage polarization to ameliorate the myocardial injury caused by diabetic cardiomyopathy. *J Transl Med.* (2019) 17:251. doi: 10.1186/s12967-019-1999-8

Németh K, Leelahavanichkul A, Yuen PS, Mayer B, Parmelee A, Doi K, et al. Bone marrow stromal cells attenuate sepsis via prostaglandin E 2-dependent reprogramming of host macrophages to increase their interleukin-10 production. *Nat Med.* (2009) 15:42. doi: 10.1038/ nm.1905

Stock SJ, Norman JE. Medicines in pregnancy. *F1000Res.* (2019) 8:911. doi: 10.12688/f1000research.17535.1

Kennedy DA, Lupattelli A, Koren G, Nordeng H. Safety classification of herbal medicines used in pregnancy in a multinational study. *BMC Complement Altern Med.* (2016) 16:102. doi: 10.1186/s12906-016-1079-z

Vishnyakova P, Elchaninov A, Fatkhudinov T, Sukhikh G. Role of the monocyte-macrophage system in normal pregnancy and preeclampsia. *Int J Mol Sci.* (2019) 20:3695. doi: 10.3390/ijms20153695

Gill M, Motta-Mejia C, Kandzija N, Cooke W, Zhang W, Cerdeira AS, et al. Placental syncytiotrophoblast-derived extracellular vesicles carry active NEP (Neprilysin) and are increased in preeclampsia. *Hypertension.* (2019) 73:1112–9. doi: 10.1161/HYPERTENSIONAHA.119.12707

Bavishi C, Messerli FH, Kadosh B, Ruilope LM, Kario K. Role of neprilysin inhibitor combinations in hypertension: insights from hypertension and heart failure trials. *Eur Heart J.* (2015) 36:1967–73. doi: 10.1093/eurheartj/ehv142

Dunlop AL, Mulle JG, Ferranti EP, Edwards S, Dunn AB, Corwin EJ. Maternal microbiome and pregnancy outcomes that impact infant health: a review. *Adv Neonatal Care.* (2015) 15:377–85. doi: 10.1097/ANC.0000000000000218

Brantsaeter AL, Myhre R, Haugen M, Myking S, Sengpiel V, Magnus P, et al. Intake of probiotic food and risk of preeclampsia in primiparous women: the Norwegian Mother and Child Cohort Study. *Am J Epidemiol.* (2011) 174:807–15. doi: 10.1093/aje/kwr168

Pelzer E, Gomez-Arango LF, Barrett HL, Nitert MD. Review: maternal health and the placental microbiome. *Placenta.* (2017) 54:30–7. doi: 10.1016/j.placenta.2016.12.003

Beckers KF, Sones JL. Maternal microbiome and the hypertensive disorder of pregnancy, preeclampsia. *Am J Physiol Heart Circ Physiol.* (2020) 318:H1–10. doi: 10.1152/ajpheart.00469.2019

Ouyang W, O'Garra A. IL-10 family cytokines IL-10 and IL-22: from basic science to clinical translation. *Immunity.* (2019) 50:871–91. doi: 10.1016/j.immuni.2019.03.020

Lai Z, Kalkunte S, Sharma S. A critical role of interleukin-10 in modulating hypoxia-induced preeclampsia-like disease in mice. *Hypertension.* (2011) 57:505–14. doi: 10.1161/HYPERTENSIONAHA.110.163329

Tinsley JH, South S, Chiasson VL, Mitchell BM. Interleukin-10 reduces inflammation, endothelial dysfunction, and blood pressure in hypertensive pregnant rats. *Am J Physiol Regul Integr Comp Physiol.* (2010) 298:R713–9. doi: 10.1152/ajpregu.00712.2009

Ostensen M, Lockshin M, Doria A, Valesini G, Meroni P, Gordon C, et al. Update on safety during pregnancy of biological agents and some immunosuppressive anti-rheumatic drugs. *Rheumatology.* (2008) 47(Suppl. 3):iii28–31. doi: 10.1093/rheumatology/ken168

Roth A, Rottinghaus ST, Hill A, Bachman ES, Kim JS, Schrezenmeier H, et al. Ravulizumab (ALXN1210) in patients with paroxysmal nocturnal hemoglobinuria: results of 2 phase 1b/2 studies. *Blood Adv.* (2018) 2:2176–85. doi: 10.1182/bloodadvances.2018020644

Patra MC, Choi S. Recent progress in the development of Toll-like receptor (TLR) antagonists. *Expert Opin Ther Pat.* (2016) 26:719–30. doi: 10.1080/13543776.2016.1185415

Smith JP, Bingaman SI, Ruggiero F, Mauger DT, Mukherjee A, McGovern CO, et al. Therapy with the opioid antagonist naltrexone promotes mucosal healing in active Crohn's disease: a randomized placebo-controlled trial. *Dig Dis Sci.* (2011) 56:2088–97. doi: 10.1007/s10620-011-1653-7

Cant R, Dalgleish AG, Allen RL. Naltrexone inhibits IL-6 and TNFalpha production in human immune cell subsets following stimulation with ligands for intracellular toll-like receptors. *Front Immunol.* (2017) 8:809. doi: 10.3389/fimmu.2017.00809

Sun J, Wang S, Wei YH. Reproductive toxicity of *Rhizoma Sparganii* (*Sparganium stoloniferum* Buch.-Ham.) in mice: mechanisms of anti-angiogenesis and anti-estrogen pharmacologic activities. *J Ethnopharmacol.* (2011) 137:1498–503. doi: 10.1016/j.jep.2011.08.026

Caputi V, Giron MC. Microbiome-gut-brain axis and toll-like receptors in Parkinson's Disease. *Int J Mol Sci.* (2018) 19:1689. doi: 10.3390/ijms19061689

Abais-Battad JM, Dasinger JH, Fehrenbach DJ, Mattson DL. Novel adaptive and innate immunity targets in hypertension. *Pharmacol Res.* (2017) 120:109–15. doi: 10.1016/j.phrs.2017.03.015

Liu M, Peng J, Tai N, Pearson JA, Hu C, Guo J, et al. Toll-like receptor 9 negatively regulates pancreatic islet beta cell growth and function in a mouse model of type 1 diabetes. *Diabetologia*. (2018) 61:2333–43. doi: 10.1007/s00125-018-4705-0

Thaxton JE, Romero R, Sharma S. TLR9 activation coupled to IL-10 deficiency induces adverse pregnancy outcomes. *J Immunol*. (2009) 183:1144–54. doi: 10.4049/jimmunol.0900788

Kuzmich NN, Sivak KV, Chubarev VN, Porozov YB, Savateeva-Lyubimova TN, Peri F. TLR4 signaling pathway modulators as potential therapeutics in inflammation and sepsis. *Vaccines*. (2017) 5:34. doi: 10.3390/vaccines5040034

Lan J, Zhao Y, Dong F, Yan Z, Zheng W, Fan J, et al. Meta-analysis of the effect and safety of berberine in the treatment of type 2 diabetes mellitus, hyperlipemia and hypertension. *J Ethnopharmacol*. (2015) 161:69–81. doi: 10.1016/j.jep.2014.09.049

Xie L, Zhang D, Ma H, He H, Xia Q, Shen W, et al. The effect of berberine on reproduction and metabolism in women with polycystic ovary syndrome: a systematic review and meta-analysis of randomized control trials. *Evid Based Complement Alternat Med*. (2019) 2019:7918631. doi: 10.1155/2019/7918631

Chu M, Ding R, Chu ZY, Zhang MB, Liu XY, Xie SH, et al. Role of berberine in anti-bacterial as a high-affinity LPS antagonist binding to TLR4/MD-2 receptor. *BMC Complement Altern Med*. (2014) 14:89. doi: 10.1186/1472-6882-14-89

National Center for Complementary and Integrative Health. *Goldenseal*. (2016) Available online at: https://www.nccih.nih.gov/health/goldenseal (accessed May 16, 2020)

Pareek A, Suthar M, Rathore GS, Bansal V. Feverfew (*Tanacetum parthenium* L.): a systematic review. *Pharmacogn Rev*. (2011) 5:103–10. doi: 10.4103/0973-7847.79105

Ernst E. Herbal medicinal products during pregnancy: are they safe? *BJOG*. (2002) 109:227–35. doi: 10.1111/j.1471-0528.2002.t01-1-01009.x

Zuurbier CJ, Abbate A, Cabrera-Fuentes HA, Cohen MV, Collino M, De Kleijn DPV, et al. Innate immunity as a target for acute cardioprotection. *Cardiovasc Res*. (2019) 115:1131–42. doi: 10.1093/cvr/cvy304

Morrison TJ, Jackson MV, Cunningham EK, Kissenpfennig A, McAuley DF, O'Kane CM, et al. Mesenchymal stromal cells modulate macrophages in clinically relevant lung injury models by extracellular vesicle mitochondrial transfer. *Am J Respir Crit Care Med*. (2017) 196:1275–86. doi: 10.1164/rccm.201701-0170OC

Tronnes JN, Lupattelli A, Nordeng H. Safety profile of medication used during pregnancy: results of a multinational European study. *Pharmacoepidemiol Drug Saf*. (2017) 26:802–11. doi: 10.1002/pds.4213

Sheffield JS, Siegel D, Mirochnick M, Heine RP, Nguyen C, Bergman KL, et al. Designing drug trials: considerations for pregnant women. *Clin Infect Dis*. (2014) 59(Suppl. 7):S437–44. doi: 10.1093/cid/ciu709

Young AN, Moyle-Heyrman G, Kim JJ, Burdette JE. Microphysiologic systems in female reproductive biology. *Exp Biol Med*. (2017) 242:1690–700. doi: 10.1177/1535370217697386

Gao W, Xiong Y, Li Q, Yang H. Inhibition of toll-like receptor signaling as a promising therapy for inflammatory diseases: a journey from molecular to nano therapeutics. *Front Physiol*. (2017) 8:508. doi: 10.3389/fphys.2017.00508

Myatt L, Roberts JM. Preeclampsia: syndrome or disease? *Curr Hypertens Rep*. (2015) 17:83. doi: 10.1007/s11906-015-0595-4

Miller CP, Shin W, Ahn EH, Kim HJ, Kim D-H. Engineering microphysiological immune system responses on chips. *Trends Biotechnol*. (2020) 38:857–72. doi: 10.1016/j.tibtech.2020.01.003

Proteomic Study of Fetal Membrane: Inflammation-Triggered Proteolysis of Extracellular Matrix May Present a Pathogenic Pathway for Spontaneous Preterm Birth

Jing Pan[1†], Xiujuan Tian[1†], Honglei Huang[2†] and Nanbert Zhong[3]*

[1] Sanya Maternity and Child Care Hospital, Sanya, China, [2] Proteomic Core Facility, Oxford University, Oxford, United Kingdom, [3] New York State Institute for Basic Research in Developmental Disabilities, Staten Island, NY, United States

*Correspondence:
Nanbert Zhong
nanbert.zhong@opwdd.ny.gov
†These authors have contributed equally to this work

Introduction: Spontaneous preterm birth (sPTB), which predominantly presents as spontaneous preterm labor (sPTL) or prelabor premature rupture of membranes (PPROM), is a syndrome that accounts for 5–10% of live births annually. The long-term morbidity in surviving preterm infants is significantly higher than that in full-term neonates. The causes of sPTB are complex and not fully understood. Human placenta, the maternal and fetal interface, is an environmental core of fetal intrauterine life, mediates fetal oxygen exchange, nutrient uptake, and waste elimination and functions as an immune-defense organ. In this study, the molecular signature of preterm birth placenta was assessed and compared to full-term placenta by proteomic profiling.

Materials and Methods: Four groups of fetal membranes (the amniochorionic membranes), with five cases in each group in the discovery study and 30 cases in each group for validation, were included: groups A: sPTL; B: PPROM; C: full-term birth (FTB); and D: full-term premature rupture of membrane (PROM). Fetal membranes were dissected and used for proteome quantification study. Maxquant and Perseus were used for protein quantitation and statistical analysis. Both fetal membranes and placental villi samples were used to validate proteomic discovery.

Results: Proteomics analysis of fetal membranes identified 2,800 proteins across four groups. Sixty-two proteins show statistical differences between the preterm and full-term groups. Among these differentially expressed proteins are (1) proteins involved in inflammation (HPGD), T cell activation (PTPRC), macrophage activation (CAPG, CD14, and CD163), (2) cell adhesion (ICAM and ITGAM), (3) proteolysis (CTSG, ELANE, and MMP9), (4) antioxidant (MPO), (5) extracellular matrix (ECM) proteins (APMAP, COL4A1, LAMA2, LMNB1, LMNB2, FBLN2, and CSRP1) and (6) metabolism of glycolysis (PKM and ADPGK), fatty acid synthesis (ACOX1 and ACSL3), and energy biosynthesis (ATP6AP1 and CYBB).

Conclusion: Our molecular signature study of preterm fetal membranes revealed inflammation as a major event, which is inconsistent with previous findings. Proteolysis may play an important role in fetal membrane rupture. Extracellular matrix s have been altered in preterm fetal membranes due to proteolysis. Metabolism was also altered in preterm fetal membranes. The molecular changes in the fetal membranes provided a significant molecular signature for PPROM in preterm syndrome.

Keywords: fetal membrane, preterm birth, prelabor premature rupture of membrane, inflammation, extracellular matrix

INTRODUCTION

Preterm birth refers to infants born alive before 37 weeks of gestation (Quinn et al., 2016). Preterm birth accounts for 5–12% of all live births worldwide (Gezer et al., 2018). As a populated country, China has about 1.17 million preterm infants birth every year (World Health Organization [WHO], 2018). In particular, since 2016, when the Chinese government relaxed the one-child policy and implemented its two-children policy, many women of high maternal age rushed to have a second child (Cheng and Duan, 2016). It has been demonstrated that pregnancy at 40 years of age and older is strongly associated with preterm birth and other disorders of pregnancy (Fuchs et al., 2018). In preterm newborns, the brain, lung, liver, and other organs are not fully developed, and there is a high incidence of brain injury, neonatal respiratory distress syndrome, bilirubin encephalopathy, and multiple organ failure (Fraser et al., 2004; Bhutani and Wong, 2013; Paton et al., 2017). It is estimated by the WHO that preterm birth is the most common cause of children's death under the age of 5 years (World Health Organization [WHO], 2018). Preterm birth brings a great economic burden to families, communities, and societies.

The placenta serves as the interface between the pregnant mother and the intrauterine fetus, with the main function of exchanging the material between the fetus and the mother, providing the oxygen and nutrients required for embryonic, as well as fetal, development, and excreting metabolic waste and CO_2 (Gude et al., 2004). In addition, the placenta also serves as a barrier to bacteria, pathogens, and drugs because of the existence of the placental barrier (Zeldovich et al., 2013). The placenta can also synthesize chorionic gonadotropin, human placental lactogen (hPL), estrogen, progesterone, cytokine, and growth factors (Costa, 2016). In addition, the placenta has immune tolerance to the fetus (Guleria and Sayegh, 2007). Therefore, abnormal placental function has a direct correlation with the occurrence of preterm birth. So far, estrogens, hPL, placenta growth factor (PLGF), human chorionic gonadotrophin (hCG), plasma protein A (PAPP-A), placental protein 13 (PP-13), pregnancy-specific glycoproteins, and progesterone metabolites have been employed as surrogate markers of placental function (Heazell et al., 2015). Despite recent progress on the study of these markers associated with function of placenta, a comprehensive and systemic understanding of the pathophysiology of the placenta is lacking, particularly little is known about the pathogenic role of fetal membrane and its involvement in the development of spontaneous preterm birth (sPTB). Here, we studied the protein expression of fetal membrane, with the aim to understand the pathophysiology of fetal membrane and to identify novel molecules associated with preterm birth in the fetal membrane. This study not only provides theoretical support for the occurrence of preterm birth, but also provides reference for the early diagnosis and early intervention of premature birth.

MATERIALS AND METHODS

Specimens

The study was approved by the Hospital Ethics Committee of Sanya Maternity and Child Care Hospital and the informed consent was obtained from pregnant women to permit the use of placentas in research studies. A retrospective study was designed to investigate the pathological alteration of protein expression with a pre-banked birth cohort of 20 placentas, which were grouped as (A): spontaneous preterm labor (sPTL), defined as a non-medical and/or non-selective spontaneous birth delivered between 20^{+1} and 36^{+6} gestational week (GW) in which regular contractions of the uterus result in changes in the cervix before 37 weeks of pregnancy, (B): prelabor premature rupture of membranes (PPROM) that occurred between 20^{+1} and 36^{+6} GW, (C): full-term birth (FTB) between 39^{+1} and 40^{+6} GW, and (D): full-term premature rupture of membrane (PROM). There were five placentas in each group. The placentas were collected from fetal membranes through full layers to the decidua. Fetal membranes were dissected within 2 cm of the edge where the membrane naturally ruptured during labor. However, if a rupture hole could be identified in the premature rupture (PPROM and PROM) cases, the membrane would be collected within 1 cm around the hole where the premature rupture occurred.

Criteria for Inclusion and Exclusion

Tissues selected from prebanked samples had to meet the following criteria: (i) age of the pregnant woman is 18–45 years, (ii) no clinically recognized infection/inflammation (INF) before and/or during pregnancy (INF is determined by phenotypically notable fever, increased counts of peripheral white blood cells, and/or increased IL6 and/or TNFα), (iii) primipara and singleton without history of miscarriage or abortion, (iv) vaginal delivery with (PPROM and PROM) or without (FTB and sPTL) premature rupture of chorioamniotic membrane,

TABLE 1 | Demographic and clinical information about placentas.

Group	A	B	C	D
Birth	sPTL	PPROM	FTB	PROM
Pregnant age (year old)	22-28	22-30	22-25	22-26
Gestational age (weeks)	29^{+3}–31^{+6}	30^{+0}–32^{+1}	40^{+0}–40^{+6}	39^{+0}–40^{+6}
Primipara	Yes	Yes	Yes	Yes
Singleton	Yes	Yes	Yes	Yes
Mode of delivery	Spontaneous	Spontaneous	Spontaneous	Spontaneous
Family history of preterm birth	No	No	No	No
Family history of birth defect	No	No	No	No
Infection history during pregnancy	No	No	No	No
Gestational complication	No	No	No	No
Use of antibiotics during pregnancy	No	No	No	No
Use of steroid	No	No	No	No
Inform consent obtained	Yes	Yes	Yes	Yes

(v) no vaginal bleeding during the pregnancy, (vi) no other pregnancy-related complication(s) and no clinical intervention with antibiotics, steroids, or tocolytics during the pregnancy, (vii) no family history of birth defects, and (viii) no consanguinity. Any cases not meeting the above criteria were excluded. Details of demographic and clinical information for the samples studied are provided in **Table 1**.

Protein Extraction From Placenta Membrane for Proteomic Analysis

The human placental amniochorionic membrane, or fetal membrane, was dissected (20- to 30-mg cross-sections) and first washed with cold PBS containing protease inhibitor (Sigma-Aldrich, United Kingdom), then placed in beads-beater tubes containing RIPA lysis buffer (Thermo Fisher Scientific, United Kingdom) to make it 50 mg/ml. Tissues were homogenized four times at 6,500 Hz for 40 s in a beads-beater (Stretton, United Kingdom) (**Figure 1**). The samples were centrifuged at 10,000 g for 5 min at 4°C to remove insoluble tissue debris. The protein concentration in the homogenates was determined by BCA assay (Thermo Fisher Scientific, United Kingdom), and 100 μg of total proteins were added to a 30-kDa filter (Merck Millipore, United Kingdom). Proteins were reduced by 10 mM Dithiothreitol (DTT) (Sigma, United Kingdom) at 37°C for 1 h and then alkylated with 40 mM iodoacetamide (IAA, Sigma, United Kingdom) for 45 min in the dark, at room temperature. Samples were centrifuged for 20 min at 14,000 g to remove DTT and IAA, followed by buffer exchange with 8 M urea twice and 50 mM ammonia bicarbonate three times. One hundred microliters of trypsin were added at a trypsin/protein ratio of 1:50 for digestion at 37°C overnight. Digested peptides were collected by upside down spin, and membrane filters were washed twice with 0.5 M NaCl and water, respectively. The peptides were purified by a SepPak C18 cartridge (Waters, United Kingdom), dried by SpeedVac centrifugation, and resuspended in buffer A (2% acetonitrile, 0.1% formic acid) for LC-MS/MS analysis.

Peptide Measurement by Mass Spectrometry

LC-MS/MS analysis was carried out by nano-ultra performance liquid chromatography tandem mass spectrometry analysis using a 75-μm-inner diameter × 25 cm C18 nanoAcquity UPLC column (1.7-μm particle size, Waters, United Kingdom). Peptides were separated with a 120-min gradient of 3–40% solvent B (solvent A: 99.9% H_2O, 0.1% formic acid; solvent B: 99.9% ACN, 0.1% formic acid) at 250 nl/min and injected into a Q Exactive High Field (HF) Hybrid Quadrupole-Orbitrap Mass Spectrometer (Thermo Fisher Scientific, United Kingdom) acquiring data in electron spray ionization (ESI) positive mode. The MS survey was set with a resolution of 60,000 FWHM, with a recording window between 300 and 2,000 m/z. A maximum of 20 MS/MS scans were triggered in data-dependent acquisition (DDA) mode.

Protein Identification and Quantification

MaxQuant software (v1.5.8.3, Max Planck Institute of Biochemistry, Germany) was used for peptide and protein identification and quantitation. Data generated from MS/MS spectra were searched against the Uniprot human database (version 2017); 20,205 entries were used for peptide homology identification. The false discovery rate (FDR) was set to 1% for protein and peptide identification. Proteins were quantified by at least one unique peptide, and match between run was selected to increase the quantifiable value cross samples (**Figure 1**). Label-free quantitation (LFQ) intensity data were used for further analysis and comparisons across the variant groups. Statistical analysis was assessed by using Persus software (version 1.5.5.3, Max Planck Institute of Biochemistry). Statistical comparisons between the groups were performed by using two-sided unpaired Student's t-test. Firstly, threshold p-value was used to define statistical significance. Secondly, permutation-based FDR was used to assess truncate data.

Validation of Differentially Expressed Proteins With Western Blot

Ten milligrams of fetal membranes or placental villi were dissected and lysed in RIPA buffer containing protease inhibitors (Roche, United States). Western blot analysis was performed by loading 15 μg of proteins on 4–12% pre-cast Bis-Tris gels (Bio-Rad, United States) and transferred to PVDF membranes (Merck Millipore, United States). Membranes were incubated with mouse anti-human MPO monoclonal antibody (Santa Cruz, United States, 1:200 diluted in 2% milk), mouse anti-human elastase, neutrophil expressed (ELANE) monoclonal antibody

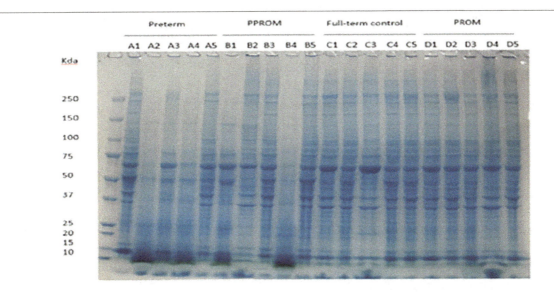

FIGURE 1 | Protein expression pattern on SDS-PAGE gel from four groups of fetal membrane. Group A: sPTL (preterm), group B: PPROM, group C: FTB, and group D: PROM. Five individual samples in each group were analyzed on an 8% SDS-PAGE stained with a dye of Instantblue.

(Santa Cruz, United States, 1:200 diluted in 2% milk), mouse anti-human GAPDH monoclonal antibody (Thermo Fisher Scientific, United Kingdom, 1:2,000 diluted in 2% milk), rabbit anti-human beta-actin antibody (Abcam, United Kingdom, 1:1,000 diluted in 2% milk). Dye-800-conjugated secondary antibodies were applied and visualized with an Odyssey Clx (Li-Cor, United States). Image studio (Li-Cor, United States) and Image J (Schneider et al., 2012) were used for Western blot quantitation, and one-way ANOVA was used for statistical significance test.

RESULTS

Quality Control of Proteins Isolated From the Fetal Membrane Tissues

Protein lysates of fetal membranes were run on SDS-PAGE and visualized with InstantBlue (**Figure 1**). Protein partial degradation was detected in samples of A2, A4 and B1, B4. The protein patterns of the rest of samples did not show a clear difference.

Differentially Expressed Proteins Identified From Mass Spectra

After LC-MS/MS measurement, Maxquant analysis identified a total of 2,880 proteins from fetal membrane samples. The hierarchical clustering analysis indicated protein abundance alteration between individual samples. In addition to comparisons of the preterm group (A + B) with the full-term control group (C + D), individual comparisons were applied to identified specific protein(s) that are associated with a specific condition (**Figure 2**). Protein differential expression was defined by the criteria of $p < 0.01$, fold change (FC) ≥ 2, and permutation-based FDR 0.05, with which, 62 (38 up-regulated and 24 down-regulated) proteins were identified to be differentially expressed (**Tables 2a,b**). Among these 62 proteins, 20 were identified to be the top-listed FC (four were down-regulated and 16 were up-regulated). The FCs of 8 of 20 up-regulated proteins were >11, among which MMP9 showed 318.64 FC as the highest (**Table 3**). All differentially expressed proteins identified from fetal membranes in sPTB (sPTL and PPROM) were subjected to Kyoto Encyclopedia of Genes and Genomes (KEGG) analysis to identify the pathways that may be associated with the sPTB. The top-scoring pathways were infection and inflammation, protein degradation and proteolysis, extracellular matrix (ECM), cell adhesion, antioxidant, glycolysis, and fatty acid (FA) oxidation (**Table 4**).

Validation of Differentially Expressed Proteins With Western Blots

Three proteins, MPO, ELANE, and GAPDH, which were shown by LC-MS/MS to be differentially expressed in fetal membrane, were randomly selected to validate the differential expression value of protein with Western blots. Westerns blot of MPO and ELANE showed the same protein expression pattern as proteome data with statistical significance. While GAPDH followed a similar increase of protein expression in fetal membrane compared to placental villi, it had a decreased expression in fetal membrane of preterm cases, including both sPTL and PPROM, compared to FTB and PROM (groups C and D) (**Figure 3**).

DISCUSSION

Placental Function and Preterm Birth

PTB plays a significant adverse impact on the increased mortality and mobility of preterm-born neonates. The etiology

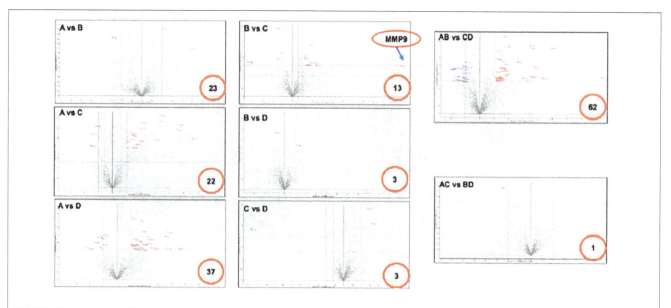

FIGURE 2 | Volcano plot of differentially expressed proteins in fetal membranes. Various comparisons identified specific protein(s) that associated with the premature condition. Number in the red circle indicates the number of differential proteins with statistical significance. X-axis indicates fold changes and Y-axis indicates p value-log Student t-test. A: sPTL, B: PPROM, C: FTB, and D: PROM.

of sPTB is multi-factorial; however, placental dysfunction has been identified as the leading cause of premature birth due to it pivotal role between the fetus and mother during pregnancy (Audette and Kingdom, 2018). As a result of the pathophysiological changes in placental dysfunction, including poor trophoblast uterine invasion and impaired transformation of the uterine spiral arteries to high capacity and low impedance vessels, which eventually leads to lower blood flow to the placenta (Ilekis et al., 2016; Cuffe et al., 2017), the placenta was unable to sustain fetal development requirements and thus preterm birth occurred. Searches for molecular markers to predict preterm birth have been conducted mainly in the maternal blood due to its richness of information and easy accessibility. It has been reported that PP-13 and PAPP-A are good predictors of preterm birth (Stout et al., 2013). Elevated maternal serum–soluble fms-like tryrosine 1 (sFlt1), inflammation marker [cysteine-rich protein (CRP)], and PIGF are associated with preterm birth (Bastek et al., 2011; Straughen et al., 2012). However, these markers have little clinical use for the prediction of preterm birth or for understanding the pathophysiology of placental dysfunction. Therefore, we conducted an unbiased proteomic analysis of the placenta in preterm birth compared to in full-term controls, followed by various comparisons to generate differentially expressed proteins specific to one single variation. Such comparisons include group B vs. group C, for example, in which the outcome of differentially expressed proteins was influenced only by premature rupture of fetal membrane in PPROM (B) vs. FTB without rupture of membrane (C). In addition, such comparisons may reduce non-specific noise, such as the comparison of group A vs. group D, in which the differentially expressed proteins would likely have resulted from the premature labor that was related to muscle contraction of uterine but not to rupture of membrane.

Proteins Involved in Infection and Inflammation

Based on molecular function, the top-scoring proteins differentially expressed in fetal membranes of sPTB have been clustered into five groups *via* their involvement in pathophysiological pathways (**Table 3**). The main pathophysiological changes in the fetal membrane from preterm birth were inflammation. Numerous studies indicated that placental intrauterine infection was strongly associated with sPTL or PPROM (Salafia et al., 1991; Helmig et al., 2002; Morgan, 2016; Pugni et al., 2016; Chisholm et al., 2018).

A study in humans demonstrated that HPGD expression in preterm-labor placenta tissues was decreased in comparison with a full-term labor group (He et al., 2015). HPGD is a member of the short-chain non-metalloenzyme alcohol dehydrogenases protein family and is responsible for the degradation of prostaglandins, hormones that modulate the inflammatory response (Aoki and Narumiya, 2012; Seo and Oh, 2017). Another study in an animal model detected high expression levels of HPGD at the beginning and at normal term of pregnancy, indicating that HPGD may play a role during the establishment and termination of gestation (von Hof et al., 2017). Our data are consistent with previously findings. The lower level of HPGD found in fetal membranes suggested a higher level of inflammatory states in the preterm group (sPTL + PPROM), possibly through negative regulation of inflammatory molecule prostaglandins.

PTPRC is a receptor-type protein tyrosine phosphatase that regulates cell growth, differentiation, and mitosis. PTPRC is

TABLE 2a | Proteins identified from fetal membranes associated with preterm birth (AB vs. CD): up-regulated.

Majority protein IDs	Protein names	Gene names	Protein family	Pathways	Functions
Q9HDC9; H0Y512; Q9HDC9-2	Adipocyte plasma membrane-associated protein	APMAP	Adipocyte plasma membrane-associated protein (PTHR10426:SF26)		
Q15904; A0A0C4DGX8	V-type proton ATPase subunit S1	ATP6AP1	V-type proton ATPase subunit S1 (PTHR12471:SF2)	Energy metabolism	ATP synthase
Q93050-1; Q93050; Q93050-3; B7Z641; B7Z2A9; F5H1T6	V-type proton ATPase 116 kDa subunit a isoform 1; V-type proton ATPase subunit a	ATP6V0A1	V-type proton ATPase 116 kDa subunit a isoform 1 (PTHR11629:SF68)	Energy metabolism	ATP synthase
F5GYQ1; P61421; J3QL14; R4GN72	V-type proton ATPase subunit d 1	ATP6V0D1	V-type proton ATPase subunit d 1 (PTHR11028:SF3)	Energy metabolism	ATP synthase
A6NC48; Q10588; H0Y984; Q10588-2	ADP-ribosyl cyclase/cyclic ADP-ribose hydrolase 2	BST1	ADP-ribosyl cyclase/cyclic ADP-ribose hydrolase 2 (PTHR10912:SF4)		
A0A0A0MSV6; D6R934; P02746; D6RGJ1	Complement C1q subcomponent subunit B	C1QB	Complement C1q subcomponent subunit B (PTHR44403:SF2)		NAD metabolism and Innate Immune System
B4DPQ0; P00736; F5H2D0	Complement C1r subcomponent; Complement C1r subcomponent heavy chain; Complement C1r subcomponent light chain	C1R	Complement C1r subcomponent (PTHR45206:SF1)		
P08571; D6RFL4	Monocyte differentiation antigen CD14; Monocyte differentiation antigen CD14, urinary form; Monocyte differentiation antigen CD14, membrane-bound form	CD14	Monocyte differentiation antigen CD14 (PTHR10630:SF3)	Toll receptor signaling pathway (P00054)	
F5GZZ9; Q86VB7-3; Q86VB7; Q86VB7-2; C9JHR8; Q86VB7-4	Scavenger receptor cysteine-rich type 1 protein M130; Soluble CD163	CD163	Scavenger receptor cysteine-rich type 1 protein M130 (PTHR19331:SF392)	Macrophages function	Acute phase-regulated receptor involved in clearance and endocytosis of hemoglobin/haptoglobin complexes by macrophages
H0YD13; P16070-18; P16070-12; P16070-14; P16070-13; P16070-11; P16070-10; P16070-16; P16070-8; P16070-17; P16070-6; P16070-4; P16070-3; P16070-7; P16070-5; P16070; H0Y2P0; H0YE40	CD44 antigen	CD44	CD44 antigen (PTHR10225:SF6)		
F8VNT9; F8VV56; F8W022; F8VWK8; P08962-3; P08962-2; P08962	Tetraspanin; CD63 antigen	CD63	CD63 antigen (PTHR19282:SF233)		
P02452	Collagen alpha-1 (I) chain	COL1A1	Collagen alpha-1(I) chain (PTHR24023:SF569)	Integrin signaling pathway (P00034)	Extracellular matrix structural constituent
P02462-2; P02462	Collagen alpha-1(IV) chain; Arresten	COL4A1	Collagen alpha-1(IV) chain (PTHR24023:SF854)	Integrin signaling pathway (P00034)	Extracellular matrix structural constituent

(Continued)

TABLE 2a | Continued

Majority protein IDs	Protein names	Gene names	Protein family	Pathways	Functions
P08311	Cathepsin G	CTSG	Cathepsin G (PTHR24271:SF13)	Protein degradation	Proteolysis
P04839	Cytochrome b-245 heavy chain	CYBB	Cytochrome b-245 heavy chain (PTHR11972:SF60)	Energy metabolism	ATP synthase/oxidase
P08246	Neutrophil elastase	ELANE	Neutrophil elastase (PTHR24257:SF16)	Protein degradation	Proteolysis/phagocytosis
A0A0D9SEN1;Q12884; B4DLR2	Prolyl endopeptidase FAP; Antiplasmin-cleaving enzyme FAP, soluble form	FAP	Prolyl endopeptidase FAP (PTHR11731:SF136)	UPS	Ubiquitin-protein ligase activity (ubiquitin proteasome system)
P98095-2; P98095	Fibulin-2	FBLN2	Fibulin-2 (PTHR44887:SF1)		
Q86UX7-2; Q86UX7;F5H1C6	Fermitin family homolog 3	FERMT3	Fermitin family homolog 3 (PTHR16160:SF1)		
P02792	Ferritin light chain	FTL	Ferritin light chain (PTHR11431:SF47)		
P11413; P11413-3; P11413-2; E9PD92; E7EM57; E7EUI8	Glucose-6-phosphate 1-dehydrogenase	G6PD	Glucose-6-phosphate 1-dehydrogenase (PTHR23429:SF0)	Glycolysis	Glycolysis
P05204; A0A087WZE9; Q15651-2; Q15651	Non-histone chromosomal protein HMG-17; High mobility group nucleosome-binding domain-containing protein 3	HMGN2;HMGN3			
P05362; K7EKL8	Intercellular adhesion molecule 1	ICAM1	Intercellular adhesion molecule 1 (PTHR13771:SF9)		Cell adhesion signaling
P11215; P11215-2	Integrin alpha-M	ITGAM	Integrin alpha-M (PTHR23220:SF120)	Inflammation mediated by chemokine and cytokine signaling pathway (P00031)/Integrin signaling pathway (P00034)	
A0A087WX80; P24043; A0A087WYF1	Laminin subunit alpha-2	LAMA2	Laminin subunit alpha-2 (PTHR10574:SF291)	Integrin signaling pathway (P00034)	Extracellular matrix linker protein receptor
P20700; E9PBF6; A0A0D9SFE5	Lamin-B1	LMNB1	Lamin-B1 (PTHR23239:SF157)	FAS signaling pathway (P00020)	Structural molecule activity
Q03252	Lamin-B2	LMNB2	Lamin-B2 (PTHR23239:SF152)	FAS signaling pathway (P00020)	Structural molecule activity
P14780	Matrix metalloproteinase-9; 67 kDa matrix metalloproteinase-9; 82 kDa matrix metalloproteinase-9	MMP9	Matrix metalloproteinase-9 (PTHR10201:SF30)	Plasminogen activating cascade (P00050)/CCKR signaling(P06959)	Collagenases (degrade collagen)
P05164-2; P05164; P05164-3	Myeloperoxidase; Myeloperoxidase; 89 kDa myeloperoxidase; 84 kDa myeloperoxidase; Myeloperoxidase light chain; Myeloperoxidase heavy chain	MPO	Myeloperoxidase (PTHR11475:SF108)		Antioxidant (GO:0016209)

(Continued)

TABLE 2a | Continued

Majority protein IDs	Protein names	Gene names	Protein family	Pathways	Functions
Q8IXM6; H0Y6T6; Q8IXM6-2	Nurim	NRM	Nurim (PTHR31040:SF1)		
Q14980-2; Q14980; A0A087WY61; Q14980-4; Q14980-3; Q14980-5	Nuclear mitotic apparatus protein 1	NUMA1	Nuclear mitotic apparatus protein 1 (PTHR18902:SF24)		
Q03405; Q03405-3; M0R0Y4; M0QYR6; M0R1I2; Q03405-2	Urokinase plasminogen activator surface receptor	PLAUR	Urokinase plasminogen activator surface receptor (PTHR10624:SF6)	Plasminogen activating cascade (P00050)/Blood coagulation (P00011)	
A2ACR1; P28065-2; P28065; A0A0G2JJA7; A2ACR0	Proteasome subunit beta type; Proteasome subunit beta type-9	PSMB9	Proteasome subunit beta type-9 (PTHR11599:SF50)	UPS	Ubiquitin proteasome system
X6R433; A0A0A0MT22; P08575-2; P08575; M3ZCP1; A0A075B788; E9PKH0	Protein-tyrosine-phosphatase; Receptor-type tyrosine-protein phosphatase C	PTPRC	Receptor-type tyrosine-protein phosphatase C (PTHR19134:SF284)	JAK/STAT signaling pathway (P00038)/B cell activation (P00010)/T cell activation (P00053)	T cell activation (P00053)
P05109	Protein S100-A8; Protein S100-A8, N-terminally processed	S100A8	Protein S100-A8 (PTHR11639:SF5)		Calmodulin signaling
P06702	Protein S100-A9	S100A9	Protein S100-A9 (PTHR11639:SF79)		Calmodulin signaling
P01011; G3V595; G3V3A0	Alpha-1-antichymotrypsin; Alpha-1-antichymotrypsin His-Pro-less	SERPINA3	Alpha-1-antichymotrypsin (PTHR11461:SF145)		Proteolysis (inhibitor)
A0A0C4DFU2; P04179; P04179-4; F5H4R2; A0A0C4DFU1; F5GYZ5; P04179-2; F5H3C5; G8JLJ2; A0A0C4DG56; P04179-3	Superoxide dismutase;Superoxide dismutase [Mn], mitochondrial	SOD2	Superoxide dismutase [Mn], mitochondrial (PTHR11404:SF6)		Antioxidant defense activity

essential to regulate T- and B-cell antigen receptor signaling by direct interaction with antigen receptor complexes or by activating Src family kinases (Pike and Tremblay, 2013). PTPRC also regulates cytokine receptor signaling by suppressing JAK kinase (Porcu et al., 2012). It has been reported that PTPRC is dysregulated in human miscarriage (Lorenzi et al., 2012). Increased levels of PTPRC in the fetal membranes of sPTB indicated activation of T- and B-cell antigen receptor signaling and suggested that sPTB may share a common pathophysiological mechanism with miscarriage.

Macrophage activation (CAPG, CD14, and CD163): CAPG is a member of the gelsolin/villin family of actin-regulatory proteins. CAPG reversibly blocks the barbed ends of F-actin filaments in a Ca^{2+}-dependent manner, thus capping the barbed ends of actin filaments and controlling actin-based motility of macrophages (Young et al., 1994). CD14 is a surface protein preferentially expressed on macrophages or monocytes. It mediates the innate immune response to bacterial lipopolysaccharide (Mogensen, 2009). A study in an animal model indicated that increased expression of TLR2 and CD14 was correlated with urea plasma parvum–induced fetal inflammatory response syndrome-like pathology (Allam et al., 2014). CD163 is a member of the scavenger receptor cysteine-rich superfamily and functions as an innate immune sensor for bacteria and an inducer of local inflammation (Fabriek et al., 2009). High levels of CD163 are associated with an increased risk of preterm delivery in pregnant women (Vogel et al., 2005). The detection of CAPG, CD14, and CD163 suggested the activation of macrophage or monocyte, even though we do not know what pathogen causes are.

Extracellular Matrix, Proteolysis, and Cell Adhesion

COL4A1, LAMA2, FBLN2, and APMAP are the ECM proteins. COL4A1 is an integral component of all basement membranes; it not only provides structural support, regulating adhesion, migration, and survival of cells, but also plays a key role in early placentation by modeling trophoblast cell invasion to remodel maternal spiral arteries and ensure sufficient blood flow to the developing fetus (Oefner et al., 2015). LAMA2 is a major component of the basement membrane and mediates the attachment and migration of cells into tissues during embryonic development by interacting with other ECMs. FBLN2 is an ECM protein belonging to the fibulin family. APMAP is a novel regulator of ECM components that may serve as a potential target to mitigate obesity-associated insulin resistance (Pessentheiner et al., 2017). The exact functions of LAMA2, FBLN2, and APMAP in the placenta are not clear; the expression level changes may indicate ECM

TABLE 2b | Proteins identified from fetal membranes associated with preterm birth (AB vs. CD): Down-regulated.

Majority protein IDs	Protein names	Gene names	Protein family	Pathways	Functions
Q15067-2; Q15067; Q15067-3	Peroxisomal acyl-coenzyme A oxidase 1	ACOX1	Peroxisomal acyl-coenzyme A oxidase 1 (PTHR10909:SF290)	Fatty acid metabolism	Fatty acid beta-oxidation
O95573	Long-chain-fatty-acid–CoA ligase 3	ACSL3	Long-chain-fatty-acid–CoA ligase 3 (PTHR43272:SF13)	Fatty acid metabolism	Fatty acid metabolic process
P09525; Q6P452	Annexin A4; Annexin	ANXA4	Annexin A4 (PTHR10502:SF28)		
P40121; P40121-2; E7ENU9	Macrophage-capping protein	CAPG	Macrophage-capping protein (PTHR11977:SF13)	FAS signaling pathway (P00020)	Macrophage function/Structural molecule activity
P21291; E9PS42; E9PND2; E9PP21	Cysteine and glycine-rich protein 1	CSRP1	Cysteine and glycine-rich protein 1 (PTHR24215:SF23)		Structural molecule activity
Q9UHQ9; H7C0R7	NADH-cytochrome b5 reductase 1	CYB5R1	NADH-cytochrome b5 reductase 1 (PTHR19370:SF74)		Oxidoreductase activity
P05108; P05108-2; E7EPP8	Cholesterol side-chain cleavage enzyme, mitochondrial	CYP11A1	Cholesterol side-chain cleavage enzyme, mitochondrial (PTHR24279:SF3)	Androgen/estrogene/progesterone biosynthesis (P02727)	
E7EQR4; P15311	Ezrin	EZR	Ezrin (PTHR23281:SF13)		Structural molecule activity
P15428; P15428-5; P15428-2; E9PBZ2; P15428-4	15-hydroxyprostaglandin dehydrogenase [NAD(+)]	HPGD	15-hydroxyprostaglandin dehydrogenase [NAD(+)] (PTHR44229:SF4)		
P40925; P40925-3; B9A041; P40925-2; B8ZZ51	Malate dehydrogenase, cytoplasmic	MDH1	Malate dehydrogenase, cytoplasmic (PTHR23382:SF3)	TCA cycle (P00051)	
E9PIY1; A0A0C4DGG1; Q9UKS6; E9PJ75; E9PNM9	Protein kinase C and casein kinase substrate in neurons protein 3	PACSIN3	Protein kinase C and casein kinase substrate in neurons protein 3 (PTHR23065:SF18)		
P30086	Phosphatidylethanolamine-binding protein 1; Hippocampal cholinergic neurostimulating peptide	PEBP1	Phosphatidylethanolamine-binding protein 1 (PTHR11362:SF28)	EGF/FGF receptor signaling pathway (P00018)	
P14618; P14618-3; B4DNK4	Pyruvate kinase PKM; Pyruvate kinase	PKM	Pyruvate kinase PKM (PTHR11817:SF15)	Glycolysis (P00024)	
P30044-2; P30044; P30044-3; P30044-4	Peroxiredoxin-5, mitochondrial	PRDX5	Peroxiredoxin-5, mitochondrial (PTHR10430:SF16)		
P61313; E7EQV9; E7ENU7; E7EX53; P61313-2	60S ribosomal protein L15; Ribosomal protein L15	RPL15	60S ribosomal protein L15 (PTHR11847:SF13)		
P62888; E5RI99; A0A0B4J213; A0A0C4DH44	60S ribosomal protein L30	RPL30	60S ribosomal protein L30 (PTHR11449:SF1)		Biosynthetic process
P46777	60S ribosomal protein L5	RPL5	60S ribosomal protein L5 (PTHR23410:SF12)		Biosynthetic process
P62277; J3KMX5	40S ribosomal protein S13	RPS13	40S ribosomal protein S13 (PTHR11885:SF6)		Biosynthetic process
P62249; M0R210; A0A087WZ27; M0R3H0; M0R1M5	40S ribosomal protein S16	RPS16;ZNF90			Biosynthetic process

TABLE 3 | Top-20 proteins identified from fetal membranes associated with preterm birth.

Gene symbol	Protein name	Function	p-value	Fold change
CSRP1	Cysteine and glycine-rich protein 1	Extracellular metrix	1.75E-03	−4.11
HPGD	15-hydroxyprostaglandin dehydrogenase [NAD (+)]	Inflammation	1.70E-03	−3.95
PKM	Pyruvate kinase	Glycolysis	1.46E-03	−3.59
ACSL3	Long-chain-fatty-acid-CoA ligase 3	Fatty acid metabolism	1.45E-03	−3.45
FBLN2	Fibulin-2	Extracellular metrix	1.36E-03	2.81
HMGN2	High mobility group nucleosomal binding domain 2	Gene transcription	2.19E-03	3.05
HMGN3	High mobility group nucleosomal binding domain 3	Gene transcription	2.19E-03	3.05
CD14	Monocyte differentiation antigen CD14	Macrophage function	1.49E-05	3.14
BST1	ADP-ribosyl cyclase/cyclic ADP-ribose hydrolase 2	B-cell growth	1.92E-03	3.25
CD163	Scavenger receptor cysteine-rich type 1 protein M130	Macrophage function	8.10E-04	3.29
LMNB1	Lamin-B1	Extracellular matrix	6.31E-05	3.47
ICAM1	Intercellular adhesion molecule 1	Cell adhesion	5.86E-04	6.07
PTPRC	Receptor-type tyrosine-protein phosphatase C	T cell activation	5.36E-05	11.24
CYBB	Cytochrome b-245 heavy chain	Energy metabolism	7.48E-05	11.24
S100A9	Protein S100-A9	Calmodulin signaling	4.82E-03	11.47
MPO	Myeloperoxidase	Oxidative stress	5.18E-03	11.99
CTSG	Cathepsin G	Protein degradation	1.22E-03	13.56
ELANE	Neutrophil elastase	Protein degradation	6.02E-03	20.22
ITGAM	Integrin alpha-M	Cell adhesion	7.61E-05	28.71
MMP9	Matrix metalloproteinase-9	Protein degradation	5.25E-03	318.64

TABLE 4 | Proteins involved in top-scored pathways in fetal membrane of sPTB.

Pathway	Up-regulated protein	Down-regulated protein
Infection and inflammation	PTPRC, BST1, CAPG, CD14, CD163, S100A9	HPGD, S100P
Protein degradation and proteolysis	CTSG, ELANE, MMP9	
Extracellular matrix	APMAP, COL4A1, LAMA2, LMNB1, LMNB2, FBLN2	
Cell adhesion	ICAM1, ITGAM	CSRP1
Antioxidant	MPO	
Glycolysis		PKM
Fatty acid beta-oxidation		ACOX1, ACSL3

degradation in PPROM and PROM. CSRP1 is a membrane of the CRP family, which may regulate cellular development and differentiation.

MMP9, ELANE, and chymotrypsin C (CTSG) are the proteins involved in proteolysis. MMP9 has been reported to break down the ECM, such as type IV and V collagens. MMP9 is mainly expressed in amnion epithelia, chorion leave trophoblast, decidua parietalis, and placental syncytiotrophoblasts. The expression level of MMP9 was increased in fetal membranes from preterm and term labor as compared to non-labors (Xu et al., 2002). Moreover, fetuses with PPROM have higher concentrations of MMP-9 than those with preterm labor with intact membrane, indicating the pathogenic role of MMP-9 during a rupture of fetal membrane in sPTB (Romero et al., 2002). The level of MMP-9 has been used as a risk factor for preterm births (Di Ferdinando et al., 2010; Sorokin, 2010). In agreement with published data, an increase in MMP-9 expression may contribute to degradation of the ECM in the fetal membrane and in placentas, thus initiating sPTB. ELANE, a multifunctional serine protease stored in azurophilic granules of mature neutrophils, is able to degrade the ECM of connective tissue during an inflammatory process. It has been implicated that PPROM, microbial invasion of the amniotic cavity, and parturition at term and preterm are associated with a significant increase in the concentration of ELANE in the amniotic fluid. Another study suggested that ELANE levels in amniotic fluid may serve as a useful marker for predicting the duration of continued pregnancy after cervical cerclage (Hatakeyama et al., 2016). CTSG is a member of the peptidase S1 protein family in azurophilic granules of neutrophilic polymorphonuclear leukocytes. CTSG has a cleavage specificity similar to chymotrypsin C and may involve connective tissue remodeling at the site of inflammation. It has been shown that intra-amniotic inflammation (IAI) is associated with increased CTSG concentration in the amniotic fluid in PPROM (Musilova et al., 2017). It has been reported that the ubiquitin–proteasome–collagen (CUP) pathway is involved in collagen degradation in PPROM (Zhao et al., 2017). In addition, the CUP pathway was epigenetically regulated by lncRNA in PROM and PPROM (Luo et al., 2015). Even though we did not identify proteins belonging to the CUP pathway, we did identify the most significant proteolytic enzymes associated with PPROM and PTB, mainly MMP-9, serine protease (ELANE), and CTSG.

Our proteome data detected over-expression of cell adhesion molecules ICAM and ITGAM in sPTB. ICAM-1 is a cell

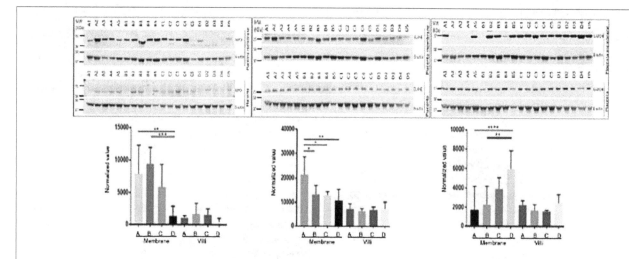

FIGURE 3 | Validation of differentially expressed proteins with placenta villi and fetal membranes. Randomly selected proteins MPO (**left panel**), ELANE (**middle panel**), and GAPDH (**right panel**) that were identified to be differentially expressed in fetal membrane (FM) vs. placental villi (PV) by MS/MS were validated with Western blots. Generally, three proteins were up-regulated in fetal membranes when compared to placental villi. MPO and ELANE were significantly increased in preterm pregnancies of sPTL (A) & PPROM (B) compared to full-term pregnancies of FTB (C) and PROM (D) fetal membranes. However, GAPDH was decreased in A + B. $*p < 0.05$, $**p < 0.01$, $***p < 0.005$, and $****p < 0.0001$. Beta-Actin was used as an internal control for normalizing the protein expression value.

surface glycoprotein expressed on endothelial cells and cells of the immune system (Egal et al., 2014). It has been reported that ICAM-1 was overexpressed in villous trophoblasts during placental infection (Juliano et al., 2006). Another study indicated that expression of ICAM-1 by the human choriodecidua was elevated with preterm birth, together with increased leukocyte infiltration (Marvin et al., 1999). ITGAM plays an important role in the adherence of neutrophils and monocytes to stimulated endothelium. The level of ITGAM was significantly elevated in the amniotic fluid of women with preterm labor with IAI compared without IAI (Romero et al., 2010). Again, increased levels of ICAM-1 and ITGAM suggest activation of white blood cells and immune response in preterm birth placenta membrane.

Oxidative Stress Proteins MPO, LMNB1, and LMNB2

MPO is a heme protein synthesized and released from activated monocytes and neutrophils. Traditionally, it was described as a microbicidal enzyme. New evidence indicates that MPO generates hypochlorite-modified proteins, activates metalloproteinase (Prokopenko et al., 2002), and oxidatively consumes endothelium-derived nitric oxide in humans during normal pregnancy as well as during pathophysiologic processes (pre-eclampsia) (Hammer et al., 2001; Gandley et al., 2008). Higher cord blood levels of MPO are associated with preterm delivery (Yang et al., 2004). LMNB1 and LMNB2 are B-type nuclear lamin located in the inner nuclear membrane and play an important role in nuclear stability, chromatin structure, and gene expression. Overexpression of LMNB1 was found through a mitochondrial reactive oxygen species (ROS) *in vitro* model to increase the proliferation rate and to delay the onset of senescence (Shimi et al., 2011). Oxidative stress was higher and antioxidant enzymes were lower in PPROM compared with sPTB (Dutta et al., 2016). Our data suggest a higher level of oxidative stress, which may induce premature cellular senescence, inflammation, and proteolysis, eventually leading to membrane rupture and PPROM.

Glycolysis, Fatty Acid Synthesis

Differentially expressed proteins involved in glycolysis and FA synthesis were down-regulated in the fetal membranes of sPTB (**Table 3**). PKM, a catalytic enzyme involved in the last step of glycolysis, is responsible for dephosphorylating phosphoenolpyruvate to pyruvate and producing ATP under hypoxic conditions. PKM is also involved in angiogenesis in embryo development. It has been reported that the expression of PKM is higher in pre-eclampsia at delivery than in normal pregnancy (Bahr et al., 2014). ADPGK is a rate-limiting enzyme within the first step of glycolysis; it catalyzes the phosphorylation of D-glucose to D-glucose 6-phosphate by using ADP as the phosphate donor. GAPDH is an enzyme responsible for glyceraldehyde dehydration in the process of glycolysis. The placenta is a main source of high lactate levels during gestation. In later gestation, the concentration of lactate can reach 10 mmol/l, as compared to 1–2 mmol/l in the newborn and 0.5 mmol/l in maternal plasma. Fatty acids are essential substances for the construction of cell membrane and development of the nervous system. The disruption of FAs' metabolism in the maternal-placental interface would result in malnutrition of the fetus and in preterm birth (Bobinski and Mikulska, 2015). Blood levels of FAs are 20 times lower in the fetal circulation than in newborns' circulation (Makinde et al., 1998). This indicates that glucose/lactate provides the main energy source in fetal development. Typically, lactate is described as a waste product catalyzed by LDH under anaerobic metabolism. A metabolism study in various cell types indicated a model whereby lactate generated in the cytosol compartment can be oxidized into pyruvate in mitochondria by LDH; pyruvate is subsequently transported into the inner membrane of the matrix and is then oxidized to acetyl CoA by pyruvate dehydrogenate (Kane, 2014). Acetyl CoA can then be fed into the TCA cycle and maintains mitochondrial function. Our data showed an increase in the level of ADPGK in the first step of glycolysis and a reduced level of PKM in the last step of glycolysis, suggesting an imbalance of glycolysis and the generation of less pyruvate through the conventional glycolysis pathway. To maintain metabolic functionality, a lactate oxidation process in mitochondria to produce pyruvate to sustain the TCA cycle is preferred. Reduction of the proteins involved in glycolysis and fatty acid synthesis may suggest that energy synthesis might be reduced in the fetal membrane tissues in sPTB. To confirm this, further investigation is needed to understand better the role of lactate's and FAs' metabolism in sPTB.

Tissue Specificity

Differential expression patterns of GAPDH were documented between the fetal membranes and placental villi. As shown in the right panel of **Figure 3**, GAPDH was found to be down-regulated in premature birth groups A and B, as compared to full-term control groups C and D with (PROM) or without (FTB) rupture of membrane in samples of fetal membrane. This finding is in agreement with the results generated from a discovery study with MS/MS. However, in the tissue of placental villi, Western blot for validation showed up-regulation, compared to FTB, which resulted in no significant change in placenta specimens between A + B vs. C + D. GAPDH is an enzyme involved in anaerobic energy metabolism through glycolysis. We speculated that the glycolysis pathway may be affected in fetal membrane and weakened the structure of fetal membrane but not in placental villi. To confirm this, further investigation should be performed to provide biochemical evidence.

CONCLUSION

By applying a proteomic approach, along with validation of proteomic results with Western blots, to study sPTL and PPROM with the capacity of distinguishing between the sPTL and PPROM groups, and of distinguishing the premature groups sPTL and PPROM from the mature groups FTB and PROM, we demonstrated a unique signature for each of the conditions, which is the strength this study. In addition, our proteomic data provide systemic insights into pathophysiological changes in the fetal membranes on the molecular level. Our data support the theory of inflammation/infection in sPTL and PPROM, even though we have not identified the source of infection. Inflammation increased the oxidative stress–triggered pyrolytic process that changes ECM structure, eventually rupturing the placental membrane and resulting in preterm birth. Metabolic function was also altered, in particular, imbalanced glycolysis and unconventional lactate oxidation, which may be associated with preterm birth. We are also aware of the limitation that applying the proteomic approach to identifying the differentially expressed protein(s) that are associated with clinical features and to identify biomarker(s) for the disease condition could be influenced by post-translational modification. Therefore, a larger sample size will need to be used for validation. In fact, studies on the inflammation-triggered proteolysis of ECM has been undertaken to verify a key pathogenic pathway for sPTB.

ETHICS STATEMENT

The study was approved by the Hospital Ethics Committee of Sanya Maternity and Child Care Hospital. Written informed consent was obtained from pregnant women to permit the use of placentas in research studies.

AUTHOR CONTRIBUTIONS

JP, XT, and HH contributed to the sample collection, processing and preparation, data acquisition, and laboratory work. NZ contributed to, and was responsible for, conceptual research design, initiating and coordinating the studies and experiments, data analysis, and drafting, finalizing, and submitting the manuscript. All authors contributed to the article and approved the submitted version.

REFERENCES

Allam, A. B., von Chamier, M., Brown, M. B., and Reyes, L. (2014). Immune profiling of BALB/C and C57BL/6 mice reveals a correlation between Ureaplasma parvum-Induced fetal inflammatory response syndrome-like pathology and increased placental expression of TLR2 and CD14. Am. J. Reprod. Immunol. 71, 241–251. doi: 10.1111/aji.12192

Aoki, T., and Narumiya, S. (2012). Prostaglandins and chronic inflammation. Trends Pharmacol Sci. 33, 304–311.

Audette, M. C., and Kingdom, J. C. (2018). Screening for fetal growth restriction and placental insufficiency. Semin. Fetal. Neonatal. Med. 23, 119–125. doi: 10.1016/j.siny.2017.11.004

Bahr, B. L., Price, M. D., Merrill, D., Mejia, C., Call, L., Bearss, D., et al. (2014). Different expression of placental pyruvate kinase in normal, preeclamptic and intrauterine growth restriction pregnancies. Placenta 35, 883–890. doi: 10.1016/j.placenta.2014.09.005

Bastek, J. A., Brown, A. G., Anton, L., Srinivas, S. K., D'addio, A., and Elovitz, M. A. (2011). Biomarkers of inflammation and placental dysfunction are associated with subsequent preterm birth. J. Matern. Fetal. Neonatal. Med. 24, 600–605. doi: 10.3109/14767058.2010.511340

Bhutani, V. K., and Wong, R. J. (2013). Bilirubin neurotoxicity in preterm infants: risk and prevention. J. Clin. Neonatol. 2, 61–69.

Bobinski, R., and Mikulska, M. (2015). The ins and outs of maternal-fetal fatty acid metabolism. Acta Biochim. Pol. 62, 499–507. doi: 10.18388/abp.2015_1067

Cheng, P. J., and Duan, T. (2016). China's new two-child policy: maternity care in the new multiparous era. *BJOG* 123(Suppl.), 7–9. doi: 10.1111/1471-0528.14290

Chisholm, K. M., Norton, M. E., Penn, A. A., and Heerema-McKenney, A. (2018). Classification of preterm birth with placental correlates. *Pediatr. Dev. Pathol.* 21, 548–560. doi: 10.1177/1093526618775958

Costa, M. A. (2016). The endocrine function of human placenta: an overview. *Reprod. Biomed. Online* 32, 14–43. doi: 10.1016/j.rbmo.2015.10.005

Cuffe, J. S. M., Holland, O., Salomon, C., Rice, G. E., and Perkins, A. V. (2017). Review: placental derived biomarkers of pregnancy disorders. *Placenta* 54, 104–110. doi: 10.1016/j.placenta.2017.01.119

Di Ferdinando, A., Patacchiola, F., Perilli, M. G., Amicosante, G., and Carta, G. (2010). Expression of matrix metalloproteinase-9 (MMP-9) in human midpregnancy amniotic fluid and risk of preterm labor. *Clin. Exp. Obstet. Gynecol.* 37, 193–196.

Dutta, E. H., Behnia, F., Boldogh, I., Saade, G. R., Taylor, B. D., Kacerovský, K., et al. (2016). Oxidative stress damage-associated molecular signaling pathways differentiate spontaneous preterm birth and preterm premature rupture of the membranes. *Mol. Hum. Reprod.* 22, 143–157. doi: 10.1093/molehr/gav074

Egal, E. S., Mariano, F. V., Blotta, M. H., Piña, A. R., Montalli, V. A., Almeida, O. P., et al. (2014). ICAM-1 expression on immune cells in chronic villitis. *Placenta* 35, 1021–1026. doi: 10.1016/j.placenta.2014.10.004

Fabriek, B. O., van Bruggen, R., Deng, D. M., Ligtenberg, A. J., Nazmi, K., Schornagel, K., et al. (2009). The macrophage scavenger receptor CD163 functions as an innate immune sensor for bacteria. *Blood* 113, 887–892. doi: 10.1182/blood-2008-07-167064

Fraser, J., Walls, M., and McGuire, W. (2004). Respiratory complications of preterm birth. *BMJ* 329, 962–965. doi: 10.1136/bmj.329.7472.962

Fuchs, F., Monet, B., Ducruet, T., Chaillet, N., and Audibert, F. (2018). Effect of maternal age on the risk of preterm birth: a large cohort study. *PLoS One* 13:e0191002. doi: 10.1371/journal.pone.0191002

Gandley, R. E., Rohland, J., Zhou, Y., Shibata, E., Harger, G. F., and Rajakumar, A. (2008). Increased myeloperoxidase in the placenta and circulation of women with preeclampsia. *Hypertension* 52, 387–393. doi: 10.1161/hypertensionaha.107.107532

Gezer, C., Ekin, A., Solmaz, U., Yildirim, A. G. S., Dogan, A., and Ozeren, M. (2018). Identification of preterm birth in women with threatened preterm labour between 34 and 37 weeks of gestation. *J. Obstet. Gynaecol.* 38, 652–657. doi: 10.1080/01443615.2017.1399990

Gude, N. M., Roberts, C. T., Kalionis, B., and King, R. G. (2004). Growth and function of the normal human placenta. *Thromb. Res.* 114, 397–407. doi: 10.1016/j.thromres.2004.06.038

Guleria, I., and Sayegh, M. H. (2007). Maternal acceptance of the fetus: true human tolerance. *J. Immunol.* 178, 3345–3351. doi: 10.4049/jimmunol.178.6.3345

Hammer, A., Desoye, G., Dohr, G., Sattler, W., and Malle, E. (2001). Myeloperoxidase-dependent generation of hypochlorite-modified proteins in human placental tissues during normal pregnancy. *Lab. Invest.* 81, 543–554. doi: 10.1038/labinvest.3780263

Hatakeyama, Y., Miura, H., Sato, A., Onodera, Y., Sato, N., Shimizu, D., et al. (2016). Neutrophil elastase in amniotic fluid as a predictor of preterm birth after emergent cervical cerclage. *Acta Obstet. Gynecol. Scand.* 95, 1136–1142. doi: 10.1111/aogs.12928

He, P., Li, Y., Ding, X., Sun, Q., Huang, Y., Gu, H., et al. (2015). Expression of 15-hydroxyprostaglandin dehydrogenase in human chorion is associated with peroxisome proliferator-activated receptor isoform expression in term labor. *Am. J. Pathol.* 185, 1981–1990. doi: 10.1016/j.ajpath.2015.03.021

Heazell, A. E., Whitworth, M., Duley, L., and Thornton, J. G. (2015). Use of biochemical tests of placental function for improving pregnancy outcome. *Cochrane Database. Syst. Rev.* 11:CD011202. doi: 10.1002/14651858.CD011202.pub2

Helmig, B. R., Romero, R., Espinoza, J., Chaiworapongsa, T., Bujold, E., Gomez, R., et al. (2002). Neutrophil elastase and secretory leukocyte protease inhibitor in prelabor rupture of membranes, parturition and intra-amniotic infection. *J. Matern. Fetal Neonatal. Med.* 12, 237–246.

Ilekis, J. V., Tsilou, E., Fisher, S., Abrahams, V. M., Soares, M. J., Cross, J. C., et al. (2016). Placental origins of adverse pregnancy outcomes: potential molecular targets: an executive workshop summary of the eunice kennedy shriver national institute of child health and human development. *Am. J. Obstet. Gynecol.* 215(Suppl.), S1–S46.

Juliano, P. B., Blotta, M. H., and Altemani, A. M. (2006). ICAM-1 is overexpressed by villous trophoblasts in placentitis. *Placenta* 27, 750–757. doi: 10.1016/j.placenta.2005.07.008

Kane, D. A. (2014). Lactate oxidation at the mitochondria: a lactate-malate-aspartate shuttle at work. *Front. Neurosci.* 8:366. doi: 10.3389/fnins.2014.00366

Lorenzi, T., Turi, A., Lorenzi, M., Paolinelli, F., Mancioli, F., La Sala, L., et al. (2012). Placental expression of CD100, CD72 and CD45 is dysregulated in human miscarriage. *PLoS One* 7:e35232. doi: 10.1371/journal.pone.0035232

Luo, X., Luo, X., Pan, J., Wang, L., Wang, P., Zhang, M., et al. (2015). -inflammation in preterm births and preterm premature rupture of membranes. *BMC Pregnancy Childbirth* 15:35. doi: 10.1186/s12884-015-0460-0

Makinde, A. O., Kantor, P. F., and Lopaschuk, G. D. (1998). Maturation of fatty acid and carbohydrate metabolism in the newborn heart. *Mol. Cell. Biochem.* 188, 49–56. doi: 10.1007/978-1-4615-5763-0_6

Marvin, K. W., Keelan, J. A., Sato, T. A., Coleman, M. A., McCowan, L. M., and Mitchell, M. D. (1999). Expression of intercellular adhesion molecule-1 (ICAM-1) in choriodecidua with labour and delivery at term and preterm. *Reprod. Fertil. Dev.* 11, 255–262.

Mogensen, T. H. (2009). Pathogen recognition and inflammatory signaling in innate immune defenses. *Clin. Microbiol. Rev.* 22, 240–273. doi: 10.1128/cmr.00046-08

Morgan, T. K. (2016). Role of the placenta in preterm birth: a review. *Am. J. Perinatol.* 33, 258–266. doi: 10.1055/s-0035-1570379

Musilova, I., Andrys, C., Drahosova, M., Soucek, O., Pliskova, L., Stepan, M., et al. (2017). Amniotic fluid cathepsin-G in pregnancies complicated by the preterm prelabor rupture of membranes. *J. Matern. Fetal. Neonatal. Med.* 30, 2097–2104. doi: 10.1080/14767058.2016.1237499

Oefner, C. M., Sharkey, A., Gardner, L., Critchley, H., Oyen, M., and Moffett, A. (2015). Collagen type IV at the fetal-maternal interface. *Placenta* 36, 59–68. doi: 10.1016/j.placenta.2014.10.012

Paton, M. C. B., McDonald, C. A., Allison, B. J., Fahey, M. C., Jenkin, G., and Miller, S. L. (2017). Perinatal brain injury as a consequence of preterm birth and intrauterine inflammation: designing targeted stem cell therapies. *Front. Neurosci.* 11:200. doi: 10.3389/fnins.2017.00200

Pessentheiner, A. R., Huber, K., Pelzmann, H. J., Prokesch, A., Radner, F., Wolinski, H., et al. (2017). APMAP interacts with lysyl oxidase-like proteins, and disruption of Apmap leads to beneficial visceral adipose tissue expansion. *FASEB J.* 31, 4088–4103. doi: 10.1096/fj.201601337r

Pike, K. A., and Tremblay, M. L. (2013). Tremblay, Regulating naive and memory CD8 T cell homeostasis–a role for protein tyrosine phosphatases. *FEBS J.* 280, 432–444. doi: 10.1111/j.1742-4658.2012.08587.x

Porcu, M., Kleppe, M., Gianfelici, V., Geerdens, E., De Keersmaecker, K., Tartaglia, M., et al. (2012). Mutation of the receptor tyrosine phosphatase PTPRC (CD45) in T-cell acute lymphoblastic leukemia. *Blood* 119, 4476–4479. doi: 10.1182/blood-2011-09-379958

Prokopenko, V. M., Aleshina, G. M., Frolova, E. V., Anan'eva, V. V., Kokriakov, V. N., and Arutiunian, A. V. (2002). [Myeloperoxidase in the human placenta at preterm labor]. *Vopr Med Khim* 48, 378–380.

Pugni, L., Pietrasanta, C., Acaia, B., Merlo, D., Ronchi, A., Ossola, M. W., et al. (2016). Chorioamnionitis and neonatal outcome in preterm infants: a clinical overview. *J. Matern. Fetal. Neonatal. Med.* 29, 1525–1529. doi: 10.3109/14767058.2015.1053862

Quinn, J. A., Munoz, F. M., Gonik, B., Frau, L., Cutland, C., Mallett-Moore, T., et al. (2016). Preterm birth: case definition & guidelines for data collection, analysis, and presentation of immunisation safety data. *Vaccine* 34, 6047–6056.

Romero, R., Chaiworapongsa, T., Espinoza, J., Gomez, R., Yoon, B. H., Edwin, S., et al. (2002). Fetal plasma MMP-9 concentrations are elevated in preterm premature rupture of the membranes. *Am. J. Obstet. Gynecol.* 187, 1125–1130. doi: 10.1067/mob.2002.127312

Romero, R., Kusanovic, J. P., Gotsch, F., Erez, O., Vaisbuch, E., Mazaki-Tovi, S., et al. (2010). Isobaric labeling and tandem mass spectrometry: a novel approach for profiling and quantifying proteins differentially expressed in amniotic fluid in preterm labor with and without intra-amniotic infection/inflammation. *J Matern Fetal Neonatal Med.* 23, 261–280. doi: 10.3109/14767050903067386

Salafia, C. M., Vogel, C. A., Vintzileos, A. M., Bantham, K. F., Pezzullo, J., and Silberman, L. (1991). Placental pathologic findings in preterm birth. *Am. J. Obstet. Gynecol.* 165(Pt 1), 934–938. doi: 10.1016/0002-9378(91)90443-u

Schneider, C. A., Rasband, W. S., and Eliceiri, K. W. (2012). NIH Image to Image J: 25 years of image analysis. *Nat. Methods* 9, 671–675. doi: 10.1038/nmeth.2089

Seo, M. J., and Oh, D. K. (2017). Prostaglandin synthases: molecular characterization and involvement in prostaglandin biosynthesis. *Prog Lipid Res.* 66, 50–68. doi: 10.1016/j.plipres.2017.04.003

Shimi, T., Butin-Israeli, V., Adam, S. A., Hamanaka, R. B., Goldman, A. E., Lucas, C. A., et al. (2011). The role of nuclear lamin B1 in cell proliferation and senescence. *Genes Dev.* 25, 2579–2593. doi: 10.1101/gad.179515.111

Sorokin, Y. (2010). Maternal serum interleukin-6, C-reactive protein, and matrix metalloproteinase-9 concentrations as risk factors for preterm birth <32 weeks and adverse neonatal outcomes. *Am. J. Perinatol.* 27, 631–640. doi: 10.1055/s-0030-1249366

Stout, M. J., Romero, R., Mele, L., Wapner, R. J., Iams, J. D., Dudley, D. J., et al. (2013). First trimester serum analytes, maternal characteristics and ultrasound markers to predict pregnancies at risk for preterm birth. *Placenta* 34, 14–19. doi: 10.1016/j.placenta.2012.10.013

Straughen, J. K., Kumar, P., and Misra, V. K. (2012). The effect of maternal soluble FMS-like tyrosine kinase 1 during pregnancy on risk of preterm delivery. *J. Matern. Fetal. Neonatal. Med.* 25, 1879–1883. doi: 10.3109/14767058.2012.666589

Vogel, I., Grove, J., Thorsen, P., Moestrup, S. K., Uldbjerg, N., and Møller, H. J. (2005). Preterm delivery predicted by soluble CD163 and CRP in women with symptoms of preterm delivery. *BJOG* 112, 737–742. doi: 10.1111/j.1471-0528.2005.00557.x

von Hof, J., Sprekeler, N., Schuler, G., Boos, A., and Kowalewski, M. P. (2017). Uterine and placental expression of HPGD in cows during pregnancy and release of fetal membranes. *Prostaglandins Other Lipid Mediat.* 12, 17–26. doi: 10.1016/j.prostaglandins.2016.12.003

World Health Organization [WHO] (2018). *Preterm Birth, Key Facts*. Geneva: WHO.

Xu, P., Alfaidy, N., and Challis, J. R. (2002). Expression of matrix metalloproteinase (MMP)-2 and MMP-9 in human placenta and fetal membranes in relation to preterm and term labor. *J. Clin. Endocrinol. Metab.* 87, 1353–1361. doi: 10.1210/jcem.87.3.8320

Yang, K. D., Wang, C. L., Huang, L. T., Chang, H., Huang, H. C., Hsu, T. Y., et al. (2004). Implication of cord blood myeloperoxidase but not of soluble p-selectin levels in preterm deliveries. *J. Perinat. Med.* 32, 49–52.

Young, C. L., Feierstein, A., and Southwick, F. S. (1994). Calcium regulation of actin filament capping and monomer binding by macrophage capping protein. *J. Biol. Chem.* 269, 13997–14002.

Zeldovich, V. B., Clausen, C. H., Bradford, E., Fletcher, D. A., Maltepe, E., Robbins, J. R., et al. (2013). Placental syncytium forms a biophysical barrier against pathogen invasion. *PLoS Pathog.* 9:e1003821. doi: 10.1371/journal.ppat.1003821

Zhao, X., Dong, X., Luo, X., Pan, J., Ju, W., Zhang, M., et al. (2017). Ubiquitin-proteasome-collagen (cup) pathway in preterm premature rupture of fetal membranes. *Front. Pharmacol.* 8:310. doi: 10.3389/fphar.2017.00310

Functional Genomics of Healthy and Pathological Fetal Membranes

Sarah J. Cunningham[1,2,3,4], Liping Feng[5], Terrence K. Allen[6] and Timothy E. Reddy[1,2,3,4]*

[1] Department of Biostatistics and Bioinformatics, Duke University, Durham, NC, United States, [2] University Program in Genetics and Genomics, Duke University, Durham, NC, United States, [3] Center for Genomic and Computational Biology, Duke University, Durham, NC, United States, [4] Center for Advanced Genomic Technologies, Duke University, Durham, NC, United States, [5] Department of Obstetrics and Gynecology, Duke University School of Medicine, Durham, NC, United States, [6] Department of Anesthesiology, Duke University Hospital, Durham, NC, United States

*Correspondence:
Timothy E. Reddy
Tim.Reddy@Duke.edu

Premature preterm rupture of membranes (PPROM), rupture of fetal membranes before 37 weeks of gestation, is the leading identifiable cause of spontaneous preterm births. Often there is no obvious cause that is identified in a patient who presents with PPROM. Identifying the upstream molecular events that lead to fetal membrane weakening presents potentially actionable mechanisms which could lead to the identification of at-risk patients and to the development of new therapeutic interventions. Functional genomic studies have transformed understanding of the role of gene regulation in diverse cells and tissues involved health and disease. Here, we review the results of those studies in the context of fetal membranes. We will highlight relevant results from major coordinated functional genomics efforts and from targeted studies focused on individual cell or tissue models. Studies comparing gene expression and DNA methylation between healthy and pathological fetal membranes have found differential regulation between labor and quiescent tissue as well as in preterm births, preeclampsia, and recurrent pregnancy loss. Whole genome and exome sequencing studies have identified common and rare fetal variants associated with preterm births. However, few fetal membrane tissue studies have modeled the response to stimuli relevant to pregnancy. Fetal membranes are readily adaptable to cell culture and relevant cellular phenotypes are readily observable. For these reasons, this is now an unrealized opportunity for genomic studies isolating the effect of cell signaling cascades and mapping the fetal membrane responses that lead to PPROM and other pregnancy complications.

Keywords: genomics, fetal membranes, transcriptomics, preterm birth, gene regulation and expression

INTRODUCTION

Preterm birth remains a major public health challenge affecting 10% of pregnancies in the United States (World Health Organization, 2016). The leading identifiable cause of preterm birth is premature preterm rupture of membranes (PPROM) (Mercer, 2010). Preeclampsia is characterized as shallow trophoblast invasion leading to incomplete spiral artery remodeling. It affects 5% of pregnancies and is an iatrogenic cause of prematurity and the leading cause of maternal and perinatal death (Souza et al., 2013).

These adverse pregnancy outcomes all have multifactorial causes incorporating genetic and environmental risk factors.

Functional genomics assays aim to define the relationships between the human genome and epigenome; the environment; and molecular, cellular, and organismal phenotypes. The past decade has been transformative for functional genomics, owing largely to high-throughput short read sequencing providing quantitative and genome-wide readout for many functional genomic assays. Such assays are particularly adept at identifying differential activity that may result from changes in the environment, such as hormone exposures or immune insults [e.g., (McDowell et al., 2018; Pulido-Salgado et al., 2018)]. Today, there are a vast array of genome-wide functional genomic technologies available to measure a wide variety of aspects of gene expression, DNA methylation, histone positioning and modifications, transcription factor binding, gene regulatory activity, other factors that indicate gene regulation (Arnold et al., 2013; Mundade et al., 2014; Finotello and Di Camillo, 2015; Tirado-Magallanes et al., 2016). Through those studies, there is now extensive information about the gene regulatory state of diverse cells and tissues.

For the purposes of this review, we define functional genomic assays as those that scan large fractions of the genome for evidence of regulatory activity. In the context of human disease studies, such regions are a promising starting point for subsequent efforts to discover causative biological mechanisms. Follow-up is then needed to evaluate the biological consequences of identified regulatory regions, both in terms of the effects on cellular and organismal phenotypes and also in terms of the effects of non-coding genetic variation on their activity.

Functional genomics studies have primarily focused on immortalized cell models, ostensibly because they are highly proliferative and robust. However, recent advances in the adaptation of functional genomics protocols for use on limited primary cells and tissues have created the potential to study more physiologically relevant cell models [e.g., (Vento-Tormo et al., 2018; Chung et al., 2019)]. In the context of preterm birth, fetal membranes are a key tissue of interest, and ideally suited for genomic analysis due to their availability and amenability to cell culture. Protocols to culture and expand amnion and chorion cells were developed in the 1980s (Burgos and Faulk, 1981). Culturing primary cells in these systems allows for interrogation of fetal membranes by genomic assays. In addition, several genomic assays are now feasible from a limited number of primary cells, and even single cells, making culturing unnecessary (Jia et al., 2018; Wang et al., 2019). Together these developments have led to a number of genomic assays comparing fetal membrane tissues from healthy pregnancies to those involved in preeclampsia, early pregnancy loss and preterm birth.

DEFINING FETAL MEMBRANE SPECIFIC REGULATORY STATE

Functional genomic assays on fetal membrane samples have been completed both by large genomics consortia such as ENCODE and Roadmap Epigenomics (The Encode Project Consortium, 2012; Roadmap Epigenomics Consortium et al., 2015), as well as by individual labs (Kim et al., 2012; Lim et al., 2012; **Table 1**). The consortia efforts have focused on amnion and chorion tissues from full term and second trimester samples. Across those samples, they have measured genome-wide gene expression using RNA-seq, cytosine methylation using whole genome bisulfite sequencing, and the locations of covalent histone modifications, indicators of active gene regulation, using ChIP-seq.

RNA-seq typically measures mRNA transcript levels that can be compared among tissue types to identify tissue specific transcription (Mortazavi et al., 2008). Bisulfite sequencing assays identify methylated cytosine that are typically thought to be related to silencing of gene activation. They do so by using sodium bisulfite treatment to convert unmethylated cytosines to uracil prior to PCR amplification and sequencing (Meissner et al., 2008). When sequencing treated and untreated DNA, the uracil bases sequence as thymine in treated samples but remain as cytosine in untreated samples (Clark et al., 1994). Finally, ChIP-seq assays use antibodies to isolate DNA-bound proteins including histones (Johnson et al., 2007; Robertson et al., 2007). ChIP-seq can detect histone subunits altered with post translational modifications that influence DNA affinity and, in turn, how accessible the DNA is to transcriptional machinery (Zhou et al., 2011). Together, these datasets can establish a baseline of gene regulatory state across among membranes from healthy pregnancies, and an assessment of the changes in gene regulation between the second and third trimester.

Additional studies have investigated the gene expression (Kim et al., 2012) of healthy term placental tissue types including fetal membranes. Transcriptomic analysis shows that placental cell types are more similar to each other when compared to other adult tissue types, but each placental cell type shows a subset of tissue type specific gene expression as well (Kim et al., 2012). The epithelial specific splice regulator ESPR1 is significantly unregulated in fetal membrane tissue, particularly the amnion, above other tissue types. In the amnion, the relative expression of ESPR1 is 50% higher than that of next highest tissue of the 16 adult tissues measured. Substantial alternative splicing and novel isoforms specific to the fetal membranes have been found by RNA-seq studied of healthy term membranes (Kim et al., 2012).

To further define healthy gene regulation in fetal membranes, microarray-based gene expression studies compared activated amnion from late term non-laboring elective Cesarean-sections, defining activation as high NF-κB protein levels similar to the levels observed in post-delivery samples (Lim et al., 2012). That activation of the amnion is an early step that stimulates the synthesis of prostaglandins, cytokines and chemokines initiating the beginning of labor. Although all the samples were non-laboring, some samples were closer to the onset of labor at the time of C-section and could be differentiated from more quiescent samples. Activation of the amnion is associated with an up regulation of a cell death and cancer associated gene network, consistent with an increase in apoptosis in activated amnion (Lim et al., 2012). An additional gene network associated with cell-to-cell signaling is also unregulated in response to activation, consistent with the role of the amnion as an early initiator of labor induction.

TABLE 1 | Published genomic analyses in fetal membrane tissues.

Source	Tissue Type	Disease State	Assay
Roadmap Epigenomics	Amnion, basal plate, chorion smooth, trophoblast, placental villi	Healthy full term and 2nd trimester c-sections	mRNA-seq, histone modification ChIP-seq
ENCODE	Amnion, basal plate, chorion, trophoblast, placental villi	Healthy full term and 2nd trimester c-sections	mRNA-seq, microRNA-seq, DNase-seq, histone modification ChIP-seq
Tromp et al., 2004	Chorioamnion	Preterm Labor, PPROM, Term in labor and term not in labor	Microarray
Montenegro et al., 2009	Chorioamnion	Term in labor and not laboring and preterm labor	microRNA microarray
Nhan-Chang et al., 2010	Amnion and Chorion	Healthy full term spontaneous rupture of membranes	Microarray
Li et al., 2011	Amnion mesenchymal cells	Healthy term c-section stimulated with IL-1B	Microarray
Kim et al., 2012	Amnion, chorion	Healthy full term c-section	RNA-seq
Kim et al., 2013	Amnion	Term in labor and not laboring and preterm labor	Illumina Methylation BeadChip
Lim et al., 2012	Amnion	Healthy full term c-section	Microarray
Kim et al., 2016	Amnion epithelial	Healthy and preeclamptic term c-section	mRNA-seq
Söber et al., 2016	Chorionic villi	Recurrent pregnancy loss and elective abortion 2nd trimester	mRNA-seq, MicoRNA-seq
Wang et al., 2017	Chorionic villi	Recurrent miscarriages and elective abortion	lncRNA microarray
Jiang et al., 2018	Chorionic trophoblasts	Healthy term c-section stimulated with LPS	RNA-seq, Whole Genome Bisulfite Sequencing
Pereyra et al., 2019	Amnion and Chorion	Severe preterm and full term spontaneous labor	RNA-seq
Yang et al., 2019	Chorionic villi	Early embryonic arrest and elective abortion 2nd trimester	mRNA-seq, MicoRNA-seq

TABLE 2 | Published genetic analyses of preterm birth.

Source	Disease State	Assay
McGinnis et al., 2017	Offspring of preeclamptic pregnancies and controls	SNP array
Modi et al., 2017	Healthy term and PPROM African American infants	Whole Exome sequencing
Modi et al., 2018	Healthy term and PPROM African American infants	Whole Exome sequencing
Liu et al., 2019	Varied gestation duration	SNP array
Tiensuu et al., 2019	Term and spontaneous preterm birth	SNP array

HEALTHY VERSUS PATHOLOGICAL FETAL MEMBRANES

Functional genomic studies are particularly powerful for identifying molecular differences between different cell states, such as between fetal membrane tissues from healthy pregnancies and those with pregnancy complications. Differentially regulated genes from these studies can identify molecular pathways that may be either causal or a downstream consequence, and in the best cases can nominate new therapeutic targets. In fetal membrane tissues, such comparative studies have been done to compare healthy tissues to those from patients with preterm birth, recurrent early pregnancy loss, and preeclampsia.

Preterm Birth and Membrane Rupture

Due to the integral role fetal membranes play in maintaining pregnancy or stimulating parturition, a substantial amount of research has been devoted to understanding changes in gene regulation that occur during the onset of parturition. RNA-seq analyses have revealed hundreds of gene expression changes that occur between the site of membrane rupture and distal membrane sites in term spontaneously ruptured membranes. For example, Nhan-Chang et al. (2010) used microarrays to identify 677 differentially expressed genes at the site of rupture compared to a distal site in the chorion (Nhan-Chang et al., 2010). The differentially expressed genes were enriched for increased expression of genes involved in complement and coagulation at the site of rupture, suggesting a role for immune activation in membrane integrity. Genes related to extracellular matrix-receptor interaction were most altered at the site of rupture, consistent with the role of the extracellular matrix in maintaining fetal membrane integrity (Bryant-Greenwood, 1998).

Because signaling cascades leading to fetal membrane rupture can be informative in identifying the causes of membrane rupture, directly comparing the gene expressed at the site of rupture in preterm and term deliveries can give more direct insight into the cause of PPROM. The gene expression patterns of term membrane samples are more internally consistent whereas preterm samples are more variable (Pereyra et al., 2019). The variability in preterm samles suggests multiple signalling cascades lead to preterm birth, distinct from those leading to term births. Despite this variability, 270 significantly differentially expressed genes with a >2-fold gene expression change were found when comparing membranes from early preterm births to membranes from term births. Several genes from the tumor necrosis factor (TNF), chemokine and voltage gated potassium channel families were significantly differentially regulated. Inflammatory and immunological pathways were also significantly up-regulated in preterm birth, consistent with a role for immune responses in the etiology of some preterm birth (Velez et al., 2008).

Functional genomic studies can also identify genes of interest for specific causes of preterm birth. In one example, comparisons of gene expression in fetal membranes between preterm labor with intact membranes and membranes from PPROM patients identified Proteinase Inhibitor 3 (PI3) having significantly decreased expression in PPROM samples (Tromp et al., 2004). Immunohistochemical staining confirmed the decreased expression levels of PI3 protein expression in fetal membranes collected from patients presenting with PPROM (Tromp et al., 2004). PI3 is an anti-proteinase that may protect the extracellular matrix from degradation by proteases, specifically Elastase 2 and Proteinase 3 (Guyot et al., 2005). In other cell types, TNFα and IL1β have been found to induce PI3 production (Pfundt et al., 2000; Bingle et al., 2001). PI3 was not previously implicated in preterm birth or PPROM specifically, but genome wide studies suggest decreased expression, due to genetic or environmental signaling, could lead to PPROM.

Functional genomic studies have also identified differential epigenetic states which may contribute to or result from such gene expression differences. Differential DNA methylation in amnion between term and preterm pregnancies in labor and term pregnancies not in labor show the majority of changes in methylation occur at the onset of labor. A large portion of the differentially methylated genes are associated with non-coding RNA and imprinted genes (Kim et al., 2013). Of the regions that show changes in methylation between preterm and term, enrichment in genes related to cation transport, cytokine production and extracellular matrix receptor interactions were observed, supporting differential expression studies demonstrating similar patterns in functional enrichment (Kim et al., 2013).

MicroRNAs, another layer of control, regulate gene expression post-transcriptionally through binding to and destabilizing mRNA molecules (Ambros, 2004). Although most miRNA lack experimentally validated targets, computational predictions can suggest genes that may be involved in biological processes (Ekimler and Sahin, 2014). Ten miRNA were specifically differentially regulated between term in labor and preterm labor membranes, all of which were down regulated (Montenegro et al., 2009). Additionally, the RNA processor Dicer was down regulated suggesting miRNAs play a key role in the parturition process at term but not preterm. Coupled with gene expression data, these studies can show regulation that occurs at the onset of labor that separates preterm and term processes.

Early Pregnancy Loss

Early embryonic arrest affects approximately 10% of pregnancies with rates increasing as the age of couples trying to conceive increases (Larsen et al., 2013). Pregnancy loss is due to factors including uterine abnormalities, abnormal chromosomes and infection pathologies but genetic factors can also lead to a pregnancy loss (Xu et al., 2016). Transcriptomic profiles from chorionic villi of early embryonic arrest samples compared to gestation age matched elective termination samples show differentially expression in PI3K-Akt signaling pathway, Jak-STAT pathway and complement and coagulation signaling cascades (Yang et al., 2019). One study looking specifically at long non-coding RNA that are differentially regulated in chorionic villi between patients with recurrent miscarriage and those undergoing an elective abortion found up regulation of steroid hormone biosynthesis and extracellular matrix interaction and well as down regulation of TGF-beta signaling and apoptosis pathways (Wang et al., 2017). An additional study comparing chorionic villi from recurrent pregnancy loss couples, defined as having five or more miscarriages, to elective termination samples shows a substantial down regulation of key small non-coding RNA as well as histone genes (Sõber et al., 2016). Those results suggest that chorionic villi cells begin repressing key cellular processes leading to loss of the pregnancy.

Preeclampsia

Preeclampsia is a common disease that is the leading cause of pregnancy associated mortality and morbidity for both the mother and child (Roberts and Cooper, 2001). Shallow trophoblast invasion and impaired remodeling of the uterine spiral arteries are associated with preeclampsia (Pennington et al., 2012). Gene expression of amnion epithelial cells from healthy and preeclamptic c-sections were compared to understand the underlying disease etiology. Functional annotation of differentially expressed genes identified pathways involved in extracellular matrix-receptor interaction and focal adhesion. Additional validation studies showed differential expression of matrix metalloproteinases that control degradation of the extracellular matrix (Kim et al., 2016).

RESPONSE TO STIMULI

Understanding signaling events that cause membrane rupture can suggest specific pathways misregulated in PPROM. Testing specific response pathways can connect early signaling events from *in vitro* stimulus response studies to *in vivo* studies that examine the progression of labor. Such *in vitro* studies can circumvent the limitation that observational studies are necessarily correlative and thus cannot differentiate between the cause and consequence. Additionally, *in vitro* stimulus-response studies can identify intermediate steps leading to the onset of phenotype that observational studies miss due to strict limits on tissue collection during pregnancy. For example, *in vitro* functional genomic studies of fetal membranes cells responding to inflammatory stimuli can reveal the direct effects of those signals on pathways related to cell proliferation, adhesion, or apoptosis that may impact the timing of membrane rupture. Indeed, studies of cultured amnion mesenchyme cells exposed to an IL1β challenge for up to 8 h showed transcriptional dynamics reflecting an immediate immune challenge compared to sustained response. The early responsive genes showed signatures of NF-κB activity, a well-documented effector of IL-1 signaling (Cogswell et al., 1994; Greten et al., 2007; Liu et al., 2017). Later responsive genes had more diverse transcription factor binding sites indicative of a cascade of downstream gene regulatory events. Those secondary factors including the AP-1 family transcription factors that were not regulated by the initial IL-1β response (Li et al., 2011). Similarly, immune challenges to chorionic trophoblast cells through lipopolysaccharide (LPS) show an increase in gene expression related to cytokine production and response, although this signaling appears to be mediated through the STAT1-STAT3 pathway

(Jiang et al., 2018). While differential DNA methylation is detected following LPS stimulation, 2 h of LPS induction may not be enough to detect significant changes in methylation. Together, these studies demonstrate the types of insights possible from functional genomic studies of fetal membrane cells after *in vitro* exposures. However, many of the common signals in pregnancy such as hormonal changes, oxidative stress and mechanical force changes remain to be investigated.

GENETIC STUDIES OF FETAL MEMBRANES

Transcriptomic and DNA methylation studies can take on additional informative power when combined with genetic association studies. Most variants identified in genome wide association studies are found in non-coding regions (Zhang and Lupski, 2015). Integration with functional genomic data sets can reveal candidate causal mechanisms, including target genes of clinical importance (Lowe and Reddy, 2015). The primary challenge is that the lead signal in a genetic association study is in linkage disequilibrium with many surrounding variants. Thus, the patterns of linkage disequilibrium in the study population limit resolution, often to >10 kb. Functional genomic datasets can suggest which variants in that LD-based region are most likely to have regulatory activity (Conde et al., 2013). That approach was used to identify a variant that abolishes a transcription factor binding site that represses interleukin 1 family members in fetal membranes (Liu et al., 2019). The variant identified was suggested to have a gene expression effect on multiple members of the interleukin 1 family including IL1A, IL36G, and IL36RN. A similar approach was also used in a genome wide association study of early preterm and term infants. Several significant variants near the gene SLIT2 were identified that overlaps regions of DNase hypersensitivity, suggesting regulatory activity, in several fetal tissues including the amnion (Tiensuu et al., 2019).

The combination of epigenomic data and genome wide association studies has also been employed for other pregnancy complications affecting the fetal membranes, including preeclampsia. A genome wide association study that incorporated both maternal and fetal DNA variants identified a variant near the gene FLT1 from the offspring of pregnancies associated with preeclampsia (McGinnis et al., 2017). The evidence for the effect of this variant was built by the fact that Roadmap Epigenomics incorporating many different epigenetic datasets, such as histone modifications and open chromatin sites, labeled this site as a putative enhancer in both amnion and trophoblast cell types.

While many genome wide association studies detect common non-coding variants from large populations, rare coding variants can also contribute to disease. In these cases, whole exome sequencing is often employed to detect these variants. A whole exome sequencing study of PPROM cases and healthy term controls in an African American population identified 10 rare variants more common in PPROM cases than term controls in native regulators of innate immunity, LPS detoxifying enzymes and antimicrobial protein genes (Modi et al., 2017). An additional follow up replication study replicated two of the variants in the genes DEFB1 and MBL2, both thought to be antimicrobial proteins in fetal membranes (Modi et al., 2018). The use of genomic sequencing technologies can detect both common and rare variants associated with fetal membranes pathologies. Studies identifying variants relevant to these pathologies are outlined in **Table 2**.

FUTURE STUDIES

While the number of studies comparing regulation between healthy and pathological membranes is growing, the data available remains sparse. Published studies have largely focused on comparing transcriptomic data or DNA methylation between cases and controls, often using microarray measurements that are noisier and have less dynamic range than sequencing-based methods (Zhao et al., 2014). In addition, few studies on fetal membranes have deposited raw data in publicly available databases, limiting benefit to other fetal membrane researchers. All together missing are assays of chromatin accessibility or histone modification in fetal membrane tissue type which can add more information about different levels of regulation and suggest transcription factors responsible for signaling that leads to pregnancy complications. Expanding studies of the response to relevant stimuli in fetal membrane tissues is a major opportunity. Studies thus far have focused on cellular responses to inflammatory stimuli but further studies looking at mechanical stress, hormone signaling and oxidative stress using *in vitro* tissue models in addition to cellular models to replicate the structural complexity of fetal membranes and cellular interaction can help add to a more complete understanding of the signaling that leads to PPROM, preterm birth, preeclampsia or early pregnancy loss.

AUTHOR CONTRIBUTIONS

SC wrote the manuscript with supervision from TR. TA and LF edited the manuscript. All authors contributed to the article and approved the submitted version.

REFERENCES

Ambros, V. (2004). The functions of animal MicroRNAs. *Nature* 431, 350–355. doi: 10.1038/nature02871

Arnold, C. D., Gerlach, D., Stelzer, C., Boryn, L. M., Rath, M., and Stark, A. (2013). Genome-wide quantitative enhancer activity maps identified by STARR-Seq. *Science* 339, 1074–1077. doi: 10.1126/science.1232542

Bingle, L., Tetley, T. D., and Bingle, C. D. (2001). Cytokine-mediated induction of the human elafin gene in pulmonary epithelial cells is regulated by nuclear factor- B. *Am. J. Respir. Cell Mol. Biol.* 25, 84–91. doi: 10.1165/ajrcmb.25.1.4341

Bryant-Greenwood, G. D. (1998). The extracellular matrix of the human fetal membranes: structure and function. *Placenta* 19, 1–11. doi: 10.1016/S0143-4004(98)90092-3

Burgos, H., and Faulk, W. P. (1981). The maintenance of human amniotic membranes in culture. *Br. J. Obstet. Gynaecol.* 88, 294–300. doi: 10.1111/j.1471-0528.1981.tb00984.x

Chung, C. Y., Ma, Z., Dravis, C., Preissl, S., Poirion, O., Luna, G., et al. (2019). Single-Cell chromatin analysis of mammary gland development reveals cell-state transcriptional regulators and lineage relationships. *Cell Rep.* 29, 495–510.e6. doi: 10.1016/j.celrep.2019.08.089

Clark, S. J., Harrison, J., Paul, C. L., and Frommer, M. (1994). High sensitivity mapping of methylated cytosines. *Nucleic Acids Res.* 22, 2990–2997. doi: 10.1093/nar/22.15.2990

Cogswell, J. P., Godlevski, M. M., Wisely, G. B., Clay, W. C., Leesnitzer, L. M., Ways, J. P., et al. (1994). NF-Kappa B regulates IL-1 beta transcription through a consensus NF-Kappa B binding site and a nonconsensus CRE-like site. *J. Immunol.* 153, 712–723.

Conde, L., Bracci, P. M., Richardson, R., Montgomery, S. B., and Skibola, C. F. (2013). Integrating GWAS and expression data for functional characterization of disease-associated SNPs: an application to follicular lymphoma. *Am. J. Hum.Genet.* 92, 126–130. doi: 10.1016/j.ajhg.2012.11.009

Ekimler, S., and Sahin, K. (2014). Computational methods for microRNA target prediction. *Genes* 5, 671–683. doi: 10.3390/genes5030671

Finotello, F., and Di Camillo, B. (2015). Measuring differential gene expression with RNA-Seq: challenges and strategies for data analysis. *Brief. Funct. Genomics* 14, 130–142. doi: 10.1093/bfgp/elu035

Greten, F. R., Arkan, M. C., Bollrath, J., Hsu, L. C., Goode, J., Miething, C., et al. (2007). NF-KB is a negative regulator of IL-1β secretion as revealed by genetic and pharmacological inhibition of IKKβ. *Cell* 130, 918–931. doi: 10.1016/j.cell.2007.07.009

Guyot, N., Zani, M. L., Maurel, M. C., Dallet-Choisy, S., and Moreau, T. (2005). Elafin and its precursor Trappin-2 still inhibit neutrophil serine proteinases when they are covalently bound to extracellular matrix proteins by tissue transglutaminase. *Biochemistry* 44, 15610–15618. doi: 10.1021/bi051418i

Jia, G., Preussner, J., Chen, X., Guenther, S., Yuan, X., Yekelchyk, M., et al. (2018). Single cell RNA-seq and ATAC-seq analysis of cardiac progenitor cell transition states and lineage settlement. *Nat. Commun.* 9:4877. doi: 10.1038/s41467-018-07307-6

Jiang, K., Wong, L., Chen, Y., Xing, X., Li, D., Wang, T., et al. (2018). Soluble inflammatory mediators induce transcriptional re-organization that is independent of Dna methylation changes in cultured human chorionic villous trophoblasts. *J. Reprod. Immunol.* 128, 2–8. doi: 10.1016/j.jri.2018.05.005

Johnson, D. S., Mortazavi, A., and Myers, R. M. (2007). Genome-wide mapping of in vivo protein-DNA interactions. *Science* 316, 1497–1503.

Kim, J., Pitlick, M. M., Christine, P. J., Schaefer, A. R., Saleme, C., Comas, B., et al. (2013). Genome-wide analysis of DNA methylation in human amnion. *Sci. World J.* 2013:678156.

Kim, J., Zhao, K., Jiang, P., Lu, Z.-X., Wang, J., Murray, J. C., et al. (2012). Transcriptome landscape of the human placenta. *BMC Genomics* 13:115. doi: 10.1186/1471-2164-13-115

Kim, M., Yu, J. H., Lee, S., Kim, A. L., and Jo, M. H. (2016). Differential expression of extracellular matrix and adhesion molecules in fetal-origin amniotic epithelial cells of preeclamptic pregnancy. *PLoS One* 11:e0156038. doi: 10.1371/journal.pone.0156038

Larsen, E. C., Christiansen, O. B., Kolte, A. M., and Macklon, N. (2013). New insights into mechanisms behind miscarriage. *BMC Med.* 11:154. doi: 10.1186/1741-7015-11-154

Li, R., Ackerman, W. E., Summerfield, T. L., Yu, L., Gulati, P., Zhang, J., et al. (2011). Inflammatory gene regulatory networks in amnion cells following cytokine stimulation: translational systems approach to modeling human parturition. *PLoS One* 6:e20560. doi: 10.1371/journal.pone.0020560

Lim, S., Macintyre, D. A., Lee, Y. S., Khanjani, S., Terzidou, V., Teoh, T. G., et al. (2012). Nuclear factor Kappa B activation occurs in the amnion prior to labour onset and modulates the expression of numerous labour associated genes. *PLoS One* 7:e34707. doi: 10.1371/journal.pone.0034707

Liu, T., Zhang, L., Joo, D., and Sun, S. C. (2017). NF-KB Signaling in inflammation. *Signal. Transduct. Target Ther.* 2:17023. doi: 10.1038/sigtrans.2017.23

Liu, X., Helenius, D., Skotte, L., Beaumont, R. N., Wielscher, M., Geller, F., et al. (2019). Variants in the fetal genome near pro-in Fl Ammatory cytokine genes on 2q13 associate with gestational duration. *Nat. Commun.* 10:3927. doi: 10.1038/s41467-019-11881-8

Lowe, W. L., and Reddy, T. E. (2015). Genomic approaches for understanding the genetics of complex disease. *Genome Res.* 25, 1432–1441. doi: 10.1101/gr.190603.115

McDowell, I. C., Barrera, A., D'Ippolito, A. M., Vockley, C. M., Hong, L. K., Leichter, S. M., et al. (2018). Glucocorticoid receptor recruits to enhancers and drives activation by motif-directed binding. *Genome Res.* 28, 1272–1284. doi: 10.1101/gr.233346.117

McGinnis, R., Steinthorsdottir, V., Williams, N. O., Thorleifsson, G., Shoote, S., Hjartardottir, S., et al. (2017). Variants in the fetal genome near FLT1 are associated with risk of preeclampsia. *Nat. Genet.* 49, 1255–1260. doi: 10.1038/ng.3895

Meissner, A., Mikkelsen, T. S., Gu, H., Wernig, M., Hanna, J., Sivachenko, A., et al. (2008). Genome-scale DNA methylation maps of pluripotent and differentiated cells. *Nature* 454, 766–770. doi: 10.1038/nature07107

Mercer, B. M. (2010). "Preterm premature rupture of the membranes," in *Preterm Birth: Prevention and Management*, Vol. 101, ed. B. M. D. Vincenzo (Washington, DC: American College of Obstetrics and Gynecologists), 217–231. doi: 10.1002/9781444317619.ch19

Modi, B. P., Parikh, H. I., Teves, M. E., Kulkarni, R., Liyu, J., Romero, R., et al. (2018). Discovery of rare ancestry-specific variants in the fetal genome that confer risk of preterm premature rupture of membranes (PPROM) and preterm birth. *BMC Med. Genet.* 12:e0174356. doi: 10.1186/s12881-018-0696-4

Modi, B. P., Teves, M. E., Pearson, L. N., Parikh, H. I., and Strauss, F. (2017). Rare mutations and potentially damaging missense variants in genes encoding fibrillar collagens and proteins involved in their production are candidates for risk for preterm premature Rupture of membranes. *BMC Med. Genet.* 19:181.

Montenegro, D., Romero, R., Kim, S. S., Tarca, A. L., Draghici, S., Kusanovic, J. P., et al. (2009). Expression patterns of MicroRNAs in the chorioamniotic membranes: a role for MicroRNAs in human pregnancy and parturition. *J. Pathol.* 217, 113–121. doi: 10.1002/path.2463

Mortazavi, A., Williams, B. A., McCue, K., Schaeffer, L., and Wold, B. (2008). Mapping and quantifying mammalian transcriptomes by RNA-Seq. *Nat. Methods* 5, 621–628. doi: 10.1038/nmeth.1226

Mundade, R., Ozer, H. G., Wei, H., Prabhu, L., and Lu, T. (2014). Role of ChIP-Seq in the discovery of transcription factor binding sites, differential gene regulation mechanism, epigenetic marks and beyond. *Cell Cycle* 13, 2847–2852. doi: 10.4161/15384101.2014.949201

Nhan-Chang, C.-L., Romero, R., Tarca, A. L., Mittal, P., Kusanovic, J. P., Erez, O., et al. (2010). Characterization of the transcriptome of chorioamniotic membranes at the site of rupture in spontaneous labor at term. *Am. J. Obstet. Gynecol.* 202:462.e1-41. doi: 10.1016/j.ajog.2010.02.045

Pennington, K. A., Schlitt, J. M., Jackson, D. L., Schulz, L. C., and Schust, D. J. (2012). Preeclampsia: multiple approaches for a multifactorial disease disease models & mechanisms. *Dis. Model. Mech.* 5, 9–18. doi: 10.1242/dmm.008516

Pereyra, S., Sosa, C., Bertoni, B., and Sapiro, R. (2019). Transcriptomic analysis of fetal membranes reveals pathways involved in preterm birth. *BMC Med. Genomics* 12:53. doi: 10.1186/s12920-019-0498-3

Pfundt, R., Wingens, M., and Bergers, M. (2000). TNF-α and serum induce SKALP / Elafin gene expression in human keratinocytes by a P38 MAP Kinase-dependent pathway. *Arch. Dermatol. Res.* 292, 180–187. doi: 10.1007/s004030050475

Pulido-Salgado, M., Vidal-Taboada, J. M., Garcia-Diaz Barriga, G., Solà, C., and Saura, J. (2018). RNA-Seq transcriptomic profiling of primary murine microglia treated with LPS or LPS + IFNγ. *Sci. Rep.* 8:16096. doi: 10.1038/s41598-018-34412-9

Roadmap Epigenomics Consortium, Kundaje, A., Meuleman, W., Ernst, J., Bilenky, M., Yen, A., et al. (2015). Integrative analysis of 111 reference human epigenomes. *Nature* 518, 317–329. doi: 10.1038/nature14248

Roberts, J. M., and Cooper, D. W. (2001). Pathogenesis and genetics of pre-eclampsia. *Lancet* 357, 53–56. doi: 10.1016/s0140-6736(00)03577-7

Robertson, G., Hirst, M., Bainbridge, M., Bilenky, M., Zhao, Y., Zeng, T., et al. (2007). Genome-wide profiles of STAT1 DNA association using chromatin immunoprecipitation and massively parallel sequencing. *Nat. Methods* 4, 651–657. doi: 10.1038/nmeth1068

Sõber, S., Rull, K., Reiman, M., Ilisson, P., Mattila, P., and Laan, M. (2016). RNA sequencing of chorionic villi from recurrent pregnancy loss patients reveals impaired function of basic nuclear and cellular machinery. *Sci. Rep.* 6:38439. doi: 10.1038/srep38439

Souza, J. P., Gülmezoglu, A. M., Vogel, J., Carroli, G., Lumbiganon, P., Qureshi, Z., et al. (2013). Moving beyond essential interventions for reduction of maternal mortality (the WHO multicountry survey on maternal and newborn health): a cross-sectional study. *Lancet* 381, 1747–1755. doi: 10.1016/S0140-6736(13)60686-8

The Encode Project Consortium (2012). An integrated encyclopedia of DNA elements in the human genome. *Nature* 489, 57–74. doi: 10.1038/nature11247

Tiensuu, H., Haapalainen, A. M., Karjalainen, M. K., Pasanen, A., Huusko, J. M., Marttila, R., et al. (2019). Risk of spontaneous preterm birth and fetal growth associates with Fetal SLIT2. *PLoS Genet.* 15:e1008107. doi: 10.1371/journal.pgen.1008107

Tirado-Magallanes, R., Rebbani, K., Lim, R., Pradhan, S., and Benoukraf, T. (2016). Whole genome DNA methylation: beyond genes silencing. *J. Cancer Res. Clin. Oncol.* 8, 5629–5637. doi: 10.1007/s00432-017-2467-6

Tromp, G., Kuivaniemi, H., Romero, R., Chaiworapongsa, T., Kim, M., Kim, R., et al. (2004). Genome-wide expression profiling of fetal membranes reveals a deficient expression of proteinase inhibitor 3 in premature rupture of membranes. *Am. J. Obstet. Gynecol.* 191, 1331–1338. doi: 10.1016/j.ajog.2004.07.010

Velez, D. R., Fortunato, S. J., Morgan, N., Edwards, T. L., Lombardi, S. J., Williams, S. M., et al. (2008). Patterns of cytokine profiles differ with pregnancy outcome and ethnicity. *Hum. Reprod.* 23, 1902–1909. doi: 10.1093/humrep/den170

Vento-Tormo, R., Efremova, M., Botting, R. A., Turco, M. Y., Vento-Tormo, M., Meyer, K. B., et al. (2018). Single-cell reconstruction of the early maternal–fetal interface in humans. *Nature* 563, 347–353. doi: 10.1038/s41586-018-0698-6

Wang, J., Rieder, S. A., Wu, J., Hayes, S., Halpin, R. A., de los Reyes, M., et al. (2019). Evaluation of ultra-low input RNA sequencing for the study of human T Cell transcriptome. *Sci. Rep.* 9:8445. doi: 10.1038/s41598-019-44902-z

Wang, L., Tang, H., Xiong, Y., and Tang, L. (2017). Differential expression profile of LONG noncoding RNAs in human chorionic villi of early recurrent miscarriage. *Clin. Chim. Acta* 464, 17–23. doi: 10.1016/j.cca.2016.11.001

World Health Organization (2016). *Preterm Birth Fact Sheet. 2016*. Geneva: World Health Organization.

Xu, Y., Shi, Y., Fu, J., Yu, M., Feng, R., Sang, Q., et al. (2016). Mutations in PADI6 cause female infertility characterized by early embryonic arrest. *Am. J. Hum. Genet.* 99, 744–752. doi: 10.1016/j.ajhg.2016.06.024

Yang, W., Lu, Z., Zhi, Z., Liu, L., Deng, L., Jiang, X., et al. (2019). High-throughput transcriptome-Seq and small RNA-Seq reveal novel functional genes and MicroRNAs for early embryonic arrest in humans. *Gene* 697, 19–25. doi: 10.1016/j.gene.2018.12.084

Zhang, F., and Lupski, J. R. (2015). Non-coding genetic variants in human disease. *Human Mol. Genet.* 24, R102–R110. doi: 10.1093/hmg/ddv259

Zhao, S., Fung-Leung, W. P., Bittner, A., Ngo, K., and Liu, X. (2014). Comparison of RNA-Seq and microarray in transcriptome profiling of activated T Cells. *PLoS One* 9:e78644. doi: 10.1371/journal.pone.0078644

Zhou, V. W., Goren, A., and Bernstein, B. E. (2011). Charting histone modifications and the functional organization of mammalian genomes. *Nat. Rev. Genet.* 12, 7–18. doi: 10.1038/nrg2905

Cholesterol Crystals and NLRP3 Mediated Inflammation in the Uterine Wall Decidua in Normal and Preeclamptic Pregnancies

Gabriela Brettas Silva[1,2], Lobke Marijn Gierman[1,2], Johanne Johnsen Rakner[1], Guro Sannerud Stødle[1], Siv Boon Mundal[1], Astrid Josefin Thaning[1], Bjørnar Sporsheim[1], Mattijs Elschot[3,4], Karin Collett[5], Line Bjørge[6,7], Marie Hjelmseth Aune[1], Liv Cecilie Vestrheim Thomsen[6,7] and Ann-Charlotte Iversen[1,2]*

[1] Centre of Molecular Inflammation Research, Department of Cancer Research and Molecular Medicine, Norwegian University of Science and Technology, Trondheim, Norway, [2] Department of Gynecology and Obstetrics, St. Olavs Hospital, Trondheim, Norway, [3] Department of Circulation and Medical Imaging, Norwegian University of Science and Technology, Trondheim, Norway, [4] Department of Radiology and Nuclear Medicine, St. Olavs Hospital, Trondheim, Norway, [5] Department of Pathology, Haukeland University Hospital, Bergen, Norway, [6] Department of Gynecology and Obstetrics, Haukeland University Hospital, Bergen, Norway, [7] Centre for Cancer Biomarkers CCBIO, Department of Clinical Science, University of Bergen, Bergen, Norway

***Correspondence:**
Ann-Charlotte Iversen
ann-charlotte.iversen@ntnu.no

Preeclampsia is a hypertensive and inflammatory pregnancy disorder associated with cholesterol accumulation and inflammation at the maternal-fetal interface. Preeclampsia can be complicated with fetal growth restriction (FGR) and shares risk factors and pathophysiological mechanisms with cardiovascular disease. Cholesterol crystal mediated NLRP3 inflammasome activation is central to cardiovascular disease and the pathway has been implicated in placental inflammation in preeclampsia. Direct maternal-fetal interaction occurs both in the uterine wall decidua and at the placental surface and these aligned sites constitute the maternal-fetal interface. This study aimed to investigate cholesterol crystal accumulation and NLRP3 inflammasome expression by maternal and fetal cells in the uterine wall decidua of normal and preeclamptic pregnancies. Pregnant women with normal ($n = 43$) and preeclamptic pregnancies with ($n = 28$) and without ($n = 19$) FGR were included at delivery. Cholesterol crystals were imaged in decidual tissue by both second harmonic generation microscopy and polarization filter reflected light microscopy. Quantitative expression analysis of NLRP3, IL-1β and cell markers was performed by immunohistochemistry and automated image processing. Functional NLRP3 activation was assessed in cultured decidual explants. Cholesterol crystals were identified in decidual tissue, both in the tissue stroma and near uterine vessels. The cholesterol crystals in decidua varied between pregnancies in distribution and cluster size. Decidual expression of the inflammasome components NLRP3 and IL-1β was located to fetal trophoblasts and maternal leukocytes and was strongest in areas of proximity between these cell types. Pathway functionality was confirmed by cholesterol crystal activation of IL-1β in cultured decidual explants. Preeclampsia without FGR was associated with increased trophoblast dependent NLRP3 and IL-1β expression, particularly in the decidual areas of trophoblast and leukocyte proximity. Our findings suggest that decidual accumulation of cholesterol crystals may activate the NLRP3 inflammasome and contribute to decidual inflammation and that this pathway is strengthened in areas with close maternal-fetal interaction in preeclampsia without FGR.

Keywords: cholesterol crystals, decidua, fetal growth restriction, NLRP3 inflammasome, inflammation, IL-1β, placenta, preeclampsia

INTRODUCTION

Pregnancy is characterized by low-grade inflammation at the maternal-fetal interface and systemically in the mother, and this is aggravated to harmful levels in the pregnancy disorder preeclampsia (1). Preeclampsia is clinically characterized in the second half of pregnancy by new onset hypertension and proteinuria or maternal organ dysfunction and/or uteroplacental dysfunction (2, 3). The disease occurs in 4–5% of pregnancies and is a leading cause of maternal and fetal morbidity and mortality, often complicating with fetal growth restriction (FGR) (4). Preeclampsia is considered a warning sign for cardiovascular disease (CVD) later in life and common pathophysiological mechanisms are shared (5, 6). Cholesterol mediated inflammation has been suggested as a link between the disorders, a theory supported by preeclamptic pregnancies being characterized by a pro-atherogenic maternal lipid profile and cholesterol accumulation at the maternal-fetal interface (7, 8).

The uterine wall decidua and the placenta are the two aligned sites for direct maternal-fetal immunological interaction throughout pregnancy. In the decidua, specialized fetal cells, called extravillous trophoblasts, invade the tissue and establish a direct molecular dialogue with resident maternal cells such as decidual stromal cells and maternal immune cells (9). Leukocytes are key cells in modulating trophoblast behavior (10). Placental cytotrophoblasts fuse together to form a multinucleated cell layer, the syncytiotrophoblast, that covers the placenta and directly interacts with maternal blood. Preeclampsia and FGR are associated with reduced trophoblast invasion and impaired artery remodeling in the uterine wall, leading to placental oxidative stress and inflammation that increase as the fetus grows (11–13). Although significant progress has been made in understanding the central role of placental inflammation for development of preeclampsia and FGR (13–15), little is known about the involvement of inflammatory mechanisms in the decidua.

Intracellular crystallization of cholesterol is a complex process that occurs upon endocytosis of oxidized low-density lipoprotein (oxLDL) and this process has been extensively studied in the arterial wall in atherosclerosis (16, 17). The cholesterol crystals promote the development of atherosclerotic lesions by activation of the potent Nod-like receptor protein (NLRP)3 inflammasome (18). The resulting interleukin (IL)-1β production from this powerful activation may lead to extensive inflammation and tissue damage (15, 19). Trophoblasts express receptors that enable cholesterol transport and uptake of oxLDL has been shown to reduce trophoblast invasiveness (20–23), but cholesterol crystals have not been investigated at the maternal-fetal interface. Dysregulated lipid transport by reduced expression of ATP-binding cassette transporter (ABCA1) has been associated with cholesterol accumulation at the placental syncytiotrophoblast layer in preeclampsia (24) and in primary extravillous trophoblasts (25). Preeclampsia is associated with increased maternal systemic inflammatory markers including total cholesterol, oxLDL, IL-1β and soluble fms-like tyrosine kinase-1 (sFlt-1) (26–28). The NLRP3 inflammasome pathway in preeclampsia has been recently reviewed and mechanistically illustrated (29). We have previously shown that the NLRP3 inflammasome is active in the placenta and associated with preeclampsia, with a central involvement of trophoblasts (28). In the decidua, increased cholesterol accumulation in preeclampsia (7) and NLRP3 inflammasome expression in cultured cells (30) has been shown. This indicates a role for cholesterol crystal mediated NLRP3 inflammasome activation across the maternal-fetal interface, but the decidual involvement still needs to be determined.

We hypothesize that cholesterol accumulation in the decidua results in formation of cholesterol crystals, which induce decidual NLRP3 inflammasome activation and influence the important dialogue between trophoblasts and maternal immune cells. This study aimed to characterize cholesterol crystal accumulation and NLRP3 inflammasome expression by maternal and fetal cells in the uterine wall decidua of normal and preeclamptic pregnancies.

METHODS

Study Participants and Decidual Biopsies

Women with normal and preeclamptic pregnancies with and without FGR were recruited at St. Olavs and Haukeland University Hospitals during 2002-2012. Preeclampsia was defined as persistent hypertension exceeding 140/90 mmHg plus proteinuria ≥0.3 g/24 h or ≥+1 by dipstick after 20 weeks of gestation. FGR was diagnosed by serial ultrasound measurements showing reduced intrauterine growth ($n = 27$), or, for neonates small for gestational age ($n = 1$), birth weight <5th percentile of Norwegian reference curves (31) combined with clinically and sonographically suspected FGR and/or postpartum defined placental pathology. Only singleton pregnancies undergoing cesarean section with no signs of labor were included. Decidua basalis tissue was collected by vacuum suction of the placental bed during cesarean section (7, 32). Tissue samples were either fixed in 10% neutral-buffered formalin and embedded in paraffin or snap frozen and stored at −80°C.

Placentas were collected from normal pregnancies after delivery by elective cesarean section for immediate isolation of decidual explants. The decidual tissue was dissected from the central region of the maternal side of the placenta. Samples were processed and cultured within 1.5 h after delivery.

Decidual Explants

Decidual tissue was washed in sterile phosphate-buffered saline, cut into pieces (explants with wet weight range of 15–33 mg) and distributed in the culture plate evenly between the different culture conditions (24 ± 2 mg, mean ± standard deviation). There were no significant differences in explant weight between the culture conditions. Explants were cultured in

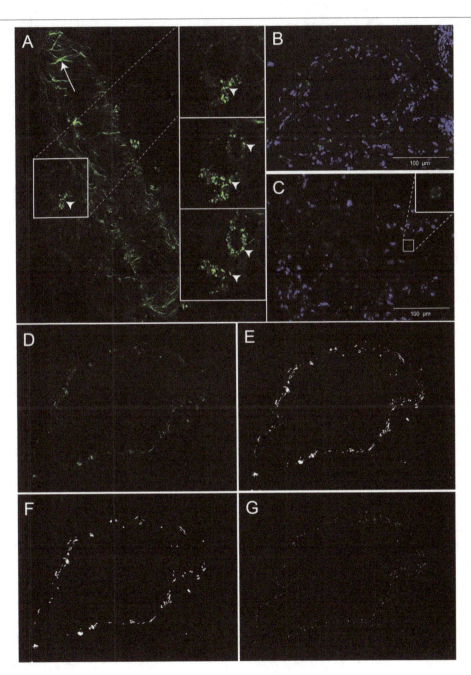

FIGURE 1 | Cholesterol crystals in decidual tissue. **(A)** Decidual tissue imaged by second harmonic generation microscopy. The arrow heads indicate cholesterol crystals and the arrow points to collagen fibers in the vessel wall. **(B,C)** Decidual tissue stained by DAPI and imaged by polarized light microscopy. Nuclei (blue) and cholesterol crystals (green) are shown near a vessel wall **(B)** and within tissue stroma **(C)**. **(D–G)** Representative images obtained by polarized light microscopy for cholesterol crystal quantification. **(D)** Unprocessed image of cholesterol crystals (green). The same image processed by MATLAB showing **(E)** total cholesterol crystals and separated into **(F)** large and **(G)** small clusters of cholesterol crystals. Scale bar 100 μM.

Ham's F12/Dulbecco's modified Eagle's medium (DMEM) with 10% fetal bovine serum and 100 mg/mL penicillin-streptomycin (Sigma-Aldrich) and incubated for 24 h at 37°C, 8% O_2 and 5% CO_2 (33). Culture medium was then replaced by fresh culture medium with or without 500 pg/ml LPS priming (#tlrl-3pelps, InvivoGen, California, United States). After 2 h, the medium was replaced by fresh culture medium with or without stimuli; 200 or 2,000 µg/ml synthetic cholesterol crystals (#C3045, Sigma-Aldrich) or the positive control 3 mM ATP (#A7699, Sigma-Aldrich). Supernatants were collected after 24 h, centrifuged and stored at −80°C. Six technical replicates for each experimental condition were combined before analysis. Tissue viability was assessed by lactate dehydrogenase (LDH) cytotoxicity assay (#04744926001, Roche, Basel, Switzerland) (**Supplementary Figure 1**). IL-1β levels in supernatants were measured undiluted in duplicate using quantitative sandwich ELISA (#557953, BD Biosciences, New Jersey, United States).

Cholesterol Crystal Imaging and Automated Quantification

To preserve cholesterol crystals, the decidual cryosections (5 µm) were analyzed untreated. DAPI mounting medium (#F6057, Sigma-Aldrich, Missouri, United States) was used to identify cellular nuclei. Cholesterol crystals in the decidual cryosections were first assessed by second harmonic generation microscopy (25X magnification Leica SP8 confocal microscope, Wetzlar; Germany). For further analysis of cholesterol crystals, three adjacent TIFF images (2,080 × 1,544 pixels) were obtained from three different regions in the decidual section using polarization filter reflected light microscopy (20X magnification, Inverted fluorescence microscope Olympus IX71, Tokyo, Japan) and defined microscope settings. The cholesterol crystals in the nine TIFF images per decidua were quantified by a customized MATLAB script (version 2018a, the MathWorks Inc., Massachusetts, United States) developed for automatic quantification of positive pixels. The total cholesterol crystal positive pixels in each decidua was determined by the sum of the positive pixels quantified in the nine pictures. The number of positive pixels in each of the nine images was used to assess the variation in cholesterol crystal tissue distribution within each decidua. To evaluate the size of the observed cholesterol crystals, aggregation of positive pixels was determined by defining small (<50 pixels) and large (≥50 pixels) cholesterol crystal clusters (representative image in **Figures 1D–G**). To verify that the crystals dissolved in alcohol, two serial decidual cryosections (5 µm) were obtained from four decidual tissue samples. One slide from each decidual sample was treated with PBS and the other slide was immersed in alcohol at room temperature for 60 s.

Immunohistochemical Staining

Immunohistochemistry staining was performed in paraffin embedded decidua. Serial sections of 3 µm were pre-treated in PT link (#PT101, Dako, Glostrup, Denmark) using Target Retrieval Solution (#K8005 or #K8004, Dako) at 97°C for 20 min, and all sections were treated with peroxidase blocking solution (#K4007, Dako) or with dual peroxidase and alkaline phosphatase blocking solution (#K5361, Dako). Decidual tissue sections were incubated overnight at 4°C with antibodies against NLRP3 (1:100, #AG-20B-0014-C100, AdipoGen, California, United States) or IL-1β (1:200, #NB600-633, Novus, Colorado, United States); or for 45 min with cytokeratin 7 (CK7) (1:300, #M0851, Dako) or 40 min with CD45 (1:150, #M0701, Dako) at room temperature. All sections were incubated for 30 min with HRP-labeled polymer (#K4007, Dako) and for 10 min with DAB+ as chromogen (1:50, #K4007 or K5361, Dako). Decidual CK7 sections were double stained with smooth muscle actin (SMA) antibodies (1:300, #M0851, Dako) using EnVision G|2 Doublestain System Rabbit/Mouse (DAB+/Permanent Red) Kit system (K#5361, Dako). Overnight staining was performed manually and otherwise by Autostainer Plus (#S3800, Dako). Sections were counterstained with hematoxylin. Negative isotype controls were included (**Figures 3G,H**). In addition to the immunohistochemical staining, a routine staining with hematoxylin (#75290, Chemi-Teknik AS, Oslo, Norway), erythrosine 239 (#720-0179, VWR, Pennsylvania, United States) and saffron (#75100, Chemi-Teknik AS) (HES) was performed for each decidua using a Sakura Tissue-Tek © Prisma StainerTM (Sakura Finetek, Oslo, Norway).

Automated Quantification of Protein Expression

Decidual tissue slides were scanned with the EVOS™ FL Auto Imaging System (Thermo Fisher Scientific, Massachusetts, United States), using 20X magnification and defined microscope settings. The large decidual scans varied in size depending on available tissue and consisted of 4 to 81 bright field TIFF images (2,048 × 1,536 pixels) per sample slide. A customized ImageJ (ImageJ$_2$) (34, 35) script was used to perform background correction (Image calculator: Difference (img1 = |img1–img2|) and tile stitching [Grid/Collection stitching plugin (36)]. Smooth muscle tissue, placental tissue, blood vessels and tissue with poor morphology were excluded by manually defining regions of disinterest. NLRP3 and IL-1β expression was automatically quantified in the large tissue section scan for each decidua by a customized MATLAB script, and the protein expression quantified with examiners blinded to pregnancy outcomes. Cell specific staining was used to select decidual regions containing trophoblasts (CK7+) and leukocytes (CD45+). A mask of patches (1,325 × 1,325 µm) defining trophoblasts, maternal leukocytes, and maternal tissue without trophoblasts, was created for each decidual sample by using serial tissue section scans of cell-specific stained trophoblasts (CK7+) and leukocytes (CD45+). These masks were used to relate NLRP3 and IL-1β expression levels to trophoblasts and maternal leukocytes in the spatially aligned NLRP3 and IL-1β images. The *expression density* of CK7, CD45, NLRP3, and IL-1β in decidual tissue was calculated as the total number of positive stained pixels divided by the total amount of tissue pixels analyzed, to account for varying amounts of tissue between the samples. The *expression intensity* of NLRP3 and IL-1β were calculated as average staining intensity of all patches using a color deconvolution algorithm based on DAB specific RGB absorption (37).

Statistical Methods

Statistical analyses were performed in SPSS (IBM SPSS Statistics 26, Illinois, United States) and GraphPad Prism (Prism8, California, United States). For clinical data, one-way ANOVA or Kruskal-Wallis with Tukey's or Dunn's multiple comparison *post hoc* test, respectively, were used for comparisons of continuous variables, and Fisher's exact test for categorical variables. Protein measurements in supernatants were analyzed by Kruskal-Wallis with Dunn's multiple comparison *post-hoc* test.

NLRP3 and IL-1β expression levels were compared between study groups using a linear mixed model with recruitment location, study group and the trophoblast and leukocyte densities implemented as fixed effects. Subject combinations and intercept were included as random effects. The cholesterol crystal analysis was performed by a linear mixed model with recruitment location and study group as fixed effect. Correlation between variables was performed by calculating Pearson's correlation coefficient. Alpha level was set to 0.05.

RESULTS

Study Material

A total of 90 women with normal ($n = 43$) and preeclamptic pregnancies with ($n = 28$) and without FGR ($n = 19$) were included to the study (**Table 1**). The preeclamptic pregnancies with and without FGR, included more primiparas, had higher systolic and diastolic blood pressure, and their infants were delivered at earlier gestation with lower placental and birth weights, compared to normal pregnancies. The gestational age at delivery, as well as placenta and birth weights, were lower in preeclamptic pregnancies complicated with FGR compared to preeclamptic pregnancies without FGR (**Table 1**).

For the three pregnancies included in the decidual explant analysis, maternal age ranged between 31 and 38 years and gestational age between 38 and 39 weeks.

Cholesterol Crystals

Decidual cryosections from 76 women with normal ($n = 34$) and preeclamptic pregnancies with ($n = 27$) and without FGR ($n = 15$) were included. A marked presence of cholesterol crystals was observed dispersed in decidual tissue by both second harmonic generation (**Figure 1A**) and polarized light microscopy (**Figures 1B–D**). The crystals appeared to be localized both intra and extracellularly and cells containing cholesterol crystals were observed close to uterine vessels (**Figure 1B**) and within the tissue stroma (**Figure 1C**). The cholesterol crystals were not uniformly dispersed within the tissue stroma but were instead aggregated in distinct areas of the tissue and the distribution of such cholesterol crystal areas varied markedly between different pregnancies (**Figure 2A**). The cholesterol crystals appeared in the decidua as clusters of different size, and the ratio between large and small clusters in normal pregnancies was about 2:3 (**Figure 2B**). The cholesterol crystals detected in the decidua dissolved after alcohol treatment for 60 s, as expected (**Supplementary Figure 2**).

No significant differences in the amount, distribution and cluster size of decidual cholesterol crystals were detected between normal pregnancies and preeclamptic pregnancies with or without FGR (**Figure 2C** and data not shown).

Decidual Tissue Composition

Morphological assessment of cells and structures in the uterine wall decidua showed presence of fetal trophoblasts (CK7+), maternal leukocytes (CD45+), decidual stroma cells and uterine blood vessels (CD31+ endothelium) (**Figures 3A–D**). Trophoblasts were observed isolated or clustered in the tissue and were either apart from or in close contact with maternal leukocytes and decidual stroma cells. Both mononucleated trophoblasts and multinucleated trophoblast giant cells were identified and included in the analysis.

Decidual NLRP3 Inflammasome Expression and Function

Paraffin embedded decidual tissue sections from 85 women with normal ($n = 41$) and preeclamptic pregnancies with ($n = 26$) and without FGR ($n = 18$) were included. From these, two pregnancies were excluded from the IL-1β and four from the NLRP3 expression analysis due to methodological errors in immunostaining or image processing. NLRP3 was strongly expressed in the cytoplasm of cells in the

TABLE 1 | Clinical characteristics of subjects included in third trimester decidual analyses ($n = 90$).

	Normal pregnancies ($n = 43$)	Preeclampsia without FGR ($n = 19$)	Preeclampsia with FGR ($n = 28$)
Baseline characteristics			
Maternal age, years	31.2 (± 5.4)*	29.3 (± 4,9)	29.5 (± 5.3)
Primiparas, n (%)	7 (16)	12 (63)*‖	17 (61)*‖
BMI†	24.8 (± 3.9)	25.7 (± 4.6)	25.4 (± 4.1)
Characteristics at time of delivery			
Systolic BP, mmHg‡	119 (± 10)	153 (± 20)‖	148 (±18)‖
Diastolic BP, mmHg‡	72 (± 8)	100 (± 12)‖	96 (± 11)‖
Severe preeclampsia, n (%)	n.a.	17 (89)	20 (69)
Early onset preeclampsia <34 weeks, n (%)	n.a.	15 (79)	21 (79)
Placental weight, g§	638 (102)	475 (128)‖	290 (101)‖#
Fetal birth weight, g	3,409 (332)	2,224 (583)‖	1,311 (469)‖#
Fetal sex, female, n (%)	23 (53.5)	8 (42.1)	16 (60.7)
Gestational age, weeks	38.6 (0.6)	33.6 (2.7)‖	31.3 (3.1)‖#

FGR, fetal growth restriction; BMI, body mass index; BP, blood pressure; n.a., not applicable.
Continuous variables listed as means (± standard deviation) or median (interquartile range), assessed for differences between groups by one-way ANOVA with Tukey's post hoc test or Kruskal-Wallis with Dunn's post hoc test. Categorical variables listed as number (percent in column), assessed for differences between groups by Fisher's exact test.
*Information missing from one woman.
†Maternal BMI in first trimester. Information is missing from five women.
‡Blood pressure from last healthcare visit before delivery. Information missing from one woman.
§Information missing from 12 women.
‖$P < 0.05$ vs. normal pregnancies.
#$P < 0.05$ vs. preeclampsia without FGR.

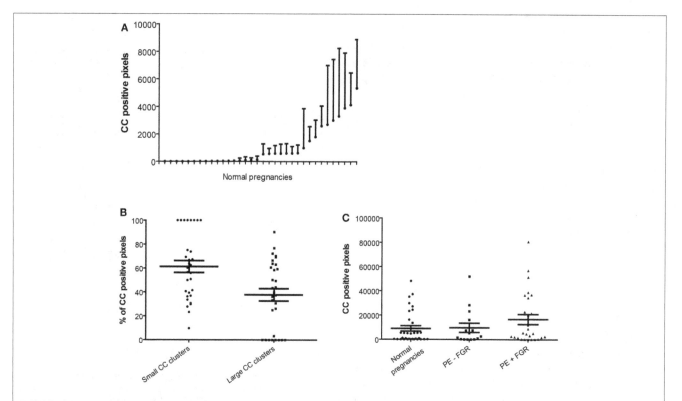

FIGURE 2 | Quantification of cholesterol crystal in decidual tissue. Cholesterol crystal (CC) quantification was performed in nine pictures per decidual cryosection (5 μm). (A) Descriptive statistics of the cholesterol crystal positive pixels, shown as estimated means with standard error of mean, per normal pregnancy. (B) Percentages of the total cholesterol crystal positive pixels corresponding to small CC clusters (<50 pixels) and large CC clusters (≥50 pixels), in normal pregnancies. (C) Total cholesterol crystal positive pixels were quantified in decidual cryosections obtained from normal ($n = 34$) and preeclamptic pregnancies with ($n = 27$) and without fetal growth restriction (FGR) ($n = 15$).

decidual tissue, including trophoblasts, maternal leukocytes, decidual stromal cells and endothelial cells (**Figure 3E**). The cell specific expression pattern of IL-1β in decidua was comparable to NLRP3 (**Figure 3F**). The cellular distribution and overall expression of NLRP3 and IL-1β in decidua of preeclamptic pregnancies appeared comparable to normal pregnancies (**Supplementary Figure 3**). The expression intensity (**Figure 4**, **Supplementary Table 1**) and density (**Supplementary Table 2**) of decidual NLRP3 and IL-1β were quantified. Preeclamptic pregnancies with normal fetal growth showed higher decidual expression intensity (**Figures 4A,B**) and density (**Supplementary Table 2**) of both NLRP3 and IL-1β compared to normal pregnancies (NLRP3 intensity $P = 0.028$ and density $P = 0.006$; IL-1β intensity $P = 0.044$, and density $P = 0.010$) and preeclamptic pregnancies complicated with FGR (NLRP3 intensity $P = 0.372$ and density $P = 0.057$; IL-1β intensity $P = 0.024$ and density $P = 0.065$, respectively). The increased decidual NLRP3 and IL-1β expression associated with preeclampsia with normal fetal growth could not be explained by differences in decidual leukocyte and trophoblast density (**Supplementary Table 2**). Preeclamptic pregnancies with FGR were associated with higher density of leukocytes, but not trophoblasts, compared to both preeclampsia with normal fetal growth and normal pregnancies (**Supplementary Table 2**).

A significant positive correlation between the decidual expression intensity of NLRP3 and IL-1β was observed in normal pregnancies ($R = 0.516$, $P = 0.01$) and pregnancies complicated with preeclampsia without FGR ($R = 0.499$, $P = 0.05$), but not in preeclamptic pregnancies with FGR ($R = 0.323$, $P = 0.116$). We have previously reported placental NLRP3 and IL-1β expression in 21 of the pregnancies included in this study (28). In this subgroup, we found no correlation between the decidual and placental expression intensity, neither in preeclampsia with ($n = 5$, NLRP3 $R = -0.329$, $P = 0.588$; IL-1β $R = -0.579$, $P = 0.306$) or without FGR ($n = 10$, NLRP3 $R = 0.096$, $P = 0.791$; IL-1β $R = -0.251$, $P = 0.484$), nor in normal pregnancies ($n = 6$, NLRP3 $R = -0.718$, $P = 0.108$; IL-1β $R = -0.059$, $P = 0.912$).

Synthetic cholesterol crystals induced NLRP3 inflammasome activation in LPS primed decidual tissue explants ($n = 3$) from normal pregnancies by significantly increasing the release of IL-1β (**Figure 5**). LDH cytotoxicity assay confirmed that the stimuli had no toxic effect on tissue viability (**Supplementary Figure 1**).

Cellular NLRP3 Inflammasome Expression in Decidua

A significant positive correlation was found between the density of trophoblasts and the expression intensity of both NLRP3 ($R = 0.244$, $P = 0.01$) and IL-1β ($R = 0.289$, $P = 0.01$)

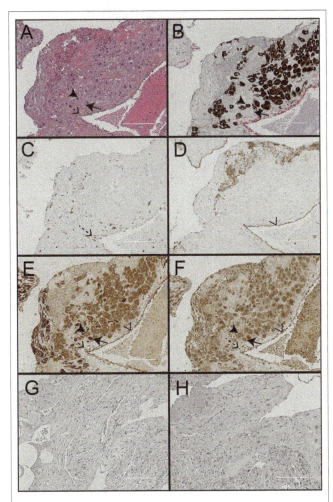

FIGURE 3 | Immunohistochemical staining of decidua from a normal pregnancy. Representative images of decidual tissue from a normal pregnancy at gestational age 40 weeks. (A) HES; (B) the trophoblast marker cytokeratin 7 (CK7); (C) the endothelium marker CD31; (D) the leukocyte marker CD45; (E) nod-like receptor protein (NLRP)3; and (F) interleukin (IL)-1β. Negative isotype control shown for (G) NLRP3; and (H) IL-1β. Black arrowheads indicate trophoblasts, black arrows indicate maternal decidual stroma cells, dashed arrows indicate maternal leukocytes and transparent arrowhead indicate endothelial cells. Scale bar 200 μM.

in decidua. In decidual areas containing trophoblasts, both the NLRP3 and IL-1β expression intensity was significantly higher in preeclamptic pregnancies with normal fetal growth compared to normal pregnancies (NLRP3 $P = 0.019$; IL-1β $P = 0.023$) (**Figures 4C,D**). Further, the IL-1β expression intensity in trophoblast-containing decidual areas was significantly higher in preeclampsia without FGR compared to preeclampsia with FGR ($P = 0.021$) (**Figure 4D**). Excluding trophoblasts from analysis abolished the significant differences between the study groups (**Supplementary Table 1**).

The maternal leukocyte density in the decidua correlated weakly with the decidual expression intensity of NLRP3 ($R = 0.044$, $P = 0.01$) and IL-1β ($R = 0.040$, $P = 0.01$). Decidual tissue containing leukocytes showed higher expression intensity of NLRP3, but not IL-1β, in preeclamptic pregnancies with normal fetal growth compared to normal pregnancies (NLRP3 $P = 0.025$ and IL-1β $P = 0.052$) (**Supplementary Table 1**).

A closer look at decidual tissue with trophoblast and maternal leukocytes in proximity showed that the expression intensity of NLRP3 and IL-1β was significantly increased in preeclampsia without FGR compared to normal pregnancies (NLRP3 $P = 0.017$ and IL-1β $P = 0.031$) (**Figures 4E,F**). A comparison between trophoblast containing areas was made to assess the influence of leukocyte presence (**Figure 6**). Significantly higher expression intensity of both NLRP3 and IL-1β expression was observed in areas containing trophoblast and maternal leukocytes in proximity, compared to areas with trophoblasts and no leukocytes, and this dependence on maternal-fetal cell proximity was apparent in all study groups (**Figure 6**).

DISCUSSION

This study is the first to reveal the presence of cholesterol crystals at the maternal-fetal interface in the uterine wall decidua, and the crystals were shown to be markedly present in both normal and preeclamptic pregnancies. The cholesterol crystal responsive NLRP3 inflammasome and IL-1β were expressed by both fetal trophoblasts and maternal leukocytes in the decidua. Pathway functionality was confirmed by cholesterol crystal mediated activation of IL-1β production in decidual explants. The expression intensity levels of NLRP3 and IL-1β correlated within the decidua but not between the two sites of the maternal-fetal interface; decidua and placenta. Preeclampsia with normal fetal growth was associated with increased expression of NLRP3 and IL-1β, particularly in decidual areas of close maternal-fetal interaction.

Normal pregnancy is characterized by elevated maternal serum cholesterol and uric acid levels (7, 28, 38), and the correlation with increased serum levels of C-reactive protein (CRP) and sFlt-1 (28) indicates a potential contribution to the elevated maternal inflammatory state of normal pregnancies. The increased serum cholesterol may contribute to accumulation of cholesterol at the maternal-fetal interface (7), eventually leading to formation of cholesterol crystals in decidual tissue, as shown in the present study. Both trophoblasts and leukocytes are equipped with receptors that enable cholesterol uptake, such as the scavenger receptor CD36 (16, 21, 22, 39). Another aspect of how cholesterol crystals may contribute to decidual inflammation is linked to atherosis formation in uterine arteries, a vascular malformation resembling early stage atherosclerosis (40). CD36 is involved in macrophage foam cell formation and atherosclerosis progression by mediating endocytosis and conversion of oxLDL into cholesterol crystals, thus promoting complement and NLRP3 inflammasome activation (16, 41–43). Oxidative stress in the decidua may induce accumulation of oxLDL and cholesterol crystal formation. A similar role for cholesterol crystals in decidual macrophage foam cell accumulation and atherosis formation is supported by our observation of cholesterol crystals around the wall of uterine vessels, but further investigation is needed. We found that

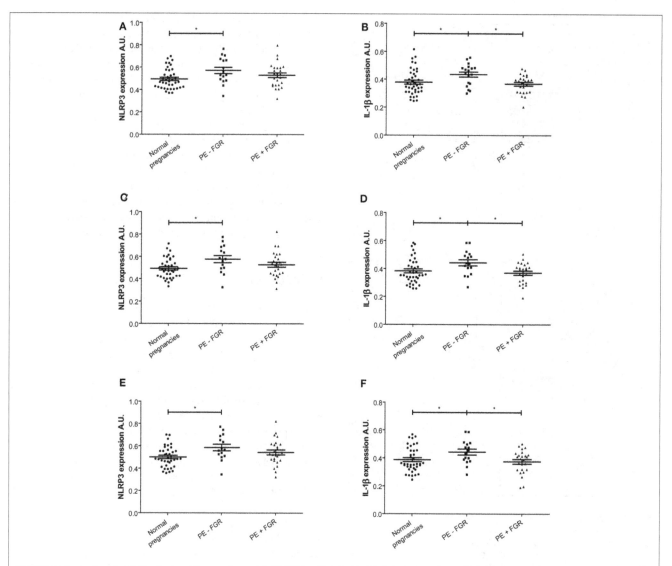

FIGURE 4 | Expression intensity levels of nod-like receptor protein (NLRP)3 and interleukin (IL)-1β in decidual tissue. **(A,C,E)** NLRP3 expression intensity in decidual tissue from normal ($n = 39$) and preeclamptic pregnancies with ($n = 26$) and without fetal growth restriction (FGR) ($n = 16$); and **(B,D,F)** IL-1β expression intensity in normal ($n = 40$) and preeclamptic pregnancies with ($n = 25$) and without FGR ($n = 18$). Expression intensity is shown for **(A,B)** decidual tissue; **(C,D)** decidual areas containing trophoblasts; and **(E,F)** decidual areas containing trophoblast and leukocytes. Data were analyzed by a linear mixed model and expression levels are shown as estimated means with standard error of mean. *$P < 0.05$. A.U. indicates arbitrary units.

cells containing cholesterol crystals appeared aggregated within decidual tissue, rather than randomly scattered, suggesting that cholesterol crystal mediated inflammation may be localized to specific regions in the decidua. Previous studies have suggested that the size of cholesterol crystals and their clusters may be an important factor in the inflammatory potential (44, 45), but this hypothesis was not substantiated for decidual inflammation in the current study. The amount and size of cholesterol crystals in the decidua did not differ between normal and preeclamptic pregnancies. Further assessment of cell specific involvement in the decidual uptake and formation of cholesterol crystals, as well as involvement of relevant priming signals, such as complement factors (46), is warranted to fully understand the inflammatory potential of cholesterol crystals at the maternal-fetal interface. It must also be determined how different pathological processes in decidua interact since oxidative stress may promote the accumulation of oxLDL and cholesterol crystal formation (16, 17). The use of established advanced microscopy methodology for cholesterol imaging learned from atherosclerosis and hepatocytes lipid droplets (47–49), combined with removal of the crystals by alcohol treatment (50), strongly support that the imaged crystals in decidua are crystalline cholesterol. Still, further verification of the chemical identity of the crystals may be performed by other advanced microscopy techniques, such as coherent anti-Stokes Raman scattering (CARS) imaging.

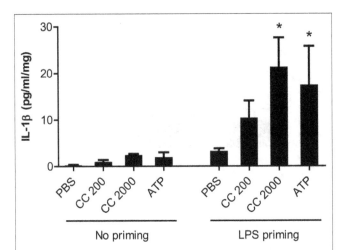

FIGURE 5 | Interleukin (IL)-1β response following cholesterol crystal stimulation of decidual explants. Decidual explants from normal pregnancies (n = 3) were primed for 2 h with or without lipopolysaccharide (LPS), before adding cholesterol crystals (CC, 200 or 2,000 µg/ml) or adenosine triphosphate (ATP) for 24 h. Six technical replicates were included for each experimental condition. Release of IL-1β to the supernatant was measured by ELISA and presented as mean with standard error of mean, relative to explant weight. Data were analyzed using Kruskal-Wallis test with Dunn's multiple comparison post-hoc test. *$P < 0.05$. PBS, phosphate-buffered saline.

This is the first demonstration of NLRP3 and IL-1β protein expression in maternal and fetal cells in the uterine wall decidua. A report of gene expression of NLRP3 inflammasome components in isolated first trimester decidual stromal cells partly supports our findings (30). Combined with our previous discovery of NLRP3 and IL-1β expression in placental trophoblasts of early and late pregnancies (28), this study clearly supports a role for NLRP3 inflammasome activation at both sites of the maternal-fetal interface throughout pregnancy. In addition, the positive correlation between decidual expression of NLRP3 and the responsive cytokine IL-1β substantiates the functionality of the NLRP3 inflammasome in decidua. Extravillous trophoblasts were here shown to be central for the decidual NLRP3 inflammasome response. This means that the characterization of placental trophoblasts and trophoblast cell lines as immunocompetent cells by their functional pattern recognition receptors (PRR) by us (28, 51, 52) and others (9, 53), has now been extended to extravillous trophoblasts in the decidua. This indicates importance for immunomodulating trophoblast activity at the maternal side of the maternal-fetal interface in the final stages of pregnancy, with dependence on the proximity and possible direct interaction between fetal and maternal cells. Supporting such maternal-fetal communication is that maternal leukocytes and trophoblasts in the decidua express complementary ligands and receptors (9, 10) and that leukocytes are key cells in modulating trophoblast behavior (54). In addition to leukocytes and trophoblasts, decidual stromal cells markedly expressed NLRP3 and IL-1β and are considered potential responders to cholesterol crystals, but further studies focused on this cell type are needed to address their inflammatory role.

Preeclampsia without FGR was associated with increased decidual expression of NLRP3 and IL-1β, suggesting that the NLRP3 inflammasome aggravates the inflammatory response and substantiates the reported shift to a pro-inflammatory profile and cell type distribution at the maternal-fetal interface in preeclampsia (9, 14, 29). The increased decidual inflammasome expression was trophoblast dependent and strongest in areas where trophoblast and leukocytes are in proximity, suggesting that NLRP3 mediated inflammation may disturb maternal-fetal communication. The novel identification of decidual cholesterol crystals combined with increased NLRP3 inflammasome expression presents a novel link between the pathophysiology of CVD and preeclampsia. NLRP3 inflammasome response may lead to extensive tissue damage and cell death and is associated with formation and progression of atherosclerotic lesions (18, 19). Correspondingly, increased formation of decidual atherosis and inflammation at the maternal-fetal interface are pathophysiological features of preeclampsia (40, 55). The NLRP3 inflammasome expression pattern in decidua further points to interesting pathophysiological differences between preeclampsia subgroups. We have previously demonstrated a placental role for the NLRP3 inflammasome in preeclampsia combined with FGR (28), while the decidual contribution presented here was apparent in preeclampsia without FGR. This points to divergent NLRP3 inflammasome activation in preeclampsia subgroups. Supporting such divergent regulation is the lack of correlation between decidual and placental expression levels of NLRP3 and IL-1β, indicating that activators in the maternal serum affect placental and decidual tissue differentially and that the local inflammatory responses in the decidua and placenta are not directly coordinated. We hypothesize that the placental tissue may be more influenced by placental dysfunction and fetal complications. FGR has been shown associated to a fetal pro-atherogenic lipid profile and placental cholesterol accumulation due to abnormal cholesterol transport (24, 56). This may lead to cholesterol accumulation and crystallization in the placenta and activation of the NLRP3 inflammasome in a process that may not influence decidual tissue. In the present study, increased decidual NLRP3 inflammasome response was observed in preeclampsia without FGR, and this could indicate that the decidual tissue may respond more to the increased maternal danger signals, including pro-atherogenic lipid profile, circulating levels of inflammatory mediators, such as HMGB1 and uric acid, and predisposition to inflammation.

Therapeutic and preventive approaches in preeclampsia are limited. A large prospective study showed limited preventive effect of administration of low-dose anti-inflammatory and antiplatelet agent aspirin on preeclampsia development (57). Pravastatin, used for treatment of dyslipidemia and prevention of CVD, is a suggested candidate for treatment and prevention of preeclampsia (58). In addition to reducing hypercholesterolemia, statins may ameliorate major pathological responses involved in preeclampsia, including inhibition of sFlt-1 release and reduction of inflammation and oxidative stress (59). Importantly, statins may inhibit formation and improve solubility of cholesterol crystals in atherosclerotic plaques (60), adding to the beneficial effects of these cholesterol-lowering drugs. Further investigation is needed to demonstrate whether a positive effect of pravastatin in preeclampsia may involve removal of cholesterol crystals at the

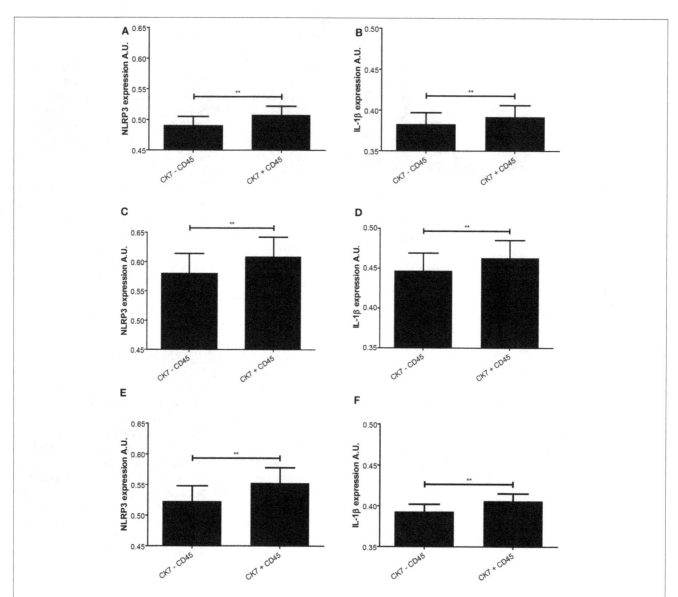

FIGURE 6 | Expression intensity levels of nod-like receptor protein (NLRP)3 and interleukin (IL)-1β in decidual tissue related to presence of trophoblast and leukocytes. NLRP3 **(A,C,E)** and IL-1β **(B,D,F)** expression was measured in normal pregnancies **(A,B)** and preeclamptic pregnancies without **(C,D)** or with **(E,F)** fetal growth restriction (FGR). The expression levels were assessed in trophoblast containing areas with (CK7 + CD45) or without (CK7 − CD45) presence of leukocytes. **$P < 0.01$. A.U. indicates arbitrary units.

maternal-fetal interface. Growing evidence supports the clinical benefits and anti-inflammatory effects of drugs targeting the NLRP3 inflammasome and IL-1β pathway in several diseases (61), but whether they are pregnancy-safe and effective in preeclampsia needs to be determined.

This study identified cholesterol crystal mediated NLRP3 inflammasome response as an inflammatory mechanism associated with maternal-fetal interaction in the uterine wall decidua in pregnancy. Cholesterol crystals were detected in considerable amounts in decidua and the expression of the NLRP3 inflammatory pathway showed importance for close interaction between fetal trophoblasts and maternal leukocytes. The increased NLRP3 inflammasome expression in preeclampsia with normal fetal growth suggests that an enhanced pro-inflammatory profile in the decidua negatively affects maternal-fetal communication and plays a role at late stages of preeclampsia pathology, possibly by intercommunication with the maternal systemic inflammatory response. The identification of decidual cholesterol crystals and increased decidual NLRP3 inflammasome expression in preeclampsia with normal fetal growth further substantiates the pathophysiological link between preeclampsia and CVD. This study showed that combined investigation of cell specific pathological mechanisms at the two sites of maternal-fetal interface may provide more comprehensive knowledge of the regulation and importance of maternal-fetal communication.

ETHICS STATEMENT

The Norwegian Regional Committee for Medical and Health Research Ethics (REC) approved the study (REC 2012/1040 and 2009/03) and written informed consent was obtained from participants. Procedures were in accordance with institutional guidelines. The patients/participants provided their written informed consent to participate in this study.

AUTHOR CONTRIBUTIONS

GBS, LG, and A-CI designed the study and all authors contributed with valuable inputs. GBS, LT, and LB collected the clinical material and information. GBS, LG, JR, SM, AT, ME, and A-CI developed the methods for image processing and automated quantification. GBS and GSS performed the decidual explant experiments. GBS, LG, and A-CI interpreted the data and wrote the manuscript. All authors contributed to the article and approved the submitted version.

ACKNOWLEDGMENTS

Immunohistochemical staining was performed by Senior Engineer Ingunn Nervik at the Cellular and Molecular Imaging Core Facility (CMIC), NTNU. CMIC is funded by the Faculty of Medicine and Health Science at NTNU and the Central Norway Regional Health Authority. We would like to thank Associate Professor Turid Follestad for statistical support and Professor Magnus Borstad Lilledahl for assistance in the second harmonic generation microscopy.

REFERENCES

Redman CWG, Sacks GP, Sargent IL. Preeclampsia: an excessive maternal inflammatory response to pregnancy. *Am J Obstetr Gynecol*. (1999) 180:499–506. doi: 10.1016/S0002-9378(99)70239-5

Staff AC, Andersgaard AB, Henriksen T, Langesæter E, Magnussen E, Michelsen TM, et al. Chapter 28 Hypertensive disorders of pregnancy and eclampsia. *Eur J Obstetr Gynecol Reprod Biol*. (2016) 201:171–8. doi: 10.1016/j.ejogrb.2016.04.001

Brown MA, Magee LA, Kenny LC, Karumanchi SA, McCarthy FP, Saito S, et al. The hypertensive disorders of pregnancy: ISSHP classification, diagnosis & management recommendations for international practice. *Preg Hypertens*. (2018) 13:291–310. doi: 10.1016/j.preghy.2018.05.004

Abalos E, Cuesta C, Grosso AL, Chou D, Say L. Global and regional estimates of preeclampsia and eclampsia: a systematic review. *Eur J Obstetr Gynecol Reprod Biol*. (2013) 170:1–7. doi: 10.1016/j.ejogrb.2013.05.005

Bellamy L, Casas J-P, Hingorani AD, Williams DJ. Pre-eclampsia and risk of cardiovascular disease and cancer in later life: systematic review and meta-analysis. *BMJ*. (2007) 335:974. doi: 10.1136/bmj.39335.385301.BE

Brown MC, Best KE, Pearce MS, Waugh J, Robson SC, Bell R. Cardiovascular disease risk in women with pre-eclampsia: systematic review and meta-analysis. *Eur J Epidemiol*. (2013) 28:1–19. doi: 10.1007/s10654-013-9762-6

Staff AC, Ranheim T, Khoury J, Henriksen T. Increased contents of phospholipids, cholesterol, and lipid peroxides in decidua basalis in women with preeclampsia. *Am J Obstetr Gynecol*. (1999) 180:587–92. doi: 10.1016/S0002-9378(99)70259-0

Adank MC, Benschop L, Peterbroers KR, Smak Gregoor AM, Kors AW, Mulder MT, et al. Is maternal lipid profile in early pregnancy associated with pregnancy complications and blood pressure in pregnancy and long term postpartum? *Am J Obstetr Gynecol*. (2019) 221:150.e151–13. doi: 10.1016/j.ajog.2019.03.025

Vento-Tormo R, Efremova M, Botting RA, Turco MY, Vento-Tormo M, Meyer KB, et al. Single-cell reconstruction of the early maternal–fetal interface in humans. *Nature*. (2018) 563:347–53. doi: 10.1038/s41586-018-0698-6

Menkhorst EM, Van Sinderen M, Correia J, Dimitriadis E. Trophoblast function is altered by decidual factors in gestational-dependant manner. *Placenta*. (2019) 80:8–11. doi: 10.1016/j.placenta.2019.03.013

Redman CWG, Sargent IL. Review article: immunology of pre-eclampsia. *Am J Reprod Immunol*. (2010) 63:534–43. doi: 10.1111/j.1600-0897.2010.00831.x

Brosens I, Pijnenborg R, Vercruysse L, Romero R. The "Great Obstetrical Syndromes" are associated with disorders of deep placentation. *Am J Obstetr Gynecol*. (2011) 204:193–201. doi: 10.1016/j.ajog.2010.08.009

Chaiworapongsa T, Chaemsaithong P, Yeo L, Romero R. Pre-eclampsia part 1: current understanding of its pathophysiology. *Nat Rev Nephrol*. (2014) 10:466–80. doi: 10.1038/nrneph.2014.102

Harmon AC, Cornelius DC, Amaral LM, Faulkner JL, Cunningham MW, Wallace K, et al. The role of inflammation in the pathology of preeclampsia. *Clin Sci*. (2016) 130:409–19. doi: 10.1042/CS20150702

Gomez-Lopez N, Motomura K, Miller D, Garcia-Flores V, Galaz J, Romero R. Inflammasomes: their role in normal and complicated pregnancies. *J Immunol*. (2019) 203:2757–69. doi: 10.4049/jimmunol.1900901

Sheedy FJ, Grebe A, Rayner KJ, Kalantari P, Ramkhelawon B, Carpenter SB, et al. CD36 coordinates NLRP3 inflammasome activation by facilitating intracellular nucleation of soluble ligands into particulate ligands in sterile inflammation. *Nat Immunol*. (2013) 14:812–20. doi: 10.1038/ni.2639

Franklin BS, Mangan MS, Latz E. Crystal formation in inflammation. *Ann Rev Immunol*. (2016) 34:173–202. doi: 10.1146/annurev-immunol-041015-055539

Duewell P, Kono H, Rayner KJ, Sirois CM, Vladimer G, Bauernfeind FG, et al. NLRP3 inflammasomes are required for atherogenesis and activated by cholesterol crystals. *Nature*. (2010) 464:1357–61. doi: 10.1038/nature08938

Grebe A, Hoss F, Latz E. NLRP3 inflammasome and the IL-1 pathway in atherosclerosis. *Circ Res*. (2018) 122:1722–40. doi: 10.1161/CIRCRESAHA.118.311362

Pavan L, Tsatsaris V, Hermouet A, Therond P, Evain-Brion D, Fournier T. Oxidized low-density lipoproteins inhibit trophoblastic cell invasion. *J Clin Endocrinol Metab*. (2004) 89:1969–72. doi: 10.1210/jc.2003-032042

Plösch T, van Straten EME, Kuipers F. Cholesterol transport by the placenta: placental liver X receptor activity as a modulator of fetal cholesterol metabolism? *Placenta*. (2007) 28:604–10. doi: 10.1016/j.placenta.2006.10.009

Duttaroy AK. Transport of fatty acids across the human placenta: a review. *Progr Lipid Res*. (2009) 48:52–61. doi: 10.1016/j.plipres.2008.11.001

Woollett LA. Review: transport of maternal cholesterol to the fetal circulation. *Placenta*. (2011) 32:S218–21. doi: 10.1016/j.placenta.2011.01.011

Baumann M, Körner M, Huang X, Wenger F, Surbek D, Albrecht C. Placental ABCA1 and ABCG1 expression in gestational disease: pre-eclampsia affects ABCA1 levels in syncytiotrophoblasts. *Placenta*. (2013) 34:1079–86. doi: 10.1016/j.placenta.2013.06.309

Vondra S, Kunihs V, Eberhart T, Eigner K, Bauer R, Haslinger P, et al. Metabolism of cholesterol and progesterone is differentially regulated in primary trophoblastic subtypes and might be disturbed in recurrent miscarriages. *J Lipid Res*. (2019) 60:1922–34. doi: 10.1194/jlr.P093427

Koçyigit Y, Atamer Y, Atamer A, Tuzcu A, Akkus Z. Changes in serum levels of leptin, cytokines and lipoprotein in pre-eclamptic and normotensive pregnant women. *Gynecol Endocrinol*. (2004) 19:267–73. doi: 10.1080/09513590400018108

Levine RJ, Lam C, Qian C, Yu KF, Maynard SE, Sachs BP, et al. Soluble endoglin and other circulating antiangiogenic factors in preeclampsia. *New Engl J Med*. (2006) 355:992–1005. doi: 10.1056/NEJMoa055352

Stødle GS, Silva GB, Tangerås LH, Gierman LM, Nervik I, Dahlberg UE, et al. Placental inflammation in pre-eclampsia by Nod-like receptor protein (NLRP)3 inflammasome activation in trophoblasts. *Clin Exp Immunol*. (2018) 193:84–94. doi: 10.1111/cei.13130

Shirasuna K, Karasawa T, Takahashi M. Role of the NLRP3 inflammasome in preeclampsia. *Front Endocrinol*. (2020) 11. doi: 10.3389/fendo.2020.00080

Pontillo A, Girardelli M, Agostinis C, Masat E, Bulla R, Crovella S. Bacterial LPS differently modulates inflammasome gene expression and IL-1β secretion in trophoblast cells, decidual stromal cells, and decidual endothelial cells. *Reprod Sci.* (2013) 20:563-6. doi: 10.1177/1933719112459240

Johnsen SL, Rasmussen S, Wilsgaard TOM, Sollien R, Kiserud T. Longitudinal reference ranges for estimated fetal weight. *Acta Obstetr Gynecol Scand.* (2006) 85:286-97. doi: 10.1080/00016340600569133

Harsem NK, Staff AC, He L, Roald B. The decidual suction method: a new way of collecting decidual tissue for functional and morphological studies. *Acta Obstet Gynecol Scand.* (2004) 83:724-30. doi: 10.1111/j.0001-6349.2004.00395.x

Miller RK, Genbacev O, Turner MA, Aplin JD, Caniggia I, Huppertz B. Human placental explants in culture: approaches and assessments. *Placenta.* (2005) 26:439-48. doi: 10.1016/j.placenta.2004.10.002

Schindelin J, Arganda-Carreras I, Frise E, Kaynig V, Longair M, Pietzsch T, et al. Fiji: an open-source platform for biological-image analysis. *Nat Methods.* (2012) 9:676-82. doi: 10.1038/nmeth.2019

Rueden CT, Schindelin J, Hiner MC, DeZonia BE, Walter AE, Arena ET, et al. ImageJ2: ImageJ for the next generation of scientific image data. *BMC Bioinform.* (2017) 18:529. doi: 10.1186/s12859-017-1934-z

Preibisch S, Saalfeld S, Tomancak P. Globally optimal stitching of tiled 3D microscopic image acquisitions. *Bioinformatics.* (2009) 25:1463-5. doi: 10.1093/bioinformatics/btp184

Ruifrok AC, Johnston DA. Quantification of histochemical staining by color deconvolution. *Anal Quant Cytol Histol.* (2001) 23:291-9.

Lippi G, Albiero A, Montagnana M, Salvagno GL, Scevarolli S, Franchi M, et al. Lipid and lipoprotein profile in physiological pregnancy. *Clin Lab.* (2007) 53:173-7.

Horne H, Holme AM, Roland MCP, Holm MB, Haugen G, Henriksen T, et al. Maternal-fetal cholesterol transfer in human term pregnancies. *Placenta.* (2019) 87:23-9. doi: 10.1016/j.placenta.2019.09.001

Alnaes-Katjavivi P, Lyall F, Roald B, Redman CWG, Staff AC. Acute atherosis in vacuum suction biopsies of decidua basalis: an evidence based research definition. *Placenta.* (2016) 37:26-33. doi: 10.1016/j.placenta.2015. 10.020

Park YM. CD36, a scavenger receptor implicated in atherosclerosis. *Exp Mol Med.* (2014) 46:e99. doi: 10.1038/emm.2014.38

Niyonzima N, Halvorsen B, Sporsheim B, Garred P, Aukrust P, Mollnes TE, et al. Complement activation by cholesterol crystals triggers a subsequent cytokine response. *Mol Immunol.* (2017) 84:43-50. doi: 10.1016/j.molimm.2016.09.019

Gravastrand CS, Steinkjer B, Halvorsen B, Landsem A, Skjelland M, Jacobsen EA, et al. Cholesterol crystals induce coagulation activation through complement-dependent expression of monocytic tissue factor. *J Immunol.* (2019) 203:853. doi: 10.4049/jimmunol.1900503

Abela GS, Kalavakunta JK, Janoudi A, Leffler D, Dhar G, Salehi N, et al. Frequency of cholesterol crystals in culprit coronary artery aspirate during acute myocardial infarction and their relation to inflammation and myocardial injury. *Am J Cardiol.* (2017) 120:1699-707. doi: 10.1016/j.amjcard.2017.07.075

Shu F, Chen J, Ma X, Fan Y, Yu L, Zheng W, et al. Cholesterol crystal-mediated inflammation is driven by plasma membrane destabilization. *Front Immunol.* (2018) 9:1163. doi: 10.3389/fimmu.2018.01163

Samstad EO, Niyonzima N, Nymo S, Aune MH, Ryan L, Bakke SS, et al. Cholesterol crystals induce complement-dependent inflammasome activation and cytokine release. *J Immunol.* (2014) 192:2837-45. doi: 10.4049/jimmunol.1302484

James J, Tanke HJ. *Biomedical Light Microscopy.* Amsterdam: Springer Science & Business Media (2012).

Suhalim JL, Chung CY, Lilledahl MB, Lim RS, Levi M, Tromberg BJ, et al. Characterization of cholesterol crystals in atherosclerotic plaques using stimulated raman scattering and second-harmonic generation microscopy. *Biophys J.* (2012) 102:1988-95. doi: 10.1016/j.bpj.2012.03.016

Ioannou GN, Subramanian S, Chait A, Haigh WG, Yeh MM, Farrell GC, et al. Cholesterol crystallization within hepatocyte lipid droplets and its role in murine NASH. *J Lipid Res.* (2017) 58:1067-79. doi: 10.1194/jlr.M072454

Nasiri M, Janoudi A, Vanderberg A, Frame M, Flegler C, Flegler S, et al. Role of cholesterol crystals in atherosclerosis is unmasked by altering tissue preparation methods. *Microsc Res Techn.* (2015) 78:969-74. doi: 10.1002/jemt.22560

Tangerås LH, Stødle GS, Olsen GD, Leknes A-H, Gundersen AS, Skei B, et al. Functional Toll-like receptors in primary first-trimester trophoblasts. *J Reprod Immunol.* (2014) 106:89-99. doi: 10.1016/j.jri.2014.04.004

Gierman LM, Stødle GS, Tangerås LH, Austdal M, Olsen GD, Follestad T, et al. Toll-like receptor profiling of seven trophoblast cell lines warrants caution for translation to primary trophoblasts. *Placenta.* (2015) 36:1246-53. doi: 10.1016/j.placenta.2015.09.004

Guleria I, Pollard JW. The trophoblast is a component of the innate immune system during pregnancy. *Nat Med.* (2000) 6:589-93. doi: 10.1038/75074

Ander SE, Diamond MS, Coyne CB. Immune responses at the maternal-fetal interface. *Sci Immunol.* (2019) 4:eaat6114. doi: 10.1126/sciimmunol.aat6114

Khong TY, Mooney EE, Ariel I, Balmus NCM, Boyd TK, Brundler M-A, et al. Sampling and definitions of placental lesions: amsterdam placental workshop group consensus statement. *Arch Pathol Lab Med.* (2016) 140:698-713. doi: 10.5858/arpa.2015-0225-CC

Barker DJ. Adult consequences of fetal growth restriction. *Clin Obstetr Gynecol.* (2006) 49:270-83. doi: 10.1097/00003081-200606000-00009

Rolnik DL, Wright D, Poon LC, O'Gorman N, Syngelaki A, de Paco Matallana C, et al. Aspirin versus placebo in pregnancies at high risk for preterm preeclampsia. *New Engl J Med.* (2017) 377:613-22. doi: 10.1056/NEJMoa1704559

Maierean SM, Mikhailidis DP, Toth PP, Grzesiak M, Mazidi M, Maciejewski M, et al. The potential role of statins in preeclampsia and dyslipidemia during gestation: a narrative review. *Exp Opin Investig Drugs.* (2018) 27:427-35. doi: 10.1080/13543784.2018.1465927

Ramma W, Ahmed A. Therapeutic potential of statins and the induction of heme oxygenase-1 in preeclampsia. *J Reprod Immunol.* (2014) 101-2:153-60. doi: 10.1016/j.jri.2013.12.120

Abela GS, Vedre A, Janoudi A, Huang R, Durga S, Tamhane U. Effect of statins on cholesterol crystallization and atherosclerotic plaque stabilization. *Am J Cardiol.* (2011) 107:1710-7. doi: 10.1016/j.amjcard.2011.02.336

Shao B-Z, Cao Q, Liu C. Targeting NLRP3 inflammasome in the treatment of CNS diseases. *Front Mol Neurosci.* (2018) 11:320. doi: 10.3389/fnmol.2018.00320

Healing Mechanism of Ruptured Fetal Membrane

Haruta Mogami[1]* and R. Ann Word[2]*

[1]Department of Gynecology and Obstetrics, Kyoto University Graduate School of Medicine, Kyoto, Japan, [2]Department of Obstetrics and Gynecology, Cecil H. and Ida Green Center for Reproductive Biology Sciences, University of Texas Southwestern Medical Center, Dallas, TX, United States

*Correspondence:
Haruta Mogami
mogami@kuhp.kyoto-u.ac.jp
R. Ann Word
ruth.word@utsouthwestern.edu

Preterm premature rupture of membranes (pPROM) typically leads to spontaneous preterm birth within several days. In a few rare cases, however, amniotic fluid leakage ceases, amniotic fluid volume is restored, and pregnancy continues until term. Amnion, the collagen-rich layer that forms the load-bearing structure of the fetal membrane, has regenerative capacity and has been used clinically to aid in the healing of various wounds including burns, diabetic ulcers, and corneal injuries. In the healing process of ruptured fetal membranes, amnion epithelial cells seem to play a major role with assistance from innate immunity. In a mouse model of sterile pPROM, macrophages are recruited to the injured site. Well-organized and localized inflammatory responses cause epithelial mesenchymal transition of amnion epithelial cells which accelerates cell migration and healing of the amnion. Research on amnion regeneration is expected to provide insight into potential treatment strategies for pPROM.

Keywords: premature rupture of membrane, fetal membrane, amnion, macrophage, wound healing

IS pPROM IRREVERSIBLE?

Preterm premature rupture of membranes (pPROM) is a leading cause of preterm birth (Menon and Richardson, 2017). Fetal membrane rupture has traditionally been regarded as an irreversible process: the mean latency period from membrane rupture to delivery is 12 days at 20–26 weeks of gestation and 4 days at 32–34 weeks of gestation (Parry and Strauss, 1998). In some cases, however, ruptured fetal membranes can spontaneously "reseal": Johnson reported that membrane resealing, defined as cessation of fluid leakage and negative nitrazine test, occurred in 24 cases of 208 pPROM patients (11.5%) in all 5,937 deliveries (Johnson et al., 1990). In addition, we know that the membrane repairs itself and heals spontaneously after amniocentesis (Borgida et al., 2000). These findings suggest that, although most women who experience pPROM deliver spontaneously within several days, the amnion has the capacity for wound healing *in vivo*.

CAUSES OF pPROM

About 30% of pPROM cases are caused by intra-amniotic infection, whereas the other 70% are unrelated to infection (Romero et al., 1988). pPROM cases that are unrelated to infection are caused by smoking, low body mass index, maternal stress or undernutrition, oxidative stresses, intrauterine bleeding, and iatrogenic factors such as amniocentesis or fetoscopy.

Romero et al. reported that intra-amniotic inflammation occurs in 37% of cases of preterm labor before 37 weeks of gestation. Interestingly, the rate of inflammation with infection was only 11%, whereas that of sterile inflammation in the absence of bacteria was 26% (Romero et al., 2014). They suggested that sterile intra-amniotic inflammation might be caused by damage-associated molecular patterns (DAMPs), such as high-mobility group box1 (HMGB1), and concluded that sterile inflammation is a more common contributor to preterm labor than bacterial infection.

DAMPs are believed to play a major role in the pathophysiology of sterile inflammation. Specifically, when a tissue is damaged, intracellular components and molecules such as HMGB1, nucleic acids, heat-shock proteins, adenosine triphosphate, hydrogen peroxide, and calcium ions are released (Kono and Rock, 2008). Uric acid and S100 proteins are associated with pPROM (Friel et al., 2007; Nadeau-Vallee et al., 2016). These DAMPs are recognized by toll-like receptors and receptor for advanced glycation end products (RAGE), leading to activation of inflammatory pathways such as NF-κB and AP-1, which yield sterile inflammation (Akira et al., 2006; Xia et al., 2017). Although DAMPs are released when tissue is damaged, they are also signals of tissue repair. Whereas pPROM initiated by bacterial infection requires immediate delivery to avoid fetal infection, the numerous pPROM cases that are unrelated to infection may be eligible for expectant management.

HEALING OF FETAL TISSUES: THE ROLES OF MACROPHAGES

The healing mechanisms of adult tissue are divided into four overlapping stages: (1) hemostasis, (2) inflammation, (3) migration and proliferation, and (4) resolution and remodeling (Sonnemann and Bement, 2011). In contrast with adult tissues, the healing of fetal tissue is much simpler (Sonnemann and Bement, 2011): inflammation is suppressed to a minimum, fetal tissue is usually not vascularized, and granulation tissue is usually not formed. These characteristics of fetal wound healing enable the tissue to heal quickly and scarlessly (Cordeiro and Jacinto, 2013). For example, when fetal skin is injured, actin and myosin proteins aggregate in the injured epidermis to form acto-myosin complexes that cause contraction of the tissue and shrinkage of the area of injury. These cellular structures stimulate migration of the epidermis and closure of the wound.

Remarkably, macrophages are recruited to injury sites to facilitate healing of fetal tissues. Circulating monocytes migrate to injury sites where they differentiate into tissue macrophages, and tissue-resident macrophages are also involved in wound healing (Jenkins et al., 2011).

Macrophages are roughly divided into two types (Murray and Wynn, 2011), classically activated macrophages (M1 macrophages) and alternatively activated macrophages (M2 macrophages) (Gordon and Martinez, 2010). Wound healing is facilitated by M2 macrophages (Murray and Wynn, 2011). These cells release growth factors, such as transforming growth factor (TGF-β) and platelet-derived growth factors (PDGF), which activate damaged epidermis and fibroblasts. TGF-β plays a major role in the differentiation of fibroblasts from myofibroblasts. These cells migrate and contract, as well as release tissue inhibitor of metalloproteinases (TIMPs), which inhibits matrix metalloproteinases (MMPs) and prevents over-destruction of tissues. Myofibroblasts also release collagen and repair damaged sites in conjunction with macrophages, which also release MMPs and TIMPs and remodel wounded tissue. Subsequently, macrophages phagocytose debris and damaged extracellular matrix (ECM) to clean the wounded tissues.

HEALING OF AMNION IN ORGAN CULTURE

In an experiment reported by Devlieger et al. (2000b), small holes were generated with a biopsy punch in the centers of human fetal membrane sample. Interestingly, increased cellularity, survival, and proliferation were limited at the tissue border and the rupture did not heal even after 12 days. This result suggests that amnion cannot heal by itself; rather, the help of other cells such as immune cells are necessary for wound healing in the amnion.

ANIMAL MODELS OF FETAL MEMBRANE HEALING

Amnion has a high tensile strength; in fact, the strength of the fetal membrane is provided exclusively by the amnion (Parry and Strauss, 1998). Although fetal membrane structures differ among mammals, humans, and several experimental animals including mice, rats, rabbits, and sheep all have similar amnion structure; they also all have amnion in the most superficial layer of the fetal membrane (Carter, 2016). Thus, animal models are useful for the study of ruptured human fetal membranes *in vivo*.

The first histological observations of the healing process in fetal membranes were conducted in rats. Pioneering work by Sopher (Sopher, 1972) demonstrated that puncturing rat gestational sacs with a 21-gauge needle on day 15 of gestation resulted in a proliferation of amnion mesenchymal cells at the edge of the amnion within 24 h. Further, she showed that the thickened edge of the amnion was covered by epithelial cells and confirmed that wound closure occurred within a few days. Similarly, in a rabbit model, amnion integrity recovered to 40% of its initial value within 30 days of puncture (Deprest et al., 1999). The healing process of rabbit pPROM involves matrix remodeling by MMPs and TIMPs (Devlieger et al., 2000a).

Using a mouse model, we investigated the mechanisms of wound healing of fetal membranes. On day 15 of pregnancy, fetal membranes were mechanically ruptured with sterile needles of various sizes through the myometrium. Ruptured fetal membranes were clearly observed after 6 h and healing began within 24 h. Our mouse study revealed that the closure of such ruptures was complete within 48–72 h (Mogami et al., 2017). Consistent with Sopher's study, we observed an aggregation of amnion mesenchymal cells at the edge of the amnion at 24 h.

Interestingly, this thickened edge was covered by a monolayer of epithelial cells. The proinflammatory cytokines IL-1β and TNF were quickly increased at the fetal membrane rupture site. When a 26-gauge needle was used to create a small rupture, this increase in proinflammatory cytokines returned to basal levels around 24 h. When a 20-gauge needle was used to create a larger rupture, the puncture-induced increases in these cytokines persisted for a longer time. At the same time, IL-10, an anti-inflammatory cytokine, increased at the ruptured site, decelerating inflammation. IL-10 assists in wound healing, as shown by the finding that overexpression of IL-10 in mice accelerates skin healing (Peranteau et al., 2008). In contrast, chronic inflammation conditions such as diabetic ulcers delay wound healing, suggesting the importance of a balance between inflammation and anti-inflammation for complete and organized wound healing. In the amnion, well-controlled switching from a pro- to an anti-inflammatory state seems to be necessary for repair.

We observed an aggregation of macrophages around the sterile ruptured amnion (Mogami et al., 2017). These macrophages were fetal-derived and were probably recruited from the amniotic fluid, although they may have been amnion-resident macrophages. These fetal-derived macrophages released IL-1β and TNF at the ruptured site. In contrast with the typical wound healing process in adults, migration of neutrophils was rarely observed. Perhaps this is not surprising given the absence of infection and the sterile nature of the inflammatory stimulus. Yet, this raises questions regarding the role of these inflammatory cytokines at the ruptured amnion. We tested the function of these cytokines through *in vitro* scratch assays using primary human amnion cells. IL-1β and TNF caused significant acceleration of amnion epithelial cell migration. They did not, however, alter amnion mesenchymal cell migration. Importantly, the shape of the amnion epithelial cells changed, assuming a more spindle-like configuration (similar to that of mesenchymal cells) at the edge of migration. These spindle-shaped cells were immunoreactive for vimentin, suggesting that these wounded epithelial cells were undergoing epithelial-mesenchymal transition (EMT). *In vivo*, similarly, vimentin-positive cells can be observed scattered in the epithelial layer of the ruptured amnion in mice, suggesting that EMT occurs *in vivo* as well. EMT is known to speed up cell migration, which in turn speeds up wound closure. Our results imply that EMT provides more mesenchymal cells to the wounded amnion, where these cells then synthesize and release extracellular matrices such as collagen to strengthen the injured site. Richardson and Menon also reported that EMT occurs during amnion healing (Richardson and Menon, 2018) and that mesenchymal-epithelial transition (MET) occurs with the help of IL-8 once amnion closure is complete. In addition, Richardson et al. also recently showed that oxidative stresses activate the p38 MAPK pathway, which causes EMT in the fetal membrane (Richardson et al., 2020). Taken together, these results suggest that EMT is a key mechanism involved in stimulating amnion healing in the presence of sterile inflammation.

There is a concern that the healing properties of the amnion differ among species. In rabbits, for example, relatively small punctures created with a 14-gauge needle spontaneously healed to 41.7% of their initial state (Deprest et al., 1999), whereas relatively large ruptures created with a 1 cm hysterotomy did not heal at all (Papadopulos et al., 1998). Similarly, in a mouse model, the amnion healed at a slower rate after being punctured with a 20-gauge needle than after being punctured with a 26-gauge needle (Mogami et al., 2017). We speculate that the reported variation in healing potential depends on the initial size of the rupture rather than on species differences.

IMPORTANCE OF "SCAFFOLDS" FOR HEALING TISSUES

ECM scaffolds have recently received attention as a fascinating mechanism involved in wound healing acceleration and tissue regeneration (Eming et al., 2014). For example, a type-1 collagen patch preserved contractility and protected cardiac tissue from injury in a mouse myocardial infarction model, accompanied by attenuated left ventricular remodeling, diminished fibrosis, and formation of a network of blood vessels within the infarct (Serpooshan et al., 2013; Wei et al., 2015). Porcine urinary bladder ECM scaffold implantation improved the regeneration of muscle in volumetric muscle loss in rodents as well as in five human patients; perivascular stem cell mobilization was seen in connection with this procedure (Sicari et al., 2014). Bioengineered biomaterials have been clinically applied to replace and restore the skin, heart valves, trachea, and tendons (Lutolf and Hubbell, 2005; Berthiaume et al., 2011).

The application of biomaterials to ruptured membranes has been attempted in such animal models as rabbits, sheep, and rats (Zisch and Zimmermann, 2008). When gelatin sponge plugs were used in ewes and rhesus monkeys, for example, rupture sites were found to be intact at term (Luks et al., 1999).

Previously, we showed that application of a collagen matrix assisted amnion healing in a mouse model of sterile pPROM (Mogami et al., 2018). In this model, a type I collagen gel was injected into mechanically-ruptured sites on murine fetal membranes immediately after puncture. The collagen gel was immediately solidified due to the animal's body temperature such that it formed a collagen matrix layer beneath the ruptured amnion (**Figure 1A**). Interestingly, macrophages were trapped in this layer of collagen (**Figure 1B**). Moreover, this injection of collagen thickened the healing site, presumably stimulating more collagen synthesis by the mesenchymal cells in the amnion. We found vimentin-positive mesenchymal cells in the wounded layer of the amnion, suggesting that EMT occurs in this situation, as we had previously reported in our mouse pPROM model. Collagen injection dramatically increased the overall healing rate to 90%, whereas an injection of phosphate buffered saline alone resulted in a healing rate of only 40%. We concluded that scaffold formation at the wounded site in the amnion stimulates wound healing through at least two mechanisms. First, the scaffold provides a base for migrating amnion cells to cover the wound. Second, the matrix scaffold traps, concentrates, and localizes wound healing macrophages.

Application of collagen to the rupture site has also been tested in a rabbit pPROM model. In that study, amnion integrity was diminished by the injection of a collagen "plug" compared

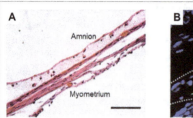
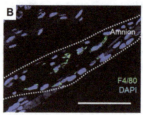

FIGURE 1 | (A) H&E staining of collagen-injected fetal membrane at ruptured site at 72 h. Note that a collagen gel layer was formed beneath the amnion, and immune cells were trapped inside the gel. **(B)** Immunofluorescence staining for F4/80 (green) and DAPI (blue) in the collagen layer at 48 h. Bars, 50 μm. All animals were handled and euthanized in accordance with the standards of humane animal care described by the National Institutes of Health Guide for the Care and Use of Laboratory Animals, using protocols approved by the Institutional Animal Care and Use Committee (IACUC) of the University of Texas Southwestern Medical Center.

to myometrial closure alone. This result is different from ours. We speculate that this is because we injected a collagen "gel" in liquid form to the rupture site using a syringe, such that the gel spreads immediately after injection around the rupture site rather than forming a "plug" as in the rabbit study (Papadopulos et al., 1998). The formation of a plug might block the migration of amnion cells. Our collagen gel, in contrast, formed a collagen layer beneath the amnion in our mouse model. This layer serves as a scaffold for migrating amnion cells and traps macrophages. Thus, it never interferes with the healing process. The form of biomaterials (liquid or solid) and the means of their application (injection or patch) may thus be as important as the material type itself.

The effectiveness of biomaterial scaffolds has been observed in other tissues. Bone and cardiac muscle-derived tissue ECM scaffolds for traumatic muscle wounds in mice improved tissue regeneration (Sadtler et al., 2016). In this study, macrophages and immune cells were increased at the injured site, allowing these immune cells to be polarized into a type 2 immune state. Therefore, providing a scaffold is a good strategy for stimulating healing of ruptured amnion. The least invasive means of accomplishing this *in vivo* remains under active investigation.

CONCLUSION

Based on several previous studies, we speculate that the amnion might be capable of healing. Several cell types coordinate and orchestrate wound healing in the fetal membranes, including amnion epithelial cells that differentiate into mesenchymal cells, migrating mesenchymal cells, differentiating resident macrophages, and recruited fetal macrophages. ECM scaffolds could support spontaneous healing of the amnion not only by promoting the migration of amnion cells but also by polarizing macrophages into a type-2 phenotype. The mechanisms by which the amnion heals itself represent a new field of study in which a great deal more research must be done to clarify how this healing process works.

AUTHOR CONTRIBUTIONS

HM and RW wrote the manuscript.

REFERENCES

Akira, S., Uematsu, S., and Takeuchi, O. (2006). Pathogen recognition and innate immunity. *Cell* 124, 783–801. doi: 10.1016/j.cell.2006.02.015

Berthiaume, F., Maguire, T. J., and Yarmush, M. L. (2011). Tissue engineering and regenerative medicine: history, progress, and challenges. *Annu. Rev. Chem. Biomol. Eng.* 2, 403–430. doi: 10.1146/annurev-chembioeng-061010-114257

Borgida, A. F., Mills, A. A., Feldman, D. M., Rodis, J. F., and Egan, J. F. (2000). Outcome of pregnancies complicated by ruptured membranes after genetic amniocentesis. *Am. J. Obstet. Gynecol.* 183, 937–939. doi: 10.1067/mob.2000.108872

Carter, A. M. (2016). IFPA senior award lecture: mammalian fetal membranes. *Placenta* 48(Suppl. 1), S21–S30. doi: 10.1016/j.placenta.2015.10.012

Cordeiro, J. V., and Jacinto, A. (2013). The role of transcription-independent damage signals in the initiation of epithelial wound healing. *Nat. Rev. Mol. Cell Biol.* 14, 249–262. doi: 10.1038/nrm3541

Deprest, J. A., Papadopulos, N. A., Decaluw, H., Yamamoto, H., Lerut, T. E., and Gratacos, E. (1999). Closure techniques for fetoscopic access sites in the rabbit at mid-gestation. *Hum. Reprod.* 14, 1730–1734. doi: 10.1093/humrep/14.7.1730

Devlieger, R., Deprest, J. A., Gratacos, E., Pijnenborg, R., Leask, R., and Riley, S. C. (2000a). Matrix metalloproteinases-2 and -9 and their endogenous tissue inhibitors in fetal membrane repair following fetoscopy in a rabbit model. *Mol. Hum. Reprod.* 6, 479–485. doi: 10.1093/molehr/6.5.479

Devlieger, R., Gratacos, E., Wu, J., Verbist, L., Pijnenborg, R., and Deprest, J. A. (2000b). An organ-culture for *in vitro* evaluation of fetal membrane healing capacity. *Eur. J. Obstet. Gynecol. Reprod. Biol.* 92, 145–150. doi: 10.1016/s0301-2115(00)00439-5

Eming, S. A., Martin, P., and Tomic-Canic, M. (2014). Wound repair and regeneration: mechanisms, signaling, and translation. *Sci. Transl. Med.* 6:265sr6. doi: 10.1126/scitranslmed.3009337

Friel, L. A., Romero, R., Edwin, S., Nien, J. K., Gomez, R., Chaiworapongsa, T., et al. (2007). The calcium binding protein, S100B, is increased in the amniotic fluid of women with intra-amniotic infection/inflammation and preterm labor with intact or ruptured membranes. *J. Perinat. Med.* 35, 385–393. doi: 10.1515/JPM.2007.101

Gordon, S., and Martinez, F. O. (2010). Alternative activation of macrophages: mechanism and functions. *Immunity* 32, 593–604. doi: 10.1016/j.immuni.2010.05.007

Jenkins, S. J., Ruckerl, D., Cook, P. C., Jones, L. H., Finkelman, F. D., van Rooijen, N., et al. (2011). Local macrophage proliferation, rather than recruitment from the blood, is a signature of TH2 inflammation. *Science* 332, 1284–1288. doi: 10.1126/science.1204351

Johnson, J. W., Egerman, R. S., and Moorhead, J. (1990). Cases with ruptured membranes that "reseal". *Am. J. Obstet. Gynecol.* 163, 1024–1030. doi: 10.1016/0002-9378(90)91117-U

Kono, H., and Rock, K. L. (2008). How dying cells alert the immune system to danger. *Nat. Rev. Immunol.* 8, 279–289. doi: 10.1038/nri2215

Luks, F. I., Deprest, J. A., Peers, K. H., Steegers, E. A., and van Der Wildt, B. (1999). Gelatin sponge plug to seal fetoscopy port sites: technique in ovine and primate models. *Am. J. Obstet. Gynecol.* 181, 995–996. doi: 10.1016/S0002-9378(99)70338-8

Lutolf, M. P., and Hubbell, J. A. (2005). Synthetic biomaterials as instructive extracellular microenvironments for morphogenesis in tissue engineering. *Nat. Biotechnol.* 23, 47–55. doi: 10.1038/nbt1055

Menon, R., and Richardson, L. S. (2017). Preterm prelabor rupture of the membranes: a disease of the fetal membranes. *Semin. Perinatol.* 41, 409–419. doi: 10.1053/j.semperi.2017.07.012

Mogami, H., Hari Kishore, A., Akgul, Y., and Word, R. A. (2017). Healing of preterm ruptured fetal membranes. *Sci. Rep.* 7:13139. doi: 10.1038/s41598-017-13296-1

Mogami, H., Kishore, A. H., and Word, R. A. (2018). Collagen type 1 accelerates healing of ruptured fetal membranes. *Sci. Rep.* 8:696. doi: 10.1038/s41598-017-18787-9

Murray, P. J., and Wynn, T. A. (2011). Protective and pathogenic functions of macrophage subsets. *Nat. Rev. Immunol.* 11, 723–737. doi: 10.1038/nri3073

Nadeau-Vallee, M., Obari, D., Palacios, J., Brien, M. E., Duval, C., Chemtob, S., et al. (2016). Sterile inflammation and pregnancy complications: a review. *Reproduction* 152, R277–R292. doi: 10.1530/REP-16-0453

Papadopulos, N. A., Van Ballaer, P. P., Ordonez, J. L., Laermans, I. J., Vandenberghe, K., Lerut, T. E., et al. (1998). Fetal membrane closure techniques after hysteroamniotomy in the midgestational rabbit model. *Am. J. Obstet. Gynecol.* 178, 938–942. doi: 10.1016/S0002-9378(98)70527-7

Parry, S., and Strauss, J. F. 3rd. (1998). Premature rupture of the fetal membranes. *N. Engl. J. Med.* 338, 663–670. doi: 10.1056/NEJM199803053381006

Peranteau, W. H., Zhang, L., Muvarak, N., Badillo, A. T., Radu, A., Zoltick, P. W., et al. (2008). IL-10 overexpression decreases inflammatory mediators and promotes regenerative healing in an adult model of scar formation. *J. Invest. Dermatol.* 128, 1852–1860. doi: 10.1038/sj.jid.5701232

Richardson, L., and Menon, R. (2018). Proliferative, migratory, and transition properties reveal metastate of human amnion cells. *Am. J. Pathol.* 188, 2004–2015. doi: 10.1016/j.ajpath.2018.05.019

Richardson, L. S., Taylor, R. N., and Menon, R. (2020). Reversible EMT and MET mediate amnion remodeling during pregnancy and labor. *Sci. Signal.* 13:eaay1486. doi: 10.1126/scisignal.aay1486

Romero, R., Miranda, J., Chaiworapongsa, T., Korzeniewski, S. J., Chaemsaithong, P., Gotsch, F., et al. (2014). Prevalence and clinical significance of sterile intra-amniotic inflammation in patients with preterm labor and intact membranes. *Am. J. Reprod. Immunol.* 72, 458–474. doi: 10.1111/aji.12296

Romero, R., Quintero, R., Oyarzun, E., Wu, Y. K., Sabo, V., Mazor, M., et al. (1988). Intraamniotic infection and the onset of labor in preterm premature rupture of the membranes. *Am. J. Obstet. Gynecol.* 159, 661–666. doi: 10.1016/S0002-9378(88)80030-9

Sadtler, K., Estrellas, K., Allen, B. W., Wolf, M. T., Fan, H., Tam, A. J., et al. (2016). Developing a pro-regenerative biomaterial scaffold microenvironment requires T helper 2 cells. *Science* 352, 366–370. doi: 10.1126/science.aad9272

Serpooshan, V., Zhao, M., Metzler, S. A., Wei, K., Shah, P. B., Wang, A., et al. (2013). The effect of bioengineered acellular collagen patch on cardiac remodeling and ventricular function post myocardial infarction. *Biomaterials* 34, 9048–9055. doi: 10.1016/j.biomaterials.2013.08.017

Sicari, B. M., Rubin, J. P., Dearth, C. L., Wolf, M. T., Ambrosio, F., Boninger, M., et al. (2014). An acellular biologic scaffold promotes skeletal muscle formation in mice and humans with volumetric muscle loss. *Sci. Transl. Med.* 6:234ra58. doi: 10.1126/scitranslmed.3008085

Sonnemann, K. J., and Bement, W. M. (2011). Wound repair: toward understanding and integration of single-cell and multicellular wound responses. *Annu. Rev. Cell Dev. Biol.* 27, 237–263. doi: 10.1146/annurev-cellbio-092910-154251

Sopher, D. (1972). The response of rat fetal membranes to injury. *Ann. R Coll. Surg. Engl.* 51, 240–249.

Wei, K., Serpooshan, V., Hurtado, C., Diez-Cunado, M., Zhao, M., Maruyama, S., et al. (2015). Epicardial FSTL1 reconstitution regenerates the adult mammalian heart. *Nature* 525, 479–485. doi: 10.1038/nature15372

Xia, C., Braunstein, Z., Toomey, A. C., Zhong, J., and Rao, X. (2017). S100 proteins as an important regulator of macrophage inflammation. *Front. Immunol.* 8:1908. doi: 10.3389/fimmu.2017.01908

Zisch, A. H., and Zimmermann, R. (2008). Bioengineering of foetal membrane repair. *Swiss Med. Wkly.* 138, 596–601. doi: 10.5167/uzh-5256

In vivo Assessment of Supra-Cervical Fetal Membrane by MRI 3D CISS

Wenxu Qi[1], Peinan Zhao[1], Wei Wang[2], Zhexian Sun[1,3], Xiao Ma[1,3], Hui Wang[1,4], Wenjie Wu[1,3], Zichao Wen[1], Zulfia Kisrieva-Ware[1], Pamela K. Woodard[2], Qing Wang[2], Robert C. McKinstry[2] and Yong Wang[1,2,3,4]*

[1] Department of Obstetrics and Gynecology, School of Medicine, Washington University in St. Louis, St. Louis, MO, United States, [2] Mallinckrodt Institute of Radiology, School of Medicine, Washington University in St. Louis, St. Louis, MO, United States, [3] Department of Biomedical Engineering, McKelvey School of Engineering, Washington University in St. Louis, St. Louis, MO, United States, [4] Department of Physics, Washington University in St. Louis, St. Louis, MO, United States, [5] Department of Electrical and Systems Engineering, Washington University in St. Louis, St. Louis, MO, United States

*Correspondence:
Yong Wang
wangyong@wustl.edu

In approximately 8% of term births and 33% of pre-term births, the fetal membrane (FM) ruptures before delivery. *In vitro* studies of FMs after delivery have suggested the series of events leading to rupture, but no *in vivo* studies have confirmed this model. In this study, we used a three-dimensional constructive interference in steady state (3D-CISS) sequence to examine the FM at the cervical internal os zone during pregnancy; 18 pregnant women with one to three longitudinal MRI scans were included in this study. In 14 women, the FM appeared normal and completely intact. In four women, we noted several FM abnormalities including cervical funneling, chorioamniotic separation, and chorion rupture. Our data support the *in vitro* model that the FM ruptures according to a sequence starting with the stretch of chorion and amnion, then the separation of amnion from chorion, next the rupture of chorion, and finally the rupture of amnion ruptures. These findings hold great promise to help to develop an *in vivo* magnetic resonance imaging marker that improves examination of the FMs.

Keywords: amnion, chorion, fetal membrane, preterm birth, premature rupture of membranes, preterm premature rupture of membranes, magnetic resonance imaging

INTRODUCTION

During pregnancy, the fetus is surrounded by amniotic fluid contained within a fetal membrane (FM). FM is composed of the amnion, which faces the fetus, and the chorion, which contacts the maternal decidua. In a healthy pregnancy, the FM is critical for maintaining a pregnancy until delivery (Parry and Strauss, 1998; Menon and Richardson, 2017). However, in about 8% of pregnancies, the FM ruptures before labor, which is called premature rupture of membranes (PROM). FM rupture before 37 weeks of gestation, termed preterm prelabor rupture of membranes (PPROM), is responsible for approximately one-third of preterm births and is the most common identifiable factor associated with preterm birth (Mathews and MacDorman, 2010; Waters and Mercer, 2011; Martin et al., 2012). Currently, there is no easy way to predict PPROM in early pregnancy, and thus the prevention is very limited.

To solve this problem, we first need to understand the mechanisms of FM rupture. Several investigators have attempted to do so by performing *in vitro* mechanical test on FM after delivery

(Artal et al., 1976; Lavery and Miller, 1979; Helmig et al., 1993; Oyen et al., 2004). For example, data from Arikat et al. and Strohol et al. suggest that FM rupture follows this sequence: (1) Amnion and chorion stretch together under load; (2) amnion separates from chorion; (3) chorion ruptures; (4) amnion distends further, non-elastically; and (5) amnion ruptures (Arikat et al., 2006; Strohl et al., 2010). Ultrasound, an imaging modality widely used clinically to monitor pregnancy *in vivo*, can detect some signs associated with PROM and PPROM, such as FM thickness (Frigo et al., 1998; Severi et al., 2008; Başaran et al., 2014; Nunes et al., 2016) and chorioamniotic separation (Devlieger et al., 2003). The FM region that appears to be most prone to rupture is near the internal cervical os (McLaren et al., 1999). However, this para-cervical weak zone is often difficult to visualize by transvaginal ultrasound because of the low contrast between the FM and the maternal decidua (Severi et al., 2008). Strong *in vivo* evidence is still absent in the literature.

Here, we proposed to visualize the FM near the internal cervical os using magnetic resonance (MR) images acquired with a sequence named three-dimensional constructive interference in steady state (3D-CISS). This sequence provides both high spatial resolution and excellent contrast between the cerebrospinal fluid (high signal from water) and tissue structures (lower signal). And thus it is commonly used in clinical procedures to evaluate fine structures, such as cranial nerves surrounded by cerebrospinal fluid (Yoshino et al., 2003; Yousry et al., 2005). In MR images, the difference of signal intensity between amniotic fluid (high signal) and the FM (low/intermediate signal) is similar to the difference of signal intensity between cerebrospinal fluid and nerves, and the FM has similar thickness as nerves. Therefore, the 3D-CISS sequence is able to visualize the FM near the internal cervical os. In our study, we performed 3D-CISS MR imaging on 18 women at one to three time points between 20 and 36 weeks of gestation. And we report the result of four women who had evidence of abnormal FM structure. Our data suggest that the *in vivo* FM rupture sequence matches what proposed from *in vitro* studies (Arikat et al., 2006; Strohl et al., 2010).

MATERIALS AND METHODS

Participants

This study was approved by the Washington University in St. Louis Institutional Review Board (protocols 201612140, 201707152). Participants were recruited by research nurses from the patient population attending the Obstetrics and Gynecology Clinic and the Women's Health Center in the Barnes-Jewish Hospital Center for Outpatient Health. Participants were included if they were 18 years of age or older and had a healthy singleton pregnancy. Participants were excluded if they had a twin pregnancy or a contraindication to MRI. Before imaging, all patients were screened for MRI safety and provided written informed consent. Age, body mass index, and other clinical information were recorded for all participants. Pregnancy outcomes were collected from the medical records. Term birth was defined as birth between 37 0/7 weeks of gestation and 42 0/7 weeks of gestation (Goldenberg et al., 2008). Preterm birth was defined as birth between 20 0/7 weeks of gestation and 36 6/7 weeks of gestation (Goldenberg et al., 2008). PROM was defined as rupture of membranes before labor. PPROM was defined as rupture of membranes followed by labor before 37 weeks of gestation (Simhan and Canavan, 2005; Goldenberg et al., 2008).

MRI Acquisition

Every patient underwent MRI examination one, two, or three times between 20 and 36 weeks of gestation. A Siemens Magnetom Vida 3T whole body MRI scanner and a 30-channel phased-array torso coil (Erlangen, Germany) were used to acquire a series of sagittal view T2 weighted images (T2WI), with a half-Fourier acquisition single-shot turbo spin echo sequence and the following parameters: repetition time, 1800 ms; echo time, 94 ms; matrix, 320 × 650; flip angle, 140°; layer thickness, 4.0 mm; slice spacing, 0.8 mm; number of layers, 25. For the 3D-CISS sequence, parameters were as follows: repetition time, 7.71 ms; echo time, 3.70 ms; flip angle, 50°; acquisition number, 1; acquisition matrix, 640 × 640; field of view, 300 mm × 300 mm; bandwidth, 460 Hz per pixel; slice thickness, 1 mm; and in-plane resolution, 0.33 mm × 0.33 mm. The total acquisition time for both T2WI and 3D-CISS was 7 min.

Image Analysis

Magnetic resonance images were independently analyzed by two radiologists (WQ and WW, with 10-year and 1-year of experience, respectively, in analyzing abdominal MR images) who were blinded to pregnancy outcomes. A consensus was reached in cases of discordance. The following imaging characteristics were evaluated: cervical funneling, chorioamniotic separation, and chorion or amnion rupture.

RESULTS

Between April 2019 and February 2020, 18 pregnant women were recruited for this study. Their mean age was 33.5 ± 12.1 years, and their mean body mass index at first prenatal visit was 23.8 ± 5.3 kg/m^2. Demographic and clinical details of the 18 women included in this study are presented in **Table 1**. A total of 43 MRI scans were performed on these 18 patients.

Fourteen patients had normal-appearing FM in which the amnion, chorion, and decidua were intact and indistinguishable from one another at all imaging time points. For example, in the patient images shown in **Figures 1A–C**, the FM was completely intact at 20, 32, and 36 weeks' gestation, though we noted some suspended FM material in the cervical canal at all three time points. None of the 14 patients with normal, intact FM had PPROM or PROM, and all 14 delivered at term.

Four patients had both cervical funneling, in which the FM protruded into the cervix, and chorioamniotic separation, in which amniotic fluid was visible between the amnion and chorion, detectable in at least one of their MRI scans.

In patient #1, the FM appeared normal at 20 weeks (**Figure 1D**). However, at 32 weeks, this patient had cervical funneling with amniotic fluid and FM protruding into the cervix

TABLE 1 | Demographic and clinical characteristics of pregnant women.

	Total (n = 18)	ROM at labor (n = 17)	PPROM (n = 1)
Age, years, median (range)	26.5 (19–35)	26 (19–35)	25
Body mass index, kg/m^2, average (range)	27.68 (18.5–39.0)	27.66 (18.5–39.0)	28.0
Race/ethnicity, n (%)			
African American	16 (88.9)	15 (88.2)	1 (100)
Caucasian	2 (11.1)	2 (11.8)	0
Asian	0	0	0
Other	0	0	0
Multiparous, n (%)	16 (88.9)	15 (88.2)	1 (100)
Nulliparity	2 (11.1)	2 (11.8)	0

(**Figure 1E**). At 36 weeks, amniotic fluid was visible between amnion and chorion, indicating chorioamniotic separation (**Figure 1F**). This patient did not have PPROM or PROM and delivered at term.

In patient #2, the FM showed cervical funneling and partial chorioamniotic separation at 32 weeks and complete chorioamniotic separation at 36 weeks (**Figures 2A,B**). This patient did not have PPROM or PROM and delivered at term.

In patient #3, the FM showed cervical funneling and partial chorioamniotic separation at 24 weeks and complete chorioamniotic separation at 32 and 36 weeks (**Figures 2C–E**). This patient did not have PPROM or PROM and delivered at term.

In patient #4, the FM showed deeper cervical funneling, chorioamniotic separation, and chorionic rupture at 36 weeks (**Figure 3**). This patient developed PPROM 6 h after the MRI scan and delivered preterm (36 2/7 weeks).

DISCUSSION

In our study, the longitudinal 3D-CISS MRI data provide the first *in vivo* evidence to support the first three steps of the model proposed by Arikat et al. regarding the sequence of events leading to FM rupture and PROM or PPROM. In the first step of their model, the FM stretches and protrudes into the cervix when the cervical internal os dilates to cause cervical funneling. This is evident in patient #1 at 32 weeks. In step 2, the amnion partially or completely separates from the chorion, as is evident in patient #1 at 36 weeks, patient #2 at 32 and 36 weeks, patient #3 at 24, 28, and 32 weeks, and patient #4 at 36 weeks. In step 3, further cervical internal os dilation leads to additional FM stretch and chorion rupture as seen in patient #4 at 36 weeks. In step 4, the amnion distends further. Finally, in step 5, the amnion ruptures, leading to PPROM or PROM. We present a schematic of the first three steps of this model in **Figure 4**.

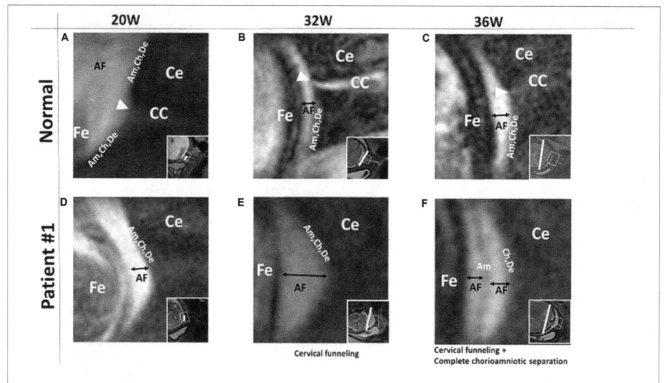

FIGURE 1 | A pregnant woman with normal FM and Patient #1. **(A–C)** 3D-CISS images from a pregnant woman with normal, intact FM at the indicated time points. The white triangle indicates FM suspended in the cervical canal region. Images from patient #1, showing normal FM at 20 weeks **(D)**, cervical funneling at 32 weeks **(E)**, and cervical funneling and complete chorioamniotic separation at 36 weeks **(F)**. Insets show T2WI images of the same regions. The white lines indicate the diameter of the cervix anatomical internal os. AF, amniotic fluid; Am, amnion; CC, cervical canal; Ce, cervix; Ch, chorion; De, decidua; Fe, fetus.

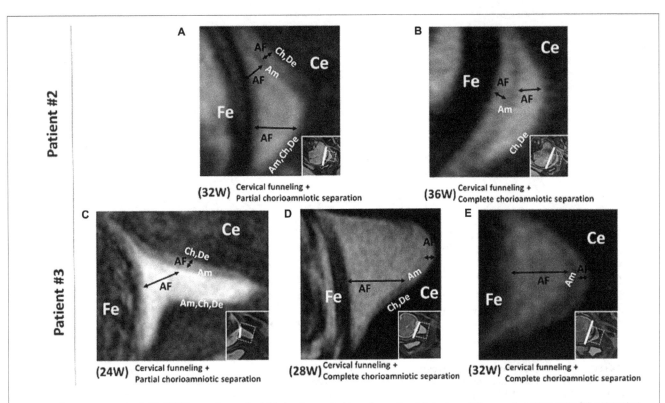

FIGURE 2 | Patients # 2 and # 3. 3D-CISS images from patient #2, showing cervical funneling and partial chorioamniotic separation at 32 weeks (A) and cervical funneling and complete chorioamniotic separation at 36 weeks (B). Images from patient #3, showing cervical funneling and partial chorioamniotic separation at 24 weeks (C) and cervical funneling and complete chorioamniotic separation at 28 weeks (D) and 32 weeks (E). Insets show T2WI images of the same regions. The white lines indicate the diameter of the cervix anatomical internal os. AF, amniotic fluid; Am, amnion; Ce, cervix; Ch, chorion; De, decidua; Fe, fetus.

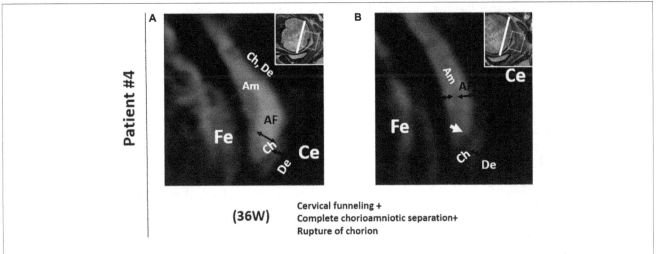

FIGURE 3 | Patient 4. 3D-CISS images from patient #4 showing cervical funneling, chorioamniotic separation, and chorionic rupture at 36 weeks. The white arrow indicates the point of chorionic rupture. Insets show T2WI images of the same regions. The white lines indicate the diameter of the cervix anatomical internal os. AF, amniotic fluid; Am, amnion; Ce, cervix; Ch, chorion; De, decidua; Fe, fetus.

Consistent with the *in vitro* studies, our *in vivo* study indicates that the stretch of FM is the first step in FM rupture. During pregnancy, outward pressure on FM from the amniotic fluid is balanced by inward pressure from the uterine wall. However, when the cervical internal os opens (cervical funneling), inward pressure on the FM overlying the cervix will decrease, and the FM will protrude into the cervical canal, causing the stretch of FM. Our longitudinal data suggest that the FM stretch in the paracervical weak zone can lead to chorioamniotic separation. Data from *in vitro* studies suggest that the mechanical force applied to FM reduces the adhesiveness between amnion and chorion, leading to chorioamniotic separation (Strohl et al., 2010). This

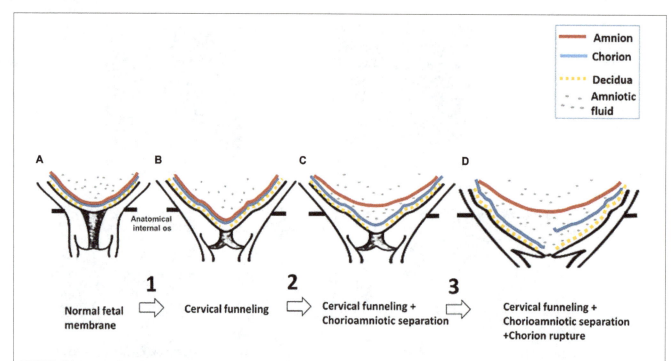

FIGURE 4 | Schematic of the first three steps of premature FM rupture detected by 3D-CISS. **(A)** After 16 weeks' gestation, the amnion (red) and chorion (blue) usually fuse, and the chorion is fused to the decidua (yellow) at the maternal–fetal interface. No amniotic fluid (gray dots) can be seen between the amnion and chorion or between the chorion and decidua. **(B)** In step 1, the FM stretches as it protrudes into the cervix when the internal cervical os dilates, causing cervical funneling. **(C)** In step 2, the amnion separates from the chorion, and amniotic fluid is detectable between the amnion and chorion. **(D)** In step 3, the FM undergoes additional stretch upon further internal cervical os dilation. This can result in chorion rupture.

result is also supported by *in vitro* second harmonic generation microscopy studies of FM, revealing that the repeated mechanical loading affects the integrity of the amnion–chorion interface and can increase the risk of FM rupture (Mauri et al., 2013).

Before 14 weeks' gestation, the chorion and amnion have not yet fused together, and the chorioamniotic separation is always normal. After 16 weeks, however, any chorioamniotic separation is identified as uncommon and anomalous (Kim et al., 2007; Bibbo et al., 2016). Such separation is dangerous, as the ultrasound-detected chorionic separation after 16 weeks is associated with adverse perinatal outcomes such as fetal extremity deformities, fetal death (Graf et al., 1997; Levine et al., 1998), and preterm delivery (Levine et al., 1998; Sydorak et al., 2002; Devlieger et al., 2003; Wilson et al., 2003). The 3D-CISS images can detect chorioamniotic separation, since the amniotic fluid lies between the chorion and amnion.

We observed that the chorioamniotic separation which occurs before FM rupture is consistent with three sets of previous data. First, in clinical observations, FM components are frequently separated at delivery after spontaneous rupture of the membranes before delivery (Strohl et al., 2010). Second, a video-recorded sequence of *in vitro* FM rupture revealed that the chorion and amnion separated before rupture (Arikat et al., 2006). Third, in *in vitro* mechanical tests, two peaks were noted in the force vs. displacement curve, suggesting that FM rupture occurs via separate rupture of the amnion and chorion (Artal et al., 1976; Lavery and Miller, 1977; Oxlund et al., 1990; Schober et al., 1994; El Khwad et al., 2005).

In patient 4, the chorion ruptured before the amnion, which is supported by *in vitro* studies (Artal et al., 1976; Lavery and Miller, 1979; Helmig et al., 1993; Oyen et al., 2004; Arikat et al., 2006). But some studies suggest that the amnion ruptures first (Artal et al., 1976; Lavery and Miller, 1979; Helmig et al., 1993; Oyen et al., 2004; Arikat et al., 2006). Our data are consistent with *in vitro* mechanical testing revealing that the amnion was consistently stronger, stiffer, and more ductile than the chorion (Arikat et al., 2006). The amnion may be stronger because it is composed of a dense layer of collagen fibrils, where the FM strength mainly comes from (Strauss, 2013).

The major strength of this work is the first ever use of 3D-CISS MRI to obtain *in vivo* images of the FM at much higher contrast and better resolution than other types of MRI or ultrasound. Clinical ultrasound is a series of 2D images acquired at several limited angles, which cannot provide a 3D description of the FM overlying the cervix. In comparison, 3D-CISS MRI is not operator dependent and can provide a high resolution, high contrast 3D spatial coverage of FM with multi-planar viewing angle capability. Therefore, 3D-CISS MRI provides a novel way to study the FM overlying the cervix. Additionally, by longitudinally imaging patients, we could define the sequences of events leading to FM rupture.

In this study, we used a 3.0 T MRI to image the FM of pregnant women. MRI has been used to evaluate obstetrical, placental, and fetal abnormalities in pregnant patients for more than 30 years, and its application during pregnancy is generally considered safe for the fetus (Patenaude et al., 2014; Radiology TACo, 2015;

Ray et al., 2016). Compared with the current commonly used fetal MRI sequence, the 3D-CISS sequence was applied without exceeding either of the specific absorption rate and acoustic noise. Additionally, 3D-CISS is a high-speed sequence (4 min) and therefore reduced the patients' exposure to the magnetic.

Our study has three main limitations. First, we had a small sample size and our data are qualitative in nature. Second, we did not measure other FM characteristics such as thickness and signal intensity. Lastly, our medical records did not separate PPROM from PTL in the history of preterm delivery.

CONCLUSION

In summary, our data support the *in vitro* model that the FM ruptures according to a sequence starting with stretch of the chorion and amnion together, then separation of the amnion from the chorion, next the rupture of the chorion, and finally the rupture of the amnion ruptures. An important next step is to conduct a larger longitudinal study to confirm these findings. If we can define an MRI marker that predicts FM rupture, we may be able to intervene to prevent PPROM.

ETHICS STATEMENT

The studies involving human participants were reviewed and approved by the Washington University in St. Louis Institutional Review Board (protocols 201612140 and 201707152). The patients/participants provided their written informed consent to participate in this study.

AUTHOR CONTRIBUTIONS

WQ and PZ designed the experiment. WQ and WiW evaluated magnetic resonance images. ZS, XM, HW, WnW, ZW, ZK-W, PW, and QW collected the data and aided in preparation of the manuscript. RM co-supervised the research. YW obtained funding for the project, supervised the work, and participated in preparation of the manuscript.

ACKNOWLEDGMENTS

We thank NIH/National Institute of Child Health and Human Development (R01HD094381 to PIs YW and AGC) and NIH/National Institute of Aging (R01AG053548 to T. Benzinger and YW) for providing funding. We also thank Dr. Molly Stout for constructive suggestions and Deborah Frank for editing the manuscript. We also thank Jessica Chubiz and Megan Steiner for coordinating the clinical team to enroll patients.

REFERENCES

Arikat, S., Novince, R. W., Mercer, B. M., Kumar, D., Fox, J. M., Mansour, J. M., et al. (2006). Separation of amnion from choriodecidua is an integral event to the rupture of normal term fetal membranes and constitutes a significant component of the work required. *Am. J. Obstet. Gynecol.* 194, 211–217. doi: 10.1016/j.ajog.2005.06.083

Artal, R., Sokol, R. J., Neuman, M., Burstein, A. H., and Stojkov, J. (1976). The mechanical properties of prematurely and non–prematurely ruptured membranes. Methods and preliminary results. *Am. J. Obstet. Gynecol.* 125, 655–659. doi: 10.1016/0002-9378(76)90788-2

Başaran, D., Özyüncü, Ö, Kara, Ö, Şahin, N., Turğal, M., and Önderoğlu, L. S. (2014). Ultrasonographic measurement of amniochorionic membrane in asymptomatic pregnant women is not a useful tool for preterm birth prediction. *J. Obstet. Gynaecol. Res.* 40, 62–66. doi: 10.1111/jog.12121

Bibbo, C., Little, S. E., Bsat, J., Botka, K. A., Benson, C. B., and Robinson, J. N. (2016). Chorioamniotic separation found on obstetric ultrasound and perinatal outcome. *AJP Rep.* 6, e337–e343. doi: 10.1055/s-0036-1593407

Devlieger, R., Scherjon, S. A., Oepkes, D., Meerman, R., Timmerman, D., and Vandenbussche, F. P. (2003). Ultrasound visualization of fetal membrane detachment at the uterine cervix: the 'moon sign'. *Ultrasound Obstet. Gynecol.* 22, 431–432. doi: 10.1002/uog.234

El Khwad, M., Stetzer, B., Moore, R. M., Kumar, D., Mercer, B., Arikat, S., et al. (2005). Term human fetal membranes have a weak zone overlying the lower uterine pole and cervix before onset of labor. *Biol. Reprod.* 72, 720–726. doi: 10.1095/biolreprod.104.033647

Frigo, P., Lang, C., Sator, M., Ulrich, R., and Husslein, P. (1998). Membrane thickness and PROM–high-frequency ultrasound measurements. *Prenat. Diagn.* 18, 333–337. doi: 10.1002/(sici)1097-0223(199804)18:4<333::aid-pd264>3.0.co;2-h

Goldenberg, R. L., Culhane, J. F., Iams, J. D., and Romero, R. (2008). Epidemiology and causes of preterm birth. *Lancet* 371, 75–84. doi: 10.1016/S0140-6736(08)60074-4

Graf, J. L., Bealer, J. F., Gibbs, D. L., Adzick, N. S., and Harrison, M. R. (1997). Chorioamniotic membrane separation: a potentially lethal finding. *Fetal Diagn. Ther.* 12, 81–84. doi: 10.1159/000264436

Helmig, R., Oxlund, H., Petersen, L. K., and Uldbjerg, N. (1993). Different biomechanical properties of human fetal membranes obtained before and after delivery. *Eur. J. Obstet. Gynecol. Reprod. Biol.* 48, 183–189. doi: 10.1016/0028-2243(93)90086-r

Kim, Y. N., Jeong, D. H., Jeong, S. J., Sung, M. S., Kang, M. S., and Kim, K. T. (2007). Complete chorioamniotic membrane separation with fetal restrictive dermopathy in two consecutive pregnancies. *Prenat. Diagn.* 27, 352–355. doi: 10.1002/pd.1673

Lavery, J. P., and Miller, C. E. (1977). The viscoelastic nature of chorioamniotic membranes. *Obstet. Gynecol.* 50, 467–472.

Lavery, J. P., and Miller, C. E. (1979). Deformation and creep in the human chorioamniotic sac. *Am. J. Obstet. Gynecol.* 134, 366–375. doi: 10.1016/s0002-9378(16)33077-0

Levine, D., Callen, P. W., Pender, S. G., McArdle, C. R., Messina, L., Shekhar, A., et al. (1998). Chorioamniotic separation after second-trimester genetic amniocentesis: importance and frequency. *Radiology* 209, 175–181. doi: 10.1148/radiology.209.1.9769829

Martin, J. A., Hamilton, B. E., Ventura, S. J., Osterman, M. J., Wilson, E. C., and Mathews, T. J. (2012). Births: final data for 2010. *Natl. Vital. Stat. Rep.* 61, 1–72.

Mathews, T. J., and MacDorman, M. F. (2010). Infant mortality statistics from the 2006 period linked birth/infant death data set. *Natl. Vital. Stat. Rep.* 58, 1–31.

Mauri, A., Perrini, M., Mateos, J. M., Maake, C., Ochsenbein-Koelble, N., Zimmermann, R., et al. (2013). Second harmonic generation microscopy of fetal membranes under deformation: normal and altered morphology. *Placenta* 34, 1020–1026. doi: 10.1016/j.placenta.2013.09.002

McLaren, J., Malak, T. M., and Bell, S. C. (1999). Structural characteristics of term human fetal membranes prior to labour: identification of an area of altered morphology overlying the cervix. *Hum. Reprod.* 14, 237–241. doi: 10.1093/humrep/14.1.237

Menon, R., and Richardson, L. S. (2017). Preterm prelabor rupture of the membranes: a disease of the fetal membranes. *Semin. Perinatol.* 41, 409–419. doi: 10.1053/j.semperi.2017.07.012

Nunes, V., Cross, J., Speich, J. E., Morgan, D. R., Strauss, J. F., and Ramus, R. M. (2016). Fetal membrane imaging and the prediction of preterm birth: a systematic review, current issues, and future directions. *BMC Pregnancy Childbirth* 16:387. doi: 10.1186/s12884-016-1176-5

Oxlund, H., Helmig, R., Halaburt, J. T., and Uldbjerg, N. (1990). Biomechanical analysis of human chorioamniotic membranes. *Eur. J. Obstet. Gynecol. Reprod. Biol.* 34, 247–255. doi: 10.1016/0028-2243(90)90078-f

Oyen, M. L., Cook, R. F., and Calvin, S. E. (2004). Mechanical failure of human fetal membrane tissues. *J. Mater. Sci. Mater. Med.* 15, 651–658. doi: 10.1023/b:jmsm.0000030205.62668.90

Parry, S., and Strauss, J. F. (1998). Premature rupture of the fetal membranes. *N. Engl. J. Med.* 338, 663–670. doi: 10.1056/NEJM199803053381006

Patenaude, Y., Pugash, D., Lim, K., Morin, L., Bly, S., Butt, K., et al. (2014). The use of magnetic resonance imaging in the obstetric patient. *J. Obstet. Gynaecol. Can.* 36, 349–363. doi: 10.1016/s1701-2163(15)30612-5

Radiology TACo, (2015). *ACR–SPR Practice Parameter for the Safe and Optimal Performance of Fetal Magnetic Resonance Imaging (MRI)*. Virginia: ACR.

Ray, J. G., Vermeulen, M. J., Bharatha, A., Montanera, W. J., and Park, A. L. (2016). Association between MRI exposure during pregnancy and fetal and childhood outcomes. *JAMA* 316, 952–961. doi: 10.1001/jama.2016.12126

Schober, E. A., Kusy, R. P., and Savitz, D. A. (1994). Resistance of fetal membranes to concentrated force applications and reconciliation of puncture and burst testing. *Ann. Biomed. Eng.* 22, 540–548. doi: 10.1007/bf02367090

Severi, F. M., Bocchi, C., Voltolini, C., Borges, L. E., Florio, P., and Petraglia, F. (2008). Thickness of fetal membranes: a possible ultrasound marker for preterm delivery. *Ultrasound Obstet. Gynecol.* 32, 205–209. doi: 10.1002/uog.5406

Simhan, H. N., and Canavan, T. P. (2005). Preterm premature rupture of membranes: diagnosis, evaluation and management strategies. *BJOG* 112(Suppl. 1), 32–37. doi: 10.1111/j.1471-0528.2005.00582.x

Strauss, J. F. (2013). Extracellular matrix dynamics and fetal membrane rupture. *Reprod. Sci.* 20, 140–153. doi: 10.1177/1933719111424454

Strohl, A., Kumar, D., Novince, R., Shaniuk, P., Smith, J., Bryant, K., et al. (2010). Decreased adherence and spontaneous separation of fetal membrane layers–amnion and choriodecidua–a possible part of the normal weakening process. *Placenta* 31, 18–24. doi: 10.1016/j.placenta.2009.10.012

Sydorak, R. M., Hirose, S., Sandberg, P. L., Filly, R. A., Harrison, M. R., Farmer, D. L., et al. (2002). Chorioamniotic membrane separation following fetal surgery. *J. Perinatol.* 22, 407–410. doi: 10.1038/sj.jp.7210753

Waters, T. P., and Mercer, B. (2011). Preterm PROM: prediction, prevention, principles. *Clin. Obstet. Gynecol.* 54, 307–312. doi: 10.1097/GRF.0b013e318217d4d3

Wilson, R. D., Johnson, M. P., Crombleholme, T. M., Flake, A. W., Hedrick, H. L., King, M., et al. (2003). Chorioamniotic membrane separation following open fetal surgery: pregnancy outcome. *Fetal Diagn. Ther.* 18, 314–320. doi: 10.1159/000071972

Yoshino, N., Akimoto, H., Yamada, I., Nagaoka, T., Tetsumura, A., Kurabayashi, T., et al. (2003). Trigeminal neuralgia: evaluation of neuralgic manifestation and site of neurovascular compression with 3D CISS MR imaging and MR angiography. *Radiology* 228, 539–545. doi: 10.1148/radiol.2282020439

Yousry, I., Moriggl, B., Schmid, U. D., Naidich, T. P., and Yousry, T. A. (2005). Trigeminal ganglion and its divisions: detailed anatomic MR imaging with contrast-enhanced 3D constructive interference in the steady state sequences. *AJNR Am. J. Neuroradiol.* 26, 1128–1135.

The Role of Danger Associated Molecular Patterns in Human Fetal Membrane Weakening

Justin G. Padron[1], Chelsea A. Saito Reis[2] and Claire E. Kendal-Wright[2,3]*

[1] Anatomy, Biochemistry and Physiology, John A. Burns School of Medicine, University of Hawai'i at Mānoa, Honolulu, HI, United States, [2] Natural Science and Mathematics, Chaminade University of Honolulu, Honolulu, HI, United States, [3] Obstetrics, Gynecology and Women's Health, John A. Burns School of Medicine, University of Hawai'i at Mānoa, Honolulu, HI, United States

*Correspondence:
Claire E. Kendal-Wright
claire.wright@chaminade.edu

The idea that cellular stress (including that precipitated by stretch), plays a significant role in the mechanisms initiating parturition, has gained considerable traction over the last decade. One key consequence of this cellular stress is the increased production of Danger Associated Molecular Patterns (DAMPs). This diverse family of molecules are known to initiate inflammation through their interaction with Pattern Recognition Receptors (PRRs) including, Toll-like receptors (TLRs). TLRs are the key innate immune system surveillance receptors that detect Pathogen Associated Molecular Patterns (PAMPs) during bacterial and viral infection. This is also seen during Chorioamnionitis. The activation of TLR commonly results in the activation of the pro-inflammatory transcription factor Nuclear Factor Kappa-B (NF-kB) and the downstream production of pro-inflammatory cytokines. It is thought that in the human fetal membranes both DAMPs and PAMPs are able, perhaps via their interaction with PRRs and the induction of their downstream inflammatory cascades, to lead to both tissue remodeling and weakening. Due to the high incidence of infection-driven Pre-Term Birth (PTB), including those that have preterm Premature Rupture of the Membranes (pPROM), the role of TLR in fetal membranes with Chorioamnionitis has been the subject of considerable study. Most of the work in this field has focused on the effect of PAMPs on whole pieces of fetal membrane and the resultant inflammatory cascade. This is important to understand, in order to develop novel prevention, detection, and therapeutic approaches, which aim to reduce the high number of mothers suffering from infection driven PTB, including those with pPROM. Studying the role of sterile inflammation driven by these endogenous ligands (DAMPs) activating PRRs system in the mesenchymal and epithelial cells in the amnion is important. These cells are key for the maintenance of the integrity and strength of the human fetal membranes. This review aims to (1) summarize the knowledge to date pertinent to the role of DAMPs and PRRs in fetal membrane weakening and (2) discuss the clinical potential brought by a better understanding of these pathways by pathway manipulation strategies.

Keywords: amnion, danger associated molecular pattern, Pattern Recognition Receptor, fetal membrane, Toll-like receptor, preterm premature rupture of fetal membrane, pathogen associated molecular pattern

UNDERSTANDING FETAL MEMBRANE RUPTURE IS IMPORTANT TO IMPROVE THE HIGH RATE OF PRETERM BIRTH

The human fetal membranes are an often-overlooked tissue by those studying the mechanisms of parturition. They are disregarded, as many consider that term fetal membranes are a dead tissue, or simply a membranous extension of the placenta. However, many researchers have successfully highlighted it's importance by culturing tissue explants (Zaga et al., 2004; Astern et al., 2012) and isolated cells (Kendal-Wright et al., 2010; Sato et al., 2016), revealing its role as a complex conduit between the mother and fetus (Hadley et al., 2018). It has a large surface area for signaling and clearly contributes to the inflammation that is an established signature of parturition (Romero et al., 2007), regardless of whether it is precipitated by infection (Gomez-Lopez et al., 2018).

Parturition involves several distinct, yet integrated, physiological events; cervical ripening and dilation, contractility of the myometrium, rupture of the membranes, placental separation and uterine involution (Christiaens et al., 2008). All of these processes need to occur in a coordinated manner for the successful delivery of the fetus at term. Thus, desynchrony or the dysregulation of these events can lead to Preterm Birth (PTB) via a number of different pathways (Goldenberg et al., 2008). Approximately 20% of all preterm deliveries are by Cesarean section for maternal or fetal indications (Christiaens et al., 2008). Of the remaining cases, around a third are caused by premature preterm rupture of the membranes (pPROM), 20–25% result from intra-amniotic infection, and the remainder due to premature uterine contractions (Christiaens et al., 2008). However, approximately 60% of all preterm deliveries still remain unexplained (Christiaens et al., 2008). Epidemiological studies have suggested that preterm delivery is a condition that clusters in families (Strauss et al., 2018), and that the incidence of pPROM and the other causes of PTB differ among ethnic groups (Manuck, 2017). Although about 50% of all PTB is due to infection, antibiotics that successfully treat the infection do not halt PTB (Gravett et al., 2007). Once the fetal membranes rupture, they are beyond rescue as there is no commonly used therapy to repair the ruptured regions, although some strategies like the Amniopatch appear promising (Deprest et al., 2011). Thus, there is a need to improve our understanding of this phenomenon, so that we can identify two groups of pPROM patients, those at risk for pPROM after infection and those at risk for non-infectious pPROM. Compounding this intricate challenge is that there are gaps in our fundamental knowledge as to how the fetal membranes weaken at the end of a normal pregnancy. Our lack of understanding of how normal membrane rupture occurs, impedes our ability to determine how this normal mechanism digresses during pPROM.

The importance of finding new therapeutic targets for the prevention of PTB, and also improving our understanding of basic parturition mechanisms, including rupture of the fetal membranes cannot be overstated. This is because much of the impact of PTB in the United States is borne by our minority populations. Americans who are members of racial and ethnic minority groups, (African Americans, American Indians and Alaska Natives, Asian Americans, Hispanics or Latinos, Native Hawaiians, and other Pacific Islanders), are more likely than Caucasians to have poor health and to die prematurely (CDC, 2020)[1]. States that have the highest rates of PTB disparity typically have large minority populations. Indeed, data from the March of Dimes mirrors this, showing that Hawai'i was ranked the 50th state in terms of PTB as a health disparity (March of Dimes Perstats[2]). The infant mortality rate is twice as high for Native Hawaiian mothers compared to whites and 43.9% of the cause of this infant mortality is PTB related (Hirai et al., 2013). Contributing to the lack of progress in Hawai'i is the lack of ethnic disaggregation, masking valuable information (Park et al., 2009; Tsark and Braun, 2009) as many established health disparities, including PTB, differentially affect ethnic groups within this population pool (Braun et al., 1996). In addition, we have no data on specific incidence of pPROM, versus other etiologies of PTB, although it is frequently seen in the clinic. It is likely that this is due to the general lack of focus on the importance of the fetal membranes in pregnancy outcomes, that is also seen in the other states. In Hawaii, like the rest of the United States, African American mothers have the highest rates of prematurity (13.8%) (March of Dimes Perstats: see text footnote 2). However, they only constitute 2.2% of the population (United States census data[3]). In other United States states African Americans constitute a much larger percentage of the population

Abbreviations: 15d-PGJ2, 15-deoxy-delta-12, 14-prostaglandin J2; a2V, V-ATPase; ADAMTS5, ADAM metallopeptidase with Thrombospondin type 1 motif 5; AEC, amnion epithelial cell; AMC, amnion mesenchymal cell; AP1, Activator protein 1; ATP, Adenosine tri-phosphate; CD, cluster differentiation; cffDNA, cell free fetal DNA; CLR, C-type lectin receptors; DAMP, Danger associated molecular pattern; DNGR1, Dendritic cell natural killer lectin group receptor-1; dsRNA, double stranded ribonucleic acid; ECM, Extracellular Matrix; ERK, extracellular-signal-regulated kinase; G-CSF, granulocyte colony stimulating factor; GIT2, ARF GTPase-activating protein; GSK, Glycogen synthase kinase 3; HBD2, b-defensin 2 HBD2; HKE, Heat killed *E. Coli*; HMGB1, high mobility group box 1; HMW, high molecular weight; HSP, Heat Shock protein; IFN, interferon; IL, Interleukin; iNOS, inducible nitric oxide synthase; IRF, IFN regulatory factors; IRF, interferon-regulatory factor; LMW, low molecular weight; LPS, Lipopolysaccharide; LRR, Leucine-rich repeats; MAL/TIRAP, MyD88 adaptor-like protein; MALP-2/FLS-1, diacyl lipopeptides; MAPK, mitogen activated protein kinase; MIP-1A, macrophage inflammatory protein; miRNA, micro ribonucleic acid; MMP, Matrix Metalloproteinase; mtDNA, mitochondrial deoxyribonucleic acid; MYD88, myeloid differentiation primary response protein 88; NF-kB, Nuclear Factor Kappa B; NLR, NOD-like receptors; NLRP3, LRR- and pyrin domain-containing protein 3; P2YR, P2 receptor; P2X7R, P2X purinoceptor 7 receptors; PAMP, Pattern associated molecular pattern; PBMC, peripheral blood mononuclear cell; PBS, phosphate buffered saline; PGE2, prostaglandin E2; PGN, peptidoglycan; Poly I:C, polyinosinic-polycytidylic; pPROM, preterm premature rupture of the membranes; PRRs, Pattern recognition receptors; PTB, Preterm birth; PTL, Preterm labor; RAGE, advanced glycation end products; RANTES, regulated upon activation, normal T expressed and secreted; RD, repressor domain; RLR, RIG-1-like receptors; ROS, reactive oxygen species; SAA1, serum amyloid A1; SAP130, sin3A associated protein 3A; SASP, senescence-associated secretory phenotype; ssRNA, single stranded ribonucleic acid; ST2, suppression of tumorigenicity 2; TIM, T-cell immunoglobulin and mucin-containing domain-3; TIR, Toll/IL1 receptor; TLR, Toll-like receptors; TNF, tumor necrosis factor; TRAM, TIR domain-containing adapter molecule 2; TRIF, TIR domain-containing adaptor-inducing IFNβ TRIF; ZAM, zone of altered morphology.

---

[1] http://www.cdc.gov/omh/AMH/dbrf.htm

[2] http://www.marchofdimes.com/peristats/Peristats.aspx (accessed May 7, 2020).

[3] https://www.census.gov/quickfacts/fact/table/HI/PST045219# (accessed May 7, 2020).

and consistently have the highest prematurity rate (Schaaf et al., 2013). These studies are typically controlled for socioeconomic and demographic confounders and therefore to improve our understanding of the underlying cause, future studies need to focus on determining the risk factors for specific ethnic groups.

THE ONSET OF FETAL MEMBRANE WEAKENING MAY BE TRIGGERED BY CELLULAR STRESS

One of the fundamental remaining questions in the field of parturition research is how the tissues of pregnancy switch from a relatively "quiescent" state that favors the maintenance of the pregnancy, to one that is "reactive" in preparation for the delivery of the fetus. Animals other than humans and non-human primates experience a drop-in progesterone level but this does not appear to happen in the same way in humans (Menon et al., 2016a). In order to increase our understanding of the differences in the mechanism, studies have focused on areas of enquiry that may lead to "functional" progesterone withdrawal, such as the role of prostaglandin receptors (Nadeem et al., 2016; Patel et al., 2018) and the minutiae of inflammation control by cytokine cascades and specific transcription factors (Lappas et al., 2008; Paulesu et al., 2010). Understating the trigger for labor onset is important for us to decipher how this may deviate in patients with PTB. It is also important to know how this labor mechanism interfaces with the trigger for the initiation of fetal membrane remodeling and weakening, another pathway that is poorly understood.

The idea that cellular stress is the trigger for both fetal membrane weakening, and labor, has been gaining traction (Menon et al., 2016b). Suggested stressors for this mechanism have included; stretch/distension (**Figure 1**) of fetal membranes (Millar et al., 2000; Joyce et al., 2016) and myometrium (Waldorf et al., 2015), and also general hypoxia/oxidative stress in all of the tissues of pregnancy. Both of these stressors are known to increase in the human fetal membranes with gestational age or labor (Chai et al., 2012; Joyce et al., 2016), and also to stimulate inflammation (Kendal-Wright, 2007; Menon and Richardson, 2017). This has been demonstrated in all of the tissues of pregnancy and pregnancy complications result from the altered levels of cell stress in these tissues (Duhig et al., 2016). Indeed, several studies have shown that oxidative stress is linked to cell aging and senescence in cells of the amnion, directly leading to increased inflammation (Menon et al., 2017; Menon, 2019). It has also been shown to lead to epithelial to mesenchymal transition in the amnion, which can also play a role in the maintenance of the integrity of this tissue (Richardson et al., 2020). Other distinct types of cellular stress that have also been the subject of study in the human fetal membranes, including, Endoplasmic Reticulum Stress (Liong and Lappas, 2014) and Mitochondrial Stress (Than et al., 2009). In addition, cells can also respond to stress in a variety of way such as initiating, the heat shock response, the unfolding protein response or a DNA damage response (Fulda et al., 2010). Therefore, there are many specific pathways and mechanisms that constitute the wide umbrella term "cell stress," these should be further investigated to elucidate their contribution to the inflammation and cellular responses seen as the fetal membranes weaken.

One of the ways in which cell stress may lead to inflammation is through the production of Danger Associated Molecular Patters (DAMPs), also known as Alarmins (Sheller-Miller et al., 2017). These molecules typically have a different specific function during normal cellular activity, but when the cell detects a stress stimulus, they are activated now functioning to signal "the alarm.". Many different molecules are classified as DAMPs, including various heat shock proteins (HSP), extracellular matrix (ECM) breakdown products, and nucleic acid fragments (**Table 1**; Patel et al., 2018). DAMPs are already known to have a role in a wide range of other diseases with strong inflammatory signatures, such as, autoimmune diseases (Systemic Lupus Erythematosus, Rheumatoid Arthritis), Osteoarthritis, cardiovascular diseases, neurodegenerative diseases and cancer (Roh and Sohn, 2018). Here, they perpetuate a positive-feedback cycle of cellular damage, inflammation and then more cellular damage (Roh and Sohn, 2018). DAMPs are known to activate various Pattern Recognition Receptors (PRRs), including the Toll-like receptor (TLRs) family (Takeda et al., 2003; Kawai and Akira, 2010) and through these receptors, they can cause the activation of the pro-inflammatory transcription factor Nuclear Factor Kappa-B (NF-κB), changes in the levels of Matrix Metalloproteinases (MMP) and stimulate apoptosis (Roh and Sohn, 2018). Due to the large number of wide-ranging biomolecules acting as DAMPs (**Table 1**) and the large number of different receptors involved, they produce their effects by working through a complex number of distinct signaling pathways.

THE WEAKENING AND SUBSEQUENT RUPTURE OF THE HUMAN FETAL MEMBRANES IS DEPENDENT ON BIOPHYSICAL AND BIOCHEMICAL CHANGE

The fetal membranes are a multilayered structure composed of various cell types and associated ECM (**Figure 1**). The normal rupture of these membranes is currently thought to be the result of both physical forces and biochemical changes. The physical properties of fetal membrane strength are known to originate from the layer closest to the fluid and fetus (**Figure 1**), the amnion (Arikat et al., 2006). The strength of this tissue is undoubtedly derived from the combination of its layers working in concert. Some of this may come from the interface between the amnion and chorion. This region in the amnion is described as a spongy layer that is ECM rich (**Figure 1**), consisting of proteoglycans, glycoproteins and type III collagen (Strauss, 2013). The interface between this and the chorion consists of a gelatinous substance made up of hyaluronan, decorin, buglycan and collagen that mediates the separation of the amnion and chorion prior to fetal membrane rupture (Meinert et al., 2001, 2007). This separation is the first step in the weakening of the fetal membranes (Arikat et al., 2006). The chorion adheres to the decidua between

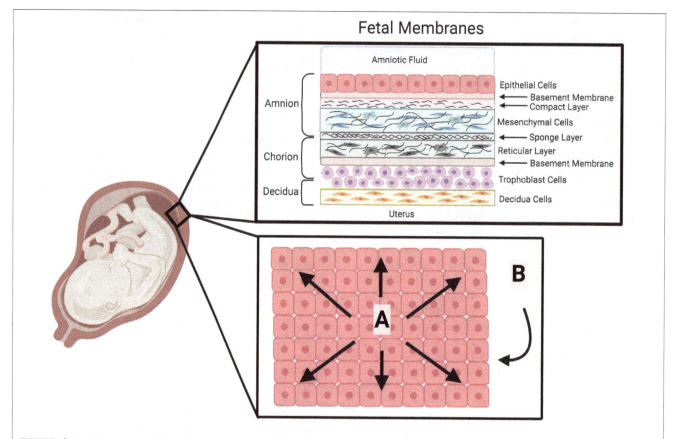

FIGURE 1 | The cellular structure of the fetal membranes and their biophysical forces. The human fetal membranes consist of a multi-layered structure which surround the fetus in utero. It is composed of the amnion, chorion and decidua (upper box). Biophysical forces are placed on these fetal membranes (lower box depicted looking down onto the apical surface of the amnion epithelium). **(A)** Linear physical forces due to multi-directional stretching of the fetal membranes adherent to the decidua. **(B)** Dynamic physical forces on the fetal membranes due to fetal movements, Braxton Hicks contractions and eventually labor. (This Figure was created using BioRender).

weeks 14 and 16 of pregnancy, by the degeneration of the capsular decidua and fusion of the chorion with the parietal decidua (Genbacev et al., 2015). Thus, this integration with the maternal tissues may also provide some strength to the tissue. However, the fetal membranes typically rupture in the region that is above the cervix (Malak and Bell, 1994; Strauss, 2013). *In vitro* it has been shown that after its separation from the amnion, this chorion layer is next to rupture (Arikat et al., 2006). Therefore, as the amnion layer is last to rupture in this sequence, after a notable period of deformation, it is widely accepted that the ECM rich compact layer containing amnion mesenchymal cells (AMC) (**Figure 1**) accounts for the strength and maintains the integrity of this tissue (Arikat et al., 2006).

An increase in apoptosis (Fortunado et al., 2000; Hsu et al., 2000; Kumagai et al., 2001) and changes in the levels of MMPs (Cockle et al., 2007) are central to the biochemical component of the changes that occur in the fetal membranes before their rupture. Although cell death in the form of apoptosis is recognized as important for the weakening process, it is thought that these cells can also die through autophagy (Shen et al., 2008; Mi et al., 2017) and perhaps necrosis (Menon and Richardson, 2017), as both of these forms of cell death are also known to be the result of cell stress (Fulda et al., 2010). In addition, it is known that necrosis can occur as the result of TLR activation in other cells (Meylan and Tschopp, 2005). Although cellular survival is obviously directly linked to the maintenance of the integrity of the amnion, its physical strength is dependent on the synthesis and degradation of the components of the ECM (El Khwad et al., 2005; Anum et al., 2009) controlled by resident cells (Parry and Strauss, 1988). Indeed, women with connective tissue disorders and related diseases are at an increased risk for complications during pregnancy, including pPROM (Anum et al., 2009). Support for this mechanism has come from several research groups as they have biochemically and mechanically identified a "zone of altered morphology" (ZAM) in the human fetal membranes (McParland et al., 2003; El Khwad et al., 2005; Osman et al., 2006; Reti et al., 2007). The ZAM constitutes a discrete zone of weakness overlying the cervix characterized by several features; an increased thickness and swelling of the connective tissue layer, a reduction in both the cytotrophoblast and decidual layers, and a reduced overall thickness of the supracervical membranes that exhibits increased ECM remodeling (Lappas et al., 2008), and apoptosis (Shen et al., 2008). It is also known that inflammation in the form of increased cytokine secretion and signaling are

TABLE 1 | Summary of key Danger Associated Molecular Patterns, their receptors and mechanisms.

Origin	DAMP	Receptor	Function (standard font = pro-inflammatory; italics = anti-inflammatory)	References
Extracellular Matrix	Aggrecan 32 mer fragment	TLR2	(iNOS), CCL2, IL-1α, IL-6, MMP12 MMP13 and ADAMTS5	Stevens et al., 2008
	Biglycan	TLR2/4	Increases levels of reactive oxygen species, CXCL-1, CCL2 and HSP70, and activates NLRP3 inflammasome by Caspase-1 and the maturation of IL-1β *Activating a TLR co-adaptor that activates IFN1 signaling*	Frey et al., 2013; Schaefer, 2014; Roedig et al., 2019
	Decorin	TLR2/4	Decreases TGFβ1 and IL-10 and increases levels of apoptosis	Merline et al., 2011
	*Fibronectin	TLR2/4	Promotes pro-inflammatory mediators and phagocytosis by macrophages	Haruta et al., 2013; Fei et al., 2018
	Fibrinogen	TLR4	Activation of monocytes	Al-Ofi et al., 2014
	LMW-HA	TLR2/4	Activates NLRP3 inflammasome by Caspase-1 and the maturation of IL-1β. Activates NF-kB	Merline et al., 2011
	HMW-HA	TLR2	*Activates a TLR co-adaptor that activates IFN1 signaling*	Scheibner et al., 2006; Frey et al., 2013
	Heparin sulfate	TLR4, RAGE	Activation of NF-kB	Xu et al., 2011
	Tenascin C	TLR4	Synthesis of pro-inflammatory cytokines	Midwood et al., 2009
	Versican	TLR2/4 CD14	IL-6, IL-1β, Il-12 and CCL2 production *Increasing IL-6 (anti-inflammatory pathways), IL-10*	Wight et al., 2014
Cytosolic	ATP	P2XR P2YR	Attracts macrophages by inflammasome activation MAPK wound healing response	Venereau et al., 2015
	Cyclophilin	CD 147	Chemotaxis and the production of pro-inflammatory factors	Burkrinsky, 2014
	F-actin	DNGR1	DNGR1 recognizes the released F-actin, which causes the uptake of damaged or dead cells	Brown, 2012
	Heat Shock Protein	TLR2/4	MyD88 dependent activation of NF-kB	Tolle and Standiford, 2013; Relja et al., 2018
	S100 proteins	TLR4, CD147 RAGE	Leads to apoptosis and activates ERK and NF-kB or AP1	Ghavami et al., 2010; Xia et al., 2018
	*Soluble amyloid beta	TLR2/4	Enhanced TNF driven inflammation	Wang et al., 2019
	Uric Acid	NLRP3	Inflammasome activation and induction of IL-1β maturation	Braga et al., 2017
Mitochondrial	mtDNA	TLR9	p38 MAPK and NF-kB activation	Zhang et al., 2010; Zhang et al., 2014; Magna and Pisetsky, 2016; Bao et al., 2016
Nuclear	*Cell free DNA	TLR9	Activation of NF-kB and AP1	Magna and Pisetsky, 2016
	Circulating Histones	TLR9	Inflammation through the activation of NF-kB	Huang et al., 2011; Kawai et al., 2016
	Extracellular self RNA	TLR7 TLR3	Sensitizes other TLR working synergistically with their other ligands MAPK, NF-κB, and IRF-5/7 pathways through MyD88 signaling	Karikó et al., 2004; Cavassani et al., 2008; Thompson et al., 2011; Noll et al., 2017; Petes et al., 2017
	*HMGB1	TLR2 TLR4 TLR9	Activation of NF-kB, and MAPK signaling though ERK and p38, release of MMPs	Qin et al., 2006; Nie et al., 2016 Menon et al., 2011; Bredeson et al., 2014; Plazyo et al., 2016
	IL-1α	IL-1R	MAPK signaling and NF-kB activation	Betheloot and Latz, 2017
	IL-33	ST2	NF-kB activation and TNF production	Isnadi et al., 2018
	SAP130	Mincle	Triggering pro-inflammatory cytokine secretion	Zhou et al., 2016; Patkin et al., 2017

* denotes has been studied in the fetal membranes or cells of the fetal membranes. ADAMTS5, ADAM metallopeptidase with Thrombospondin type 1 motif 5; AP-1, Activator protein 1; CD, Cluster Differentiation; DNGR1, Dendritic cell natural killer lectin group receptor-1; ERK, extracellular-signal-regulated kinase; HSP, Heat Shock protein; IFN1, Interferon; IL, Interleukin; iNOS, Inducible Nitric Oxide; IRF, Interferon regulatory factors; MMP, Matrix Metalloproteinase; MyD88, myeloid differentiation primary response protein 88; NF-kB, Nuclear Factor Kappa B; NLRP3, LRR- and pyrin domain-containing protein 3; RAGE, advanced glycation end products; ST2, suppression of tumorigenicity 2; TGF, Transforming growth factor; TLR, Toll-like receptor; TNF, Tumor Necrosis Factor.

also involved in the initiation and progression of membrane rupture both at term and preterm. This is particularly evident when associated with intrauterine infection and chorioamnionitis (Bowen et al., 2002). However, it is important to note that inflammation in the absence of infection, in the form of what has been coined "sterile inflammation," leads to pPROM and normal rupture of the membranes (Shim et al., 2004).

Roles for several key pro-inflammatory cytokines; Interleukin 1β (IL-1β), IL-6, IL-8, and Tumor Necrosis Factor-α (TNF-α) in parturition are apparent. Their increase in abundance in gestationally advanced fetal membranes is not only associated with labor (Keelan et al., 1999) but they have also all been demonstrated to independently increase the synthesis of MMPs (Bowen et al., 2002). Additionally, many of these cytokines can cause the translocation of the pro-inflammatory transcription factor NF-κB thus leading to further increases in inflammatory mediators. This provides a pathway of pro-inflammatory self-induction (Christiaens et al., 2008) that is thought to terminate with delivery of the fetus. This can be exemplified by the chemokine IL-8, which leads to the increased infiltration of polymorphonuclear leukocytes, which can further contribute to the increase in inflammation in a feed-forward manner and can lead to birth. In further support of a central role for cytokine-induced cascades in membrane weakening, TNF-α and IL-1β have been shown to directly cause significant weakening of fetal membranes, inducing the biochemical markers characteristic of the ZAM (Kumar et al., 2006).

In addition to the polymorphonuclear leukocytes that are attracted to the tissue by chemokines, an infectious inflammatory response leads also leads to the recruitment of macrophages. These produce cytokines, MMPs, and prostaglandins, which increase the risk of pPROM (Parry and Strauss, 1988). In addition, stimulated monocytes in human chorionic cells produce the inflammatory cytokines IL-1α and TNFα, which result in the increased expression of MMP-1 and MMP-3 (Katsura et al., 1989; So et al., 1992). In fetal membranes with chorioamionitis, adhesive granulocytes have also been noted adjacent to apoptotic amnion epithelial cells (AECs) near the rupture site (Leppert et al., 1996). Together these data illustrate how immune cells promote cellular changes within the fetal membranes by driving inflammation, and breaking down ECM through the production of MMPs, predisposing the tissue for rupture. However, more recently it has been demonstrated that immune cells may also have fetal membrane healing properties through the migration of macrophages from the amniotic fluid to a rupture site in the amnion (Mogami et al., 2017). These cells were seen to induce wound healing by secreting IL-1β and TNFα and stimulating epithelial to mesenchymal transition (Mogami et al., 2017).

It is thought that the forces produced by the cell stressor distension, may be the link between the biochemical and biophysical changes seen in the fetal membranes toward term. This was originally based on the observation that human pregnancies with more than one fetus often result in premature delivery (Keith and Oleszczuk, 2002). The insertion and subsequent slow inflation of a balloon above the cervix in humans is also known to induce labor (Manabe et al., 1985). This led to the study of the distension of the uterus to discern the resultant biochemical changes and how they might lead to the activation of uterine contraction (Shynlova et al., 2009). Less work has been performed studying the effect of distension on the fetal membranes although it has been clearly shown that they are massively stretched *in vivo* at term (Millar et al., 2000; Joyce et al., 2016). It is assumed that this is the result of the combination of their adherence to the uterine wall and the termination of cellular proliferation, halting their further growth, at the beginning of the third trimester (**Figure 1**). Work performed stretching both the uterus, pieces of fetal membranes (Nemeth et al., 2000) or cells of the amnion (Kendal-Wright et al., 2008, 2010) show that this stimulus is able to induce pro-inflammatory cytokine production and secretion, and can also regulate apoptosis (Kendal-Wright et al., 2008; Poženel et al., 2019). Thus, the distension of the fetal membranes in normal term pregnancies and its over distension in PTB, can lead to its inflammatory signature. This distension also constitutes a significant source of cellular stress through physical strain. Interestingly, our recently collected data confirms that cellular distension of cells of the amnion *in vitro* can indeed act as a cell stressor, increasing the secretion of the DAMP, High mobility group box 1 (HMGB1) (Norman Ing et al., 2019).

DANGER ASSOCIATED MOLECULAR PATTERNS ARE A LARGE GROUP OF BIOMOLECULES WITH DISTINCT CELLULAR COMPARTMENTALIZATION

Danger Associated Molecular Patterns are a wide-ranging group of biomolecules, originating from various cellular compartments. These molecules were classified as DAMPs when released, activated or secreted in response to tissue injury, and by damaged or dying cells (Schaefer, 2014). They can originate from nuclear or intracellular location, or cleaved from ECM. They have a wide range of effects resultant from their interaction with PRR on both immune cells and endogenous cells of organs (**Table 1**). The intention here is not to discuss an exhaustive list of all those that have been identified to date, but to briefly highlight the distinct origins of DAMPs and discuss what is known about them in the fetal membranes (**Table 1**).

The ECM has an important role in shaping the innate immune response, it is dynamic, not simply a static network that provides tissue integrity and strength. The majority of DAMPs coming from the ECM are derived from proteoglycan or glycoprotein (**Table 1**), and are typically released by the cleavage by MMPs, Hyaluronidase, and Heparanase (Gaudet and Popovich, 2014). However, they can also be *de novo* synthesized or released by unfolding due to mechanical stimulation (Smith et al., 2007). When released, they function to trigger sterile inflammation or prolong pathogen-induced responses by "fine-tuning" the production of inflammatory mediators (Frevert et al., 2018). Some are known to promote inflammation, whereas others are also anti-inflammatory (Frevert et al., 2018). These diverging roles are dependent on the activation of specific signaling profiles working through specific PRRs. Thus, these DAMPs work to modulate inflammation by their interaction with a range of receptors including; TLRs (TLR2 and TLR4), RIG-1-like receptors (RLRs), NOD-like receptors (NLRs), receptor for advanced glycation end products (RAGE), integrins and cluster differentiation 44 (CD44). Although their role has not been directly studied in the fetal membranes, it is reasonable, given that the amnion that provides the strength of the tissue is ECM rich (**Figure 1**) and is subject to cell stress in the form of distension toward term, that these molecules could have a key role in driving the weakening mechanisms of this tissue toward the end of gestation.

A wide range of DAMPs from various intracellular origins have also been characterized (**Table 1**). They can be cytosolic, endoplasmic, or they can also be released from granules or the plasma membrane. However, one of the most important unifying characteristics of this group of DAMPs is that when "activated" by cell stress, they typically change cellular compartment and lead to differential signaling events, compared to those seen during their normal biological role in "unstressed" conditions. In addition, various proteins and nucleic acids from the nucleus and mitochondria have been widely studied for their DAMP roles (**Table 1**). This group of DAMPs include but are not limited to; HMGB1, circulating histones, various interleukins, Free DNA, mitochondrial DNA, and self-extracellular RNA. The variety of DAMPs provide a range of receptor specificity and pro/anti-inflammatory functionality (**Table 1**).

DANGER ASSOCIATED MOLECULAR PATTERNS AND PATHOGEN ASSOCIATED MOLECULAR PATTERNS ACTIVATE PATTERN RECOGNITION RECEPTORS

It is clear that DAMPs cause inflammation in other tissues, therefore we believe they could be the key regulators that begin the weakening of the fetal membranes by driving inflammation during this process too. They elicit their effects through numerous receptors known as PRRs. One of the largest groups of receptors that belong to this group is the TLRs. They are a distinct class of germline-encoded PPRs that initiate the innate immune response for the initial detection of a pathogen (West et al., 2006). They are located on cell surfaces or within endosomes and generally have a conserved function to protect against pathogens via activation of downstream signaling pathways (Kawai and Akira, 2010). Several roles of TLRs have been identified including the clearance of pathogenic microbes, protection of endogenous threats, and regulation of the innate and adaptive immune response (Hug et al., 2018). There are ten TLR isoforms (TLR1–10) in humans that are expressed on immune and non-immune cells including macrophages, fibroblasts, epithelial cells, and endothelial cells (Kumar et al., 2009). TLR1, TLR2, TLR4, TLR5, and TLR6 are expressed on the cell surface, whereas TLR3, TLR7, TLR8, and TLR9 are expressed in endosomes (Takeda, 2004; Kumar et al., 2009). TLR10 is a distinct receptor, in that it is the only TLR known to act as inhibitory protein through the induction of anti-inflammatory cytokine IL-1Ra (Oosting et al., 2014).

The cell surface TLRs mainly recognize PAMPs generated from cell wall components and flagellin from gram positive and gram-negative bacteria, yeast, and fungi (Chaturvedi and Pierce, 2009). Interestingly, the recognition of DAMPs by these cell surface TLRs are shown to require different co-receptors and accessory molecules to the PAMPs. The endogenous ligands of these receptors appear to be limited, perhaps to help constrain TLR responses so that they can sufficiently function for pathogenic recognition, without causing detrimental responses to the host (Miyake, 2007). The intracellular TLRs (TLR3, 7, 8, 9) function within endolysosomal compartments and detect foreign nucleic acids that are signatures often belonging to invading viruses and microbes (Blasius and Beutler, 2010). Generally, it is thought that the endosomal TLRs are able to distinguish between host and foreign nucleic acids, although there is mounting evidence that some TLRs may not have this ability, and cannot discriminate between the nucleic acid molecules of host and microbial origin (Blasius and Beutler, 2010). It is known that endogenous mRNA and RNA from necrotic cells can also activate the intracellular TLR mediated pathway (Karikó et al., 2004; Cavassani et al., 2008; Thompson et al., 2011), resulting in an antiviral and pro-inflammatory response via Interferon (IFN) and cytokine induction (Perales-Linares and Navas-Martin, 2013).

Although the family of TLRs were originally identified for their abilities to recognize and mediate signaling pathways for a variety of microbial components (Poltorak, 1998; Takeuchi et al., 1999, 2001, 2002; Hemmi et al., 2000; Alexopoulou et al., 2001; Hayashi et al., 2001; Lund et al., 2004) many studies have shown that they are important in the detection of endogenous DAMP molecules (**Table 1**; Beg, 2002; Wallin et al., 2002). This is where the function of PAMPs and DAMPs differ, as DAMPs are also necessary for tissue repair. Further exploration into the exogenous (PAMP) and endogenous (DAMP) ligand activation of the TLR family may provide new and effective therapies to mediate the negative effects of TLR-driven inflammation.

Several PRRs and co-receptors other than the family of TLR have also been shown to be important for the function of DAMPs and PAMPs (Takeuchi and Akira, 2010). These include, but are not limited to, RLRs, NLRs, RAGE, C-type lectin receptors (CLRs), P2X purinoceptor 7 receptors (P2X7Rs), LRR- and pyrin domain-containing protein 3 (NLRP3) inflammasome, and distinct members of the cluster differentiation receptor family. Similarly, to TLRs, all of these receptors are responsible for triggering distinct inflammatory cascades of the immune response. Some literature suggests that the intervention of DAMP and PAMP driven inflammation through these receptors, and their specific signaling signatures, may ablate the negative effects of associated pathologies (**Figure 2**).

DANGER ASSOCIATED MOLECULAR PATTERNS AND PATTERN ASSOCIATED MOLECULAR PATTERNS IN THE FETAL MEMBRANES

There is a growing body of evidence demonstrating that DAMPs and PAMPs work via a similar set of PRRs to guide the responses of innate immune system. However, much of what we understand about the potential of DAMPs to cause fetal membrane weakening and pPROM comes from work studying

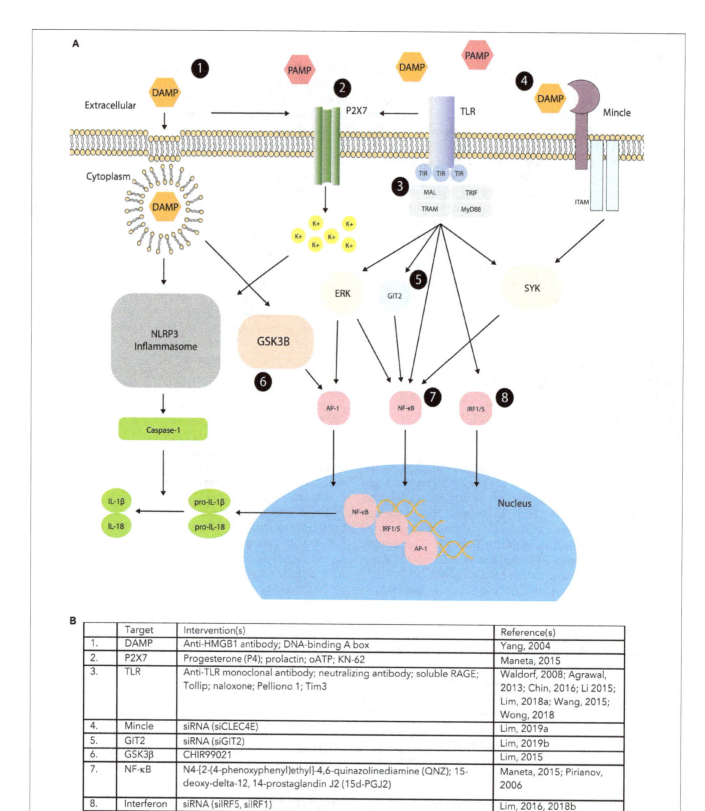

FIGURE 2 | DAMP/PAMP PPR pathway manipulation. (A) TLR, Mincle, and P2X7 receptor activation regulated by DAMP and PAMP signaling have been shown to stimulate downstream pathways involving various modulatory proteins (ERK, GSK3B, GIT2, SYK). This may activate AP-1, NFkB, IRF1/5, or inflammasome activation that leads to induction of pro-inflammatory cytokines. Studies have demonstrated different areas of modulation (1–8) that can manipulate DAMP/PAMP mediated inflammation associated with PTB. (B) The supporting table lists several interventions that demonstrate the manipulation of the DAMP/PAMP mediated pathways that correspond to the different areas of modulation.

the effect of PAMPs in this and other tissues. However, it cannot be assumed that the signaling events and downstream outcomes between these two groups of biomolecules (DAMPs and PAMPs), are identical, even during their activation of the same receptor. Regardless, work on the role of PAMPs in the fetal membranes has been able to provide us with insights as to how DAMPs may also function, providing foundational data that can guide our understanding of their potential as directors of fetal membrane weakening. There is a clear link between fetal membrane weakening and PAMP driven inflammation in PTB with pPROM. Indeed, TLR-mediated PTB in response to PAMPs have been studied and extensively reviewed elsewhere (Thaxton et al., 2010). Thus, the intention of this review is to discuss the work most relevant to and that was performed in the fetal membranes.

PAMP Activation of Inflammation in the Fetal Membranes

Inflammation initiated by bacterial infection causes PTB by preterm labor and pPROM. The initiation of this inflammation is caused by different PAMPs upon their interaction with their specific TLR; for example, lipopolysaccharide (LPS) with TLR4. To determine the role of PAMP ligands specifically in fetal membranes, numerous *ex-vivo* tissue explant studies have been completed. Under normal physiological conditions the fetal membranes express all of the TLR isoforms (1-10) that could be activated and lead to specific pro-inflammatory signatures. Indeed, the treatment of fetal membrane explants with bacterial TLR agonists; peptidoglycan (TLR2), LPS (TLR4), and flagellin (TLR5) all produce a pro-inflammatory response with increased production of various cytokines, including; IL-1β, IL-6, IL-8, IL-10, granulocyte colony stimulating factor (G-CSF), macrophage inflammatory protein (MIP-1A) and Regulated upon Activation Normal T Expressed and Secreted (RANTES) (Hoang et al., 2014).

Not only do bacterial ligands lead to infection driven inflammation but they also lead to increases in the receptors that detect them. This was demonstrated in normal human fetal membranes, where the levels of TLR expression changed upon exposure to various bacteria associated with PTB pPROM. Specifically, treatment with the bacterial stimuli *Mycoplasma hominis* lead to increased expression of TLR 4, 6, and 8. Increased expression of TLR8 was also seen with *Ureaplasma parvum* and increased expression of TLR7 upon treatment with *Porphyromonas gingivalis*. Interestingly, gram negative *E. Coli* significantly decreased TLR10 expression rather than increase TLR expression as demonstrated by the other bacterial stimuli. This is of note as TLR10 is still considered an orphan receptor and therefore its function is not well understood. These data suggest that fetal membranes vary their TLR expression levels upon treatment with bacterial ligands. This observation may be used in the future to indicate the severity of infection and differences in the receptor expression level will likely further direct the magnitude of an inflammatory immune response (Abrahams et al., 2013). In further support of the bacterial ligands affecting the levels of the TLRs, fetal membranes with chorioamnionitis, have also been shown to have differential expression of TLRs. The increased expression of *TLR1* at the gene level in preterm fetal membranes with histological chorioamnionitis has been described (Waring et al., 2015), as have increases in TLR1, TLR2, TLR4, and TLR6 in chorioamniotic fetal membranes (Moco et al., 2013). Together these data suggest a role for these receptors not only in the surveillance of bacteria in this tissue but also that they adapt to the bacterial challenge.

Chorioamnionitis is not the only route to bacterial infection in the fetal membranes. Periodontal disease is a chronic inflammatory disease caused by multiple strains of bacteria, several of which have been detected in amniotic fluid, placenta and fetal membranes. It is now accepted that there is a link between these bacterial and several pregnancy complications including PTB. *P. gingivalis* has been detected in chorionic tissue and LPS derived from it, used to treat chorion derived cells. This resulted in increased expression of TLR2 causing the increased production of IL-6 and IL-8. To further study this relationship, TLR-2 gene-silenced chorionic derived cells demonstrated a reduction in IL-6 and IL-8 secretion. Taken together this suggests an important role for TLR2 in periodontic bacterial signaling in the fetal membranes (Hasegawa-Nakamura et al., 2011). In support of this, the periodontal bacteria *Fusobacterium nucleatum* has also been detected in chorionic tissue from high-risk pregnant women. Similarly, to the previous study, it was then used to treat chorionic cells where it was also able to increase inflammation by increasing IL-6 and corticotrophin-releasing hormone (CRH) secretion via TLR2 and TLR4 activation (Tateishi et al., 2012). These data indicate that periodontal bacteria act similarly to other PAMPs in these tissues as they find their way into the amniotic fluid, placenta and fetal membranes, where they activate the TLR system and downstream inflammation.

Although humans are not thought to experience the sharp drop in progesterone that is thought to initiate the onset of parturition in other animals (Menon et al., 2016a), its administration is used to maintain pregnancy and lower the risk of PTB (Chenung et al., 2020) as it is thought that humans may experience a "functional" progesterone withdrawal (Nadeem et al., 2016). Progesterone (P4) has been shown to have a protective role in fetal membranes by reducing pro-inflammatory cytokine production upon LPS treatment (Flores-Espinosa et al., 2014). It does this in part by significantly reducing TLR4 expression upon LPS treatment. This directly results in the reduced secretion of the pro-inflammatory cytokines TNFα, IL-6, and β-defensin 2 (HBD2) (Flores-Espinosa et al., 2014). Therefore, this intriguing mechanism could be a way for progesterone to decrease the ability of this tissue to detect DAMPs until its functional levels decrease toward the end of gestation.

Animal models have also been used to determine how PAMPs induce inflammation leading to different pregnancy complications. They have also provided models of PTB that can be used to test novel therapeutic targets. In humans, the histological assessment of preterm fetal membranes detected TLR4 expression in the fundus and low segment suggesting a role in PTB (Choi et al., 2012). This receptor's role was further investigated in an infection, LPS-induced PTB mouse model. The TLR4 antagonist (+)-naloxone, was able to suppress the expression the inflammatory cytokines IL-1β, IL-6, TNFα, and IL-10 and prevent PTB. Another study also established the role for TLR4 in PTB by using a mouse model by inducing infection with an LPS variant, heat killed *E. Coli* (HKE). HKE treatment induced PTB in all TLR4 normal mice compared to none of the TLR4 mutant mice. In addition, another study induced PTB in CD1 mice by administering intrauterine injections of saline, peptidoglycan (PGN, TLR2 agonist) or polyinosinic-polycytidylic acid (Poly I:C, TLR3 agonist) (Jaiswal et al., 2013). The regulation of a2 isoform of V-ATPase (a2V) has a role in pregnancy and was assessed post exposure to these two ligands, PGN and Poly I:C. This led to significantly decreased expression of a2V in the fetal membranes and play a role in the induction of PTB in mice (Jaiswal et al., 2013).

Collectively, several mouse studies have provided evidence that demonstrate the importance of bacterial PAMP/TLR driven inflammation to cause PTB. Providing model systems that can be continued to be used to study future therapies to address PTB by these pathways. Indeed, models activating TLRs by ligand injection (Kaga et al., 1996; Wang and Hirsch, 2003) or placental stimulation (Liu et al., 2007; Koga et al., 2009) are also models for PTB.

PAMP Stimulation of Amnion Epithelial Cells Isolated From Fetal Membranes

Human AECs form the most superficial layer of the fetal membranes functioning as an immunological barrier for the fetus against intra-amniotic infection. Their response to pregnancy specific PAMP ligands has been studied to help us understand the contribution of these cells to inflammation in the fetal membranes but also to their production of pro-inflammatory signaling molecules that may also communicate with the growing fetus. Under normal physiological conditions, these cells express TLR 1-10 and can be activated by the PAMPs that reach them. TLR5 and TLR 2/6 activation by PAMP the ligands, Flagellin and macrophage-activating lipopeptide-2 (MALP-2), respectively, significantly increase the secretion of IL-6 and IL-8 (Gillaux et al., 2011). They also cause the nuclear translocation of NF-κB subunit p65, thus inducing a pro-inflammatory response. The activation of TLR4 by LPS, however, has also been demonstrated to induce apoptosis and decrease cell viability of these cells (Gillaux et al., 2011). However, the activation of this receptor also increases Transforming Growth factor beta 1 (TGFβ1) and prostaglandin E2 (PGE2), TNFα and IL-1β production (Motedayyen et al., 2019), which has been confirmed for TGFβ1 and PGE2 but not for IL-1β, IL-6, and IL-10 (Taheri et al., 2018). Taken together these data suggest that not only does the activation of this PAMP TLR mechanism mediate an immunological response to PAMPs in AEC, but it could contribute to the inflammation seen in the fetal membranes with PTB and may also signal to the fetus when an infection was detected. It is possible that AMC respond similarly to AEC to PAMP stimulation, however, there has been a lack of focus on this system in AMC. In addition, differences in the fundamental functions of these cells in the fetal membranes make it difficult to evaluate similarities between them. Thus, it is challenging to know how similar the pathway signaling is in this cell type, that functions to maintain the integrity of ECM in the fetal membranes.

PAMP Stimulation of Amnion Mesenchymal Cells Isolated From Fetal Membranes

Human AMCs are located within the ECM rich layer of the amnion that is closest to the chorion in the of fetal membranes (**Figure 1**). This layer is responsible for the maintenance of the strength and integrity of the whole tissue. Our work has shown that the human AMCs isolated from human fetal membranes express all ten TLR isoforms (Sato et al., 2016). This suggests that similarly to AECs, AMC are able to detect PAMPs and produce a pro-inflammatory signature. However, as their location and function are different to that of AEC, the downstream consequences may also be different. We have also been able to show that indeed the TLR2/6 ligand MALP-2, could increase the pro-inflammatory cytokines and NF-κB translocation, it did not increase levels of apoptosis.

Viral PAMP Activation of the Fetal Membranes

In addition to bacterially derived PAMPs, viral infection also elicits an immune response through the activation of TLRs. This is typically through the release and subsequent detection of viral nucleic acids. TLR 3, 7, 8, and 9 are all nucleic acid ligand response receptors that are activated upon exposure to viral nucleic acid ligands. Thus, fetal membrane explants treated with viral double stranded RNA (dsRNA) and viral single stranded RNA (ssRNA) activate TLR 3 and TLR8, respectively, and induce downstream pro-inflammatory cytokine production that result in two different distinct antiviral response profiles (Bakaysa et al., 2014). Those explants treated with Poly (I:C) (TLR3), or the viral ligands, imiquimod (TLR7), and ssRNA40 (TLR8) also caused the production of pro-inflammatory cytokines IL-6 and IL-8 (Bryant et al., 2017). Although there is little data on the response of the fetal membranes to viral PAMPs, these data support the idea that all of the viral, as well as bacterial TLR receptors are able to be activated on cells of the fetal membranes and that they could result in inflammation, potentially leading to fetal membrane weakening and rupture.

DAMPS and Fetal Membranes

Work studying the direct effect of DAMPs or DAMP production by the fetal membranes is limited. Indeed, so far to our knowledge only four have been directly tested in the fetal membranes (**Table 1**). However, others that have also been shown to play a role in pregnancy are, HMGB1, cell-free fetal DNA (cffDNA), uric acid and IL-1. Little is known about the specific roles of any of these molecules in fetal membranes, and their potential as novel therapeutic targets and biomarkers in the pathologies of pregnancy.

High mobility group box 1 is the most comprehensively studied DAMP in the fetal membranes and has been shown to be a critical regulator throughout different stages of pregnancy. It activates TLRs to initiate an inflammatory immune response in a sterile environment, but it is also released by PAMP stimulation of TLRs. This was confirmed by its presence in the Amniotic fluid from preterm mothers with damaged fetal membranes due to intra-amniotic infection (Baumbusch et al., 2016). Its increase in levels also correlate with increases in IL-6 and with infection in amniotic fluid but its does not seem to increase with gestational age in this compartment. HMGB1 levels are also elevated in chorioamniotic membrane extracts from preterm labor compared to term labor (Plazyo et al., 2016) and it has been seen that this increase contributes to increased expression of pro-inflammatory cytokines (Plazyo et al., 2016). It also increases *MMP-9* gene expression and active-MMP-9 levels in chorioamniotic fetal membrane explants, compared to control treated fetal membranes (Plazyo et al., 2016). These data suggest that HMGB1 induction of MMP-9 could directly promote fetal membrane weakening. Pregnant mice treated with intra-amniotic injections of HMGB1 resulted in increased pup mortality, PTL and PTB compared to pregnant mice treated with PBS (Gomez-Lopez et al., 2016). This study did not asses the role of HMGB1 in the fetal membranes, but these data suggest HMGB1 has an important role in promoting PTB. Fetal membranes treated with exogenous HMGB1 increase TLR2 and TLR4 expression and activation of the inflammatory immune response regulator, p38 Mitogen Activated Protein Kinases (MAPK) which also leads to a senescent phenotype consistent with a sterile inflammatory response (Bredeson et al., 2014). Moreover, term fetal membranes have a phenotype consistent with senescent cells, reduced telomeres, increased activation of p38 MAPK and increased in senescence-associated beta (SA-B) galactosidase and senescence-associated secretory phenotype (SASP) gene expression found a senescent phenotype (Menon et al., 2016b). HMGB1, oxidative stress and apoptosis is also increased in normal fetal membrane explants exposed to cigarette smoke extract compared to control treated fetal membrane explants (Menon et al., 2011). In a study that also linked HMGB1 with fetal membrane weakening, fetal membranes from women who had preterm labor or pPROM were found to have increased levels of HMGB1 in their serum (Qiu et al., 2017). This suggests that HMGB1 could also be a potential biomarker for PTB. Immunofluorescent labeling of fetal membranes delivered preterm with chorioamnionitis also showed HMGB1 localized AECs, with more diffuse labeling in the myofibroblast and macrophages compared to term fetal membranes delivered at term (Romero et al., 2011). Interestingly, another study has demonstrated that microRNA 548 (miRNA) regulates the expression of HMGB1 in fetal membrane tissues with very minimal expression in preterm chorioamniotic fetal membranes (Son et al., 2019). Induced expression of miRNA 548 in isolated epithelial cells from fetal membranes decreased HMGB1 levels and pro-inflammatory cytokine levels. Together these data strongly suggest that although HMGB1 secretion is increased during the cellular stress of infection it may also have a role in a sterile immune response working in autocrine and paracrine ways that could contribute to PTB.

A possible role for serum amyloid A1 (SAA1) in ECM remodeling was assessed in amnion fetal membrane explants. Human amnion fetal membrane explants treated with SAA1 showed increased protein expression of MMP-1, MMP-8, and MMP-13 compared to control treatment (Wang et al., 2019). The increased expression of MMPs suggest a potential role for SAA1 in ECM remodeling in fetal membranes after rupture.

TLR9 recognizes unmethylated CpG-containing DNA sequences in addition to bacterial and viral DNA to activate an immune response, similarly to all the other DAMPs. cffDNA is one of the few nucleic acid DAMPs that have been studied in the context of a placental source of cffDNA. It is thought that cffDNA released from the placenta can circulate in the maternal plasma to activate TLR9 on leukocytes and macrophages. This then can induce a pro-inflammatory immune response that triggers labor, which ultimately leads to birth (Phillippe, 2014). A study in support of the importance of this group of DAMPs, demonstrated that TLR9 is expressed on fetal membranes from term placentas in the presence and absence of labor (Beck et al., 2019). Indeed, its levels are highly expressed in AEC (Gillaux et al., 2011; Sato et al., 2016) and AMC (Sato et al., 2016). Exosomes from senescent AECs are known to package cffDNA and HMGB1 that could also to signal within the fetal membranes acting as a trigger for parturition (Sheller-Miller et al., 2017). In further support of this, human peripheral blood mononuclear cells (PBMCs) treated with fetal DNA or CpG DNA increased IL-6 secretion and pregnant Bagg Albino (BALB/c) mice injected with fetal DNA, CpG DNA or LPS increased the number of resorbed fetuses. In addition, TLR9 knockout mice treated with fetal DNA showed decreased numbers of resorbed mice, whereas those treated with the TLR9 inhibitor Chloroquine reduced fetal resorptions and IL-6 production. This suggests a role for TLR9 in promoting PTB upon cffDNA treatment (Scharfe-Nugent et al., 2012). More studies are needed to show the mechanism by which cffDNA could contribute to the activation of parturition and also what role it has in the fetal membranes where the expression of its detection receptors is high in AEC and AMC (Sato et al., 2016).

To our knowledge only one study has specifically tested the activation of AMC by DAMPs. In this study the authors elegantly show that the TLR4 receptor is present and able to be activated by the DAMP, fetal fibronectin, on AMC (Haruta et al., 2013) resulting in the increase in the activity of MMP-1 and MMP-9.

It is clear that due to the high incidence of infection driven PTB, including those with pPROM, the role of TLR and their ligands in the fetal membranes with and without chorioamnionitis has been the subject of some study. To date, only a few papers have produced data linking DAMPs (as opposed to PAMPs) and the fetal membranes. These have mostly focused on the production of HMGB1, which has been confirmed to increase in amniotic fluid of human fetal membranes with pPROM (Romero et al., 2011), and is induced by intrauterine infection with LPS, in sheep (Regan et al., 2016). Even though much of the current work that is focused on DAMPs in the fetal membranes is AEC centric, the data provides strong evidence that DAMP production by AMC would produce inflammation, perhaps in an autocrine fashion, and this would likely influence the integrity of the amnion. In addition, DAMPs are produced by many of the other cells important for the maintenance of pregnancy (Phillippe, 2014; Nadeau-Vallee et al., 2016). They could also activate AMC in a paracrine fashion and contribute to the increase in inflammation and MMPs, which could ultimately lead to membrane rupture.

DAMP/PAMP PRR PATHWAY MANIPULATION: POTENTIAL THERAPEUTIC STRATEGIES FOR FETAL MEMBRANE MAINTENANCE

There are a multitude of developing therapies based on PRRs recognition of their ligands for the resolution of diseases with an inflammatory signature. Indeed, in other disease and disorder fields like sepsis for example, DAMP manipulation is being tested by the antagonism of HMGB1 (Yang et al., 2005). Although this body of work is expansive, it will not be focused on here as it would warrant its own focused review article. Here we aim to describe the studies that have been specifically focused on the manipulation of this pathway in the tissues of pregnancy, including the fetal membranes where possible, and therefore show promise for future development of strategies to address the maintenance of the integrity of this tissue (**Figure 2**).

Signaling events activated by the DAMP and PAMP ligands are numerous, and complex, with an ever-expanding repertoire of players. Some of these molecules overlap between pathways, while others are more specific. This broad network provides numerous potential targets for manipulation and his has been explored due to their potential for other causes of PTB, but rarely for their direct effects on the fetal membranes. This is because it is highly likely that DAMPs and PAMPs working through their PRRs also have a role in myometrial activation and cervical ripening. This body of work has provided some exciting data (**Figure 2**) that may be used to help us discern the ability for some of the already tested strategies, or develop novel ones, that could be used to help manipulate the timing of membrane rupture too.

It has been suggested that anti-TLR monoclonal antibodies could be good therapeutic target to decrease inflammation driven adverse perinatal outcomes (Wong et al., 2018) and thus it should be considered whether they may also serve as good PTB therapies. Indeed, neutralizing antibodies against TLR4 reduce the percentages of decidual invariant natural killer cells, decreasing inflammation (Li et al., 2015). Soluble TLRs have also been suggested as potential markers or treatment sites for those conditions where they are understood to have a key role (Abrahams et al., 2013). However, it still remains to see their effects elsewhere in the other tissues when pregnant. An alternative strategy in the same vein has been to use soluble RAGE as a therapeutic tool to decrease inflammation. Pretreatment with these inhibited LPS-induced preterm uterine contractility, cytokines, and prostaglandins in Rhesus monkeys (Waldorf et al., 2008), supporting the premise that this approach has merit for further exploration in pregnancy.

An alternate approach designed to target pathways more specifically has been to knockdown downstream signaling for the PRRs. Interferon regulatory factor (IRF) 5 knockdown leads to less inflammation in myometrium (Lim et al., 2018) and thus inhibitors for IRF1 have also been suggested as a therapeutic strategy due to their direct role in TLR signaling (Lim et al., 2016). Other studies testing the potential of TLR4 inhibitors have been successful at decreasing levels of inflammation associated with its activation. Indeed, levels of Tollip, an inhibitor of TLR4 that is known to correlate with PE severity (Nizyaeva et al., 2019) and the TLR4 antagonist (+)-naloxone (Chin et al., 2016) were shown to suppress cytokine expression. Although these studies were performed in the placenta and myometrium/decidua, respectively, they provide promising data for developing this approach in fetal membranes.

Other work has focused specifically on PAMP stimulated TLR response manipulation. Thus, several different biomolecules have been shown to inhibit inflammation or PTB in animal models due to their ability to decrease TLR ligand induced responses. Surfactant-A intrauterine injection was found to significantly decrease TLR ligand induced inflammation and inhibit preterm delivery via TLR2 (Agrawal et al., 2014). As GSK3 α and β activity is increased in fetal membranes after labor, the GSK3β inhibitor CHIR99021 was tested and found to decrease LPS stimulated pro-inflammatory cytokines, TNFα, IL-1β, IL-6, IL-8, prostaglandins and MMP-9 in myometrial cells and fetal membranes cells (Lim and Lappas, 2015). In addition, the protein Pellino 1 was shown to regulate TLR and TNF signaling, by decreasing TLR2/6, TLR3, TLR5 and the pro-inflammatory cytokines IL-8, IL-1β, and IL-6 (Lim et al., 2018). When the addition of Tim3 was tested, it was found to protect decidual cells from TLR extracellular signal-regulated protein kinase 1 and 2 (ERK1/2) dependent apoptosis and inflammation (Wang et al., 2015).

Decreases in TLR signaling by the removal of their key partners or decreasing receptor numbers have also been studied. The elimination of Mincle, a sensor for lipids, was shown to lead to decreased effect of TLR ligands to cause inflammation in uterus (Lim and Lappas, 2019). In addition, GIT2 knockdown, in myometrial and amnion cells also lead to decreased inflammation in response to TLR ligands (Lim and Lappas, 2019). The P2X7 receptor, which has been shown to regulate IL-1β release from gestational tissues working in concert with TLRs has also been studied. The inflammation it produced on stimulation with a specific receptor agonist, was inhibited by the progesterone, prolactin and an NF-κB inhibitor (Maneta et al., 2015). Finally, treatment with 15-deoxy-delta-12, 14-prostaglandin J2 (15d-PGJ2) affected TLR4 by blocking its NF-κB induced inflammation, reducing preterm labor in a mouse model (Pirianov et al., 2009).

It remains to be seen how the further development of these potential therapeutic targets will continue. With such a large number of signaling pathways, receptors and ligands involved, there are many other targets that are yet to be investigated. However, which of the manipulated mechanisms will have too many unwanted effects, or that have an unwanted global biological effect on other organs and the fetus, remains to be determined. Regardless, interest in these pathways is gathering momentum due to their potential to increase our understanding of the mechanisms at play and to prevent the rupture of the membranes. Due to their central role in infection and non-infection driven inflammation, they also have enormous potential for treatments for the other etiologies of PTB (Ekman-Ordeberg and Dubicke, 2012).

SUMMARY

The trigger that initiates tissue remodeling in preparation for parturition remains elusive. This missing stimulus includes that which activates the weakening cascade of the fetal membranes in preparation for its rupture. Understanding this is not only important to determine what happens in normal pregnancy but also because the timing of this event is crucial for healthy pregnancy outcomes. If rupture does not occur in a timely fashion it can result in pROM or pPROM leaving the fetus vulnerable to infection and distress. It can also precipitate PTB, as pPROM is evident in approximately one third of all cases of premature delivery. It is currently thought that the change that may switch on the process of membrane weakening is an increase in cellular stress. This is already known to increase toward the end of gestation in the form of physical distension of the fetal membrane tissue and also the build-up of ROS. It is well established that DAMPs are generated by many forms of cell stress and their general biological function is to raise the alarm within tissues. They do this by producing a number of pro-inflammatory cytokines, MMPs and often lead to apoptosis. They accomplish this through their interaction with numerous PRRs and their downstream signaling pathways, often achieving their influence on inflammation by activating the transcription factor NF-κB. Much of what we understand about the role of DAMPs, especially in the fetal membranes, comes from work in other tissue types or from consideration of data from PAMP ligand action. This is because these ligands also work through many of the same PRRs. However, these data should be viewed with caution; PAMPs and DAMPs have been seen to result in differential signaling through the same PRR. Despite this, numerous similarities that have been described in their actions. PAMPs are well established to cause infection driven membrane rupture, and so it is tempting to postulate that the DAMP counterparts are also able to do this. These molecules could therefore be the link between the biophysical and biochemical changes that happen toward term to weaken the fetal membranes. This idea has been least studied from the perspective of understanding the ECM DAMPs. Perhaps this is because they are one of the more difficult molecules to study in this tissue, given that most researchers are working on it at in term state when much of the ECM has already started to breakdown. Thus, we need to build new models to study the interaction and generation of ECM DAMPs with the AMC within this layer of the amnion. There have been several studies that have focused on understanding the potential of the manipulation of the DAMP, PAMP, PRR system, with an eye to future therapies for various PTB etiologies. Although still in their infancy, it is tempting to speculate that more work focused in this vein will indeed not only solidify the key role of these molecules in parturition, but provide much needed prevention and identification biomolecular targets to help us address the high rates of PTB in the United States.

AUTHOR CONTRIBUTIONS

JP contributed to all the written sections focused on the different receptors and also drew and annotated **Figure 1**. CS contributed to the PAMPs and DAMPs written sections and assisted with editing. CK-W contributed to all sections, tables, and figures.

REFERENCES

Abrahams, V. M., Potter, J. A., Bhat, G., Peltier, M. R., Saade, G., and Menon, R. (2013). Bacterial modulation of human fetal membrane Toll-like receptor expression. *Am. J. Reprod. Immunol.* 69, 33–40. doi: 10.1111/aji.12016

Agrawal, V., Jaiswal, M. K., Ilievski, V., Beaman, K. D., Jilling, T., and Hirsch, E. (2014). Platelet-activating factor: a role in preterm delivery and an essential interaction with Toll-like receptor signaling in mice. *Biol. Reprod.* 91:119. doi: 10.1095/biolreprod.113.116012

Alexopoulou, L., Holt, A. C., Medzhitov, R., and Flavell, R. A. (2001). Recognition of double-stranded RNA and activation of NF-κB by Toll-like receptor 3. *Nature* 413, 732–738. doi: 10.1038/35099560

Al-Ofi, E., Coffelt, S. B., and Anumba, D. O. (2014). Fibrinogen, an endogenous ligand of toll-like receptor 4, activates monocytes in pre-eclamptic patients. *J. Reprod. Immunol.* 103, 23–28. doi: 10.1016/j.jri.2014.02.004

Anum, E., Hill, L., Pandya, A., and Straus, J. (2009). Connective tissue and related disorders and preterm birth: clues to genes contributing to prematurity. *Placenta* 30, 207–215. doi: 10.1016/j.placenta.2008.12.007

Arikat, S., Novince, R. W., Mercer, B. M., Kumar, D., Fox, J. M., Mansour, J. M., et al. (2006). Separation of amnion from choriodecidua is an integral event to the rupture of normal term fetal membranes and constitutes a significant component of the work required. *Am. J. Obstet. Gynecol.* 194, 211–217. doi: 10.1016/j.ajog.1005.06.083

Astern, J. M., Collier, A. C., and Kendal-Wright, C. E. (2012). Pre-B cell colony enhancing factor (PBEF/NAMPT/Visfatin) and vascular endothelial growth factor (VEGF) cooperate to increase the permeability of the human placental amnion. *Placenta* 34, 42–49. doi: 10.1016/j.placenta.2012.10.008

Bakaysa, S. L., Potter, J. A., Hoang, M., Han, C. S., Guller, S., Norwitz, E. R., et al. (2014). Single- and double-stranded viral RNA generate distinct cytokine and antiviral responses in human fetal membranes. *Mol. Hum. Reprod.* 20, 701–708. doi: 10.1093/molehr/gau028

Bao, W., Xia, H., Liang, Y., Ye, Y., Lu, Y., Xu, X., et al. (2016). Toll-like receptor 9 can be activated by endogenous mitochondrial dna to induce podocyte apoptosis. *Sci. Rep.* 6:22579. doi: 10.1038/srep22579

Baumbusch, M. A., Buhimschi, C. S., Oliver, E. A., Zhao, G., Thung, S., Rood, K., et al. (2016). High mobility group box 1 (HMGB1) levels are increased in amniotic fluid of women with intra-amniotic inflammation-determined preterm birth, and the source may be the damaged fetal membranes. *Cytokine* 81, 82–87. doi: 10.1016/j.cyto.2016.02.013

Beck, S., Buhimschi, I. A., Summerfield, T. L., Ackerman, W. E., Guzeloglu-Kayisli, O., Kayisli, U. A., et al. (2019). Toll-like receptor 9, maternal cell-free DNA and myometrial cell response to CpG oligodeoxynucleotide stimulation. *Am. J. Rerod. Immunol.* 81, 1–12. doi: 10.1111/aji.13100

Beg, A. (2002). Endogenous ligands of Toll-like receptors: implications for regulating inflammatory and immune responses. *Trends Immunol.* 23, 509–512. doi: 10.1016/s1471-4906(02)02317-7

Betheloot, D., and Latz, E. (2017). HMGB1, IL-1alpha, IL-33 and S100 proteins: dual-function alarmins. *Cell. Mol. Immunol.* 14, 43–64. doi: 10.1038/cmi.2016.34

Blasius, A. L., and Beutler, B. (2010). Intracellular toll-like receptors. *Immunity* 32, 305–315. doi: 10.1016/j.immuni.2010.03.012

Bowen, J. M., Chamley, L., Keelan, J. A., and Mitchell, M. D. (2002). Cytokines of the placenta and extra-placental membranes: roles and regulation during human pregnancy and parturition. *Placenta* 23, 257–273. doi: 10.1053/plac.2001.0782

Braga, T. T., Forni, M., Correa-Costa, M., Ramos, R. N., Barbuto, J. A., Branco, P., et al. (2017). Soluble uric acid activates the NLRP inflammasome. *Sci. Rep.* 7:39884. doi: 10.1038/srep39884

Braun, K. L., Look, M. A., Yang, H., Onaka, A. T., and Horiuchi, B. Y. (1996). Native Hawaiian mortality, 1980 and 1990. *Am. J. Public Health* 86, 888–889.

Bredeson, S., Papaconstantinou, J., Deford, J. H., Kechichian, T., Syed, T. A., Saade, G. R., et al. (2014). HMGB1 promotes a p38MAPK associated non-infectious inflammatory response pathway in human fetal membranes. *PLoS One* 9:e113799. doi: 10.1371/journal.pone.0113799

Brown, G. D. (2012). Immunology: actin' dangerously. *Nature* 485, 589–590. doi: 10.1038/485589a

Bryant, A. H., Menzies, G. E., Scott, L. M., Spencer-Harty, S., Davies, L. B., Smith, R. A., et al. (2017). Human gestation-associated tissues express functional cytosolic nucleic acid sensing pattern recognition receptors. *Clin. Exp. Immunol.* 189, 36–46. doi: 10.1111/cei.12960

Burkrinsky, M. (2014). Extracellular cyclophilins in health and disease. *Biochim. Biophys. Acta* 1850, 2087–2095. doi: 10.1016/j.bbagen.2014.11.013

Cavassani, K. A., Ishii, M., Wen, H., Schaller, M. A., Lincoln, P. M., Lukacs, N. W., et al. (2008). TLR3 is an endogenous sensor of tissue necrosis during acute inflammatory events. *J. Exp. Med.* 205, 2609–2621. doi: 10.1084/jem.20081370

CDC (2020). *Centers for Disease Control and Prevention*. Available online at: http://www.cdc.gov/omh/AMH/dbrf.htm (accessed May 7, 2020).

Chai, M., Barker, G., Menon, R., and Lappas, M. (2012). Increased oxidative stress in human fetal membranes overlying the cervix from term non-labouring and post labour deliveries. *Placenta* 33, 604–610. doi: 10.1016/j.placenta.2012.04.014

Chaturvedi, A., and Pierce, S. K. (2009). How location governs toll-like receptor signaling. *Traffic* 10, 621–628. doi: 10.1111/j.1600-0854.2009.00899.x

Chenung, K. W., Seto, M. T. Y., and Ng, E. H. Y. (2020). Early universal use of oral progesterone for prevention of preterm births in singleton pregnancy (SINPRO study): protocol of a multicenter, randomized, double-blind, placebo-controlled trial. *Trials* 21:121. doi: 10.1186/s13063-020-4067-z

Chin, P. Y., Dorian, C. L., Hutchinson, M. R., Olson, D. M., Rice, K. C., Moldenhauer, L. M., et al. (2016). Novel toll-like receptor-4 antagonist (+)-naloxone protects mice from inflammation-induced preterm birth. *Sci. Rep.* 6:36112. doi: 10.1038/srep36112

Choi, S. J., Jung, S. H., Eom, M., Han, K. H., Chung, I. B., and Kim, S. K. (2012). Immunohistochemical distribution of toll-like receptor 4 in preterm human fetal membrane. *J. Obstet. Gynaecol. Res.* 38, 108–112. doi: 10.1111/j.1447-0756.2011.01626.x

Christiaens, I., Zaragoza, D., Guilbert, L., Roberston, S. A., Micthell, B. F., and Olson, D. M. (2008). Inflammatory processes in preterm and term parturition. *J. Reprod. Immunol.* 79, 50–57. doi: 10.1016/j.jri.2008.04.002

Cockle, J., Gopichandran, N., Walker, J., Levene, M. I., and Orsi, N. M. (2007). Matrix metalloproteinases and their tissue inhibitors in preterm perinatal complications. *Reprod. Sci.* 14, 629–645. doi: 10.1177/1933719107304563

Deprest, J., Emonds, M. P., Richter, J., DeKoninck, P., Van Mieghem, T., Van Schoubroeck, D., et al. (2011). Amniopatch for iatrogenic rupture of the fetal membranes. *Prenat. Diagn.* 31, 661–666. doi: 10.1002/pd.2780

Duhig, K., Chappell, L. C., and Shennan, A. H. (2016). Oxidative stress in pregnancy and reproduction. *Obstet. Med.* 9, 113–116. doi: 10.1177/1753495X16648495

Ekman-Ordeberg, G., and Dubicke, A. (2012). Preterm Cervical Ripening in humans. *Facts Views Vis. Obgyn.* 4, 245–253.

El Khwad, M., Stetzer, B., Moore, R., Kumar, D., Mercer, B., Arikat, S., et al. (2005). Term human fetal membranes have a weak zone overlying the lower uterine pole and cervix before onset of labor. *Biol. Reprod.* 72, 720–726. doi: 10.1095/biolreprod.104.033647

Fei, D., Meng, X., Yu, W., Yang, S., Song, N., CaO, Y., et al. (2018). Fibronectin (FN) cooperated with TLR2/TLR4 receptor to promote innate immune responses of macrophages via binding to integrin β1. *Virulence* 9, 1588–1600. doi: 10.1080/21505594.2018.1528841

Flores-Espinosa, P., Pineda-Torres, M., Vega-Sanchez, R., Estrada-Gutierrez, G., Espejel-Nunez, A., Flores-Pliego, A., et al. (2014). Progesterone elicits an inhibitory effect upon LPS-induced innate immune response in pre-labor human amniotic epithelium. *J. Reprod. Immunol.* 71, 61–72. doi: 10.1111/aji.12163

Fortunado, S., Menon, R., Bryant, C., and Lombardi, S. (2000). Programmed cell death (apoptosis) as a possible pathway to metalloproteinase activation and fetal membrane degradation in premature rupture of membranes. *Am. J. Obstet. Gynecol.* 182, 1468–1476. doi: 10.1067/mob.2000.107330

Frevert, C. W., Felgenhauer, J., Wygrecka, M., Nastase, M. V., and Schaefer, L. J. (2018). Danger-associated molecular patterns derived from the extracellular matrix provide temporal control of innate immunity. *Histochem. Cytochem.* 66, 213–227. doi: 10.1369/0022155417740880

Frey, H., Schroeder, N., Manon-Jensen, T., Iozzo, R. V., and Schaefer, L. (2013). Biological interplay between proteoglycans and their innate immune receptors in inflammation. *FEBS J.* 280, 2165–2179. doi: 10.1111/febs.12145

Fulda, S., Gorman, A. M., Hori, O., and Samali, A. (2010). Cellular stress responses: cell survival and cell death. *Int. J. Cell Biol.* 2010:214074. doi: 10.1155/2010/214074

Gaudet, A. D., and Popovich, P. G. (2014). Extracellular matrix regulation of inflammation in the healthy and injured spinal cord. *Exp. Neurol.* 258, 24–34. doi: 10.1016/j.expneurol.2013.11.020

Genbacev, O., Vicovac, L., and Larcoque, N. (2015). The role of chorionic cytotrophoblasts in the smooth chorion fusion with parietal decidua. *Placenta* 36, 716–722. doi: 10.1016/j.placenta.2015.05.002

Ghavami, S., Eshragi, M., Ande, S. R., Chazin, W. J., Klonisch, T., Halayko, A. J., et al. (2010). S100A8/A9 induces autophagy and apoptosis via ROS-mediated cross-talk between mitochondria and lysosomes that involves BNIP3. *Cell Res.* 20, 314–331. doi: 10.1038/cr.2009.129

Gillaux, C., Mehats, C., Vaiman, D., Cabrol, D., and Breuiller-Fouche, M. (2011). Functional screening of TLRs in human amniotic epithelial cells. *J. Immunol.* 187, 2766–2774. doi: 10.4049/jimmunol.1100217

Goldenberg, R. L., Culhane, J. F., Iams, J. D., and Romero, R. (2008). Epidemiology and causes of preterm birth. *Lancet* 371, 75–84. doi: 10.1016/S0140-6736(08)60074-4

Gomez-Lopez, N., Romero, R., Panaitescu, B., Leng, Y., Xu, Y., Tarca, A. L., et al. (2018). Inflammasome activation during spontaneous preterm labor with intra-amniotic infection or sterile intra-amniotic inflammation. *Am. J. Reprod. Immunol.* 80:e13049. doi: 10.1111/aji.13049

Gomez-Lopez, N., Romero, R., Plazyo, O., Panaitescu, B., Furcron, A. E., Miller, D., et al. (2016). Intra-amniotic administration of HMGB1 induces spontaneous Preterm Labor and Birth. *Am. J. Reprod. Immunol.* 75, 3–7. doi: 10.1111/aji.12443

Gravett, M., Adams, K., Sadowsky, D., Grosvenor, A. R., Witkin, S. S., Axthelm, M. K., et al. (2007). Immunomodulator plus antibiotics delay preterm delivery after experimental intraamniotic infection in a nonhuman primate model. *Am. J. Obstet. Gynecol.* 197, 518.e1–518.e8. doi: 10.1016/j.ajog.2007.03.064

Hadley, E. E., Sheller-Miller, S., Saade, G., Salomon, C., Mesiano, S., Taylor, R. N., et al. (2018). Amnion epithelial cell-derived exosomes induce inflammatory changes in uterine cells. *Am. J. Obstet. Gynecol.* 219, 478.e1–478.e21. doi: 10.1016/j.ajog.2018.08.021

Haruta, M., Kishore, A. H., Shi, H., Keller, P. W., Akgul, Y., and Word, R. A. (2013). Fetal fibronectin signaling induces matrix metalloproteases and cyclooxygenase-2 (COX-2) in amnion cells and preterm birth in mice. *J. Biol. Chem.* 288, 1953–1966. doi: 10.1074/jbc.M112.424366

Hasegawa-Nakamura, K., Tateishi, F., Nakamura, T., Nakajima, Y., Kawamata, K., Douchi, T., et al. (2011). The possible mechanism of preterm birth associated with peridontopathic porphyromonas gingivalis. *J. Periodontal Res.* 46, 497–504. doi: 10.1111/j.1600-0765.2011.01366.x

Hayashi, F., Smith, K. D., Ozinsky, A., Hawn, T. R., Yi, E. C., Goodlett, D. R., et al. (2001). The innate immune response to bacterial flagellin is mediated by Toll-like receptor 5. *Nature* 410, 1099–1103. doi: 10.1038/35074106

Hemmi, H., Takeuchi, O., Kawai, T., Kaisho, T., Sato, S., Sanjo, H., et al. (2000). A Toll-like receptor recognizes bacterial DNA. *Nature* 408, 740–745. doi: 10.1038/35047123

Hirai, A. H., Hayes, D. K., Taualii, M. M., Singh, G. K., and Fuddy, L. J. (2013). Excess infant mortality among native hawaiians: identifying determinants for preventative action. *Am J Public Health.* 103, e88–e95. doi: 10.2105/AJPH.2013.301294

Hoang, M., Potter, J. A., Gysler, S. M., Han, C. S., Guller, S., Norwitz, E. R., et al. (2014). Human fetal membranes generate distinct cytokine profiles in response to bacterial toll-like receptor and nod-like receptor agonists. *Biol. Reprod.* 90:39. doi: 10.1095/biolreprod.113.115428

Hsu, C., Meaddough, E., Bacherra, H., Harirah, H., and Lu, L. (2000). Increased apoptosis in human amnion is associated with labor at term. *Am. J. Reprod. Immunol.* 43, 255–258. doi: 10.1111/j.8755-8920-2000.430502.x

Huang, H., Evanovich, J., Yan, W., Nace, G., Zhang, L., Ross, M., et al. (2011). Endogenous histones function as alarmins in sterile inflammatory liver injury, through Toll-like receptor 9 in mice. *Hepatology* 54, 999–1008. doi: 10.1002/hep.24501

Hug, H., Mohajeri, M. H., and La Fata, G. (2018). Toll-like receptors: regulation of the immune response in the human gut. *Nutrients* 10:203. doi: 10.3390/nu10020203

Isnadi, M. F. A. R., Chin, V. K., Majid, R. A., Lee, T. Y., Abdullah, M. A., Omenesa, R. B., et al. (2018). Critical Roles of IL-33/ST2 Pathway in Neurological Disorders. *Mediators Inflamm.* 2018:5346413. doi: 10.1155/2018/5346413

Jaiswal, M. K., Agrawal, V., Mallers, T., Gilman-Sachs, A., Hirsch, E., and Beaman, K. D. (2013). Regulation of apoptosis and innate immune stimuli in inflammation-induced preterm labor. *J. Immunol.* 191, 5702–5713. doi: 10.4049/jimmunol.1301604

Joyce, E. M., Diaz, P., Tamarkin, S., Moore, R., Strohl, A., Stetzer, B., et al. (2016). In-vivo stretch of term human fetal membranes. *Placenta* 38, 57–66. doi: 10.1016/j.placenta.2015.12.011

Kaga, N., Katsuki, Y., Obata, M., and Shibutani, Y. (1996). Repeated administration of low-dose lipopolysaccharide induces preterm delivery in mice: a model for human preterm parturition and for assessment of the therapeutic ability of drugs against preterm delivery. *Am. J. Obstet. Gynecol.* 174, 754–759. doi: 10.1016/s0002-9378(96)70460-x

Karikó, K., Ni, H., Capodici, J., Lamphier, M., and Weissman, D. (2004). mRNA is an endogenous ligand for toll-like receptor 3. *J. Biol. Chem.* 279, 12542–12550. doi: 10.1074/jbc.M310175200

Katsura, M., Ito, A., Hirakawa, S., and Mori, Y. (1989). Human recombinant interleukin-1alpha increases biosynthesis of collagenase and hyaluronic acid in cultured human chorionic cells. *FEBS Lett.* 224, 315–318. doi: 10.1016/0014-5793(89)80553-8

Kawai, C., Kotani, H., Miyao, M., Ishida, T., Jemail, L., Abiru, H., et al. (2016). Circulating extracellular histones are clinically Relevant mediators of multiple organ injury. *Am. J. Pathol.* 186, 829–843. doi: 10.1016/j.ajpath.2015.11.025

Kawai, T., and Akira, S. (2010). The role of pattern-recognition receptors in innate immunity: update on Toll-like receptors. *Nat. Immunol.* 11, 373–384. doi: 10.1038/ni.1863

Keelan, J. A., Marvin, K. W., Sato, T. A., Coleman, M., McCowan, L. M., and Mitchell, M. D. (1999). Cytokine abundance in placental tissues: evidence of inflammatory activation in gestational membranes with term and preterm parturition. *Am. J. Obstet. Gynecol.* 181, 1530–1536. doi: 10.1016/s0002-9378(99)70400-x

Keith, L. G., and Oleszczuk, J. J. (2002). Triplet births in the United States. An epidemic of high-risk pregnancies. *J. Reprod. Med.* 47, 259–265.

Kendal-Wright, C. E. (2007). Stretching, mechanotransduction and proinflammatory cytokines in the fetal membranes. *Reprod. Sci.* 14, 35–41. doi: 10.1177/1933719107310763

Kendal-Wright, C. E., Hubbard, D., and Bryant-Greenwood, G. D. (2008). Chronic stretching of amniotic epithelial cells increases pre-B cell colony-enhancing factor (PBEF/Visfatin) expression and protects them from apoptosis. *Placenta* 29, 255–265. doi: 10.1016/j.placenta.2007.12.008

Kendal-Wright, C. E., Hubbard, D., Gowin-Brown, J., and Bryant-Greenwood, G. D. (2010). Stretch and inflammation-induced Pre-B cell colony-enhancing factor (PBEF/Visfatin) and Interleukin-8 in amniotic epithelial cells. *Placenta* 3, 665–674. doi: 10.1016/j.placenta.2010.06.007

Koga, K., Cardenas, I., Aldo, P., Abrahams, V. M., Peng, B., Fill, S., et al. (2009). Activation of TLR3 in the trophoblast is associated with preterm delivery. *Am. J. Reprod. Immunol.* 61, 196–212. doi: 10.1111/j.1600-0897.2008.00682.x

Kumagai, K., Otsuki, Y., Ito, Y., Shibata, M. A., Abe, H., and Ueki, M. (2001). Apoptosis in the normal human amnion at term, independent of Bcl-2 regulation and onset of labour. *Mol. Hum. Reprod.* 7, 681–689. doi: 10.1093/molehr/7.7.681

Kumar, D., Fung, W., Moore, R., Pandey, V., Fox, J., Stetzer, B., et al. (2006). Proinflammatory cytokines found in amniotic fluid induce collagen remodeling, apoptosis and biophysical weakening of cultured human fetal membranes. *Biol. Reprod.* 74, 29–34.

Kumar, H., Kawai, T., and Akira, S. (2009). Pathogen recognition in the innate immune response. *Biochem. J.* 420, 1–16. doi: 10.1042/BJ20090272

Lappas, M., Odumetse, T., Riley, C., Reti, N. G., Holdsworth-Carson, S. J., Rice, G. E., et al. (2008). Pre-labor fetal membranes overlying the cervix display alterations in inflammation and NF-kappaB signaling pathways. *Placenta* 29, 995–1002. doi: 10.1016/j.placenta.2008.09.010

Leppert, P. C., Takamoto, N., and Yu, S. Y. (1996). Apoptosis in fetal membranes may predispose them to rupture. *J. Soc. Gynecol. Invest.* 3:128A.

Li, L., Yang, J., Jiang, Y., Tu, J., and Schust, D. J. (2015). Activation of decidual invariant natural killer T cells promotes lipopolysaccharide-induced preterm birth. *Mol. Hum. Reprod.* 21, 369–381. doi: 10.1093/molehr/gav001

Lim, R., Barker, G., and Lappas, M. (2018). Pellino 1 is a novel regulator of TNF and TLR signaling in human myometrial and amnion cells. *J. Reprod. Immunol.* 127, 24–35. doi: 10.1016/j.jri.2018.04.003

Lim, R., and Lappas, M. (2015). A novel role for GSK3 in the regulation of the processes of human labour. *Reproduction* 149, 189–202. doi: 10.1530/REP-14-0493

Lim, R., and Lappas, M. (2019). Expression and function of macrophage-inducible c-type lectin (mincle) in inflammation driven parturition in fetal membranes and myometrium. *Clin. Exp. Immunol.* 197, 95–110. doi: 10.1111/cei.13281

Lim, R., Tran, H. T., Liong, S., Barker, G., and Lappas, M. (2016). The transcription factor interferon regulatory factor-1 (IRF1) plays a key role in the terminal effector pathways of human preterm labor. *Biol. Reprod.* 94:32. doi: 10.1095/biolreprod.115.134726

Liong, S., and Lappas, M. (2014). Endoplasmic reticulum stress is increased after spontaneous labor in human fetal membranes and myometrium where it regulates the expression of prolabor mediators. *Biol. Reprod.* 91:70. doi: 10.1095/biolreprod.114.120741

Liu, H., Redline, R. W., and Han, Y. W. (2007). Fusobacterium nucleatum induces fetal death in mice via stimulation of TLR4-mediated placental inflammatory response. *J. Immunol.* 179, 2501–2508. doi: 10.4049/jimmunol.179.4.2501

Lund, J. M., Alexopoulou, L., Sato, A., Karow, M., Adams, N. C., Gale, N. W., et al. (2004). Recognition of single-stranded RNA viruses by Toll-like receptor 7. *Proc. Natl. Acad. Sci. U.S.A.* 101, 5598–5603. doi: 10.1073/pnas.0400937101

Magna, M., and Pisetsky, D. S. (2016). The alarmin properties of DNA and DNA-associated nuclear proteins. *Clin. Ther.* 38, 1029–1041. doi: 10.1016/j.clinthera.2016.02.029

Malak, T. M., and Bell, S. C. (1994). Structural characteristics of term human fetal membranes: a novel zone of extreme morphological alteration within the rupture site. *Br. J. Obstet. Gynecol.* 101, 375–386. doi: 10.1111/j.1471-0528.1994.tb11908.x

Manabe, Y., Yoshimura, S., Mori, T., and Aso, T. (1985). Plasma levels of 13,14-dihydro-15-keto prostaglandin F2 alpha, estrogens, and progesterone during stretch-induced labor at term. *Prostaglandins* 30, 141–152.

Maneta, E., Warren, A. Y., Hay, D. P., and Khan, R. N. (2015). Caspase-1-mediated cytokine release from gestational tissues, placental and cord blood. *Front. Physiol.* 6:186. doi: 10.3389/fphys.2015.00186

Manuck, T. A. (2017). Racial and ethnic differences in preterm birth. *Semin. Perinatol.* 41, 511–518. doi: 10.1053/j.semperi.2017.08.010

McParland, P., Taylor, D., and Bell, S. (2003). Mapping of zoned of altered morphology and chorionic connective tissue phenotype in human fetal membranes (amniochorion and decidua) overlying the lower uterine pole and cervix before labor at term. *Am. J. Obstet. Gynecol.* 189, 1481–1488.

Meinert, M., Eriksen, G. V., Peterson, A. C., Helmig, R. B., Laurent, C., Uldbjerg, N., et al. (2001). Proteoglycans and hyaluronan in fetal membranes. *Am. J. Obstet. Gynecol.* 184, 679–685. doi: 10.1067/mob.2001.110294

Meinert, M., Malmstrom, A., Tufvesson, E., Westergren-Thorsson, G., Peterson, A. C., Laurent, C., et al. (2007). Labour induces increased concentrations of biglycan and hyaluronan in human fetal membranes. *Placenta* 28, 482–486. doi: 10.1016/j.placenta.2006.09.006

Menon, R. (2019). Initiation of human parturition: signaling from senescent fetal tissues via extracellular vesicle mediated paracrine mechanism. *Obstet. Gynecol. Sci.* 62, 199–211. doi: 10.5468/ogs.2019.62.4.199

Menon, R., Bonney, E. A., Condon, J., Messiano, S., and Taylor, R. N. (2016a). Novel concepts on pregnancy clocks and alarms: redundancy and synergy in human parturition. *Hum. Reprod. Update* 22, 535–560. doi: 10.1093/humupd/dmw022

Menon, R., Behnia, F., Polettini, J., Saade, G. R., Campisi, J., and Velarde, M. (2016b). Placental membrane aging and HMGB1 signaling associated with human parturition. *Aging* 8, 216–230. doi: 10.18632/aging.100891

Menon, R., Fortunato, S. J., Yu, J., Milne, G. L., Sanchez, S., Drobek, C. O., et al. (2011). Cigarette smoke induced oxidative stress and apoptosis in normal term fetal membranes. *Placenta* 32, 317–322. doi: 10.1016/j.placenta.2011.01.015

Menon, R., Mesiano, S., and Taylor, R. N. (2017). Programmed fetal membrane senescend and exosome-mediated signaling: a mechanism associated with timing of human parturition. *Front. Endocrinol.* 8:196. doi: 10.3389/fendo.2017.00196

Menon, R., and Richardson, L. S. (2017). Preterm prelabor rupture of the membranes: a disease of the fetal membranes. *Semin. Perinatol.* 41, 409–419. doi: 10.1053/j.semperi.2017.07.012

Merline, R., Moreth, K., Beckmann, J., Nastase, M. V., Zeng-Brouwers, J., Tralhao, J. G., et al. (2011). Signaling by the matrix proteoglycan decorin controls inflammation and cancer through PDCD4 and microRNA-21. *Sci. Signal.* 4:ra75. doi: 10.1126/scisignal.2001868

Meylan, E., and Tschopp, J. (2005). The RIP kinases: crucial integrators of cellular stress. *Trends Biochem. Sci.* 30, 151–159. doi: 10.1016/j.tibs.2005.01.003

Mi, Y., Wang, W., Zhang, W., Liu, C., Jiangwen, L., Li, W., et al. (2017). Autophagic degradation of Collagen 1A1 by Cortisol in Human Amnion Fibroblasts. *Endocrinology* 158, 1005–1014.

Midwood, K., Sacre, S., Piccinini, A. M., Inglis, J., Trebaul, A., Chan, E., et al. (2009). Tenascin-C is an endogenous activator of toll-like receptor 4 that is essential for maintaining inflammation in arthritic joint disease. *Nat. Med.* 15, 774–780. doi: 10.1038/nm

Millar, L. K., Stollberg, J., DeBuque, L., and Bryant-Greenwood, G. (2000). Fetal membrane distension: determination of the intrauterine surface area and distention of the fetal membranes preterm and at term. *Am. J. Obstet. Gynecol.* 182, 128–134. doi: 10.1016/s0002-9378(00)70501-1

Miyake, K. (2007). Innate immune sensing of pathogens and danger signals by cell surface Toll-like receptors. *Semin. Immunol.* 19, 3–10. doi: 10.1016/j.smim.2006.12.002

Moco, N. P., Martin, L. F., Pereira, A. C., Polettini, J., Peracoli, J. C., Coelho, K. I., et al. (2013). Gene expression and protein localization of TLR-1, -2, -4, and -6 in amniochorion membranes of pregnancies complicated by histological chorioamnionitis. *Eur. J. Obstet. Gynecol. Reprod. Biol.* 171, 12–17. doi: 10.1016/j.ejogrb.2013.07.036

Mogami, H., Hari Kishore, A., Akgul, Y., and Word, R. A. (2017). Healing of preterm ruptured fetal membranes. *Sci. Rep.* 7:13139. doi: 10.1038/s41598-017-13296-1

Motedayyen, H., Fathi, F., Fasihi-Ramandi, M., Sabzghabaee, A. M., and Taheri, R. A. (2019). Toll-like receptor 4 activation on human amniotic epithelial cells is a risk factor for pregnancy loss. *J. Res. Med. Sci.* 24:1. doi: 10.4103/jrms.JRMS_463_18

Nadeau-Vallee, M., Obari, D., Palacois, J., Brien, M. E., Duval, C., Chemtob, S., et al. (2016). Sterile Inflammation and pregnancy complications: a review. *Reproduction* 152, R277–R292. doi: 10.1530/REP-16-0453

Nadeem, L., Shynlova, O., Matysiak-Zablocki, E., Mesiano, S., Dong, X., and Lye, S. (2016). Molecular evidence of functional progesterone withdrawal in human myometrium. *Nat. Commun.* 7:11565. doi: 10.1038/ncomms11565

Nemeth, E., Millar, L. K., and Bryant-Greenwood, G. (2000). Fetal membrane distention: II. Differentially expressed genes regulated by acute distention in vitro. *Am. J. Obstet. Gynecol.* 182, 60–67. doi: 10.1016/s0002-9378(00)70491-1

Nie, Y., Yang, D., and Oppenhiem, J. J. (2016). Alarmins and antitumor immunity. *Clin. Ther.* 38, 1042–1053. doi: 10.1016/j.clinthera.2016.03.021

Nizyaeva, N. V., Kulikova, G. V., Nagovitsyna, M. N., and Shchegolev, A. I. (2019). Peculiarities of the expression of TLR4 and inhibitor of TLR-cascade tollip in the placenta in earlyand late-onset Preeclampsia. *Bull. Exp. Biol. Med.* 166, 507–511. doi: 10.1007/s10517-019-04383-6

Noll, F., Behnke, J., Leiting, S., Trodi, K., Alves, G. T., Muller-Redetzky, H., et al. (2017). Self-extracellular RNA acts in synergy with exogenous danger signals to promote inflammation. *PLoS One* 12:e0190002. doi: 10.1371/journal.pone.0190002

Norman Ing, N., Baker, H., Ignacio, V., Song, C. and Kendal-Wright, C. E. (2019). "Stretch increases high-mobility group box 1 (HMGB1) secretion from human epithelial cells," in *Proceedings of the 66th Annual Society for Reproductive Investigation Meeting* (Paris: Reproductive Biology F019).

Oosting, M., Cheng, S.-C., Bolscher, J. M., Vestering-Stenger, R., Plantinga, T. S., Verschueren, I. C., et al. (2014). Human TLR10 is an anti-inflammatory pattern-recognition receptor. *Proc. Natl. Acad. Sci. U.S.A.* 111, E4478–E4484. doi: 10.1073/pnas.1410293111

Osman, I., Young, A., Jordon, F., Greer, I. A., and Norman, J. E. (2006). Leukocyte density and proinflammatory mediator expression in regional human fetal membranes and decidua before and during labor at term. *J. Soc. Gynecol. Investig.* 13, 97–103. doi: 10.1016/j.jsgi.2005.12.002

Park, C. B., Braun, K. L., Horiuchi, B. Y., Tottori, C., and Onaka, A. T. (2009). Longevity disparities in multiethnic Hawaii: an analysis of 2000 life tables. *Public Health Rep.* 124, 579–584. doi: 10.1177/003335490912400415

Parry, S., and Strauss, J. F. (1988). Premature rupture of the fetal membranes. *N. Engl. J. Med.* 338, 663–670. doi: 10.1056/NEJM199803053381006

Patel, B., Peters, G. A., Skomorovska-Prokvolit, Y., Yi, L., Tan, H., Yousef, A., et al. (2018). Control of progesterone receptor-A transrepressive activity in myometrial cells: implications for the control of human parturition. *Reprod. Sci.* 25, 214–221. doi: 10.1177/1933719117716775

Patkin, E. C., Orr, S. J., and Schaible, U. E. (2017). Macrophage inducible C-type Lectin as a multifunctional player in immunity. *Front. Immunol.* 8:861. doi: 10.3389/fimmu.2017.00861

Paulesu, L., Bhattacharjee, J., Bechi, N., Romagnoli, R., Jantra, S., and Ietta, F. (2010). Pro-inflammatory cytokiens in animal and human gestation. *Curr. Pharm. Des.* 16, 3601–3615. doi: 10.2174/138161210793797933

Perales-Linares, R., and Navas-Martin, S. (2013). Toll-like receptor 3 in viral pathogenesis: Friend or foe? *Immunology* 140, 153–167. doi: 10.1111/imm.12143

Petes, C., Odoardi, N., and Gee, K. (2017). The toll for trafficking: toll-like receptor 7 delivery to the endosome. *Front. Immunol.* 8:1075. doi: 10.3389/fimmu.2017.01075

Phillippe, M. (2014). Cell-free fetal DNA—a trigger for parturition. *N. Engl. J. Med.* 370, 2534–2536. doi: 10.1056/NEJMcibr1404324

Pirianov, G., Waddington, S. N., Lindstrom, T. M., Terzidou, V., Mehmet, H., and Bennett, P. R. (2009). The cyclopentenone 15-deoxy-delta 12,14-prostaglandin J(2) delays lipopolysaccharide-induced preterm delivery and reduces mortality in the newborn mouse. *Endocrinology* 150, 699–706. doi: 10.1210/en.2008-1178

Plazyo, O., Romero, R., Unkel, R., Balancio, A., Mial, T. N., Xu, Y., et al. (2016). HMGB1 induces an inflammatory response in the chorioamniotic membranes that is partially mediated by the inflammasome. *Biol. Reprod.* 95, 1–14. doi: 10.1095/biolreprod.116.144139

Poltorak, A. (1998). Defective LPS signaling in C3H/HeJ and C57BL/10ScCr mice: mutations in Tlr4 gene. *Science* 282, 2085–2088. doi: 10.1126/science.282.5396.2085

Poženel, L., ALindenmair, A., Schmidt, K., Kozlov, A. V., Grillari, J., Wolbank, S., et al. (2019). Critical impact of human amniotic membrane tension on mitochondrial function and cell viability in vitro. *Cells* 2019:1641. doi: 10.3390/cells8121641

Qin, S., Wang, H., Yuan, R., Li, H., Ochani, M., Ochani, K., et al. (2006). Role of HMGB1 in apoptosis-mediated sepsis lethality. *J. Exp. Med.* 203, 1637–1642. doi: 10.1084/jem.20052203

Qiu, X. Y., Sun, L., Han, X. L., Chang, Y., Cheng, L., and Yin, L. R. (2017). Alarmin high mobility group box-1 in maternal serum as a potential biomarker of chorioamnionitis-associated preterm birth. *Gynecol. Endocrinol.* 33, 128–131. doi: 10.1080/09513590.2016.1214260

Regan, J. K., Kannan, P. S., Kemp, M. W., Kramer, B. W., Newnham, J. P., Jobe, A. H., et al. (2016). Damage-associated molecular pattern and fetal membrane vascular injury and collagen disorganization in lipopolysaccharide-induced intra-amniotic inflammation in fetal sheep. *Reprod. Sci.* 23, 69–80. doi: 10.1177/1933719115594014

Relja, B., Mors, K., and Marzi, I. (2018). Danger signals in Trauma. *Eur. J. Trauma Emerg. Surg.* 44, 301–316. doi: 10.1007/s00068-018-0962-3

Reti, N., Lappas, M., Riley, C., Wlodek, M. E., Permezel, M., Walker, S., et al. (2007). Why do membranes rupture at term? Evidence of increased cellular apoptosis in the supracervical fetal membranes. *Am. J. Obstet. Gynecol.* 196, 484.e1–484.e10. doi: 10.1016/j.ajog.2007.01.021 484e1-10,

Richardson, L. S., Taylor, R. N., and Menon, R. (2020). Reversible EMT and MET mediate amnion remodeling during pregnancy and labor. *Sci. Signal.* 13:618. doi: 10.1126/scisignal.aay1486

Roedig, H., Nastase, M. V., Wygrecka, M., and Schaefer, L. (2019). Breaking down chronic inflammatory diseases: the role of biglycan in promoting a switch between inflammation and autophagy. *FEBS J.* 286, 2965–2979. doi: 10.1111/febs.14791

Roh, J. S., and Sohn, D. H. (2018). Damage-Associated molecular patterns in inflammatory disease. *Immune Netw.* 18:e27. doi: 10.4110/in.2018.18.e27

Romero, R., Chaiworapongsa, T., Alpay Savasan, Z. A., Xu, Y., Hussein, Y., Dong, Z., et al. (2011). Damage-associated molecular patterns (DAMPs) in preterm labor with intact membranes and preterm PROM: a study of the alarmin HMGB1. *J. Matern. Fetal Neonatal Med.* 24, 1444–1455. doi: 10.3109/14767058.2011.591460

Romero, R., Espinoza, J., Gonçalves, L. F., Kusanovic, J. P., Friel, L., and Hassan, S. (2007). The role of inflammation and infection in preterm birth. *Semin. Reprod. Med.* 25, 21–39. doi: 10.1055/s-2006-956773

Sato, B. L., Collier, E. S., Vermudez, S. A., Junker, A. D., and Kendal-Wright, C. E. (2016). Human amnion mesenchymal cells are pro-inflammatory when activated by the toll-like recetor 2/6 ligand, macrophage-activating lipoprotein-2. *Placenta* 44, 69–79. doi: 10.1016/j.placenta.2016.06.005

Schaaf, J. M., Liem, S. M. S., Mol, B. W. J., Abu-Hanna, A., and Ravelli, A. C. J. (2013). Ethnic and racial disparities in the risk of preterm birth: a systematic review and meta-analysis. *Am. J. Perinatol.* 30, 433–450.

Schaefer, L. (2014). Complexity of danger: the diverse nature of damage-associated molecular patterns. *J. Biol. Chem.* 289, 35237–35245. doi: 10.1074/jbc.R114.619304

Scharfe-Nugent, A., Corr, S. C., Carpenter, S. B., Keogh, L., Doyle, B., Martin, C., et al. (2012). TLR9 provokes inflammation in response to fetal DNA: mechanism for fetal loss in preterm birth and preeclampsia. *J. Immunol.* 188, 5706–5712. doi: 10.4049/jimmunol.1103454

Scheibner, K. A., Lutz, M. A., Boodoo, S., Fenton, M. J., Powell, J. D., and Horton, M. R. (2006). Hyaluronan fragments act as an endogenous danger signal by engaging TLR2. *J. Immunol.* 177, 1272–1281. doi: 10.4049/jimmunol.177.2.1272

Sheller-Miller, S., Urrabaz-Garza, R., Saade, G., and Menon, R. (2017). Damage-associated molecular pattern markers HMGB1 and cell-free fetal telomere fragments in oxidative-stressed amnion epithelial cell-derived exosomes. *J. Reprod. Immunol.* 123, 3–11. doi: 10.1016/j.jri.2017.08.003

Shen, Z., Li, E., Lu, S., Shen, J., Cai, Y. M., Wu, Y. E., et al. (2008). Autophagic and apoptotic cell death in amniotic epithelial cells. *Placenta* 29, 956–961. doi: 10.1016/j.placenta.2008.09.001

Shim, S., Romero, R., Hong, J., Park, C. W., Jun, J. K., Kim, B. I., et al. (2004). Clinical significance of intra-amniotic inflammation in patients with preterm premature rupture of membranes. *Am. J. Obstet. Gynecol.* 191, 1339–1345. doi: 10.1016/j.ajog.2004.06.085

Shynlova, O., Tsui, P., Jaffer, S., and Lye, S. (2009). Integration of endocrine and mechanical signals in the regulation of myometrial functions during pregnancy and labour. *Eur. J. Obstet. Gynecol. Reprod. Biol.* 144, S2–S10. doi: 10.1016/j.ejogrb.2009.02.044

Smith, M. L., Gourdon, D., Little, W. C., Kubow, K. E., Eguiluz, R. A., Luna-Morris, S., et al. (2007). Force-induced unfolding of fibronectin in the extracellular matrix of living cells. *PLoS Biol.* 5:e268. doi: 10.1371/journal.pbio.0050268

So, T., Ito, A., Sato, T., Mori, Y., and Hirakawa, S. (1992). Tumor necrosis factor alpha stimulates the biosynthesis of matrix metalloproteinases and plasmogen activator in cultured human chorionic cells. *Biol. Reprod.* 46, 772–778. doi: 10.1095/biolreprod46.5.772

Son, G. H., Kim, Y., Lee, J. J., Ham, H., Song, J. E., Park, S. T., et al. (2019). MicroRNA-548 regulates high mobility group box-1 expression in patients with preterm birth and chorioamnionitis. *Sci. Rep.* 9:19746. doi: 10.1038/s41598-019-56327-9

Stevens, A. L., Wheeler, C. A., Tannenbaum, S. R., and Grodzinsky, A. J. (2008). Nitric oxide enhances aggrecan degradation by aggrecanase in response to TNF-α but not IL-1β treatment at a post-transcriptional level in bovine cartilage explants. *Osteoarthritis Cartilage* 16, 489–497. doi: 10.1016/j.joca.2007.07.015

Strauss, J. F. III (2013). Extracellular matrix dynamics and fetal membrane rupture. *Reprod. Sci.* 20, 140–153. doi: 10.1177/1933719111424454

Strauss, J. F. III, Romero, R., Gomez-Lopez, N., Haymond-Thornburg, H., Modi, B. P., Teves, M. E., et al. (2018). Spontaneous preterm birth: advances toward the discovery of genetic predisposition. *Am. J. Obstet. Gynecol.* 218, 294–314.e2. doi: 10.1016/j.ajog.2017.12.009

Taheri, R. A., Motedayyen, H., Ghotloo, S., Masjedi, M., Mosaffa, N., Mirshafiey, A., et al. (2018). The effect of lipopolysaccharide on the expression level of immunomodulatory and immunostimulatory factors of human amniotic epithelial cells. *BMC Res. Notes* 11:343. doi: 10.1186/s13104-018-3411-9

Takeda, K. (2004). Toll-like receptors in innate immunity. *Int. Immunol.* 17, 1–14. doi: 10.1093/intimm/dxh186

Takeda, K., Kaisho, T., and Akira, S. (2003). Toll-like receptors. *Annu. Rev. Immunol.* 21, 335–376. doi: 10.1146/annurev.immunol.21.120601.141126

Takeuchi, O., and Akira, S. (2010). Pattern recognition receptors and inflammation. *Cell* 140, 805–820. doi: 10.1016/j.cell.2010.01.022

Takeuchi, O., Hoshino, K., Kawai, T., Sanjo, H., Takada, H., Ogawa, T., et al. (1999). Differential roles of TLR2 and TLR4 in recognition of gram-negative and gram-positive bacterial cell wall components. *Immunity* 11, 443–451. doi: 10.1016/s1074-7613(00)80119-3

Takeuchi, O., Kawai, T., Mühlradt, P. F., Morr, M., Radolf, J. D., Zychlinsky, A., et al. (2001). Discrimination of bacterial lipoproteins by Toll-like receptor 6. *Int. Immunol.* 13, 933–940. doi: 10.1093/intimm/13.7.933

Takeuchi, O., Sato, S., Horiuchi, T., Hoshino, K., Takeda, K., Dong, Z., et al. (2002). Cutting edge: role of toll-like receptor 1 in mediating immune response to microbial lipoproteins. *J. Immunol.* 169, 10–14. doi: 10.4049/jimmunol.169.1.10

Tateishi, F., Hasegawa-Nakamura, K., Nakamura, T., Oogai, Y., Komatsuzawa, H., Kawamata, K., et al. (2012). Detection of *fusobacterium nucleatum* in chorionic tissues of high-risk pregnant women. *J. Clin. Periodontal.* 39, 417–424. doi: 10.1111/j.1600-051X.2012.01855.x

Than, G. N., Romero, R., Tarca, A. L., Draghici, T. S., Erez, O., and Chaiworapongsa, T. (2009). Mitochondrial manganese superoxide dismutase mRNA expression in human chorioamniotic membranes and its association with labor, inflammation and infection. *J. Matern. Fetal Neonatal Med.* 22, 1000–1013. doi: 10.3109/14767050903019676

Thaxton, J. E., Nevers, T. A., and Sharma, S. (2010). TLR-mediated preterm birth in response to pathogenic agents. *Infect. Dis. Obstet. Gynecol.* 2010:378472. doi: 10.1155/2010/378472

Thompson, M. R., Kaminski, J. J., Kurt-Jones, E. A., and Fitzgerald, K. A. (2011). Pattern recognition receptors and the innate immune response to viral infection. *Viruses* 3, 920–940. doi: 10.3390/v3060920

Tolle, L. B., and Standiford, T. J. (2013). Danger-associated molecular patterns (DAMPs) in acute lung injury. *J. Pathol.* 229, 145–156. doi: 10.1002/path.4124

Tsark, J., and Braun, K. L. J. (2009). Eyes on the Pacific: cancer Issues of Native Hawaiians and Pacific Islanders in Hawai'i and the US-Associated Pacific. *J. Cancer Educ.* 24, S68–S69. doi: 10.1080/08858190903404619

Venereau, E., Ceriotti, C., and Bianchi, M. E. (2015). DAMPs from cell death to new life. *Front. Immunol.* 18:422. doi: 10.3389/fimmu.2015.00422

Waldorf, A. K. M., Persing, D., Novy, M. J., Sadowsky, D. W., and Gravett, M. G. (2008). Pretreatment with toll-like receptor 4 antagonist inhibits lipopolysaccharide-induced preterm uterine contractility, cytokines, and prostaglandins in rhesus monkeys. *Reprod. Sci.* 15, 121–127. doi: 10.1177/1933719107310992

Waldorf, A. K. M., Singh, N., Mohan, A. R., Young, R. C., Ngo, L., Das, A., et al. (2015). Uterine overdistention induces preterm labor mediated by inflammation: observations in pregnant women and nonhuman primates. *Am. J. Obstet. Gynecol.* 213, 830.e1–830.e19. doi: 10.1016/j.ajog.2015.08.028

Wallin, R. P. A., Lundqvist, A., Moré, S. H., von Bonin, A., Kiessling, R., and Ljunggren, H.-G. (2002). Heat-shock proteins as activators of the innate immune system. *Trends Immunol.* 23, 130–135. doi: 10.1016/s1471-4906(01)02168-8

Wang, H., and Hirsch, E. (2003). Bacterially-induced preterm labor and regulation of prostaglandin-metabolizing enzyme expression in mice: the role of toll-like receptor 4. *Biol. Reprod.* 69, 1957–1963. doi: 10.1095/biolreprod.103.019620

Wang, S., Cao, C., Piao, H., Li, Y., Tao, Y., Zhang, X., et al. (2015). Tim-3 protects decidual stromal cells from toll-like receptorr-mediated apoptosis and inflammatory reactions and promotes Th2 bias at the maternal-fetal interface. *Sci. Rep.* 5:9013. doi: 10.1038/srep09013

Wang, Y. W., Wang, W. S., Wang, L. Y., Bao, Y. R., Lu, J. W., Lu, Y., et al. (2019). Extracellular matrix remodeling effects of serum amyloid A1 in the amnion: implications for fetal membrane rupture. *Am. J. Reprod. Immunol.* 81:e13073. doi: 10.1111/aji.13073

Waring, G. J., Robson, S. C., Bulmer, J. N., and Tyson-Capper, A. J. (2015). Inflammatory signaling in fetal membranes: increased expression levels of TLR1 in the presence of preterm histological chorioamnionitis. *PLoS One* 10:e0124298. doi: 10.1371/journal.pone.0124298

West, A. P., Koblansky, A. A., and Ghosh, S. (2006). Recognition and signaling by toll-like receptors. *Annu. Rev. Cell Dev. Biol.* 22, 409–437. doi: 10.1146/annurev.cellbio.21.122303.115827

Wight, T. N., Kang, I., and Merrilees, M. J. (2014). Versican and the control of inflammation. *Matrix Biol.* 35, 152–161. doi: 10.1016/j.matbio.2014.01.01

Wong, Y. P., Tan, G. C., Wong, K. K., Anushia, S., and Cheah, F. C. (2018). Gardnerella vaginalis in perinatology: an overview of the clinicopathological correlation. *Malays J. Pathol.* 40, 267–286.

Xia, C., Braunstein, Z., Toomey, A. C., Zhong, J., and Rao, X. (2018). S100 proteins as a important regulator of macrophage inflammation. *Front. Immunol.* 8:1908. doi: 10.3389/fimmu.2017.01908

Xu, D., Young, J., Song, D., and Esko, J. D. (2011). Heparan sulfate is essential for high mobility group protein 1 (HMGB1) receptor signaling by the receptor for advanced glycation end products (RAGE). *J. Biol. Chem.* 286, 41736–41744. doi: 10.1074/jbc.M111.299685

Yang, H., Wang, H., Czura, C. J., and Tracey, K. J. (2005). The cytokine activity of HMGB1. *J. Leukoc. Biol.* 78, 1–8.

Zaga, V., Estrada-Gutierrez, G., Beltran-Montoya, J., Maida-Claros, R., Lopez-Vancell, R., and Vadillo-Ortega, F. (2004). Secretions of interleukin-1beta and tumor necrosis factor alpha by whole fetal membranes depend on initial interactions of amnion or choriodecidua with lipopolysaccharide or group B Streptococci. *Biol. Rep.* 71, 1296–1302. doi: 10.1095/biorepord.104.028621

Zhang, J. Z., Liu, Z., Liu, J., Ren, J. X., and Sun, T. S. (2014). Mitochondrial DNA induces inflammation and increases TLR9/NF-κB expression in lung tissue. *Int. J. Mol. Med.* 33, 817–824. doi: 10.3892/ijmm.2014.1650

Zhang, Q., Kiyoshi, I., and Carl, H. J. (2010). Mitochondrial dna is released by shock and activates neutrophils via p38 map kinase. *Shock.* 34, 55–59. doi: 10.1097/SHK.0b013e3181cd8c08

Zhou, H., Yu, M., Zhao, J., Martin, B. N., Roychowdhury, S., McMullen, M. R., et al. (2016). IRAKM-Mincle axis links cell death to inflammation: pathophysiological implications for chronic alcoholic liver disease. *Hepatology* 64, 1978–1993. doi: 10.1002/hep.28811

Permissions

All chapters in this book were first published by Frontiers; hereby published with permission under the Creative Commons Attribution License or equivalent. Every chapter published in this book has been scrutinized by our experts. Their significance has been extensively debated. The topics covered herein carry significant findings which will fuel the growth of the discipline. They may even be implemented as practical applications or may be referred to as a beginning point for another development.

The contributors of this book come from diverse backgrounds, making this book a truly international effort. This book will bring forth new frontiers with its revolutionizing research information and detailed analysis of the nascent developments around the world.

We would like to thank all the contributing authors for lending their expertise to make the book truly unique. They have played a crucial role in the development of this book. Without their invaluable contributions this book wouldn't have been possible. They have made vital efforts to compile up to date information on the varied aspects of this subject to make this book a valuable addition to the collection of many professionals and students.

This book was conceptualized with the vision of imparting up-to-date information and advanced data in this field. To ensure the same, a matchless editorial board was set up. Every individual on the board went through rigorous rounds of assessment to prove their worth. After which they invested a large part of their time researching and compiling the most relevant data for our readers.

The editorial board has been involved in producing this book since its inception. They have spent rigorous hours researching and exploring the diverse topics which have resulted in the successful publishing of this book. They have passed on their knowledge of decades through this book. To expedite this challenging task, the publisher supported the team at every step. A small team of assistant editors was also appointed to further simplify the editing procedure and attain best results for the readers.

Apart from the editorial board, the designing team has also invested a significant amount of their time in understanding the subject and creating the most relevant covers. They scrutinized every image to scout for the most suitable representation of the subject and create an appropriate cover for the book.

The publishing team has been an ardent support to the editorial, designing and production team. Their endless efforts to recruit the best for this project, has resulted in the accomplishment of this book. They are a veteran in the field of academics and their pool of knowledge is as vast as their experience in printing. Their expertise and guidance has proved useful at every step. Their uncompromising quality standards have made this book an exceptional effort. Their encouragement from time to time has been an inspiration for everyone.

The publisher and the editorial board hope that this book will prove to be a valuable piece of knowledge for researchers, students, practitioners and scholars across the globe.

List of Contributors

Jossimara Polettini
Universidade Federal da Fronteira Sul (UFFS), Programa de Pós Graduação em Ciências Biomédicas, Faculdade de Medicina, Campus Passo Fundo, Brazil

Marcia Guimarães da Silva
Universidade Estadual Paulista (UNESP), Faculdade de Medicina, Departamento de Patologia, Botucatu, Brazil

Cecilia Beatrice Chighizola, Paola Adele Lonati, Pier Luigi Meroni and Francesco Tedesco
Experimental Laboratory of Immunological and Rheumatologic Researches, Istituto Auxologico Italiano, IRCCS, Milan, Italy

Laura Trespidi
Department of Obstetrics and Gynaecology, Fondazione Cà Granda, Ospedale Maggiore Policlinico, Milan, Italy

Héléna Choltus, Marilyne Lavergne and Corinne Belville
CNRS, INSERM, GReD, Université Clermont Auvergne, Clermont-Ferrand, France

Régine Minet-Quinard and Vincent Sapin
CNRS, INSERM, GReD, Université Clermont Auvergne, Clermont-Ferrand, France
CHU de Clermont-Ferrand, Biochemistry and Molecular Genetic Department, Clermont-Ferrand, France

Julie Durif
CHU de Clermont-Ferrand, Biochemistry and Molecular Genetic Department, Clermont-Ferrand, France

Ippei Yasuda
Department of Obstetrics and Gynecology, University of Toyama, Toyama, Japan
Laboratory of Immunology, Faculty of Pharmacy, Osaka Ohtani University, Osaka, Japan

Tomoko Shima
Department of Obstetrics and Gynecology, University of Toyama, Toyama, Japan

Taiki Moriya, Yutaka Kusumoto and Michio Tomura
Laboratory of Immunology, Faculty of Pharmacy, Osaka Ohtani University, Osaka, Japan

Ryoyo Ikebuchi
Laboratory of Immunology, Faculty of Pharmacy, Osaka Ohtani University, Osaka, Japan
Research Fellow of Japan Society for the Promotion of Science, Tokyo, Japan

Damien Bouvier
Biochemistry and Molecular Genetic Department, Centre Hospitalier Universitaire (CHU) Clermont-Ferrand, Clermont-Ferrand, France
Faculty of Medicine, CNRS 6293, INSERM 1103, GReD, Université Clermont Auvergne, Clermont-Ferrand, France

Yves Giguère and Jean-Claude Forest
Centre de Recherche du Centre Hospitalier Universitaire (CHU) de Québec-Université Laval, Québec City, QC, Canada
Department of Molecular Biology, Medical Biochemistry and Pathology, Faculty of Medicine, Université Laval, Québec City, QC, Canada

Loïc Blanchon
Faculty of Medicine, CNRS 6293, INSERM 1103, GReD, Université Clermont Auvergne, Clermont-Ferrand, France

Emmanuel Bujold
Centre de Recherche du Centre Hospitalier Universitaire (CHU) de Québec-Université Laval, Québec City, QC, Canada
Department of Obstetrics and Gynecology, Faculty of Medicine, Université Laval, Québec City, QC, Canada

Bruno Pereira
Biostatistics Unit Direction de la Recherche Clinique et des Innovations (DRCI), Centre Hospitalier Universitaire (CHU) Clermont-Ferrand, Clermont-Ferrand, France

Nathalie Bernard
Centre de Recherche du Centre Hospitalier Universitaire (CHU) de Québec-Université Laval, Québec City, QC, Canada

Denis Gallot
Faculty of Medicine, CNRS 6293, INSERM 1103, GReD, Université Clermont Auvergne, Clermont-Ferrand, France
Department of Obstetrics and Gynecology, Centre Hospitalier Universitaire (CHU) Clermont-Ferrand, Clermont-Ferrand, France

List of Contributors

Tamas Zakar
Department of Maternity & Gynaecology, John Hunter Hospital, New Lambton Heights, NSW, Australia
School of Medicine and Public Health, Faculty of Health and Medicine, The University of Newcastle, Callaghan, NSW, Australia
Priority Research Centre for Reproductive Science, The University of Newcastle, Callaghan, NSW, Australia
Hunter Medical Research Institute, New Lambton Heights, NSW, Australia

Jonathan W. Paul
School of Medicine and Public Health, Faculty of Health and Medicine, The University of Newcastle, Callaghan, NSW, Australia
Priority Research Centre for Reproductive Science, The University of Newcastle, Callaghan, NSW, Australia
Hunter Medical Research Institute, New Lambton Heights, NSW, Australia

Wang-Sheng Wang and Kang Sun
Center for Reproductive Medicine, Ren Ji Hospital, School of Medicine, Shanghai Jiao Tong University, Shanghai, China
Shanghai Key Laboratory for Assisted Reproduction and Reproductive Genetics, Shanghai, China

Chun-Ming Guo
School of Life Sciences, Yunnan University, Kunming, China

Mackenzie L. Wheeler and Michelle L. Oyen
Department of Engineering, East Carolina University, Greenville, NC, United States

Sean M. Harris and Rita Loch-Caruso
Department of Environmental Health Sciences, School of Public Health, University of Michigan, Ann Arbor, MI, United States

Erica Boldenow
Department of Biology, Calvin College, Grand Rapids, MI, United States

Steven E. Domino
Department of Obstetrics and Gynecology, University of Michigan Medical School, Ann Arbor, MI, United States

Regina Hoo and Roser Vento-Tormo
Wellcome Sanger Institute, Cambridge, United Kingdom
Centre for Trophoblast Research, University of Cambridge, Cambridge, United Kingdom

Annettee Nakimuli
Wellcome Sanger Institute, Cambridge, United Kingdom
Department of Obstetrics and Gynecology, School of Medicine, Makerere University, Kampala, Uganda

Yosuke Ono and Shinichiro Wada
Department of Obstetrics and Gynecology, Teine Keijinkai Hospital, Sapporo, Japan

Osamu Yoshino, Takehiro Hiraoka and Erina Sato
Department of Obstetrics and Gynecology, Kitasato University School Medicine, Tokyo, Japan,

Yamato Fukui, Yasushi Hirota and Yutaka Osuga
Department of Obstetrics and Gynecology, Faculty of Medicine, University of Tokyo, Tokyo, Japan

Akemi Ushijima, Akitoshi Nakashima and Shigeru Saito
Department of Obstetrics and Gynecology, Faculty of Medicine, University of Toyama, Toyama, Japan

Allah Nawaz
Department of Molecular and Medical Pharmacology, Faculty of Medicine, University of Toyama, Toyama, Japan

Kazuyuki Tobe
First Department of Internal Medicine, University of Toyama, Toyama, Japan

William Marinello and Terrence K. Allen
Department of Anesthesiology, Duke University Hospital, Durham, NC, United States

Liping Feng
Department of Obstetrics and Gynecology, Duke University Hospital, Durham, NC, United States
Department of Obstetrics and Gynecology, Duke University School of Medicine, Durham, NC, United States

Eman Mosaad, Hassendrini N. Peiris, Isabella Morean Garcia and Murray D. Mitchell
School of Biomedical Science, Institute of Health and Biomedical Innovation – Centre for Children's Health Research, Faculty of Health, Queensland University of Technology, Brisbane, QLD, Australia

Olivia Holland
School of Biomedical Science, Institute of Health and Biomedical Innovation – Centre for Children's Health Research, Faculty of Health, Queensland University of Technology, Brisbane, QLD, Australia
School of Medical Science, Griffith University, Southport, QLD, Australia

Ingrid Aneman, Dillan Pienaar and Lana McClements
Faculty of Science, School of Life Sciences, University of Technology Sydney, Sydney, NSW, Australia

Sonja Suvakov and Vesna D. Garovic
Division of Nephrology and Hypertension, Department of Internal Medicine, Mayo Clinic, Rochester, MN, United States

Tatjana P. Simic
Faculty of Medicine, Institute of Medical and Clinical Biochemistry, University of Belgrade, Belgrade, Serbia
Department of Medical Sciences, Serbian Academy of Sciences and Arts, Belgrade, Serbia

Jing Pan and Xiujuan Tian
Sanya Maternity and Child Care Hospital, Sanya, China

Honglei Huang
Proteomic Core Facility, Oxford University, Oxford, United Kingdom

Nanbert Zhong
New York State Institute for Basic Research in Developmental Disabilities, Staten Island, NY, United States

Sarah J. Cunningham and Timothy E. Reddy
Department of Biostatistics and Bioinformatics, Duke University, Durham, NC, United States
University Program in Genetics and Genomics, Duke University, Durham, NC, United States
Center for Genomic and Computational Biology, Duke University, Durham, NC, United States
Center for Advanced Genomic Technologies, Duke University, Durham, NC, United States

Gabriela Brettas Silva, Lobke Marijn Gierman and Ann-Charlotte Iversen
Centre of Molecular Inflammation Research, Department of Cancer Research and Molecular Medicine, Norwegian University of Science and Technology, Trondheim, Norway
Department of Gynecology and Obstetrics, St. Olavs Hospital, Trondheim, Norway

Johanne Johnsen Rakner, Guro Sannerud Stødle, Siv Boon Mundal, Astrid Josefin Thaning, Bjørnar Sporsheim and Marie Hjelmseth Aune
Centre of Molecular Inflammation Research, Department of Cancer Research and Molecular Medicine, Norwegian University of Science and Technology, Trondheim, Norway

Mattijs Elschot
Department of Circulation and Medical Imaging, Norwegian University of Science and Technology, Trondheim, Norway
Department of Radiology and Nuclear Medicine, St. Olavs Hospital, Trondheim, Norway

Karin Collett
Department of Pathology, Haukeland University Hospital, Bergen, Norway

Line Bjørge and Liv Cecilie Vestrheim Thomsen
Department of Gynecology and Obstetrics, Haukeland University Hospital, Bergen, Norway
Centre for Cancer Biomarkers CCBIO, Department of Clinical Science, University of Bergen, Bergen, Norway

Haruta Mogami
Department of Gynecology and Obstetrics, Kyoto University Graduate School of Medicine, Kyoto, Japan

R. Ann Word
Department of Obstetrics and Gynecology, Cecil H. and Ida Green Center for Reproductive Biology Sciences, University of Texas Southwestern Medical Center, Dallas, TX, United States

Wenxu Qi, Peinan Zhao, Zichao Wen and Zulfia Kisrieva-Ware
Department of Obstetrics and Gynecology, School of Medicine, Washington University in St. Louis, St. Louis, MO, United States

Wei Wang, Pamela K. Woodard, Qing Wang and Robert C. McKinstry
Mallinckrodt Institute of Radiology, School of Medicine, Washington University in St. Louis, St. Louis, MO, United States

Zhexian Sun, Xiao Ma and Wenjie Wu
Department of Obstetrics and Gynecology, School of Medicine, Washington University in St. Louis, St. Louis, MO, United States
Department of Biomedical Engineering, McKelvey School of Engineering, Washington University in St. Louis, St. Louis, MO, United States

Hui Wang
Department of Obstetrics and Gynecology, School of Medicine, Washington University in St. Louis, St. Louis, MO, United States
Department of Physics, Washington University in St. Louis, St. Louis, MO, United States

List of Contributors

Yong Wang
Department of Obstetrics and Gynecology, School of Medicine, Washington University in St. Louis, St. Louis, MO, United States
Mallinckrodt Institute of Radiology, School of Medicine, Washington University in St. Louis, St. Louis, MO, United States
Department of Biomedical Engineering, McKelvey School of Engineering, Washington University in St. Louis, St. Louis, MO, United States
Department of Physics, Washington University in St. Louis, St. Louis, MO, United States

Justin G. Padron
Anatomy, Biochemistry and Physiology, John A. Burns School of Medicine, University of Hawai'i at Mānoa, Honolulu, HI, United States

Chelsea A. Saito Reis
Natural Science and Mathematics, Chaminade University of Honolulu, Honolulu, HI, United States

Claire E. Kendal-Wright
Natural Science and Mathematics, Chaminade University of Honolulu, Honolulu, HI, United States
Obstetrics, Gynecology and Women's Health, John A. Burns School of Medicine, University of Hawai'i at Mānoa, Honolulu, HI, United States

Index

A

Alarmins, 21-22, 24, 28-31, 207, 218-220

Amniocentesis, 56, 193, 196, 203

Amniochorion, 90, 220

Amnion, 6, 9, 21-31, 46, 52-59, 61-68, 70-76, 81, 83-84, 88, 90-91, 117-122, 124-127, 132-133, 137-138, 169, 175-179, 193-208, 210, 214-222

Amniotic Fluid, 5-7, 22, 31-32, 46, 52, 56, 68, 70, 75, 78-79, 81, 84, 87, 89-90, 92, 95, 118, 127-128, 138-139, 149, 158, 169-170, 172, 193, 198-202, 210, 213, 215, 218-219

Angiogenesis, 11, 13-14, 18, 41, 108, 116, 134-135, 142-143, 148, 154-155, 157-159, 170

Anti-phospholipid Syndrome, 10, 14-16, 19

B

Basement Membrane, 15, 68, 167

C

Cardiovascular Disease, 143, 155, 181-182, 191

Cell Culture, 22, 54, 73, 119-121, 124, 174

Cell Migration, 14, 18, 29, 44, 134, 139, 157, 193, 195

Cellular Stress, 205, 207, 210, 215, 218

Cholesterol Crystals, 181-192

Chorioamnion, 77-79, 81, 89, 176

Chorion, 22, 54-56, 58-62, 67-68, 72-75, 83-84, 89, 91, 95, 125-126, 132, 138, 169, 172, 175-176, 198-203, 207-208, 213-214, 218

Chromatin Modifications, 54, 61

Cluster Differentiation, 206, 209-211

Collagen, 22, 57, 67, 70-71, 73-76, 83-84, 118, 124, 126-127, 150, 158, 165-166, 169, 172-173, 183, 193-197, 202, 207, 219-221

Cytokine, 11, 16, 21-24, 28-31, 43, 52, 55, 58, 72, 74, 87-88, 90-91, 104, 117-118, 124-126, 128, 133, 146, 148, 150, 156-157, 161, 166-167, 177, 179-180, 189, 192, 195, 207-211, 213-220, 222

D

Decidua, 6, 12-14, 17, 22, 43, 54-56, 59-63, 65-66, 68, 71, 73, 75-76, 84, 87, 90, 92-95, 97-101, 104, 116, 127, 132-133, 146-149, 156, 158, 161, 169, 181-182, 184-192, 198-202, 207-208, 216, 218, 220

Dendritic Cells, 33-34, 43-44, 97, 103-105, 139, 155, 157

Diphtheria-toxin Receptor, 107

Distal Target Cells, 134-135

E

Eicosanoids, 129-133, 135-139

Endosomes, 134-135, 211

Endothelial Dysfunction, 14, 139, 141-143, 147-148, 158-159

Epithelial Cells, 9, 29, 55, 63, 68, 72, 75-76, 84, 88, 95, 97-98, 103, 107-110, 114, 116, 118-119, 124-126, 177, 179, 193-196, 205, 210-211, 215, 218-221

Exosomes, 5-6, 8-9, 46, 51-53, 129-130, 133-140, 146, 215, 218, 221

Extracellular Matrix, 13, 57, 67, 70-71, 73, 76, 91, 118, 160-161, 163, 165-167, 176-177, 179, 194, 204, 206-207, 218, 221

Extracellular Vesicles, 45-47, 49-51, 53, 129, 133, 136, 139, 141, 146, 155, 158-159

F

Fetal Development, 6, 75, 91, 93, 100, 105, 129, 139, 141, 151-152, 164

Fetal Growth Restriction, 142, 171, 181-182, 185-186, 188, 190, 192

Fetal Membranes, 1-8, 21-22, 25-32, 46, 51-54, 56, 59, 61, 63, 66-77, 79, 81-86, 89-92, 117-118, 124-129, 132, 136, 138-139, 160-165, 167-171, 173-180, 193-194, 196-197, 203-211, 213-222

Feto-maternal Interface, 18, 34, 43, 76, 148

Feto-maternal Tolerance, 33-34, 41

Fibroblast Growth Factor, 107-108

Fibroblasts, 2-4, 9, 60-61, 63, 68, 70-72, 74-76, 83, 97-98, 100, 105, 194, 211, 220

Flagellin, 44, 211, 213-214, 219

G

Gene Regulation, 54, 57, 63, 65, 126, 174-175

Gestation, 1, 6, 11, 13-14, 17-18, 22, 24, 28, 45-47, 54-59, 61-62, 65, 68-75, 77, 79, 82-85, 93, 98, 101, 104-105, 127, 129, 132-134, 137-138, 141-143, 146-150, 154, 161, 164, 170, 172, 174, 176-177, 182, 185, 192-194, 196, 198-199, 202, 211, 213, 217-218, 220

Glucocorticoid Receptor, 74-76, 117-118, 124, 126-128, 179

Glucocorticoids, 67-76, 118, 124-125

Glycation, 21-22, 31-32, 45-50, 52-53, 194, 206, 209-210, 222

H

Healthy Pregnancy, 12, 83, 101, 146, 153, 155, 198

Homeostasis, 5, 22, 44, 67, 108, 116, 172

Hypertension, 14-15, 19-20, 56, 65, 137, 141-143, 146-148, 152, 154-159, 172, 182

I

Immune Cells, 6, 9, 17, 34, 83-84, 87, 92-94, 96-97, 100, 125, 138, 141-143, 146-148, 150, 152-155, 172, 182, 194, 196, 210

Inflammasome, 5, 8-9, 32, 46, 52, 100, 105, 181-182, 185-187, 189-192, 209, 211-212, 218, 220

Innate Immunity, 31, 92, 104, 141, 151-152, 159, 178, 193, 196, 218, 221

Intra-amniotic Infection, 88, 93, 127, 137-138, 172, 193, 196, 206, 214-215, 218

L
Late-onset Preeclampsia, 19, 141-142, 157, 220

M
Macrophage, 5, 8, 30, 85, 90, 95, 107, 116, 137, 143-144, 146-147, 150-151, 156-158, 160, 167-169, 172-173, 187, 193, 196-197, 206, 213-214, 219-222

Magnetic Resonance Imaging, 198, 204

O
Obstetric Complications, 10-11, 13-14, 65

Oxidative Stress, 1-5, 7-9, 51, 55, 83-85, 90, 118, 125, 147, 169-172, 178, 182, 187-189, 207, 215, 218, 220

P
Parturition, 1-9, 22, 32, 46, 52, 54, 64-65, 67-76, 83-84, 87, 90-91, 103, 126-127, 129-130, 132-133, 135-140, 157, 169, 172, 176-177, 179, 205-207, 209, 213, 215, 217-220

Pathophysiology, 1, 10, 104, 118, 128, 137-138, 154-156, 161, 164, 189, 191, 194

Pattern Recognition Receptors, 22, 97, 105, 157, 205-206, 218, 221

Phenotype, 4, 9, 18, 33-34, 37-38, 41, 43, 54-55, 59-63, 90, 134-135, 142-143, 146-148, 150, 152-153, 155, 177, 196, 206, 215, 220

Placenta, 1-2, 5-10, 12-14, 17-20, 28-29, 31-32, 51, 58, 63-66, 68-69, 73-76, 82-83, 85, 87-106, 124, 127-129, 132, 134, 137-139, 143-150, 153-162, 164, 167, 170-173, 179, 182-183, 185, 187, 189, 191-192, 196, 203-204, 206, 213, 215-221

Preeclampsia, 1, 5, 7, 10, 14, 18-20, 31, 43, 46, 52, 64-66, 81, 133, 136, 138-139, 141-159, 172, 174, 176-179, 181-182, 185-187, 189-192, 220-221

Prelabor Premature Rupture, 160-161

Premature Rupture, 1, 3, 5, 7-9, 21, 31-32, 45-50, 52, 64, 66, 70, 74-75, 77-79, 81, 83, 88-91, 117-118, 126-128, 160-161, 164, 172-173, 179-180, 193, 197-198, 204-205, 218, 220-221

Preterm Birth, 7-9, 14, 19-20, 22, 28, 31, 46, 52, 58-59, 62-66, 69, 76-78, 80-82, 88-91, 95, 105, 118, 126-127, 133, 136-138, 142, 151, 157, 160-165, 168-180, 193, 198, 203-204, 206, 217-221

Preterm Labor, 5, 8, 14, 29, 31-32, 46, 52-53, 56, 59, 65-66, 70, 75, 82, 84, 88-89, 91, 95, 118, 127-130, 133, 136, 160-161, 169-170, 172, 176-177, 194, 197, 206, 213, 215-216, 218-219, 222

Preterm Premature Rupture, 3, 5, 7-9, 21, 31, 45-50, 52, 64, 66, 70, 74, 89-91, 117-118, 126-128, 172-173, 179, 193, 198, 204-205,

Progesterone, 58, 60, 62, 64-66, 72, 75, 90, 107-113, 115-121, 124-128, 132, 136-139, 145, 150, 156, 161, 168, 191, 207, 213, 216, 218-220

Progestins, 117-118, 121, 124, 126-127

Prostaglandins, 5, 8, 55, 67, 71-76, 78, 83-84, 129-130, 133, 136-139, 158, 164, 171, 173, 175, 210, 216, 219, 222

Proteinuria, 14, 16-17, 56-57, 141-142, 182

Proteolysis, 160-161, 163, 166-167, 169-171

R
Replicative Senescence, 2-3, 9

Rheumatic Diseases, 10, 18

S
Signaling Pathways, 7, 83-84, 88, 104, 117, 146, 172, 207, 211, 216-217, 219

Soluble Receptor, 32, 46-50, 52

Sterile Inflammation, 7, 9, 21-22, 28-29, 32, 45-46, 51, 194-195, 197, 205, 209-210, 220

Systemic Lupus Erythematosus, 10, 15-16, 18-20, 152, 207

T
Telomere Shortening, 1-9

Tissue Remodeling, 12-13, 18, 62, 108, 143, 146, 169, 205, 217

Toll-like Receptor, 31, 65, 104, 145, 157, 159, 192, 205, 207, 209, 217-222

Toxicant Pathogen, 82

Transcriptomics, 65, 101, 105-106, 174

Trichloroethylene, 82, 84, 86-91

Trophoblast, 5, 10, 12-15, 18-19, 68, 74-75, 92-95, 98-99, 101-106, 134, 137-139, 142, 146-149, 151, 154-155, 157, 164, 167, 169, 174, 176-178, 181-182, 185-192, 219

U
Uterine-placental Interface, 92-93, 100-103

V
Vertical Transmission, 92-97, 100-103

W
Wound Healing, 11, 18, 193-196, 209-210

Printed in the USA
CPSIA information can be obtained
at www.ICGtesting.com
JSHW062346180324
59442JS00004B/29